Progress in

Obstetrics and Gynecology

Progress in Obstetrics and Gynecology

VOLUME 18

Edited by

John Studd
Professor of Gynaecology, Imperial College, London University
Chelsea and Westminster Hospital, London, UK

Seang Lin Tan
James Edmund Dodds Professor and Chairman
Department of Obstetrics and Gynaecology, McGill University
Royal Victoria Hospital, Montreal, Canada

Frank A. Chervenak
Given Foundaton Professor and Chairman
Department of Obstetrics and Gynaecology
New York Weill Cornell Medical Center, New York, USA

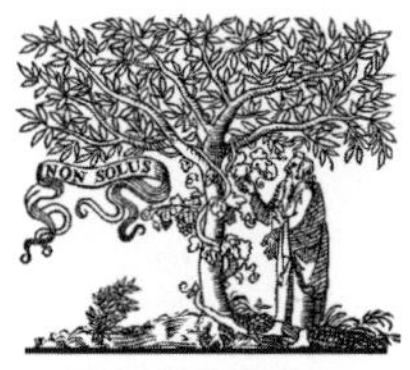

ELSEVIER

EDINBURGH LONDON NEW YORK OXFORD PHILADELPHIA St LOUIS SYDNEY TORONTO 2008

ELSEVIER

First published 2008

ISBN: 978-0-443-06923-9

British Library Cataloguing in Publication Data
A catalogue record for this book is available from the British Library

Library of Congress Cataloging in Publication Data
A catalog record for this book is available from the Library of Congress

Note
Knowledge and best practice in this field are constantly changing. As new research and experience broaden our knowledge, changes in practice, treatment and drug therapy may become necessary or appropriate. Readers are advised to check the most current information provided (i) on procedures featured or (ii) by the manufacturer of each product to be administered, to verify the recommended dose or formula, the method and duration of administration, and contraindications. It is the responsibility of the practitioner, relying on their own experience and knowledge of the patient, to make diagnoses, to determine dosages and the best treatment for each individual patient, and to take all appropriate safety precautions. To the fullest extent of the law, neither the Publisher nor the Editors assumes any liability for any injury and/or damage to persons or property arising out or related to any use of the material contained in this book.

Commissioning Editor – Pauline Graham
Development Editor – Gill Haddock
Project Manager – Andrew Palfreyman
Senior Designer – Sarah Russell
Editorial and Typesetting services – BA & GM Haddock
Printed in China

The publisher's policy is to use **paper manufactured from sustainable forests**

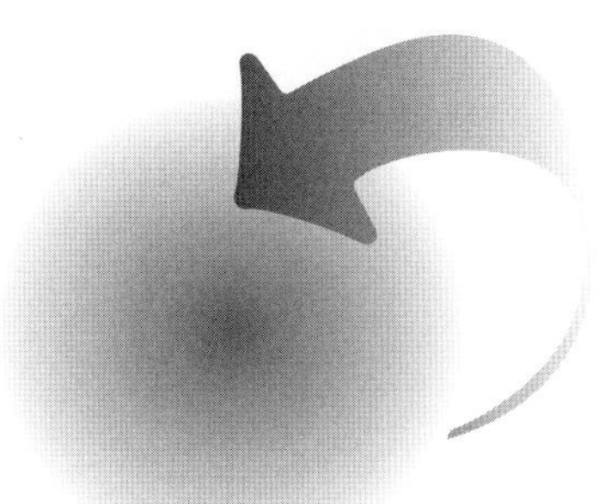

Contents

GYNECOLOGY

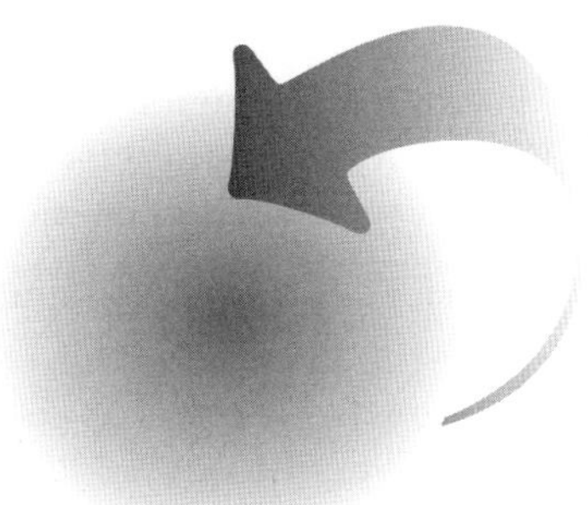

Contributors

Sharifa Al Mahrizi MD
Fellow of Reproductive Endocrinology and Infertility, McGill University, Montréal, Québec, Canada

Jesus R. Alvarez MD
Third Year Maternal-Fetal Medicine Fellow, Department of Obstetrics, Gynecology and Women's Health, UMDNJ–New Jersey Medical School, Newark, New Jersey, USA

Joseph J. Apuzzio MD
Professor of Obstetrics, Gynecology and Radiology; Director, Division of Maternal-Fetal Medicine, Department of Obstetrics, Gynecology and Women's Health, UMDNJ–New Jersey Medical School, Newark, New Jersey, USA

Anga S. Arunkalaivanan MD MRCOG
Honorary Senior Lecturer at University of Birmingham and Consultant Urogynaecologist and Obstetrician, City Hospital, Birmingham, UK

Hugh Barber MD
Professor Emeritus, Weill Medical College of Cornell University, New York, USA *(Deceased)*

Maya Basu MBBS BSc(Hons)
Specialist Registrar, Department of Obstetrics and Gynaecology, Medway Maritime Hospital, Gillingham, Kent, UK

Isaac Blickstein MD
Hadassah-Hebrew University School of Medicine, Jerusalem, and Professor, Department of Obstetrics and Gynecology, Kaplan Medical Center, Rehovot, Israel

Kristi Borowski MD
Fellow, Division of Maternal-Fetal Medicine, Department of Obstetrics and Gynecology, University of Iowa Hospitals and Clinics, Iowa City, Iowa, USA

Robert L. Brent MD PhD
Head, Clinical and Environmental Teratology Research Laboratory, Alfred I. duPont Hospital for Children, and Professor of Pediatrics, Radiology and Pathology, Thomas Jefferson Univeristy, Wilmington, Delaware, USA

Richard Brown MBBS DFFP FRCOG, Director of Ultrasound and Assistant Professor of Obstetrics and Gynaecology, Department of Obstetrics & Gynaecology & Division of Maternal and Fetal Medicine, McGill University, Montréal, Québec, Canada

William Buckett MD FRCOG
Assistant Professor, Department of Obstetrics and Gynecology, McGill University, Hôpital Royal Victoria, Montréal, Québec, Canada

Celia Burrell MRCOG
Senior Specialist Registrar, Department of Obstetrics and Gynaecology, Hinchingbrooke Hospital, Huntingdon, Cambridgeshire, UK

Raydeen Busse MD FACOG
Assistant Professor, Department of Obstetrics and Gynecology and Women's Health, John A. Burns School of Medicine, University of Hawaii, Kapiolani Medical Center for Women and Children, Honolulu, Hawaii, USA

Thomas A. Caputo MD
Professor of Obstetrics and Gynecology, Department of Obstetrics and Gynecology, Division of Gynecologic Oncology, New York Presbyterian Hospital-Weill Medical College of Cornell University, New York, USA

Ri-Cheng Chian MSc PhD
Assistant Professor, Department of Obstetrics and Gynecology, McGill University Royal Victoria Hospital, Montréal, Québec, Canada

Lachlan de Crespigny MBBS MD FRCOG FRACOG DDU COGU
Associate Professor, Department Obstetrics & Gynaecology, University of Melbourne, Honorary Fellow, Murdoch Children's Research Institute, Obstetrician Sonologist, Mercy Hospital for Women and Melbourne Ultrasound for Women, Melbourne, Australia

Ezgi Demirtas MD
Clinical/Resarch Fellow in Reproductive Endocrinology and Infertility, Department of Obstetrics and Gynecology, McGill University Royal Victoria Hospital, Montréal, Québec, Canada

Jonathan R.A. Duckett FRCOG
Consultant Urogynaecologist, Medway Maritime Hospital, Gillingham, Kent, UK

Shai E. Elizur MD
Clinical/Resarch Fellow in Reproductive Endocrinology and Infertility, Department of Obstetrics and Gynecology, McGill University Royal Victoria Hospital, Montréal, Québec, Canada

Gillian Fowler MRCOG
Specialist Registrar in Obstetrics and Gynaecology, Warrington District General Hospital, Croft Warrington, UK

Lubna Ghani
Medical Student, King's College London, London, UK

Yariv Gidoni MD
Clinical/Resarch Fellow in Reproductive Endocrinology and Infertility, Department of Obstetrics and Gynecology, McGill University Royal Victoria Hospital, Montréal, Québec, Canada

Kevin M. Holcomb MD
Associate Professor, Department of Obstetrics and Gynecology, Weill Medical College of Cornell University, New York, USA

Nigel Holland MD FRCOG DipVen
Consultant Obstetrician and Gynaecologist, Warrington District General Hospital, Warrington, UK

Hananel E.G. Holzer MD
Assistant Professor, Department of Obstetrics and Gynecology, McGill University Royal Victoria Hospital, Montréal, Québec, Canada

Marilyn Huang MD
Department of Obstetrics and Gynecology, Division of Gynecologic Oncology, New York Presbyterian Hospital-Weill Medical College of Cornell University, New York, USA

Laurie Montgomery Irvine MD(Lond) FRCOG
Consultant Obstetrician and Gynaecologist, West Hertfordshire Hospitals NHS Trust, Watford General Hospital, Watford, UK

Sean Keeler MD
Fellow, Division of Maternal Fetal Medicine, Department of Obstetrics and Gynecology, New York University School of Medicine, New York, USA

Nina Khazaezadeh MSc BSc
Public Health Consultant Midwife, Guy's and St Thomas's NHS Foundation Trust, London, UK

Robert C. Knapp MD
Professor Emeritus, Harvard Medical School, Boston, Massachusetts, USA

Suresh Kumar MBBS MD MRCOG
General Practitioner, Sun Lane Surgery, Hythe, Kent, UK

William J. Ledger MD
Professor and Chairman Emeritus, Department of Obstetrics and Gynecology, Weill Medical College of Cornell University, New York, USA

Boon H. Lim FRCOG FRANZCOG
Consultant Obstetrician and Gynaecologist, Department of Obstetrics and Gynaecology, Hinchingbrooke Hospital, Huntingdon, Cambridgeshire, UK

Gunilla Lindmark MD(Uppsala) FRCOG
Professor, Department of Women's and Children's Health, Section of International Maternal and Child Health, Uppsala University, Uppsala, Sweden

Franz Majoko MB ChB PhD(Uppsala) FRCOG
Consultant, Department of Obstetrics and Gynaecology, Singleton Hospital, Swansea, UK

Sujit Mukhopadya MRCOG
Specialist Registrar in Obstetrics & Gynaecology, King's Mill Hospital, Sutton-in-Ashfield, Mansfield, UK

Stephen P. Munjanja MD(Birm) FRCOG
Senior Lecturer, Department of Obstetrics and Gynaecology, College of Health Sciences, University of Zimbabwe, Zimbabwe

Mini S. Nair MBBS MD MRCOG
Specialist Registrar, Department of Obstetrics and Gynaecology, Medway Maritime Hospital, Gillingham, Kent, UK

Jennifer R. Niebyl MD
Professor and Head, Department of Obstetrics and Gynecology, University of Iowa Hospitals and Clinics, Iowa City, Iowa, USA

Eugene Oteng-Ntim MBBS MRCOG
Consultant Obstetrician, St Thomas's Hospital, London, UK

Nagy M Rafla MRCOG MOG
Consultant Obstetrician and Gynaecologist, Queen Elizabeth the Queen Mother Hospital, Margate, Kent, UK

Maha Ragunath MRCOG MSc
Senior Registrar in Obstetrics & Gynaecology, Queen's Medical Centre, Derby Road, Nottingham, UK

Katherine Shaio Sandhu MD
Fellow, Division of Urogynecology, Department of Obstetrics and Gynecology, Albert Einstein College of Medicine, Bronx, New York, USA

Vicki Seltzer MD
The Edie and Marvin H. Schur Professor of Obstetrics & Gynecology and Women's Health, Albert Einstein College of Medicine, Vice President for Women's Health Services, North Shore-LIJ Health System, and Chairman, Obstetrics and Gynecology, North Shore University Hospital and Long Island Jewish Medical Center, New York, USA

David E. Seubert MD JD
Director, Division of Maternal Fetal Medicine and Assistant Professor, Department of Obstetrics and Gynecology, New York University Medical Center, New York, USA

Jai B. Sharma MD DNB FRCOG MFFP MAMS FICOG FIMSA
Assistant Professor of Obstetrics and Gynaecology, All India Institute of Medical Sciences, New Delhi, India

Brian M. Slomovitz MD MS
Assistant Professor, Department of Obstetrics and Gynecology, Division of Gynecologic Oncology, New York Presbyterian Hospital-Weill Medical College of Cornell University, New York, USA

Olanrewaju Sorinola MRCOG MMedSc
Consultant Obstetrician and Gynaecologist, Honorary Associate Professor University of Warwick, Obstetrics and Gynaecology Department, Warwick Hospital, Warwick, UK

John Studd DSc MD FRCOG
Professor of Gynaecology, Chelsea and Westminster Hospital, London, UK

Seang Lin Tan MBBS FRCOG FRCSC FACOG MMed(O&G) MBA
James Edmund Dodds Professor and Chairman, Department of Obstetrics and Gynecology, McGill University Royal Victoria Hospital, Montréal, Québec, Canada

Togas Tulandi MD MHCM FRCSC FACOG
Professor of Obstetrics and Gynecology and Milton Leong Chair in Reproductive Medicine, McGill University, Montréal, Québec, Canada

Padma Vanga MBBS
Specialist Registrar, City Hospital, Birmingham, UK

Jean-Claude Veille MD
Former Professor and Chair, Division of Maternal Fetal Medicine, Albany Medical Center, Albany, New York, USA

Swati Vyas MBBS
Senior SHO, St Thomas's Hospital, London, UK

Susan J. Ward FRCOG MD
Consultant in Obstetrics and Gynaecology, King's Mill Hospital, Sutton-in-Ashfield, Mansfield, UK

Susan M. White MBBS FRACP
Clinical Geneticist, Genetic Health Services Victoria, Murdoch Children's Research Institute, Royal Children's Hospital, Parkville, Australia

Ivica Zalud MD PhD FACOG FAIUM
Associate Professor and Chief, Obstetrics and Gynecology Imaging Division, Department of Obstetrics and Gynecology and Women's Health, John A. Burns School of Medicine, University of Hawaii, Kapiolani Medical Center for Women and Children, Honolulu, Hawaii, USA

Vicki Seltzer

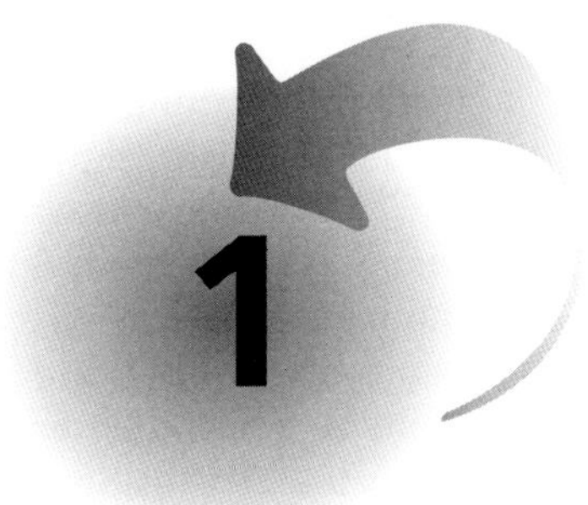

Women's health

During the last century there have been dramatic improvements in the status of women's health and life expectancy, particularly in developed countries. Yet, both in developed and in developing countries, women continue to suffer needless disability and to die prematurely of preventable causes. For instance, in the US, approximately one-half of premature deaths, one-third of acute disabilities, and one-half of chronic disabilities are preventable.[1]

Obstetrician-gynecologists provide extremely sophisticated specialty and subspecialty care. Because there have been so many important advances in the discipline, the scope of the obstetrician-gynecologist's practice responsibilities within the specialty and the time required to maintain cutting-edge practice skills continue to grow. However, obstetrician-gynecologists can play a dramatic role in reducing the incidence of premature morbidity and mortality for their patient population without an overly burdensome additional time commitment.

Obstetrician-gynecologists have already made major contributions in the area of prevention and early detection. Some examples of this success include cytology screening and colposcopy, mammography screening, rubella vaccination, and blood sugar control of the pregnant diabetic.

By examining the causes of premature mortality in women, strategies for prevention and early detection become clearer. Although many of the issues in this chapter are focused on the needs of women in developed countries, there is in many instances overlap with the needs of women in developing countries.

The American College of Obstetricians and Gynecologists has published tables on the leading causes of morbidity and mortality for women in the US, divided by age groups.[2] Although there will be a fair amount of variation from

Vicki Seltzer MD
The Edie and Marvin H. Schur Professor of Obstetrics & Gynecology and Women's Health, Albert Einstein College of Medicine, Vice President for Women's Health Services, North Shore-LIJ Health System, and Chairman, Department of Obstetrics and Gynecology, North Shore University Hospital and Long Island Jewish Medical Center, 270–05 76th Avenue, Suite 1100, New Hyde Park, NY 11040, USA.
E-mail: vseltzer@lij.edu

country to country, there is considerable overlap for the developed countries, and certain preventive strategies become readily apparent.

The leading causes of mortality for women in the US aged 19–39 years are: motor vehicle and other accidents, cancer, HIV infections, heart disease, homicide and suicide.[2] The leading causes of mortality for women in the US aged 40–64 years are cancer, heart disease, cerebrovascular disease, motor vehicle and other accidents, chronic obstructive pulmonary disease, and diabetes.[2] The leading causes of mortality for women in the US aged 65 years and older are heart disease, cancer, cerebrovascular disease, chronic obstructive pulmonary disease, pneumonia and influenza, diabetes, and motor vehicle and other accidents.[2]

In reviewing these lists, clear themes emerge for how the obstetrician-gynecologist can reduce premature mortality and morbidity for their patients by placing some emphasis on prevention and early detection. It is important to acknowledge that, for many obstetrician-gynecologists in a variety of practice settings and in most countries, the amount of time that can be spent with an individual patient has been decreasing while the sophistication and variety of the care that needs to be provided for the patient has been increasing. Still, most of what can be done for our patients regarding preventive care can be done without the expenditure of enormous amounts of time, and often with the assistance of other healthcare personnel.

In most developed countries, two of the leading causes of death in women are cardiovascular disease and cancer. For these two categories of disease there is much that can be accomplished in disease prevention, delay of onset of disease, and early detection to reduce morbidity and mortality.

In the US, cardiovascular disease is the leading cause of death in women, and cancer is the second leading cause. However, when looking at ways to reduce premature mortality this aggregate statistic is somewhat deceptive. When looking at causes of death for women aged 35–54 years and also for women aged 55–74 years, cancer was the leading cause of death and cardiovascular disease the second leading cause of death.[3] It is not until women are in their mid-sixties that cardiovascular disease overtakes cancer as the leading cause of death. Aggressive preventive and early detection strategies should be undertaken for both diseases.

CANCER

The largest preventable contributor to premature death and disability for women in many developed countries is cigarette smoking. In the US alone, between 1980 and 2000 approximately 3 million women died prematurely from smoking-related disorders, and these women lost an average of 14 years of life each. Unfortunately, cigarette smoking is becoming more common for women in the developing world as well.[4] It has been estimated that, world-wide, more than 200 million women smoke (100 million in developing countries and 100 million in developed countries),[5] and that by 2025 if current world-wide smoking rates persist, 9% of the world's deaths and disabilities will be related to tobacco use.[6]

Since cigarette smoking is a prime contributor to both cancer mortality and cardiovascular mortality in women, aggressive programs focused on abstinence from smoking would have a positive effect on both. During the past two decades there have been substantial advances in pharmacotherapy to assist in smoking cessation programs. It has been demonstrated that a combination of counseling and pharmacotherapy is most effective in helping smokers to quit and to remain abstinent.[4] Currently, the most commonly used pharmacotherapies are nicotine replacement and bupropion.

The US Public Health Service recommends that clinicians adopt a program of the 5A's to help reduce smoking rates. The components of this program take minimal time and can save many lives.

1. ASK about use of tobacco at every visit and record as a vital sign.
2. ADVISE patients that tobacco is a major hazard to their health and that as their physician you advise that they do not smoke or use tobacco products.
3. ASSESS the patient's willingness to quit. If they are willing, provide assistance and/or referral. If they are not willing to quit, conduct a brief motivational intervention.
4. AID the patient in quitting.
5. ARRANGE for follow-up.[7]

It has been estimated that cancer mortality for women in many developed countries could be reduced by as much as 25% in the next quarter century by focusing on prevention and early detection. One might explore why this could theoretically be an achievable goal by looking at the etiology of cancer deaths for women in the US. Of the deaths, 25% are attributable to cancer of the lung and bronchus, 16% are from breast cancer, 11% are from cancer of the colon and rectum, and 5% are from ovarian cancer.[3]

About 90% of lung cancer deaths and 30% of all cancer deaths are related to smoking.[3] With aggressive efforts by the healthcare community both to prevent and to treat this addiction, cancer incidence and mortality will decline. Since the etiology of cancer of the lung and oropharynx for the majority of affected individuals is clear, prevention would be the optimal avenue to reduce lung cancer mortality. However, in addition, lung cancer is usually diagnosed when the disease is at an advanced stage, and lung cancer cure rates are better when the disease is diagnosed early. For the past several years, efforts have been underway to evaluate the value of screening high-risk individuals with chest CT. It has been demonstrated that chest CT screening will identify smaller cancers, and cancers which are more likely to be Stage I.[8] On the other hand, there is concern about false positives, the morbidity and mortality related to intervention, over-diagnosis, and cost.[9] The 2005 Consensus Statement on CT screening for lung cancer concluded that: 'there is insufficient evidence to justify recommending CT screening for lung cancer, including those at high risk for lung cancer'.[9] A minority opinion was issued, which concluded that if a high-risk, asymptomatic individual wants to be screened and has been fully informed of the implications of screening and the treatment that may result, it is reasonable for that individual to decide to be screened by a suitably defined CT regimen.[8]

Breast cancer is one of the leading causes of cancer death in women in many countries. Screening mammography has been demonstrated to result in earlier detection and reduced mortality,[10–12] including in women aged 40–49 years.[13,14] Yet, not all women who are eligible avail themselves of this important diagnostic tool. The role of breast MRI is also being further defined, and the American College of Radiology (ACR) issued guidelines for its use in 2004.[15] In those guidelines, screening breast MRI was not recommended for the general population of asymptomatic women. However, breast MRI has many important indications which were identified by the ACR.

Both Tamoxifen and Raloxifene have been demonstrated to reduce the incidence of breast cancer in women who are at high risk of developing the disease. Tamoxifen has been demonstrated to reduce the incidence of estrogen-receptor positive breast cancers and carcinoma *in situ* in both pre- and post-menopausal women. Raloxifene has been demonstrated to reduce the incidence of estrogen-receptor positive breast cancer, and is used only in women who are post-menopausal. Preliminary data from the STAR trial appear to indicate that Tamoxifen has a higher likelihood of serious side effects than Raloxifene. However, both drugs are associated with the potential for serious side effects; therefore, consideration of their use as preventive agents should only be for women at high risk of developing breast cancer. In the very near future, the results of the STAR trial will be published, and will provide further clarification on the benefits and risks of these two drugs.

Also, more women at high risk for carrying the BRCA-1 and BRCA-2 gene mutations which are associated with very high risk of developing breast and ovarian cancer are being tested for these mutations, and are often electing to undergo preventive strategies (including surgery) to reduce their risk of developing these malignancies.

Colorectal cancer is the third leading cause of cancer death for women in the US, representing 11% of cancers and 11% of cancer deaths.[3] Many of these cancer deaths, and many of the cancers, could be preventable if women were screened.

The adenomatous polyp is the precursor lesion of colorectal cancer. Approximately 10% of adenomatous polyps will become malignant over 10 years, and about 20% will become malignant over 15 years. Ideally, colorectal cancer can be prevented by identifying and removing adenomatous polyps. If that has not been achieved, identifying colorectal cancer in its earliest stages by screening will still substantially improve survival.

There are a variety of modalities available to screen a woman for colorectal cancer. The American Cancer Society recommends screening the average risk woman from age 50 years onward, with screening initiated earlier for higher risk women. Of course, any woman at any age who has rectal bleeding or other symptoms should have a thorough evaluation and a diagnosis made.

Of the available screening modalities, colonoscopy is expensive, but its advantage is that it permits evaluation of the entire colon plus removal of any polyps identified, all in one process. Virtual colonoscopy (a radiological procedure in which the lining of the colon is very well visualized) is less expensive and does not require i.v. sedation; however, if a lesion is identified, colonoscopy still needs to be performed as a second stage procedure to obtain a tissue diagnosis and to remove the lesion. Barium enema is less sensitive than colonoscopy or virtual colonoscopy, and requires a second procedure if an abnormality is found; however, it is less expensive. Sigmoidoscopy is much less expensive. Flexible sigmoidoscopy will identify 40–60% of women with adenomatous polyps and colon cancer; however, a significant percentage of lesions will not be within the range of the sigmoidoscopic evaluation. Fecal occult blood testing is the least costly screening methodology. Although it has a high false-positive rate and is less likely to identify the presence of pre-malignant lesions than more sophisticated studies such as colonoscopy, it has been demonstrated to reduce mortality from colorectal cancer.[16] In some colon cancer screening programs, a combination of modalities is used.

Of the gynecological malignancies, cervical cancer is the leading cause of cancer death world-wide. It is, in fact, the second most common cancer in women world-wide, with 471,000 cases diagnosed, and 233,000 deaths.[17] Approximately 80% of cervical cancers occur in less developed countries, where women have a life-time risk of cervical cancer of 2%, and 15% of cancers in women are cancer of the cervix.[17] Cytology screening (and now HPV testing) have produced dramatic results in reducing cervical cancer incidence and mortality in those countries in which screening has been affordable for the population. The HPV vaccine will have an important future role in reducing the incidence of cervical cancer.

Ovarian cancer survival has been significantly increased by improved surgery and chemotherapy. In addition, genetic testing for women at high risk for carrying BRCA-1 and BRCA-2 mutations, with subsequent prophylactic surgery, can benefit women who are carriers of this genetic mutation. However, the most important goal – early identification of disease – has not yet been reached for the vast majority of affected women. Screening with CA-125 and ultrasound studies has not resulted in dramatic changes. Identification of early disease via proteomics is currently being evaluated, and may be promising.

Uterine cancer affected 189,000 women last year, with the majority of cases occurring in developed countries.[17] By prevention (treatment for anovulation, treatment of premalignant disease) and early detection (evaluation of abnormal bleeding), as well as by sophisticated therapy, mortality from uterine cancer can be further reduced.

In summary, as pertains to reducing cancer incidence and mortality in women, the obstetrician-gynecologist can have a major impact. For many women, there is a long-standing and trusting relationship with their obstetrician-gynecologist, who may be the only physician that they see. By addressing smoking cessation, recommending screening for breast and colorectal cancers, recommending genetics counseling and testing for high-risk women (with subsequent preventive treatments as appropriate), and of course continuing to screen and treat women for premalignant and malignant cervical disease, we can affect the overall health of our patients.

CARDIOVASCULAR DISEASE

One of the other most common etiologies of premature death and disability in women in developed countries is cardiovascular disease. Here too, the obstetrician-gynecologist can have a dramatic impact in reducing death and disability for women, and again this can be achieved in collaboration with other healthcare providers, and within the framework of a very busy obstetric-gynecologic practice.

Some of the most important factors that lead to premature cardiac death and disability can be readily addressed by focusing on prevention and screening. Once the problem has been identified, the obstetrician-gynecologist will often refer the patient for treatment.

Hypertension is a leading contributor to cardiovascular death and disability in women. Yet, it is known that, in the US, only 41% of people with hypertension are receiving treatment, and only one-third are controlled to a blood pressure below 140/90.[18] There is a continuous and consistent relationship between blood pressure and myocardial infarction, stroke, heart failure, and kidney disease. Beginning at 115/75, cardiovascular disease risk doubles for every increment of 20/10.[18] In addition, isolated systolic hypertension, particularly after age 50 years, is a potent cardiovascular disease risk factor.

The obstetrician-gynecologist can improve the health of their patients by identifying hypertensives and pre-hypertensives, educating patients regarding prevention and lifestyle modification (exercise, diet, *etc.*), making certain that their hypertensive patients are receiving adequate treatment, and making certain that the treatment is controlling the blood pressure to an acceptable range (140/90, or 130/80 in patients with diabetes or chronic kidney disease).[18]

More than two-thirds of hypertensive patients will require more than one drug to control their blood pressure adequately; for some women, three or more antihypertensive agents may be required. In most countries and most practice settings, the primary management of the non-gravid hypertensive is not done by the obstetrician-gynecologist. However, the obstetrician-gynecologist can play a very important role in reducing cardiovascular morbidity and mortality for their patients by focusing on the very straightforward and simple issues addressed in the prior paragraph.

Smoking is another major contributor to cardiovascular death and disability. Smoking has a profound effect on cardiovascular disease for women at all ages; it is estimated that smoking is responsible for 55% of the cardiovascular deaths in women under the age of 65 years.

Making certain that patients are appropriately educated regarding diet, ideal weight, and exercise, and that they understand how important their physician feels these issues are to their overall health is another substantial contribution that obstetrician-gynecologists can make in reducing morbidity and mortality. In many developed countries, obesity and inadequate exercise are major contributors to premature morbidity and mortality in women. Obesity, inappropriate diet, and lack of exercise are substantial contributors to cardiovascular disease and diabetes, as well as several other very common disorders in women.

Untreated hyperlipidemia is another major contributor to cardiovascular disease in women. The recommendation of the US National Cholesterol Education Program (NCEP) Adult Treatment Panel III (ATP III) is that all individuals aged 20 years or older should have a fasting lipoprotein profile (total cholesterol, LDL, HDL, and triglycerides), and that if it is normal it should be repeated every 5 years.[19] ATP III defines the optimal LDL cholesterol level as < 100, and high LDL beginning at 160. It defines desirable total cholesterol as < 200, and high as ≥ 240. High HDL (good) cholesterol is defined as ≥ 60, and low as < 40. ATP III defines a normal triglyceride as < 150, and high as ≥ 200.[19]

Elevated LDL cholesterol is a major risk factor for cardiovascular disease. The primary target of cholesterol-lowering therapy is LDL, and LDL lowering therapy has been demonstrated to reduce cardiovascular risk. In 2004, the NCEP Coordinating Committee made recommendations which built further on ATP III, and were based on 5 major clinical trials.[20] They recommended that for high-risk people the LDL goal should be < 100, and that in very high-risk individuals it should be < 70. Other components of the lipid profile, such as very high triglycerides, may require additional treatment. In most countries and most practice settings, the obstetrician-gynecologist is not likely to be the primary physician treating hyperlipidemia. However, given the fact that it is such a substantial contributor to premature cardiovascular morbidity and mortality, the obstetrician-gynecologist can have a major impact just by making certain that these bloods are being drawn and that abnormal results are being addressed.

In the US, and in many developed countries, more than half of all deaths in adult women are due to cancer and cardiovascular disease.[21] By just focusing on the aforementioned simple steps, the obstetrician-gynecologist can have a dramatic role in reducing premature morbidity and mortality in their patients from these two causes. However, there are many other important, equally simple, contributions that the obstetrician-gynecologist can make, which also do not require large amounts of time, and which can have enormous impact.

INFECTIOUS DISEASE

Prevention of infectious diseases is another area in which the obstetrician-gynecologist can play a role in preventing death and disability. Both in developed and in developing countries, large numbers of women continue to die each year from vaccine- preventable diseases. Depending upon the practice setting, obstetrician-gynecologists may: (i) decide to vaccinate their patients for all vaccine-preventable infectious diseases for which their patient population is at risk; (ii) identify only certain vaccine-preventable infectious diseases with referral for vaccination for others; or (iii) they may just inform their patients of the necessary vaccination schedule, urge their patients to be vaccinated according to the recommended schedule, and make certain that their patients have a venue for vaccination (family practitioner, internist, public health clinic, *etc.*).

Common vaccine-preventable infectious diseases for which women should be vaccinated will depend upon where they live and their travel and work circumstances and exposure risk.

Vaccination programs may include many or all of the following:

Influenza	*Pneumonia*
Tetanus and diphtheria	*Measles, mumps, rubella*
Varicella	*Polio*
Hepatitis B	*Hepatitis A*
Meningococcal meningitis	

Other vaccines are also available, and will be appropriate for subgroups of women depending upon their risk of exposure. There are currently more than 50 types of vaccines. Not only are vaccination programs cost-effective, but they also prevent unnecessary and premature death and disability.

Prevention of transmission of the human immunodeficiency virus has been an important contribution of the obstetrician-gynecologist. The incidence of vertical transmission to newborns has been substantially reduced in many countries. In addition, obstetrician-gynecologists have been at the forefront in educating women about protecting themselves and their offspring.

DIABETES

Diabetes is another important contributor to premature death and disability. It substantially increases a woman's risk of coronary artery disease, stroke, renal failure, blindness, peripheral vascular disease, and other problems. Uncontrolled blood sugar also is associated with a substantially increased risk of congenital anomalies. The obstetrician-gynecologist can contribute greatly to reducing disease burden by focusing on prevention (exercise, diet), screening and detection, and emphasizing to patients the importance of euglycemia to prevent end organ damage and morbidity and mortality.

ACCIDENTS

Accidents are a major contributor to premature death and disability for women in both developed and developing countries, although the types of accidents may be different. In the US, accidents are the leading cause of death for women between the ages of 19–39 years, and the fourth leading cause of death for women between the ages of 40–64 years.[2] Automobile-associated fatalities (often related to alcohol and/or drug use and failure to use seatbelts) are largely preventable. Obstetrician-gynecologists and their staffs can discuss accident prevention with women during routine visits. They can also use simple screening questions for alcohol and drug use (with counseling and/or referral as appropriate).

REDUCING MORBIDITY

In addition to focusing on prevention, screening, and early detection of the major causes of mortality in women, the obstetrician-gynecologist can make substantial contributions to reducing morbidity as well. The obstetrician-gynecologist already focuses on many of the preventable and correctable major causes of morbidity in women and, by doing so, has a profoundly positive impact on their patients' quality of life. For instance, urinary incontinence in women often results in a significant curtailment of activities; by diagnosing and treating this problem, the obstetrician-gynecologist enables their patients to resume previously enjoyed activities.

Osteoporosis is another very serious problem which is increasingly common in women as they age. By focusing on prevention beginning when patients are young, and subsequently, as well on early diagnosis and treatment, the obstetrician-gynecologist may be able to reduce the incidence of fractures, pain, and impaired mobility and function.

The obstetrician-gynecologist, of course, is also involved in preventing morbidity from a wide variety of other causes by being involved in programs for such problems as the early detection of exposure to tuberculosis, prevention and treatment of sexually transmitted diseases, identification of women with eating disorders, *etc.*

Table 1 Criteria for diagnosis of a major depressive episode[22]

1.	Sad or irritable mood
2.	Decreased pleasure in previously pleasurable events and activities
3.	Decreased energy
4.	Decreased interest in one's usual activities
5.	Difficulty concentrating
6.	Withdrawal from social relationships
7.	Psychomotor retardation or agitation
8.	Changes in sleep
9.	Changes in appetite and weight
10.	Loss of libido
11.	Helplessness and hopelessness
12.	Feelings of worthlessness and guilt
13.	Thoughts of death and/or suicide

The mental health and safety of patients are other very important issues. In many countries, the obstetrician-gynecologist has taken an increasingly active role in identifying problems related to mental health and to abuse (sexual abuse, elder abuse, domestic violence, *etc.*), and in working with, or making referrals to, available resources in the community.

Depression is an illness which is 2–3 times more common in women than men. Obstetrician-gynecologists have played an increasing role in screening women for depression, and either treating their patients or referring them for treatment. Table 1 presents the criteria for diagnosis of a major depressive episode.[22] To diagnose a major depressive episode in a patient, the woman must have at least five of the thirteen signs and symptoms (one of which must be #1 or #2), and they must be present most of the day every day for at least 2 weeks.

Obstetrician-gynecologists have become increasingly involved in making certain that their patients are screened for depression. They will then usually refer the patients who they have identified for pharmacotherapy and/or psychotherapy or counseling. However, some obstetrician-gynecologists do treat their patients who have mild depression.

In addition to identifying those women who are depressed, identifying those who may be suicidal and getting them immediate help is essential, especially since suicide is one of the ten leading causes of death in certain age groups in some countries.

In addition to identifying women who are depressed, by identifying patients with other psychiatric disorders and significant psychosocial problems, the obstetrician-gynecologist can dramatically improve the lives of their patients.

During the past half century, obstetrician-gynecologists have made profound contributions to the health of their patients by: reducing perinatal mortality; reducing maternal mortality; treating infertility; diagnosing and treating sexually transmitted diseases; diagnosing and treating symptomatic disorders of the pelvic floor; and preventing, diagnosing, and treating gynecologic malignancies. These contributions to women's health by focusing on specialty and subspecialty care have been spectacular, and dramatic advances continue to be made.

In addition, obstetrician-gynecologists have made substantial contributions to the overall health of their patients by focusing on general women's wellness, prevention, screening, and early detection. By emphasizing to their patients issues related to cancer screening, cardiac prevention, bone health, diet, exercise, and smoking cessation, obstetrician-gynecologists have prevented premature morbidity and mortality from problems not always traditionally considered a part of the specialty of obstetrics and gynecology.

For most obstetrician-gynecologists their practices are busy and the time that they can spend with each patient must have some limitations. However, by either personally (or by having office staff or even literature or other media) focusing some attention on prevention, screening, and early detection of some of the main contributors to premature morbidity and mortality in the patient population they serve, obstetrician-gynecologists can further contribute to the well-being of their patients.

References

1 Seltzer VL. Prevention. In: Seltzer VL, Pearse WH. (eds) Women's Primary Health Care, 2nd edn. New York: McGraw-Hill, 2000

2 American College of Obstetricians and Gynecologists. Primary Care Review for the Obstetrician-Gynecologist, Primary and Preventive Care. Washington, DC: ACOG, 1997

3 Seltzer V. Cancer in women: prevention and early detection. J Women's Health 2000; 9: 483–488

4 Seltzer V. Smoking as a risk factor in the health of women. Int J Gynecol Obstet 2003; 82: 393–397

5 World Health Organization. Tobacco or health: A global status report. Geneva: WHO, 1997

6 Cole HM. A future without tobacco. JAMA 1999; 282: 1284

7 A clinical practice guideline for treating tobacco use and dependence. A US public health service report. JAMA 2000; 293: 3244–3254

8 Henschke CI, Austin JHM, Berlin N *et al.* Minority opinion. CT screening for lung cancer. J Thorac Imaging 2005; 20: 324–325

9 Swensen S, Aberle D, Kazerooni EA *et al.* Consensus Statement: CT screening for lung cancer. J Thorac Imaging 2005; 20: 321

10 Duffy SW, Tabar L, Chen HH *et al.* The impact of organized mammography service screening on breast carcinoma mortality in seven Swedish counties. Cancer 2002; 95: 458–469

11 Chu KC, Smart CR, Tarone RE. Analysis of breast cancer mortality and stage distribution by age for the health insurance plan clinical trial. J Natl Cancer Inst 1998; 80: 1125–1132

12 Smith RA, Duffy SW, Gabe R *et al.* The randomized trials of breast cancer screening. What have we learned? Radiol Clin North Am 2004; 42: 793–806

13 Hendrick RE, Smith RA, Rutledge JH *et al.* Benefit of screening mammography in women aged 40–49: A new meta-analysis of randomized controlled trials. Monogr Natl Cancer Inst 1997; 22: 87–92

14 Bjurstam N, Bjorneld L, Duffy SW *et al.* The Gothenburg breast screening trial. Cancer 1997; 80: 2091–2099

15 American College of Radiology. ACR practice guidelines for the performance of magnetic resonance imaging (MRI) of the breast. ACR Practice Guideline 2004; 341–346

16 Markowitz AJ, Winawer SJ. Screening and surveillance for colorectal cancer. Semin Oncol 1999; 26: 485–498

17 Parkin DM. Global cancer statistics in the year 2000. Lancet Oncol 2001; 2: 533–543

18 Chobanian AV, Bakris GL, Black HR *et al.* Seventh report of the joint national committee on prevention, detection, evaluation, and treatment of high blood pressure. Hypertension 2003; 42: 1206–1252

19 US National Cholesterol Education Program (NCEP) Adult Treatment Panel III (ATP III). Executive summary of the third report of the National Cholesterol Education Program (NCEP) expert panel on detection, evaluation, and treatment of high blood cholesterol in adults (Adult Treatment Panel III) JAMA 2001; 285: 2486–2497

20 Grundy SM, Cleeman JL, Merz CNB *et al.* Implications of recent clinical trials for the national cholesterol guidelines. Circulation 2004; 110: 227–239

21 Misra D. (ed) The Women's Health Data Book, 3rd edn. Washington, DC and Menlo Park, CA: Jacobs Institute of Women's Health and Henry J. Kaiser Family Foundation, 2001

22 American Psychiatric Association. Diagnostic and Statistical Manual of Mental Disorders, 4th edn. Washington, DC: American Psychiatric Press, 1994

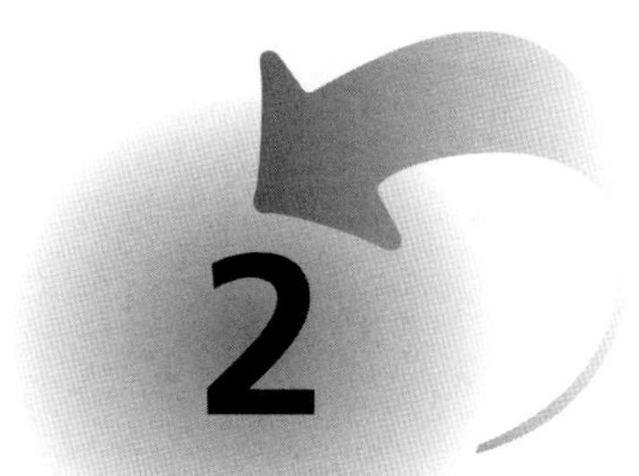

Swati Vyas Lubna Ghani Nina Khazaezadeh
Eugene Oteng-Ntim

Pregnancy and obesity

Obesity has reached epidemic proportions globally, with more than one billion adults overweight – at least 300 million of them clinically obese – and is a major contributor to the global burden of chronic disease and disability <http://www.who.int/nut/#obs>. The prevalence of obesity in the UK has trebled since 1980 and continues to rise. In the UK, 22% of men, 24% of women,[1] and 10% of children are obese. In the US, the prevalence of overweight and obesity now exceeds more than 60% among adults and, alarmingly, a similar trend is increasingly observed in children and adolescents. The latest data from the US National Center for Health Statistics show that 30% of adults (over 60 million people aged 20 years and older) are obese. It is classed as sixth most important risk factor contributing to overall burden of disease is attributed to 30,000 deaths in the UK per year. The World Health Organization (WHO) describes obesity as: 'one of the most blatantly visible, yet most neglected, public-health problems that threatens to overwhelm both more and less developed countries'. A recent study showed that 1 in 5 women booking for antenatal care in 2002–2004 were obese.[2]

A generally accepted definition of obesity is a body mass index (BMI) > 30 kg/m^2 (Table 1). Obesity is known to be associated with serious obstetric complications. Studies have reported an increased incidence of gestational

Swati Vyas MB BS
Senior SHO, St Thomas's Hospital, London, UK

Lubna Ghani
Medical Student, King's College London, London, UK

Nina Khazaezadeh BSc MSc
Public Health Consultant Midwife, Guy's and St Thomas' NHS Foundation Trust, London, UK

Eugene Oteng-Ntim MBBS MRCOG (for correspondence)
Consultant Obstetrician, St Thomas's Hospital, Lambeth Palace Road, London SE1 7EH, UK
E-mail: eugene.oteng-ntim@gstt.nhs.uk

Table 1 Definition of obesity

BMI (kg/m^2)	Weight status
< 18.5	Underweight
18.5–24.9	Normal
25.0–29.9	Overweight
> 30.0	Obese

Adapted from <http://www.who.int/nut/#obs> (accessed 21 November 2005)

diabetes, gestational hypertension and pre-eclampsia, fetal macrosomia, shoulder dystocia and cesarean section. Increased obesity rates among pregnant women are a significant public health concern with various implications for prenatal care and supervision of delivery. In pregnancy, BMI is calculated using prepregnant weight. If this is unknown, the first weight measurement at prenatal care is used.[3]

The increased risk of complications in obese women during pregnancy and delivery coupled with the rising epidemic of obesity among women emphasise the need for the specialists involved in treating obese women to be aware of the risks and complications and their management.

This article will review these obesity-related, adverse-pregnancy outcomes with a brief outline of the possible physiological mechanisms involved, followed by a discussion of the best practise in managing obese mothers from pregravid to postpartum and their effectiveness in reducing the risk of the obesity-related, adverse outcomes in pregnancy.

OBESITY-RELATED ADVERSE OUTCOMES IN PREGNANCY

The impact of obesity on pregnancy is a major problem. Obesity can be a barrier to reproduction as there is an association between high BMI and infertility. Furthermore, obese women commonly present with higher incidences of menstrual disorders and miscarriage.

Linsten *et al.*[4] showed that a high BMI is related to a lower live birth rate and a higher incidence of early pregnancy loss among women undergoing *in vitro* fertilisation or intracytoplasmic sperm injection. This is mainly due to an increased risk of early pregnancy loss in obese women. In addition, an impaired response to ovarian stimulation in obese women was also observed. These results suggest that subfertility treatment is dependent on BMI and interventions to reduce weight would be beneficial in the treatment of subfertility and subsequently during pregnancy.

Interestingly, studies have shown that the fat distribution may play a significant role in fertility. Central obesity appears to be detrimental to ovarian function because it is associated with higher levels of fasting insulin, luteinizing hormone, estrone and androstenedione than the same body mass with a peripheral fat distribution.[5]

The major maternal complications associated with obesity during pregnancy include:[6]

1. Diabetes (pregestational and gestational).
2. Hypertensive disease (chronic hypertension and pre-eclampsia).

3. Thrombo-embolic disease.
4. Respiratory disorders (asthma and sleep apnoea).
5. Infections (urinary tract infections, wound infections and endometritis).

Gestational diabetes mellitus

Gestational diabetes mellitus is defined by the American Diabetes Association as:[7] 'any degree of glucose intolerance with onset or first recognition during pregnancy'. Factors related to the development of gestational diabetes mellitus are ethnicity, prepregnancy weight, previous gestational diabetes mellitus, age, parity and family history of diabetes.[7]

Approximately 1–3% of women, compared to 17% of obese women, develop gestational diabetes mellitus during pregnancy.[8] Several studies have shown that there is a strong correlation between obesity and gestational diabetes mellitus. Therefore, it is pertinent to identify women at risk of developing gestational diabetes mellitus as this increases the risk of hypertensive disorders in pregnancy, macrosomia in the infant and predisposes the women to a higher risk of developing type 2 diabetes mellitus in later life. Furthermore, obese mothers with gestational diabetes mellitus have twice the risk of delivering children with chromosomal defects than those without.[9]

Linne *et al.*[10] followed up 28 women with gestational diabetes mellitus and a control group ($n = 52$) for 15 years and found that women with gestational diabetes mellitus who developed type 2 diabetes mellitus gained significantly more weight (15.1 kg) following the birth of their first child compared to both women without gestational diabetes mellitus and women with gestational diabetes mellitus who did not develop type 2 diabetes mellitus. Thus, active strategies for weight control and life-style advice after delivery with regular follow-up is needed for the management of women with gestational diabetes mellitus[10] to prevent type 2 diabetes mellitus and the associated morbidity and mortality.

Hypertensive disease

The majority of studies show that maternal obesity is an important factor for gestational hypertension.[3] However there is controversy regarding pre-eclampsia and BMI. The systemic review of O'Brien *et al.*[12] demonstrated a consistently strong positive association between maternal prepregnancy BMI and the risk of pre-eclampsia. The risk of pre-eclampsia typically doubled with each 5–7 kg/m^2 increase in prepregnancy BMI. Overall, the literature shows that obese pregnant women have a 14–25% incidence of pre-eclampsia.[6] Although maternal BMI is strongly correlated with the risk of pre-eclampsia, no correlation has been found with the incidence of hemolysis, elevated liver enzymes and low platelet count (HELLP) syndrome.[3]

Women who have had pre-eclampsia die from cardiovascular disease (RR = 8.1) and stroke (RR = 5.1), thus preventative measures need to be taken.[9] Recent research has revealed that a low level of sex hormone-binding globulin, a marker of insulin resistance in obese women, is an early predictor of pre-eclampsia, allowing preventive treatment.[9] Further research into the sensitivity and specificity of this test is needed for it to be routinely used in obese pregnant women.

Thrombo-embolic complications

Venous thrombo-embolic complications are a leading cause of maternal mortality in the developed world. Pregnancy-associated death from thrombo-embolism occurs once in around 70,000 pregnancies, a 12-fold increase compared to the non-pregnant state, where the risk is around one in a million.[13] The Royal College of Obstetricians and Gynaecologists report[14] on maternal deaths concluded that obesity is the most common risk factor for thrombo-embolism.[3] Pregnancy increases the risk of venous thrombo-embolism through venous stasis, changes in blood coagulability and damage to vessels.

Therefore, it seems important to identify obese women who are at increased risk of venous thrombo-embolism, who might also have other risk factors present. Low molecular weight heparin is an effective thromboprophylaxis in pregnancy.[13]

Many studies have suggested that an elevation of procoagulant factors is a possible mechanism by which obesity leads to increased thrombotic risk; however, other researchers have not found this.[15]

Respiratory complications

There is limited research looking at the effects of obesity in pregnancy on the respiratory system. Obesity has been shown to have a causal association with sleep apnoea and asthma. Sahota *et al.*[16] showed that obese women in early pregnancy had increased rates of sleep-related apnoea, snoring and 4% oxygen desaturation compared to non-obese pregnant women. However, there is a lack of evidence showing the long-term outcomes of these finding in pregnancy.[6,16]

Sleep apnoea

The mechanical effects of bulky fatty tissue around the neck induce an obstruction to breathing, particularly during sleep, leading to sleep apnoea. A neck circumference of 43.0 cm or more in men or 40.5 cm or more in women is associated with episodes of disrupted breathing, recurring up to 30 times a night. Observers describe loud snoring, followed by a pause of 10 s or longer in breathing, then a loud grunt and resumption of normal respiration. About 3% of middle-aged people in more developed countries are affected, with a male to female ratio of 4:1. Sleep apnoea can lead to pulmonary hypertension, right heart failure, drug-resistant hypertension, stroke, and arrhythmias, but the main risk is accidents caused by day-time somnolence, for example, when driving.

Infections

A recent population-based observational study found an increased incidence of urinary tract infections in obese women supporting existing literature. However, there was no increase in the incidence of genital or wound infections in obese women as previously reported. This difference could be a result of exclusion of women with diabetes or to the practice of giving antibiotic prophylaxis at cesarean section.[17]

Metabolic syndrome

Metabolic syndrome is defined by the US National Cholesterol Education Program as the presence of any three of the following conditions:[46]

1. Excess weight around the waist (waist measurement of more than 40 inches for men and more than 35 inches for women).
2. High levels of triglyceride (150 mg/dl or higher).
3. Low levels of high density lipid, or 'good' cholesterol (below 40 mg/dl for men and below 50 mg/dl for women).
4. High blood pressure (130/85 mmHg or higher).
5. High fasting blood glucose levels (110 mg/dl or higher)

Metabolic syndrome predisposes individuals to diabetes and cardiovascular disease. Metabolic syndrome is defined as the association of obesity, insulin resistance, glucose intolerance, hypertension, and a characteristic dyslipidemia. Boney *et al.*[11] suggested that obese mothers who do not fulfil the clinical criteria for gestational diabetes mellitus might still have metabolic factors that affect fetal growth and postnatal outcomes. This is of interest as the study of Boney *et al.*[11] showed that children exposed to maternal obesity were at increased risk of developing metabolic syndrome, an observation with grave implications for subsequent generations.

OBESITY-RELATED ADVERSE OUTCOMES IN LABOR

Obese women have increased incidences of labor induction. The estimated increase is 1.7–2.2-fold, which remains significant after adjusting for associated antepartum complications. The evidence regarding labor induction is conflicting, with some investigators reporting higher incidences of prolonged labor and failure to progress. A better understanding of the relationship between obesity and labor mechanism is needed to prevent the high rates of intervention during labor.[18]

Cesarean sections

Maternal obesity is an independent risk factor for cesarean sections. Sheiner *et al.*[19] investigated the pregnancy outcome of obese patients not suffering from hypertensive disorders or diabetes mellitus. They found that the association between obesity and cesarean section remained significant after controlling for variables recognised to co-exist with obesity. It was suggested that this might be because of care-giver bias. Similarly, Sebire *et al.*[20] showed that the cesarean section rate for obese women was over 20% compared to nearer 10% for normal-weight women.

Sheiner *et al.*[19] also found that, after the exclusion of hypertensive disorders and diabetes mellitus, maternal obesity was not found to be associated with an increased rate of adverse perinatal outcome, which is often used as a reason for cesarean section in obese women.

Table 2 shows that there were no significant differences found regarding low Apgar scores, perinatal mortality, congenital malformations, preterm delivery, *etc.*, contrary to evidence in the literature.

Table 2 Perinatal and maternal outcomes of obese and non-obese patients

Characteristic	Obese (n = 1769)	Non-obese (n = 124,311)	OR	95% CI	P-value
Apgar 1 min < 7	4.4%	4.3%	1.0	0.8–1.3	0.93
Apgar 5 min < 7	0.6%	0.6%	1.0	0.5–1.8	0.94
Perinatal mortality	1.7%	1.3%	1.3	0.9–1.8	0.18
Shoulder dystocia	0.3%	0.2%	1.6	0.7–4.0	0.25
Congenital malformations	4.0%	3.9%	1.0	0.8–1.3	0.74
Postpartum hemorrhage	0.5%	0.4%	1.0	0.5–2.1	0.89
Packed-cells transfusion	1.8%	1.3%	1.4	0.9–1.9	0.09
Peripartum fever	0.9%	0.6%	1.6	0.9–2.6	0.06

Adapted from Sheiner *et al.*[19]

In support of this, Sheiner *et al.*[19] suggest that the increased risk of perinatal complications associated with obesity may be due to the 'significant contribution of diabetes mellitus and hypertension, and not obesity *per se*, to the adverse perinatal outcome'.

In light of this evidence and the known increased risk for anesthesia-related complications for the obese mother including peri-operative thrombo-embolic events, postoperative infection, risks and difficulty with anesthesia, and increased risk of mortality, the increased tendency to perform cesarean sections in obese mothers needs to be weighed against the risk of cesarean sections to the mother.[19]

However, Chauhan *et al.*[21] found that, in women weighing more than 136.3 kg, vaginal delivery after previous cesarean section was successful in only 13% of cases, which is lower than that cited for the general population at 60–80%. The commonest reason for morbidly obese women failing a trial of labor was a non-reassuring fetal heart rate tracing. In support of this, Sheiner *et al.*[19] found that obese women were more likely to have labor induction, failure to progress during the first stage of labor, meconium-stained amniotic fluid, malpresentations and cesarean sections than non-obese women (Table 3).

In obese women with prior cesarean delivery, the infectious morbidity was 53% higher when attempting a trial of labor than having a repeat elective cesarean section. Implications of this are that the low success rate and greater than 50% chance of infectious morbidity associated with trial of labor calls for

Table 3 Pregnancy and labour complications of obese and non-obese parturients

Characteristic	Obese (n = 1769)	Non-obese (n = 124,311)	OR	95% CI	P-value
Labour induction	18.3%	8.7%	2.3	2.1–2.6	< 0.0001
Placental abruption	0.3%	0.7%	0.4	0.2–1.2	0.08
Placenta previa	0.3%	0.4%	0.8	0.4–1.9	0.65
Failure to progress 1st stage	6.0%	1.6%	4.0	3.2–4.9	< 0.001
Failure to progress 2nd stage	1.5%	1.7%	0.9	0.6–1.3	0.67
Meconium-stained amniotic fluid	21.5%	16.2%	1.4	1.2–1.6	< 0.0001
Malpresentation	9.2%	5.9%	1.6	1.3–1.9	< 0.0001
Cesarean delivery	27.8%	10.8%	3.2	2.9–3.5	< 0.0001

Adapted from Sheiner *et al.*[19]

the health professional to be aware that obese patients may not be ideal candidates for attempting vaginal birth after previous cesarean section.[21]

Usha *et al.*[17] reported the effect of maternal obesity on pregnancy complications with minimal confounding bias. The study supports existing evidence that woman with a BMI > 30 kg/m^2 have a 1–2-fold higher risk of cesarean section. The researchers advocate that this may be an effect of the increased rate of large for gestational age infants leading to disproportion during labor. Furthermore, they suggest that it may be possible that uterine contractility may be suboptimal in a subgroup of obese women, or there may be increased fat deposition in the soft tissues of the pelvis. However, it is possible that the higher rates of cesarean section are because obese women have a higher incidence of post-term and difficulty with induction leading to other interventions.[17]

Shoulder dystocia

Shoulder dystocia is defined as a delivery in which additional manoeuvres are required to deliver the fetus after normal gentle downward traction has failed. It occurs when the fetal anterior shoulder impacts against the maternal symphysis following delivery of the vertex.[22] Shoulder dystocia complicates 0.13–2.1% of all deliveries and is associated with adverse pregnancy outcome (Table 4).

Relevant risk factors have included fetal macrosomia, maternal diabetes, post-term pregnancy, prolonged second stage of labor, history of a previous macrosomic infant, instrumental delivery, advanced maternal age, multiparity, and maternal obesity.

Controversy exists regarding maternal obesity as a risk factor for shoulder dystocia. It has been argued this association could be related to the correlation of obesity with diabetes mellitus. A case control study by Robinson *et al.*[23] showed that the strongest predictors of shoulder dystocia are related to fetal macrosomia. Furthermore, they found that for obese non-diabetic women carrying fetuses whose weights are estimated to be within normal limits, there is no increased risk of shoulder dystocia. Therefore, for obese women, the predictors of shoulder dystocia are similar to those of non-obese women.

Table 4 Complications of shoulder dystocia

Maternal
Postpartum hemorrhage
Rectovaginal fistula
Symphyseal separation or diathesis, with or without transient femoral neuropathy
Third- or fourth-degree episiotomy or tear
Uterine rupture
Fetal
Brachial plexus palsy
Clavicle fracture
Fetal death
Fetal hypoxia, with or without permanent neurological damage
Fracture of the humerus

Adapted from Baxley and Gobbo.[22]

However, the study in Israel by Sheiner *et al.*[19] was unable to verify this as, after excluding patients with diabetes mellitus, no association was found despite higher rates of fetal macrosomia in the study population. Conversely, two different ethnic groups with different life-styles were studied which could have resulted in conflicting reports.

Postpartum complications

Evidence has shown that obese women tend to have higher rates of postpartum hemorrhage; the increased incidence of cesarean sections among obese women has been implicated as a causal factor. However, Usha et al.[17] showed the increased rate of cesarean section might not be the only factor influencing the blood loss in this group. Obese women who had a vaginal delivery had a greater than 500 ml blood loss compared to those with a BMI of 20–30 kg/m^2.[17]

Moreover, Sebire *et al.*[20] noted a 44% increased risk for a major postpartum hemorrhage in gravidas with a BMI > 30 kg/m^2 even after accounting for predisposing factors, *i.e.* cesarean section. They suggested this might be explained by excess bleeding from the relatively larger area of implantation of the placenta usually associated with a large for gestational age fetus. Nuthalapaty and Rouse[18] considered the possibility that the relatively large volume of distribution related to obesity and the resultant decreased bioavailability of uterotonic agents could be an additional factor related to the increased risk.

Other postpartum complications

Lactate dysfunction

Obesity is associated with increased risk of failure to initiate lactation and decreased duration of lactation; however, there is conflicting evidence regarding this. Maternal obesity is implicated in altering the hypothalamic–pituitary–gonadal axis and fat metabolism, resulting in lactate dysfunction; however, the exact mechanism remains to be determined.[18]

Aftercare

In the postpartum period, obese women are found to have a significantly higher incidence of hospitalisation for more than 4 days compared to non-obese women. This has significant health resource implications and studies are needed to prevent the high hospitalisation rate among obese women in postpartum.[18]

OBESITY-RELATED ADVERSE OUTCOMES ON THE FETUS

Neural tube defects

Neural tube defects are serious malformations affecting approximately 1 per 1000 births, yet the mechanisms by which they arise are unknown. There is an extensive list of neural tube defect risk factors, including race/ethnicity of parents, maternal age, socio-economic status, and maternal disorders such as functional vitamin deficiencies (for example, folic acid).

Recently, there has been evidence to support the association between maternal obesity and the increased risk of neural tube defects. The Atlanta

Birth Defect Risk Factor surveillance study, a population-based, control study found that for every incremental unit increase in BMI the risk of neural tube defect increased by 7%.[24]

The mechanism for the observed association between obesity and neural tube defect is not known, but several possible explanations have been proposed. Hendricks *et al.*[25] showed that hyperinsulinemia is a strong risk factor for neural tube defects and may be the driving force for the observed risk in obese women. However, this study needs to be interpreted with caution as the patient cohort were Mexican-American women, who tend to have lower intakes of supplemental folic acid than the general American population (3–9% compared with 25%) and are genetically disposed to diabetes mellitus; moreover, 54% of the control women had elevated insulin levels (> 10 μIU/ml). Nevertheless, Hendricks *et al.*[25] showed that hyperinsulinemia was an independent risk factor for neural tube defects but, even after adjustment for hyperinsulinemia, obesity continued to be a modest risk factor.

Other possible mechanisms implicated in the association between obesity and neural tube defects include increased triglycerides, uric acid and endogenous estrogen levels in addition to insulin resistance.[26] It has been speculated that obese women may have poor quality diets and or dieting behavior resulting in nutritional deficits, contributing to the increased risk of congenital defects. However, multivitamin and folic acid intake has been shown to be similar among obese and non-obese women. This raises the possibility that other nutrients not recognised as causing birth defects could be involved.[24]

However, there is evidence to suggest that the association between neural tube defects and obese women could be due to that the fact that such women require higher intakes of folic acid. Werler *et al.*[27] compared maternal prepregnancy weight in two groups of fetuses or infants: 604 with a neural tube defect and 1658 controls with other major malformations. Folate consumption was found to be associated with a reduced risk for neural tube defects among women < 70 kg weight, but not among heavier women. They concluded that the risk of neural tube defects increased with increasing prepregnant weight, independent of the effects of folate intake.[27] This emphasises the importance of efforts to reduce weight in obese women before pregnancy due to the failure of the protective action of folate against neural tube defects.

Recently, Ray *et al.*[28] examined whether the risk of open neural tube defect, in relation to maternal obesity, changed after the introduction of Canada's folic acid fortification program. Overweight women are at increased risk for fetal neural tube defects, but they also naturally eat more than normal-weight women and are, as a result, likely to consume more fortified flour. Table 5 shows that a prefortification maternal weight of Q4 (> 73.6 kg) was associated with a slightly increased risk of neural tube defect (adjusted OR 1.4; 95% CI 1.0–1.8). However, after fortification, the risk was more pronounced (adjusted OR 2.8; 95% CI 1.2–6.6). This study emphasises that, despite the introduction of folic acid flour fortification, women of increased weight have remained at significantly higher risk of neural tube defect compared women in Q1–-Q3.[28]

The physiological mechanism(s) behind obesity and birth defects are unknown. In light of the results of Ray et al.[28] and Watkins *et al.*,[24] it seems

Table 5 Risk of open neural tube defects in relation to elevated maternal weight and folic acid flour fortification

Maternal weight by quartile (kg)	Adjusted OR* (95% CI) Prefortification (n = 316,064)	Postfortification (n = 90,127)
Q1–Q3 ≤ 73.6	1.0 (reference)	1.0 (reference)
Q4 > 73.6	1,4 (1.0–1.8)	2.8 (1.2–6.6)

OR, odds ratio; CI, confidence interval; Q, quartile.
*Adjusted for maternal age, ethnicity and presence of pregestational diabetes mellitus from Ray *et al.*[28]

unethical to await the elucidation of such mechanisms in obese women and great emphasis needs to be placed on ensuring that reproductive-aged women are of healthy weight preconceptionally.[24]

Small for gestational age, intra-uterine death

Cnatinguis *et al.*[29] studied a large, population-based cohort of Swedish women and found that the risk of delivering a small for gestational age baby decreased with increasing BMI among parous women. The study of Cedergren[30] also supports this; however, after excluding women with pre-eclampsia, this increased risk was no longer statistically significant (adjusted OR 1.23; 95% CI 0.94–1.60; Table 6).

The study of Sebire *et al.*[20] showed that obese parous women had a significantly increased risk of late fetal death relative to women of normal weight (BMI 20–25 kg/m^2) after adjustment for obesity-related diseases in pregnancy. Also, Cedergren[30] found that morbidly obese women (BMI > 40 kg/m^2) had an almost 3-fold increased risk of antepartum stillbirth.

Nohr *et al.*[31] suggested that the increased risk of stillbirth could be related to rapid fetal growth due to fetal hyperglycemia, which may place the fetus at risk of death, by hypoxia if the placenta cannot transfer sufficient oxygen for metabolic requirements. Yet, the Danish National Birth Cohort study found

Table 6 Risk of delivering a small or large for gestational age infant in singleton pregnancies among obese and morbidly obese women

Maternal BMI (kg/m^2)	AGA	SGA < 2 SD	Adjusted OR* (95% CI)	LGA > 2 SD	Adjusted OR* (95% CI)
19.8–26	486,783	10,981	Reference	26,339	Reference
29.1–35	58,738	1257	0.98 (0.93–1.04)	7744	2.20 (2.14–2.26)
35.1–40	10,260	234	1.02 (0.90–1.17)	1848	3.11 (2.96–3.27)
> 40	2675	79	1.37 (1.09–1.71)	610	3.82 (3.50–4.16)

SGA, small for gestational age; LGA, large for gestational age; AGA, appropriate for gestational age; SD, standard deviation; OR, odds ratio; CI, confidence interval.
*Adjustments were made for maternal age, parity, smoking in early pregnancy, and year of birth from Cedergren.[30]

that when gestational age was taken into account, the birth weights of unexplained intra-uterine deaths among obese women were typically lower than the median birth weights of all live births.[31] They proposed that the presence of some intra-uterine growth restriction rather than excess fetal growth is the causative factor. The mechanism behind maternal obesity and stillbirth is unclear. However, studies seem to show that the degree of obesity plays a significant role in the association.[30]

Preterm births

A recent prospective study by Hendler *et al.*,[32] the Maternal-Fetal Medicine Units Network, Preterm Prediction study found that prepregnancy obesity, (BMI ≥ 30 kg/m^2), was associated with fewer total preterm births and spontaneous preterm births. Conversely, a significantly high percentage of the preterm births in obese women were found often in association with pre-eclampsia, compared to preterm births of thin women. Of note, maternal thinness was associated with an increased incidence of spontaneous preterm births. There is some evidence to suggest that malnutrition could be a causative factor for spontaneous preterm birth, which might explain the low incidence of spontaneous preterm birth in obese compared to lean women who may have lower intakes of nutrients.[32]

However, data regarding the relationship of preterm birth in obese women is contradictory. Overall, it seems that, in obese women, the increased risk of preterm birth is associated with obesity-related medical and antenatal complications and not some intrinsic predisposition to spontaneous preterm birth.[18]

Macrosomia

Macrosomia has been associated with multiple factors, including maternal age and weight. However, increased maternal prepregnancy weight and decreased prepregnancy insulin sensitivity are strongly correlated with fetal growth, in particular fat mass at birth. It is thought that, in early pregnancy, increased maternal insulin resistance may be related to altered placental function, in addition to increased fetoplacental availability of glucose, free fatty acids and amino acids; however, the mechanism behind his unknown.[33]

Catalano[33] reported a significant increase in neonatal fat mass in birth weights of infants born to women with gestational diabetes mellitus. The strongest predictor of fat mass in infants of women with gestational diabetes mellitus was found to be maternal fasting glucose levels. This neonatal obesity is proposed to be a significant risk factor for adolescent/adult obesity.[33] More importantly, obese female neonates have been shown to have higher rates of gestational diabetes mellitus;[9] thus, a vicious cycle is created. Figure 1 shows the potential long-term effects of fetal overgrowth.

Life-style treatment of obesity has varying rates of success. In light of this evidence showing an abnormal metabolic state *in utero* in obese women, there seems a potential for *in utero* therapy/intervention to prevent the effects of maternal obesity on subsequent generations.[33] In a recent review, Beall *et al.*[34] suggested that there may be opportunities to prevent fetal programming for adult obesity. Studies on rats have shown that administration of leptin to the

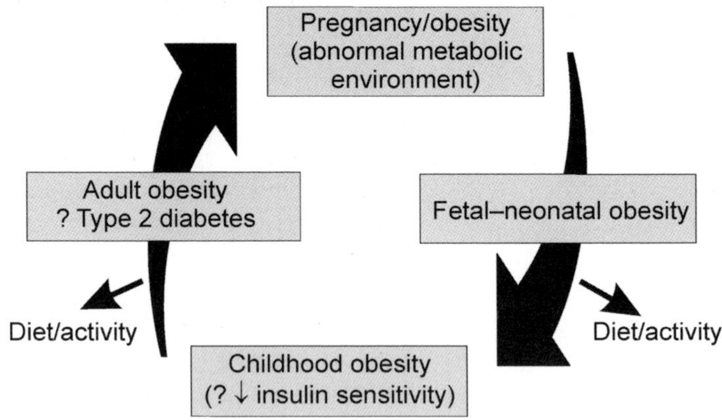

Fig. 1 Potential long-term implications of fetal overgrowth. Adapted from Catalano.[33]

mother during pregnancy resulted in less body fat in the adult offspring in both the normally fed and protein-restricted rats.[34] Currently, there is extensive research into developmental programming of the metabolic syndrome by maternal nutritional imbalance in animal models[35] and how this can be reversed and applied to humans.

Childhood obesity

There is a lack of evidence to support a relationship between birth weight and adolescent obesity. However, maternal obesity results in infants at birth having an increased degree of adiposity, yet these infants are not significantly more obese compared to controls at 6 months of age but at 12 months of age there is a significant difference.[18] Nevertheless, obesity beyond 12 years of age has been shown to develop into adult obesity in > 80% of cases.[9]

Recent data from the Avon Longitudinal Study of Parents and Children, a prospective birth cohort study, assessed potential risk factors for obesity (> 95% BMI) in 7758 7-year-old children. It was shown that, after adjustment for confounding variables, maternal BMI > 30 kg/m^2 (OR 4.25), paternal BMI > 30 kg/m^2 (OR 2.54), birth weight (OR 1.05/100 g) and weight gain in the first 12 months of life (OR 1.06/100 g) were factors associated with obesity in childhood.[36] Interestingly, data from the 1970 British Cohort Study, on adult outcomes of childhood obesity, demonstrated that childhood obesity had little effect on future economic, educational, and social well-being.[47] However, there is evidence showing that elevated antepartum plasma levels of maternal free fatty acids, a hallmark of obesity and insulin resistance, correlate inversely with the intelligence of offspring at 2–5 years of age.[9]

Barker's fetal origin of adult disease hypothesis showed that low-weight babies have an increased risk of developing cardiovascular disease and diabetes. This is of importance as obese mothers often deliver premature, underweight babies. However, there is some evidence to suggest that developing obesity and type 2 diabetes mellitus is also a risk factor for infants born at the upper end of the birth weight curve, *i.e.* the risk is U-shaped.[33,37]

MANAGING OBESE MOTHERS FROM PREGRAVID TO POSTPARTUM

Preconception counselling

More women are obese (21%) compared to men (17%), having greater health and socio-economic implications. Stringent anti-obesity measures need to be implemented in women, due to the detrimental effect of obesity on pregnancy and transgenerational outcomes. In particular, obesity prevention/intervention strategies need to be targeted in childhood, to prevent the complications of obesity in the reproductive years.

Nutritional education, behavior modification, drug treatment and dieting have not been successful in reducing weight in obese adults. In women in whom these strategies have been unsuccessful, Kral[9] advocated that bariatric surgery should be considered, as this is the only treatment proven to maintain medically significant weight loss effectively in the majority of treated patients for 5 years or more. In support of this, a recent meta-analysis showed that bariatric surgery is more effective than non-surgical treatment for weight loss and control of some co-morbid conditions such as diabetes in patients with a BMI of 40 kg/m^2 or greater.[38]

Furthermore, there are studies comparing pregnancy outcomes before bariatric surgery to outcomes after surgery in the same women, which have revealed significant improvements in pregnancy outcomes.[9] A recent study with the largest number of pregnancies after bariatric surgeries (n = 298) to date showed that previous bariatric surgery is not associated with adverse perinatal outcome.[39]

However, pregnancies after bariatric surgery were found to be associated with an increased risk of anemia because of iron, folate, and vitamin B_{12} deficiencies.[39] Hence, there is potential for fetal undernutrition in mothers post bariatric surgery. The data in the literature are conflicting, perhaps reflecting the different types of surgery and other confounding factors.[9] Further research is needed into the long-term effects of surgery on the infants and their mothers as this group of patients is growing with very little information available to healthcare providers on management of such cases.

Optimal weight gain in obese pregnant women

Gestational weight gain greater than that recommended by the Institute of Medicine is associated with complications in pregnancy (Table 7). Figure 2 shows the association between birth weight and pregnancy weight gain. The graph illustrates that high birth weight (> 4.5 kg) did not increase significantly until pregnancy weight gains exceeded the upper limit of the Institute of Medicine range (16 kg).[40]

Table 7 Acceptable amounts of weight gain in pregnancy.

Weight-for-height category	Recommended total gain (kg)
Low (BMI < 19.8 kg/m^2)	12.5–18
Normal (BMI 19.8–26.0 kg/m^2)	11.5–16
High (BMI > 26.0 kg/m^2)	7–11.5

Derived from Abrams *et al.*[40]

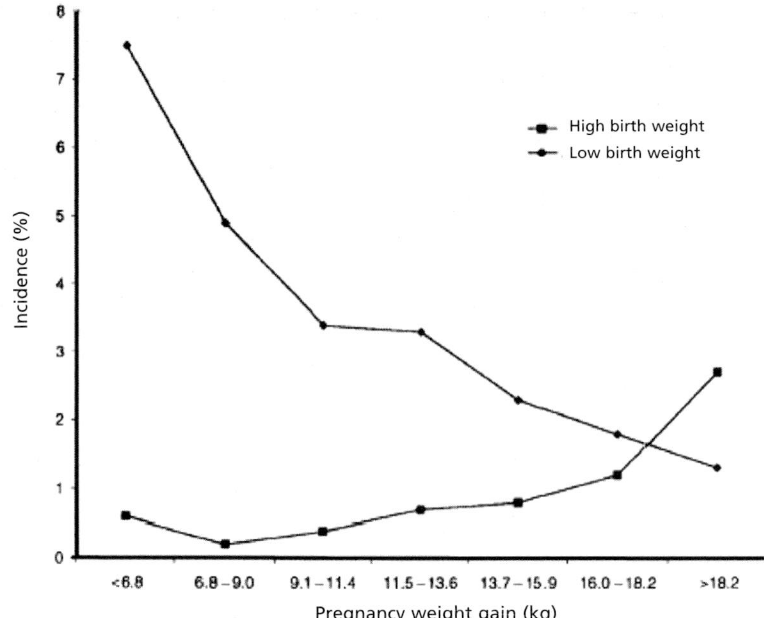

Fig. 2 Incidence of low and high birth weight by pregnancy weight gain in normal weight women. Adapted from Abrams *et al.*[40]

It is not recommended that obese women lose weight during pregnancy due to the increased risk of ketosis. However, interventions in early pregnancy for obese and overweight women, to keep weight gain within the recommended limits during pregnancy, may reduce the incidence of complications associated with obesity. Rode *et al.*[41] suggested that patient compliance is highest during early pregnancy as results from smoking campaigns suggest that women are more motivated at this point.

Postpartum

During pregnancy, 2–10 kg of fat is stored in women's bodies. About 14–20% of women are unable to lose this weight, on average gaining 5 kg or more post-pregnancy. This should not be considered as a 'benign effect of pregnancy' as obesity is associated with prenatal complications in pregnancy and chronic illnesses such as cardiovascular disease and type 2 diabetes mellitus.[42]

However, in obese and overweight women, it remains to be determined whether reduced gestational weight gain can reduce the number of complications during pregnancy and delivery.[41]

Nevertheless, there is a positive relationship between gestational weight gain and weight retained during the postpartum period; therefore, the risk of weight-related complications increases in the subsequent pregnancies. Of note, postpartum weight retention is unrelated to maternal age, parity, gestational length, infant sex, breast-feeding and infant birth weight.[42]

Siega-Riz *et al.*[43] stressed that few studies have examined determinants of excessive weight gain and postpartum weight retention. Furthermore, these studies were not comprehensive in assessing diet, physical activity and psychosocial factors and suffer from small sample sizes. Moreover, there is limited data available regarding pregnant women's perceptions about eating and gaining weight. Additionally, little is known regarding eating habits and what psychosocial factors influence behavior during pregnancy and in the postpartum period.[43] Such information would be valuable in drafting intervention policies to tackle excessive weight gain in pregnancy.

Walker *et al.*[42] underlined the importance of measures to prevent child-bearing becoming a transitional event for obesity and weight gain. They advocate that greater nursing intervention is needed in identifying women at risk of obesity and educating and supporting obese women whatever their reproductive status, especially as half of pregnancies are unplanned.

Olson *et al.*[44] evaluated the efficacy of an intervention, which was that healthcare providers monitored the participants gestational weight gain. Additionally, participants received patient education directed at preventing excessive gestational weight gain by mail. The intervention appeared to reduce the risk of excessive gestational weight gain only in the low-income subgroup. This finding is important because low-income women have been found to be at substantially increased risk for excessive gestational weight gain.

This study has clinical relevance in that the intervention carried out can be integrated into clinical practice as minimal time is required by the healthcare provider to monitor and discuss the importance of appropriate gestational weight gain and to encourage women to self-monitor weight gain. The more time-consuming task of general patient education on diet and exercise was conducted through posted newsletters.[44] This had the advantage of allowing the patient to read the information as many times as she likes and to share the information with friends and family.

Finally, in the postpartum period, contraception needs to be chosen according to maternal relative weight and possible concomitant metabolic or vascular disorders. Women with gestational diabetes mellitus need to be given life-style and dietary advice in order to prevent the occurrence of type 2 diabetes mellitus and be screened for type 2 diabetes mellitus.[45]

CONCLUSIONS

At present in the UK, 1 in 5 women at booking are obese. As mentioned above, obesity in pregnancy has numerous potential detrimental effects on the mother and baby, including gestational diabetes, pre-eclampsia and eclampsia, increased risk of congenital abnormalities, preterm fetal loss, still-birth and complicated delivery, often requiring cesarean section. Greater awareness of these adverse effects needs to be made to healthcare professionals who can target obese and/or overweight women of child-bearing age. Such women should be informed of the risks associated with obesity and pregnancy and receive appropriate dietary and life-style advice. Hence, effective anti-obesity strategies are needed at a national and international level to stop this growing problem.

Finally, the health and economic impact of rising obesity rates in women of reproductive years is of significant public health importance as obesity is an important modifiable risk factor for adverse pregnancy outcome. Further research is needed into the mechanisms by which obesity adversely affects pregnancy and how this can be modified in obese pregnant women, as obesity is proving difficult to curb and rising significantly. In the meantime, greater significance and awareness needs to be placed on the importance of normal weight before conception.

KEY POINTS FOR CLINICAL PRACTICE

- Obesity is an urgent growing health epidemic.
- Obese pregnant women are at an increased risk of almost every complication of pregnancy.
- Obese mothers are more likely to develop metabolic syndrome later on in life thus posing a significant health and economic burden world wide.
- Greater awareness is needed by the health professionals who can target obese women of childbearing age.
- Research is needed into the creation of an effective, affordable, and acceptable community-based program for obese pregnant women and those planning a pregnancy.

ACKNOWLEDGEMENT

The authors would like to thank Simon Wheeler for his guidance and help.

References

1 Vlad I. Obesity costs UK economy £2bn a year. BMJ 2003; 327: 1308
2 Kanagalingam MG, Forouhi NG, Greer IA, Sattar N. Changes in booking body mass index over a decade: retrospective analysis from a Glasgow Maternity Hospital. Br J Obstet Gynaecol 2005; 112: 1431–1433
3 Andreasen KR, Anderen ML, Schantz AL. Obesity and pregnancy. Acta Obstet Gynecol Scand 2004; 83: 1022–1029. doi:10.1111/j.0001-6349.2004.00624.x
4 Lintsen AM, Pasker-de Jong PC, de Boer EJ *et al*. Effects of subfertility cause, smoking and body weight on the success rate of IVF. Hum Reprod 2005; 20: 1867–1875
5 van der Spuy ZM, Dyer SJ. The pathogenesis of infertility and early pregnancy loss in polycystic ovary syndrome. Best Pract Res Clin Obstet Gynaecol 2004; 18: 755–771
6 Castro L, Avina R. Maternal obesity and pregnancy outcomes. Curr Opin Obstet Gynecol 2002; 14: 601–606
7 American Diabetes Association. Gestational diabetes mellitus. Diabetes Care 2003; 26 (Suppl 1): S103–S105
8 Linne Y et al. 2004 Effects of obesity on women's reproduction and complications during pregnancy. Obes Rev 2004; (August) 5: 137–143.
9 Kral JG. Preventing and treating obesity in girls and young women to curb the epidemic. Obes Res 2004; 12: 1539–1546
10 Linne Y, Barkeling B, Rossner S. Natural course of gestational diabetes mellitus: long term follow up of women in the SPAWN study. Br J Obstet Gynaecol 2002; 109: 1227–1231
11 Boney CM, Verma A, Tucker R, Vohr BR. Metabolic syndrome in childhood: association with birth weight, maternal obesity, and gestational diabetes mellitus. Pediatrics 2005; 115: e290–e296

12 O'Brien TE, Ray JG, Chan WS. Maternal body mass index and the risk of preeclampsia: a systematic overview. Epidemiology 2003; 14: 368–374
13 Drife J. Thromboembolism. Br Med Bull 2003; 67: 177–190
14 Royal College of Obstetricians and Gynaecologists. CEMD 2001 Report
15 Abdollahi M, Cushman M, Rosendaal FR. Obesity risk of venous thrombosis and the interaction with coagulation factor levels and oral contraceptive use. Thromb Haemost 2003; 89: 493–498
16 Sahota PK, Jain SS, Dhand R. Sleep disorders in pregnancy. Curr Opin Pulmon Med 2003; 9: 477–483
17 Usha KTS, Hemmadi S, Bethel J, Evans J. Outcome of pregnancy in a woman with an increased body mass index. Br J Obstet Gynaecol 2005; 112: 768–772.
18 Nuthalapaty FS, Rouse DJ. The impact of obesity on obstetrical practice and outcome. Clin Obstet Gynecol 2004; 47: 898–913
19 Sheiner E, Levy A, Menes TS, Silverberg D, Katz M, Mazor M. Maternal obesity as an independent risk factor for caesarean delivery. Paediatr Perinat Epidemiol 2004; 18: 196–201
20 Sebire NJ, Jolly M, Harris JP *et al*. Maternal obesity and pregnancy outcome: a study of 287 213 pregnancies in London. Int J Obes 2001; 25: 1175–1182
21 Chauhan SP, Magann EF, Carroll CS, Barrilleaux PS, Scardo JA, Martin Jr JN. Mode of delivery for the morbidly obese with prior cesarean delivery: vaginal versus repeat cesarean section. Am J Obstet Gynecol 2001; 185: 349–354
22 Baxley EG, Gobbo RW. Shoulder dystocia. Am Fam Phys 2004; 69: 1707–1714
23 Robinson H, Tkatch S, Mayes DC, Bott N, Okun N. Is maternal obesity a predictor of shoulder dystocia? Obstet Gynecol 2003; 101: 24–27
24 Watkins ML, Rasmussen SA, Honein MA, Botto LD, Moore CA. Maternal obesity and risk for birth defects. Pediatrics 2003; 111: 1152–1158
25 Hendricks KA, Nuno OM, Suarez L, Larsen R. Effects of hyperinsulinemia and obesity on risk of neural tube defects among Mexican Americans. Epidemiology 2001; 12: 630–635
26 Hall LF, Neubert AG. Obesity and pregnancy. Obstet Gynecol Surv 2005; 60: 253–260
27 Werler MM, Louik C, Shapiro S, Mitchell AA. Prepregnant weight in relation to risk of neural defects. JAMA 1996; 275(14): 1089–1092
28 Ray JG, Wyatt PR, Vermeulen MJ, Meier C, Cole DEC. Greater maternal weight and the ongoing risk of neural tube defects after folic acid flour fortification. Obstet Gynecol 2005; 105: 261–265
29 Cnattingius S, Bergstrom R, Lipworth L, Kramer MS. Prepregnancy weight and the risk of adverse pregnancy outcomes. N Engl J Med 1998; 338: 147–152
30 Cedergren MI. Maternal morbid obesity and the risk of adverse pregnancy outcome. Obstet Gynecol 2004; 103: 219–224
31 Nohr EA, Bech BH, Davies MJ, Frydenberg M, Henriksen TB, Olsen J. Prepregnancy obesity and fetal death: a study within the Danish National Birth Cohort. Obstet Gynecol 2005; 106: 250–259
32 Hendler I, Goldenberg RL, Mercer BM *et al*. The Preterm Prediction Study: association between maternal body mass index and spontaneous and indicated preterm birth. Am J Obstet Gynecol 2005; 192: 882–886
33 Catalano PM, Kirwan JP, Haugel-de Mouzon S, King J. Gestational diabetes and insulin resistance: role in short- and long-term implications for mother and fetus. J Nutr 2003; 133(Suppl 2): 16745–16835
34 Beall MH, El Haddad M, Gayle D, Desai M, Ross MG. Adult obesity as a consequence of *in utero* programming (Review). Clin Obstet Gynecol 2004; 47(4): 957–966 (discussion 9801)
35 Armitage JA, Khan IY, Taylor PD, Nathanielsz PW, Poston L. Developmental programming of the metabolic syndrome by maternal nutritional imbalance: how strong is the evidence from experimental models in mammals? J Physiol 2004; 561: 355–377
36 Reilly JJ, Armstrong J, Dorosty AR *et al*. Early life risk factors for obesity in childhood: cohort study. BMJ 2005; 330: 1357–1364
37 Pettitt DJ, Jovanovic L. Birthweight as a predictor of type 2 diabetes mellitus: the U-shaped curve. Curr Diab Report 2001; 1: 78–81

38 Maggard MA, Shugarman LR, Suttorp M *et al*. Meta-analysis: surgical treatment of obesity. Ann Intern Med 2005; 142: 547–559
39 Sheiner E, Levy A, Silverberg D *et al*. Pregnancy after bariatric surgery is not associated with adverse perinatal outcome. Am J Obstet Gynecol 2004; 190: 1335–1340
40 Abrams B, Altman SL, Pickett KE. Pregnancy weight gain: still controversial. Am J Clin Nutr 2000; 71 (Suppl): 1233S–1241S
41 Rode L, Nilas L, Wojdemann K, Tabor A. Obesity-related complications in Danish single cephalic term pregnancies. Obstet Gynecol 2005; 105: 537–542
42 Walker LO, Sterling BS, Timmerman GM. Retention of pregnancy-related weight in the early postpartum period: implications for women's health services. J Obstet Gynecol Neonatal Nurs 2005; 34: 418–427
43 Siega-Riz AM, Evenson KR, Dole N. Pregnancy-related weight gain – a link to obesity? Nutr Rev 2004; 62: S105–S111
44 Olson CM, Strawderman MS, Reed RG. Efficacy of an intervention to prevent excessive gestational weight gain. Am J Obstet Gynecol 2004; 191: 530–536
45 Galtier-Dereure F, Boegner C, Bringer J. Obesity and pregnancy: complications and cost. Am J Clin Nutr 2000; 71 (Suppl): 1242S–1248S
46 National Cholesterol Education Program. Third Report of the Expert Panel on Detection, Evaluation, and Treatment of High Blood Cholesterol in Adults (Adult Treatment Panel III). Bethesda, MD: National Heart, Lung, and Blood Institute, National Institutes of Health, 2001
47 Viner RM, Cole TJ. Adult socioeconomic, educational, social, and psychological outcomes of childhood obesity: a national birth cohort study. BMJ 2005; 330: 1354–1359

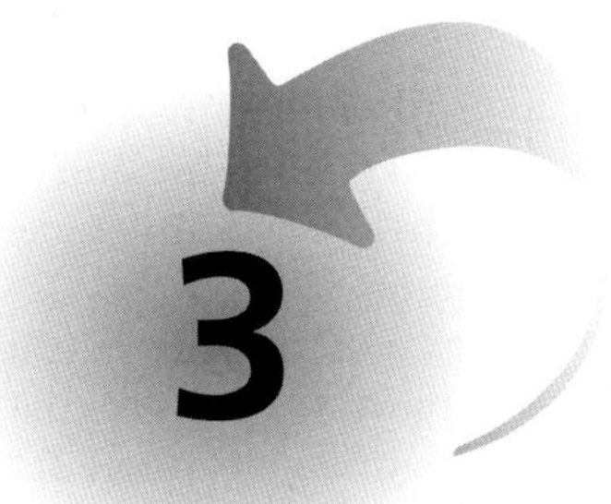

Nagy Rafla Mini S. Nair Suresh Kumar

Exercise in pregnancy

Pregnancy is perceived to be an opportunity for introducing women to healthier life-style choices such as cessation of smoking, avoidance of alcohol and introduction of physical activity.[1] The benefits of regular exercise in maintaining health has been well established. Many women who are physically active prior to their pregnancy are keen to continue exercising in pregnancy but are constrained by concerns about adverse outcome to the pregnancy.

Advice given to women regarding exercising in pregnancy has changed over time. From advising women to maintain sedentary life-styles, gradually, increasing levels of exercise has been deemed safe for pregnant women. The American College of Obstetrics and Gynecology (ACOG) guidelines published in 1985 recommend that heart rate during exercise should not exceed 140 beats/min and that women should limit the duration of any strenuous activities to 15 min.[2] The revised guidelines in 1994 did not specify an upper limit to the heart rate but suggested that the exercise should be limited by maternal symptoms.[3] An update published in 2002 suggested that pregnant women accumulate 30 min or more of moderate exercise most or all days of the week, similar to the advice given to non-pregnant individuals.[4]

Nagy M. Rafla MRCOG MOG
Consultant Obstetrician and Gynaecologist, Queen Elizabeth the Queen Mother Hospital, St Peter's Road, Margate, Kent CT9 4AN, UK

Mini S. Nair MBBS MD MRCOG (for correspondence)
Specialist Registrar, Department of Obstetrics and Gynaecology, Medway Maritime Hospital, Windmill Road, Gillingham, Kent ME7 5NY, UK
E-mail: mininair@hotmail.co.uk

Suresh Kumar MBBS MD MRCOG
General Practitioner, Sun Lane Surgery, Hythe, Kent CT21 5JY, UK

Pregnant women have physiological and physical changes, which might make it harder and riskier for them to indulge in certain physical activities. There is continuous weight gain in pregnancy. Pregnancy hormones make the joints lax and gravid uterus causes lumbar lordosis and shifts the center of gravity making the pregnant woman clumsier and increasing the risk of injuries. There is a physiological rise in basal heart rate. Temperature regulation is altered, leading to reduced tolerance of strenuous activity. There are concerns regarding safety of the fetus with increased core temperatures attained during exercise. There is also the worry that physical activity would set off preterm labor.

There are questions regarding the types of exercise regimens that are safe for pregnant women and their fetus. Can women who have a very active lifestyle maintain their fitness by continuing their regimens in pregnancy without fear of adverse outcome? Are there specific advantages in pregnancy and labor for women who are physically active in pregnancy? We aim to examine the evidence regarding these issues relating to exercising in the pregnant state.

PHYSIOLOGY OF EXERCISE IN PREGNANCY

Energy expenditure during exercise

Exercising results in energy expenditure above that of the resting stage. Stored fat and carbohydrates are converted into energy by the muscular tissue in the presence of oxygen. Various physiological changes, including cardiovascular and respiratory, occur at the beginning of exercise to increase the oxygen uptake. Physiological adaptations to pregnancy modify these changes in the pregnant woman. This affects not only the way pregnant women respond to exercise but also the interpretation of the changes that occur in response. The physiological changes brought about by exercise can be quantified in many ways, such as by measuring changes in oxygen uptake, minute ventilation, heart rate, stroke volume and blood pressure.

Exercise can be weight bearing (walking, treadmill) and non-weight bearing (swimming, cycling). Oxygen consumption is higher in weight bearing as compared to non-weight bearing exercise, which is relevant due to increasing weight during pregnancy. This increase is due to energy costs in counteracting the pull of gravity. Thus, many day-to-day activities such as walking require higher energy expenditure in pregnancy, particularly with increasing gestation. The energy expenditure for non-weight bearing exercises increases at the same rate as the increase in resting energy expenditure; however, the weight bearing exercises result in increasing energy expenditure with advancing pregnancy.[5] There is also evidence that glucose is used at a higher rate during pregnancy than in the non-pregnant state particularly in non-weight bearing exercises.[6,7]

Energy expenditure can be estimated from the amount of oxygen consumed during the activity. Each litre of oxygen consumed results in the release of approximately 5 kcal of energy. Resting caloric expenditure, which has been estimated to be about 1 kcal/min, can go up by as much as 15 times during exercise.[8]

Although the oxygen cost of an activity is dependent on the workload, several factors may influence the absolute amount of oxygen consumed. The economical use of oxygen by an individual is termed metabolic efficiency. Biomechanical factors as well as the type of exercise can affect efficiency. The literature on energy efficiency during pregnancy is contradictory. If there is a decrease in efficiency, the reason is not clearly understood; increased work of breathing and greater myocardial oxygen consumption could play a part.[8]

The energy costs are also affected by the intensity. Exercise that does not require maximal effort is referred to as sub maximal exercise. This can be expressed as a percentage of the maximal effort, for example, 70% of maximal effort. The relative intensity of an activity for an individual can be ascertained by measuring the percentage of maximum heart rate or maximal oxygen consumption achieved. Energy expenditure to perform the same relative intensity of exercise may be different for different individuals.[5]

Respiratory changes

There are several significant changes to the respiratory system in pregnancy. Effective CO_2 exchange between fetus and mother requires that the pCO_2 in the fetus is higher than in the mother. This is achieved by resetting of the respiratory centers in the mother, which make women extremely sensitive to CO_2 in pregnancy. The resulting increase in ventilation is mostly due to increase in tidal volume and not respiratory frequency. However, owing to the changes in the mechanics of breathing (flaring of ribs and the rise of diaphragm) and the increase in tidal volume, there is reduction in the functional residual capacity.[9] The oxygen consumption at rest is higher for pregnant as compared to non-pregnant women. Women also feel dyspnoeic at rest and during exercise in pregnancy.[10]

Increase in oxygen requirement during exercise is achieved in pregnancy by an increase in minute ventilation and tidal volume; this increase is disproportionately high for the work achieved as compared to the non-pregnant state.[10] During pregnancy, minute volume is increased by 23–26% during a given level of sub maximal exercise as compared to non-pregnant individuals.[11] Because of the increased resting oxygen requirements and the increased work of breathing caused by pressure of the enlarged uterus on the diaphragm, there is decreased oxygen availability for the performance of aerobic exercise during pregnancy. Thus, both subjective workload achievable and maximum exercise performance are decreased.

Cardiac changes

Cardiac output increases in pregnancy and at least 60% of this rise has occurred by 8–10 weeks. There is an increase of 10% in the stroke volume while the pulse rate goes up by 10–15%. There is enlargement of the left ventricle. There is a fall in diastolic blood pressure and peripheral vascular resistance.[9]

In non-pregnant individuals, the stroke volume increases with exercise intensity up to 40–50% of maximal capacity, then stops. Heart rate increases linearly with oxygen uptake up to maximal capacity. With increasing exercise, systolic blood pressure rises, mostly due to increasing cardiac output. Diastolic blood pressure may increase, decrease, or stay the same. Blood flow is selectively directed towards areas of higher metabolic activity (such as muscles) and away from splanchnic and renal vascular beds. Most studies show that cardiac output, stroke volume and heart rate are increased in pregnancy during exercise in comparison to non-pregnant responses.[12] Increases in cardiac output are reported in both cycle ergometry and treadmill walking, though the changes are higher for the latter possibly due to the weight gain of pregnancy. Blood pressure changes are unchanged or slightly decreased from the non-pregnant state. As pregnancy advances, increases in stroke volume and cardiac output are reduced with little change in exercise heart rate. This could be due to venous pooling and decreased venous return. It is possible that, although maximal cardiac output and stroke volume are increased during pregnancy, maximal heart rates achieved are lower due to blunted response to catecholamine.[13,14] If this is the case, heart rate cannot be used as the means to predict exercise intensity while prescribing exercise in pregnancy.

Uteroplacental blood flow

Uterine blood flow increases in pregnancy from 50 ml/min in the first trimester to 500 ml/min at term. There is massive vasodilatation in skeletal muscles during exercise leading to diversion of blood flow towards the working muscles. Doppler studies of uterine and umbilical vessels have been performed during exercise. Rafla and Etokowo[15] found transient decreased resistance in uterine artery flow after an episode of stationary cycling lasting 5 min in 101 subjects in the second half of pregnancy. Other studies confirm these findings in women in the third trimester;[16,17] however, Morrow *et al.*[18] found no change in a group of eight women between 16–28 weeks' gestation. In spite of reduction of flow in the uterine artery, umbilical artery flow appears well maintained with moderate exercise even in the third trimester.[16–19] Rauramo and Forss[20] showed that there was no alteration in intervillous placental blood flow after sub maximal exercise lasting for 6 min in late pregnancy.

There may also be a protective response from the hemoconcentration noticed during acute exercise in animal and human studies.[21,22] Examination of placental function and morphology reveals adaptations to improve placental perfusion and transfer function by early to mid-pregnancy in regularly exercising women.[23]

TEMPERATURE RISE WITH EXERCISE

Working muscles can generate heat that can raise maternal body temperature during exercise. As the exercise progresses, thermoregulatory mechanisms come into play and heat is lost from the body by radiation into the atmosphere, convection and evaporation of sweat. If the ambient temperature is high or evaporation of sweat hampered by high levels of humidity, the process of thermoregulation may become impaired resulting in increased core temperature. Trained athletes have better thermoregulatory mechanisms and are better able to maintain circulation to both working muscles and to the peripheral blood vessels to aid dissipation of heat. They generally have a lower resting core temperature and heart rate, and are better able to sustain long periods of exercise before their core temperature increases.

Heart rate and core temperature increase are more closely linked to the relative intensity of exercise rather than the workload or energy expenditure. As pregnancy advances, women gain weight and the same amount of absolute work would represent higher relative work and hence core temperature and heart rate would be higher. Fetal temperature is about 0.5°C higher than the maternal core temperature, to maintain a gradient to assist dissipation of heat produced by fetal metabolic processes. An increase in maternal core temperature can reverse this gradient.

There is no direct evidence that exercise in pregnancy results in fetal hyperthermia or that fetal hyperthermia following exercise is teratogenic in humans. Animal studies indicate an increase in the risk of congenital anomalies following maternal hyperthermia in early pregnancy.[24,25] Hyperthermia in human pregnancies has also been shown to be associated with congenital malformations such as neural tube defects; however, hyperthermia was induced by causes other than exercise.[26]

Several studies on pregnant women at various stages of pregnancy examined the core body temperature attained during and after exercise.[27–30] Clapp[28] monitored rectal temperature in 18 recreational athletes before, during, and after 20 min of continuous exercise before conception and every 6–8 weeks during pregnancy. Larsson and Lindqvist[29] studied 40 pregnant women and 11 controls participating in low-impact aerobic exercise before, at maximum-exercise level, and after exercise with regard to core temperature and other parameters. O'Neill[30] reported on 11 healthy women with low-risk pregnancies who completed three separate upright cycling tests at 34–37 weeks' gestation. None of these studies showed a peak value of greater than 39°C on sub-maximal exercise at 60–80% of predicted maximal heart rate.

There seem to be maternal adaptations to pregnancy designed to protect the fetus by reducing the magnitude of temperature changes in response to exercise. These studies suggest that women can continue moderate-intensity exercise safely in pregnancy without risk of hyperthermia.

NUTRITIONAL NEEDS OF PHYSICALLY ACTIVE, PREGNANT WOMEN

Nutritional needs of active pregnant women have not been studied. Sedentary pregnant women are estimated to need on an average 300 kcal/day more than non-pregnant women. However, heavy physical activity can result in expenditure of energy, which, in turn, may deprive the fetus of energy required for growth. Weight-bearing activities such as walking require more energy particularly in later gestation as compared to the non-pregnant state due to increasing weight gain. Hence, pregnant women who are active need to have extra caloric intake to compensate for the extra expenditure. This extra intake depends upon the type and intensity of activity. It is difficult to make general recommendations and 500 kcal of extra energy during the day can be recommended for a start to women who maintaining a 30-min exercise program.[31] Active women can be advised to eat to their appetite and adequate calorific intake monitored by monitoring the rate of weight gain.

EXERCISE AND UTERINE ACTIVITY

One of the concerns regarding exercising in pregnancy is that it will lead to uterine activity precipitating labor. Alternately, it is also said that well-conditioned women have shorter labor.

There may be an increase in uterine activity during exercise at term as shown by Spinnewijn *et al.*[32] in a study involving moderate exercise in 30 women at term admitted for elective induction; the activity recovered on resting. Durak *et al.*[33] evaluated the effect of five aerobic exercise machines on uterine activity during the third trimester of pregnancy. Uterine activity correlated with the type of exercise, but not with the level of exertion. At equivalent workloads, the bicycle ergometer led to uterine activity in 50% of sessions, the treadmill in 40%, the rowing ergometer in 10%, recumbent bicycle in 0%, and the upper arm ergometer in 0% of women in late pregnancy.[33]

Two large observational studies showed no difference in the length of pregnancy in women regardless of whether they indulged in regular leisure-time physical activity during pregnancy. Hatch *et al.*[34] followed a cohort of 557 pregnant patients until delivery. No association was found between low-to-moderate exercise and gestational length. Heavier exercise appeared to reduce, rather than raise, the risk of preterm birth.[34] In a survey of 9089 women, Leiferman and Evenson[35] showed no significant relationship between regular leisure time physical activity (RLPA) and timeliness of delivery.

Regular activity in the antenatal period appears to have favorable effects on labor. Clapp[36] compared the outcome of pregnancy in two groups of recreational athletes. Of these women, 87 continued to exercise throughout pregnancy at or above 50% of preconceptual levels, whereas 44 of the women stopped after the first trimester. The incidence of preterm labor was the same in the two groups. Women in the exercising group had an early onset of labor, lower incidence of abdominal and operative vaginal delivery. Active labor was shorter in women who delivered vaginally.[36]

Beckman *et al.*[37] reported a shorter first and second stage in primiparous women who exercised as compared to those who did not. They also observed a higher spontaneous vaginal delivery rate and a lower cesarean section rate in this group of regularly exercising primiparous women.[37] Kardel and Kase[38] reported no difference in labor characteristics among well-conditioned women continuing exercise in pregnancy regardless of whether they indulged in high-intensity or medium-intensity exercise.

It is possible that women with a past history of adverse pregnancy events, such as preterm labor, have been left out of these studies due to failure to volunteer participation in such studies.

EFFECT OF MATERNAL EXERCISE ON THE FETUS

Changes to the fetal heart

Exercising during pregnancy has the potential to compromise the fetus by diverting the blood flow away from the uterus. A number of studies have looked at the effect of exercise on fetal heart rate parameters. The methodology and monitoring techniques vary widely. However, no fetal adverse effects have been described following moderate exercise at any gestation in healthy pregnancies.

In healthy women, exercise is followed by a significant, but short-lasting, increase in base-line fetal heart rate.[39–42] This effect is not modified by the physical condition of the women, although the exercise output is higher for well-conditioned women.[43] A drop in fetal heart rate has also been reported in the immediate post exercise period even if transient.[43] Bradycardia is much more likely following strenuous exercise and in high-risk pregnancies.[40,44] Manders *et al.*[45] also reported a reduction in fetal heart rate variability and body movement.

Changes in fetal heart rate during exercise are more difficult to monitor and Doppler studies during exercise have shown bradycardia as well as tachycardia.[41,43,46] However, when monitoring with two-dimensional ultrasound (to reduce artefacts), researchers found no change in the fetal heart during exercise.[44]

Pregnancies, in which women who were previously sedentary started a regimen of regular exercise, also had a normal outcome.[47]

Fetal growth

Maintaining physical training as well as introducing a regular regimen of exercise can affect the growth and the development of the fetus. The effect depends upon the intensity and frequency of exercise and the period of gestation up to which exercise is maintained. A review of the effect of exercise on birth weight found that there was no significant difference in birth weight in women reporting low or moderate amounts of exercise compared to sedentary controls even when exercise was continued throughout pregnancy.[48]

The introduction of exercise can result in the birth of babies with higher birth weights. Clapp *et al.*[49] reported on 46 women who did not exercise regularly and were randomly assigned at 8 weeks either to no exercise (n = 24) or to weight-bearing exercise (n = 22) 3–5 times a week for the remainder of the pregnancy. The group of 22 previously sedentary women introduced to a regimen of moderately strenuous, regular exercise showed an increase in birth weight and an increase in placental volume as compared to the 24 women who remained sedentary.[49] However, women who exercised regularly prior to the pregnancy and continued to maintain the high volume of moderate intensity exercise throughout pregnancy had babies that were significantly lighter than women who reduced the volume of exercise after 20 weeks. The latter women also had larger placental volumes.[50] These results are confirmed by Bell *et al.*,[51] who found that women who continued regular vigorous exercise after 25 weeks of pregnancy had significantly lighter babies compared to women who did not exercise regularly. This difference in birth weight was also seen in women undergoing endurance training at or near preconceptual levels throughout pregnancy and those who stopped at 28 weeks.[52] However, Kardel *et al.*[38] found that birth weight was similar whether women indulged in moderate or high intensity exercise.

It appears that moderate-to-vigorous exercise carried out at frequencies of more than three times a week in the last trimester can result in birth of babies with lower birth weight than less active controls. The reduction in body weight of the neonate has been shown to be mostly due to a loss of body fat, with no difference in head circumference or Ponderal index (birth weight/height x 100).[49,53] Clapp *et al.*[54] studied the offspring of 52 women who exercised in their pregnancy with 52 controls who were similar in terms of other variables. At birth, the neonates weighed less in the group that exercised; however, at 1 year of age, morphometric and neuorodevelopmental parameters were similar in both groups.[54] In another study comparing children 5 years after birth between a group of women who exercised to another who were physically active, Clapp[55] found similar results.

HIGH-RISK PREGNANCY AND EXERCISE

Diabetes and exercise

Gestational diabetes mellitus (GDM) is defined as any degree of glucose intolerance with onset or first recognition during pregnancy. Traditionally, the management is by monitoring of blood glucose levels, modification of diet, and introduction of insulin if changes in diet alone fail to maintain normoglycemia. A recent Cochrane review[56] found that addition of exercise as a therapeutic intervention in type 2 diabetics significantly improved glycemic control. However, its role in prevention and treatment of gestational diabetes is still unclear. Introduction of exercise regimens are more complex in type I diabetics since they are more prone to develop hypoglycemia and ketoacidosis.

In women with gestational diabetes, addition of exercise along with diet control may delay or reduce the need for insulin. Addition of exercise to diet control in treating women with GDM may potentially improve glycemic control and delay the requirement for insulin therapy. It may also control weight gain and reduce the risk of developing diabetes mellitus after GDM, which can vary between 2.8–70% within 6 weeks to 18 years after pregnancy.[57]

Exercise as therapeutic intervention in gestational diabetes

Brankston *et al.*[58] studied the effect of diet control versus diet and resistance exercise in a group of 32 women with GDM. There was no difference in the number of women who required insulin in the two groups. However, women on exercise training with diet, required less insulin and required initiation of insulin treatment at a later stage than women on diet alone. Moreover, there was a subgroup of overweight women on diet control and exercise, who showed a lower incidence of insulin use.[58]

Bung *et al.*,[59] in a randomised controlled trial, found that women with gestational diabetes requiring insulin enrolled into a program of diet control and regular exercise 3 times a week remained normoglycemic without insulin as compared to a group of similar women on diet control. Gestational age at delivery, premature delivery, still-birth, neonatal death, macrosomia, birth weight, small for date, respiratory distress syndrome, congenital malformation, 5-min Apgar < 7, neonatal hypoglycemia, preterm labor, induction of labor, cesarean section, instrumental delivery were similar in both groups.[59]

These results were also confirmed in a small study, which showed that glycosylated hemoglobin and blood glucose levels were lower in women with gestational diabetes who exercised regularly along with diet control as opposed to women who only controlled their diet.[60]

In contrast, Avery *et al.*[61] failed to find any difference in daily fasting and postprandial blood glucose levels, hemoglobin A1C, incidence of exogenous insulin therapy, and incidence of newborn hypoglycemia in two groups of women with gestational diabetes who had been randomly assigned to regular exercise or no exercise.

To date, there are no large, well-controlled studies looking at the effect of exercise as a therapeutic adjunct in the management of diabetic control. However, the data available appear to show that addition of regular low-to-medium intensity exercise to the management strategy of these women is of some benefit in maintaining glycemic control, without any adverse effects.

Exercise and prevention of GDM

Benefits of regular physical activity in prevention of type 2 diabetes are well documented. Epidemiological studies suggest that this beneficial effect can be seen for gestational diabetes as well. In a survey of 12,799 women in New York, Dye and colleagues[62] found that women with a body mass index of over 33 kg/m^2 had a significantly reduced risk of developing GDM if they engaged in any exercise during their pregnancy; they also observed that a higher socio-economic factor was a significant risk factor among these obese women pointing to a role of diet.

Dempsey *et al.*[63] explored the relationship between recreational physical activity performed during the year before, and during the first 20 weeks of, pregnancy and the risk of GDM. They found that among 155 GDM cases and 386 normotensive, non-diabetic pregnant controls, women who participated in any recreational physical activity during the first 20 weeks of pregnancy, as compared with inactive women, experienced a 48% reduction in risk of GDM. Beneficial effect was most pronounced in women who had engaged in physical activity in the year before pregnancy as well as in the first 20 weeks of pregnancy.[63]

Oken *et al.*[64] assessed the duration and intensity of physical activity and time spent viewing television both before and during pregnancy among 1805 women and found that physical activity, especially vigorous activity before pregnancy and at least light-to-moderate activity during pregnancy, may reduce the risk for abnormal glucose tolerance and GDM.

Pre-eclampsia and exercise

Prevention of pre-eclampsia

In 2006, a Cochrane Database review of randomised controlled trials concluded that there is insufficient evidence to show the effect of exercise on prevention of pre-eclampsia.[65] Yet, some epidemiological studies seem to show some value of recreational physical activities in reducing the risk of developing pre-eclampsia. Sorenson *et al.*[66] showed that women who were physically active in early pregnancy and in the year before becoming pregnant had a lower incidence of pre-eclampsia compared to sedentary women. Light-to-moderate as well as vigorous activities resulted in a decreasing trend of risk of pre-eclampsia. These results are similar to those of Marcoux *et al.*[67] who showed reduction in the risk of pre-eclampsia in women engaging in regular physical activity with moderate-to-high calorie expenditure in early pregnancy. In contrast, a study looking at the impact of work activity on risk of pre-eclampsia found that moderate-to-high physical activity at work seems to increase the risk of severe pre-eclampsia.[68]

In a review, Wolfe *et al.*[69] postulated that exercise could reduce the risk of developing pre-eclampsia by counteracting the inadequate placental development seen in early pregnancy in women who later develop pre-eclampsia. They also proposed, since exercise is well known to reduce oxidative stress, this perhaps attenuates the development of vascular endothelial dysfunction that results from oxidative stress in pre-eclampsia. Finally, they suggest that it may be possible to correct existing endothelial damage, since circulatory shear stress associated with exercise enhances endothelial function and has been reported to improve endothelial functions in patients with existing vascular disease.[69]

Prediction

Exercise testing has been assessed for its efficiency in predicting pre-eclampsia. Umbilical artery Doppler and blood pressure response following cycle ergometry showed low positive predictive values for the development of pre-eclampsia.[70,71] For this reason, it is not recommended as a screening tool to identify women at risk of pre-eclampsia who want to engage in an exercise program in pregnancy.

Safety of exercise for women with pre-eclampsia

Rafla[74] documented a significant rise in the mean systolic pressure after exercise in pregnant women with PIH in the last trimester of pregnancy. Umbilical artery Doppler showed significantly raised S/D ratio before and after exercise when maternal blood pressure rose to 180–190 mmHg after an exercise test. Nevertheless, there were no sustained ill effects in any of the mothers and their fetuses. Hackett *et al.*[73] found increased uteroplacental resistance in normal and abnormal pregnancies tested following supine cycling and postulated that this might be harmful in women who already have abnormal resistance in the resting state such as pre-eclampsia and IUGR. Studies evaluating safety of exercise in women with pre-eclampsia have tended to assess the response to brief episodes of physical activity; thus, it is unknown whether a regular program of exercise will have a deleterious effect in pre-eclampsia patients in the long term. Similar findings were noted by the first author in unpublished data.

IUGR

Exercise in women with normal pregnancies results in transient fetal tachycardia and recovery. Rafla[74] performed umbilical artery Doppler in 18 women with IUGR in the last trimester of their pregnancy while they exercised to 65% of their predicted capacity. The umbilical artery pulsatility index (PI), after an initial decrease, showed a 12% rise at 8, 16 and 30 min of recovery.[74] Another study, comparing two groups of women with and without uteroplacental vascular insufficiency, exercising at 10–55% of maximum between 22–26 weeks, documented transient absence of end diastolic flow in the umbilical artery in three of the 12 pregnancies with UPVI 75.

However Nabeshima *et al.*[76] found no significant change in the S/D ratio of umbilical artery in pregnancies with or without IUGR, following exercise at term. Ertan *et al.*[77] also found no change in uterine and umbilical artery Doppler following sub-maximal exercise in 10 women with IUGR. They did find increased resistance in fetal aorta and fetal cerebral vasodilatation. To date, there are no studies looking at long-term effects of exercise on pregnancies with IUGR.

OBESITY AND PREGNANCY

Increasing obesity is becoming a public health problem in the UK. The incidence of obesity in pregnant women has also increased over the last 15 years.[78] Maternal obesity in pregnancy is associated with increased maternal and fetal risks. Miscarriage occurs three times more commonly and the risk of operative delivery increases. Pre-eclampsia, thrombo-embolism and gestational diabetes are also more prevalent in this group. There is also an increase in perinatal mortality and macrosomia in the fetus.[79] Exercising in pregnancy may prevent excess weight gain.[80] It may also benefit obese women by reducing the risks of gestational diabetes and pre-eclampsia.

Excess weight gain during pregnancy and failure to lose weight afterwards is also an important predictor of long-term obesity.[81] Introduction of life-style changes may facilitate loss of the pregnancy weight gain in the postpartum period.

EXERCISE PRESCRIPTION

Exercise programs are commonly intended to result in expenditure of 150–300 kcal/day. This can be achieved in non-pregnant women by the equivalent of a 1.5–3 mile walk or run each day. Caloric cost of walking a mile is estimated to be approximately 80–120 kcal, depending on weight. Speed is relatively unimportant in terms of calorie expenditure and faster work rates only increase caloric expenditures by 6–10%.[8]

It is important to assess a women's general medical and obstetric status to ensure that there are no contra-indications to exercising, particularly in women who were previously sedentary. The contra-indications to exercising as recommended by ACOG are given in Tables 1 and 2.[4] The following are considered absolute contra-indications: incompetent cervix, serious cardiac disorder, pregnancy-induced hypertension, placenta previa and ruptured membranes or premature labor. Caution is recommended in cases of IUGR,

Table 1 Absolute contra-indications to aerobic exercise during pregnancy

- Hemodynamically significant heart disease
- Restrictive lung disease
- Incompetent cervix/cerclage
- Multiple gestation at risk for premature labor
- Persistent second or third trimester bleeding
- Placenta previa after 26 weeks' gestation
- Premature labor during the current pregnancy
- Ruptured membranes
- Pregnancy induced hypertension

Reproduced with permission of American College of Obstetricians and Gynecologists.[4]

Table 2 Relative contra-indications to aerobic exercise during pregnancy

- Severe anemia
- Unevaluated maternal cardiac arrhythmia
- Chronic bronchitis
- Poorly controlled type I diabetes
- Extreme morbid obesity
- Extreme underweight (body mass index < 12 kg/m^2)
- History of extremely sedentary life-style
- Intra-uterine growth restriction in current pregnancy
- Poorly controlled hypertension/pre-eclampsia
- Orthopedic limitations
- Poorly controlled seizure disorder
- Poorly controlled thyroid disease
- Heavy smoker

Reproduced with permission of American College of Obstetricians and Gynecologists.[4]

extremes of weight, in extremely sedentary women and cardiovascular disease. ACOG also warns of certain signs to terminate exercise (Table 3).

Canadian National Guidelines for exercise during pregnancy and postpartum recommend initiation of an exercise program in previously sedentary women in the second trimester rather than the first, due to the minor ailments of first trimester as well due to possible deleterious effect of maternal hyperthermia on fetus.[82]

Type of exercise

A variety of activities appears to be safe and is recommended during pregnancy such as cycling, swimming, walking, and low impact aerobics. Level of activity is best decided based on the physical fitness of the women when becoming pregnant. For women who were sedentary, non-weight bearing exercises such as cycling or swimming would be a good way of introducing increased physical activity. However, weight-bearing activities such as walking and low-impact aerobics are also suitable. In addition, resistance training to improve musculoskeletal fitness is also important and beneficial as part of an exercise program.[82]

Table 3 Warning signs to terminate exercise while pregnant

Warning signs to terminate exercise while pregnant
Vaginal bleeding
Dyspnoea before exertion
Dizziness
Headache
Chest pain
Muscle weakness
Calf pain or swelling (need to rule out thrombophlebitis)
Preterm labor
Decreased fetal movement
Amniotic fluid leakage

Reproduced with permission of American College of Obstetricians and Gynecologists.[4]

Sports with risks of abdominal trauma, falling or orthopedic injuries such as skiing, horseback riding gymnastics, tennis, and contact sports may be best avoided due to the musculoskeletal changes associated with pregnancy, which impair co-ordination.

During pregnancy, scuba diving is not recommended since the fetus is at risk from decompression problems and can suffer malformations and gas embolism. However, snorkelling can still be practised in pregnancy.[83]

Duration and frequency of exercise

ACOG recommends 30 min or more of moderate-intensity exercise to be undertaken for most, if not all, days of the week. Previously, sedentary women may work up to this level of activity over weeks, from shorter sessions of 15 min.

Women who exercised regularly prior to pregnancy may maintain their routine during the first trimester though they may find that with advancing gestation their exercise intensity gradually reduces.

Canadian guidelines recommend initiation of exercise regimens at 3 times a week gradually increasing in frequency to 4–5 times per week.[84]

Intensity guidelines – target heart rate (THR) range and estimated rate of perceived exertion (RPE)

The maximal intensity that can be safely achieved in pregnancy has not been established. The intensity recommended would depend upon the fitness level of the pregnant women prior to pregnancy. Exercise intensity can be assessed and tailored to individual requirements in many ways. Target heart rate, Borg Rating of Perceived Exertion (RPE) and the talk test are the commonly used methods. The best method of monitoring exercise intensity in pregnancy is still controversial.

Maximal oxygen uptake is closely correlated with the age adjusted maximal heart rate (220-age). Heart rate is commonly used in non-pregnant women for prescribing exercise intensity. Target heart rates of 60–80% of the age-adjusted maximal level are recommended as a measure of moderate intensity exercise. This recommendation is appropriate in pregnant women as well. However, in pregnancy, resting heart rate increases and there is evidence to show that maximal heart rate response is blunted, which may make it unsuitable. A modified scale may be used by reducing the upper end of the heart rate target zone by 5 beats/min for each decade.[84]

Ratings of perceived exertion have been suggested as an alternative or an addition to the target heart rate for monitoring intensity. Perceived exertion is based on the physical perception of the individual of changes due to exercise such as heart rate, respiration, sweating, fatigue and provides a fairly good estimate of actual heart rate during the activity. Borg's scale of perceived exertion (Table 4) is recommended with a rating of 12–14 as appropriate for pregnancy.[85]

Canadian guidelines also retain the talk test as a final check to avoid overexertion. A person engaging in moderate-intensity exercise should be able comfortably to carry on a conversation.

Table 4 Borg's rating of perceived exertion[85]

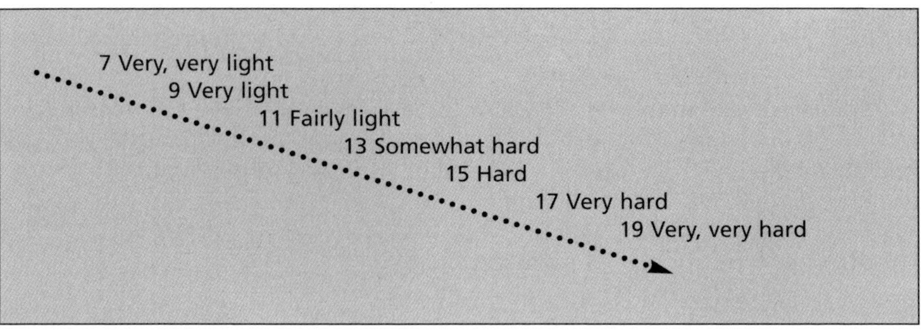

CONCLUSIONS

There is much research on the effect of exercise in pregnancy. However, studies are generally small with inconsistent designs and the researchers are limited by the difficulty of exercising pregnant women to exhaustion without adequate safety data. Most of the studies are on fit, low-risk Caucasian women. Within these constraints, the available data seem to suggest that it is safe for active women with normal pregnancies to continue moderate levels of activity throughout pregnancy. Previously sedentary women can be safely introduced to gradually increasing levels of activity from the second trimester.

Regular leisure-time physical activity may be beneficial not just in promoting health but may also shorten labor, reduce the risk of pre-eclampsia and gestational diabetes mellitus. There could also be a role in management of gestational diabetes mellitus. Nevertheless, we still need to be cautious in advising exercise in women with high-risk pregnancies such as pre-eclampsia and IUGR. Large, randomised, controlled studies are required to assess the beneficial and adverse effects that exercising can have in pregnancy.

KEY POINTS FOR CLINICAL PRACTICE

- It is safe for active women with normal pregnancies to continue moderate levels of activity throughout pregnancy.
- Regular leisure-time physical activity may be beneficial, not just in promoting health but may also reduce the risk of excess weight gain and gestational diabetes mellitus.
- 30 min or more of moderate-intensity exercise is recommended for most, if not all, days of the week.

References

1 Kaiser LL, Allen L, American Dietetic Association. Position of the American Dietetic Association: nutrition and lifestyle for a healthy pregnancy outcome. Am Diet Assoc 2002; 102: 1479–1490

2 American College of Obstetricians and Gynecologists. Exercise During Pregnancy and the Postnatal Period. Washington, DC: ACOG, 1985

3 American College of Obstetricians and Gynecologists. Technical Bulletin No. 173. Women and Exercise. Washington, DC: ACOG, 1994
4 American College of Obstetricians and Gynecologists. Exercise During Pregnancy and the Postpartum Period ACOG Committee. Opinion no. 267: exercise during pregnancy and the postpartum period. Obstet Gynecol 2002; 99: 171–173
5 O'Toole ML. Physiological aspects of exercise in pregnancy. Clin Obstet Gynaecol 2003; 46: 379–389
6 Soultanakis HN, Artal R, Wiswell RA. Prolonged exercise in pregnancy: glucose homeostasis, ventilatory and cardiovascular responses. Semin Perinatol 1996; 20: 315–327
7 Artal R, Masaki DI, Khodiguian N *et al*. Exercise prescription in pregnancy: weight-bearing versus non-weight-bearing exercise. Am J Obstet Gynecol 1989; 161: 1464–146–9
8 Wiswell RA. Exercise physiology. In Mittelmark RA, Wiswell RA, Drinkwater BL. (eds) Exercise in Pregnancy, 2nd edn. New York: Williams & Wilkins, 1991; 141–155
9 McFadyen IR. Maternal physiology in pregnancy. In Chamberlain G. (ed) Turnbull's Obstetrics, 2nd edn. Edinburgh: Churchill Livingstone, 1992; 115–142
10 Mittelmark RA, Greenspoon JS, Wiswell RA, Romam Y. Pulmonary responses to exercise in pregnancy. In Mittelmark RA, Wiswell RA, Drinkwater BL. (eds) Exercise in Pregnancy, 2nd edn. New York: Williams & Wilkins, 1991; 185–194
11 Khodiguian N, Jaque-Fortunato SV *et al*. A comparison of cross-sectional and longitudinal methods of assessing the influence of cardiac function during exercise. Semin Perinatol 1996; 20: 232–241
12 Wallace JP, Wiswell RA. Maternal cardiovascular response to exercise in pregnancy. In Mittelmark RA, Wiswell RA, Drinkwater BL. (eds) Exercise in Pregnancy, 2nd edn. New York: Williams & Wilkins, 1991; 185–194
13 Lotgering FK, van Doorn MB, Struijk PC, Pool J. Wallenburg HC. Maximal aerobic exercise in pregnant women: heart rate, O_2 consumption, CO_2 production, and ventilation J Appl Physiol 1991; 70: 1016–1023
14 Avery ND, Wolfe LA, Amara CE, Davies GAL, McGrath MJ. Effects of human pregnancy on cardiac autonomic function above and below the ventilatory threshold. J Appl Physiol 2001; 90: 321–328
15 Rafla NM, Etokowo GA. The effect of maternal exercise on uterine artery velocimetry waveforms. J Obstet Gynaecol 1998; 18: 14–17
16 Kennelly MM, Geary M, McCaffrey N, McLoughlin P, Staines A, McKenna P. Exercise-related changes in umbilical and uterine artery waveforms as assessed by Doppler ultrasound scans. Am J Obstet Gynecol 2002; 187: 661–666
17 Erkkola RU, Pirhonen JP, Kivijarvi AK. Flow velocity waveforms in uterine and umbilical arteries during submaximal bicycle exercise in normal pregnancy. Obstet Gynecol 1992; 79: 611–615
18 Morrow RJ, Ritchie JW, Bull SB. Fetal and maternal hemodynamic responses to exercise in pregnancy assessed by Doppler ultrasonography. Am J Obstet Gynecol 1989; 160: 138–140
19 Rafla NM. Umbilical artery flow velocity waveforms following maternal exercise. J Obstet Gynaecol 1999; 19: 385–389
20 Rauramo I, Forss M. Effect of exercise on maternal hemodynamics and placental blood flow in healthy women. Acta Obstet Gynecol Scand 1988; 67: 21–25
21 Lotgering FK, Gilbert RD, Longo LD. Exercise responses in pregnant sheep: oxygen consumption. Uterine blood flow and blood volume. J Appl Physiol 1983; 55: 834–841
22 Jovanovic L, Kessler A, Peterson CM. Human maternal and fetal response to graded exercise. J Appl Physiol 1985; 58: 1719–1722
23 Jackson MR, Gott P, Lye SJ, Ritchie JW, Clapp 3rd JF. The effects of maternal aerobic exercise on human placental development: placental volumetric composition and surface areas. Placenta 1995; 16: 179–191
24 Germain MA, Webster WS, Edwards MJ. Hyperthermia as a teratogen: parameters determining hyperthermia-induced head defects in the rat. Teratology 1985; 31: 265–272
25 Kimmel CA, Cuff JM, Kimmel GL *et al*. Skeletal development following heat exposure in the rat. Teratology 1993; 47: 229–242
26 Moretti ME, Bar-Oz B, Fried S, Koren G. Maternal hyperthermia and the risk for neural

tube defects in offspring: systematic review and meta-analysis. Epidemiology 2005; 16: 216–219
27 Lindqvist PG, Marsal K, Merlo J, Pirhonen JP. Thermal response to submaximal exercise before, during and after pregnancy: a longitudinal study. J Matern Fetal Neonat Med 2003; 13: 152–156
28 Clapp 3rd JF. The changing thermal response to endurance exercise during pregnancy. Am J Obstet Gynecol 1991; 165: 1684–1689
29 Larsson-L, Lindqvist P-G. Low-impact exercise during pregnancy – a study of safety. Acta Obstet Gynecol Scand 2005; 84: 34–38
30 O'Neill ME. Maternal rectal temperature and fetal heart rate responses to upright cycling in late pregnancy. Br J Sports Med 1996; 30: 32–35
31 Butterfield G, King JC. Nutritional needs of physically active pregnant women. In Mittelmark RA, Wiswell RA, Drinkwater BL. (eds) Exercise in Pregnancy, 2nd edn. New York: Williams & Wilkins, 1991; 185–194
32 Spinnewijn WE, Lotgering FK, Struijk PC, Wallenburg HC. Fetal heart rate and uterine contractility during maternal exercise at term. Am J Obstet Gynecol 1996; 174: 43–48
33 Durak EP, Jovanovic-Peterson L, Peterson CM. Comparative evaluation of uterine response to exercise on five aerobic machines. Am J Obstet Gynecol 1990; 162: 754–756
34 Hatch M, Levin B, Shu XO, Susser M. Maternal leisure-time exercise and timely delivery. Am J Public Health 1998; 88: 1528–1533
35 Leiferman JA, Evenson KR. The effect of regular leisure physical activity on birth outcomes. Matern Child Health J 2003; 7: 59–64
36 Clapp 3rd JF. The course of labor after endurance exercise during pregnancy. Am J Obstet Gynecol 1990; 163: 1799–1805
37 Beckmann CRB, Beckmann CA. Effects of a structured antepartum exercise program on pregnancy and labor outcome in primiparas. J Reprod Med 1990; 35: 704–709
38 Kardel KR, Kase T. Training in pregnant women: effects on fetal development and birth. Am J Obstet Gynecol 1998; 178: 280–286
39 Kennelly MM, McCaffrey N, McLoughlin P, Lyons S, McKenna P. Fetal heart rate response to strenuous maternal exercise: not a predictor of fetal distress. Am J Obstet Gynecol 2002; 187: 811–816
40 Rafla NM, Cook JR. The effect of maternal exercise on fetal heart rate. J Obstet Gynaecol 1991; 19: 381–384
41 Clapp 3rd JF, Little KD, Capeless EL. Fetal heart rate response to sustained recreational exercise. Am J Obstet Gynecol 1993; 168: 198–206
42 van Doorn MB, Lotgering FK, Struijk PC, Pool J, Wallenburg HC. Maternal and fetal cardiovascular responses to strenuous bicycle exercise. Am J Obstet Gynecol 1992; 166: 854–859
43 Webb KA, Wolfe LA, McGrath MJ. Effects of acute and chronic maternal exercise on fetal heart rate. J Appl Physiol 1994; 77: 2207–2213
44 Carpenter MW, Sady SP, Hoegsberg B *et al*. Fetal heart rate response to maternal exertion. JAMA 1988; 259: 3006–3009
45 Manders MSM, Sonder GJB, Mulder EJH, Visser GH. The effects of maternal exercise on fetal heart rate and movement patterns. Early Hum Dev 1997; 48: 237–247
46 Artal R, Romem Y, Paul RH, Wiswell R. Fetal bradycardia induced by maternal exercise. Lancet 1984; 2: 258–260
47 Brenner IK, Wolfe LA, Monga M, McGrath MJ. Physical conditioning effects on fetal heart rate responses to graded maternal exercise. Med Sci Sports Exerc 1999; 31: 792–799
48 Leet T, Flick L. Effect of exercise on birthweight. Clin Obstet Gynecol 2003; 46: 423–431
49 Clapp 3rd JF, Kim H *et al*. Beginning regular exercise in early pregnancy: effect on fetoplacental growth. Am J Obstet Gynecol 2000; 183: 1484–148
50 Clapp 3rd JF, Kim H *et al*. Continuing regular exercise during pregnancy: effect of exercise volume on fetoplacental growth. Am J Obstet Gynecol 2002; 186: 142–147
51 Bell RJ, Palma SM, Lumley JM. The effect of vigorous exercise during pregnancy on birth-weight. Aust NZ J Obstet Gynaecol 1995; 35: 46–51
52 Clapp 3rd JF, Dickstein S. Endurance exercise and pregnancy outcome. Med Sci Sports Exerc 1984; 16: 556–562
53 Clapp 3rd JF, Capeless EL. Neonatal morphometrics after endurance exercise during pregnancy. Am J Obstet Gynecol 1990; 163: 1805–1811

54 Clapp 3rd JF, Simonian S, Lopez B, Appleby-Wineberg S, Harcar-Sevcik R. The one-year morphometric and neurodevelopmental outcome of the offspring of women who continued to exercise regularly throughout pregnancy. Am J Obstet Gynecol 1998; 178: 594–599
55 Clapp JF. Morphometric and neurodevelopmental outcome at age five years of the offspring of women who continued to exercise regularly throughout pregnancy. J Pediatr 1996: 129: 856–863
56 Thomas DE, Elliott EJ, Naughton GA. Exercise for type 2 diabetes mellitus. Cochrane Database Syst Rev 2006; 19; 3: CD002968
57 Kim C, Newton KM, Knopp RH. Gestational diabetes and the incidence of type 2 diabetes: a systematic review. Diabetes Care 2002; 25: 1862–1868
58 Brankston GN, Mitchell BF, Ryan EA, Okun NB. Resistance exercise decreases the need for insulin in overweight women with gestational diabetes mellitus. Am J Obstet Gynecol 2004; 190: 188–193
59 Bung P, Artal R, Khodiguian N, Kjos S. Exercise in gestational diabetes. An optional therapeutic approach? Diabetes 1991; 40 (Suppl 2): 182–185
60 Jovanovic-Peterson L, Durak EP, Peterson CM. Randomized trial of diet versus diet plus cardiovascular conditioning on glucose levels in gestational diabetes. Am J Obstet Gynecol 1989; 161: 415–419
61 Avery M, Leon K. To examine the effectiveness of a partially homebased, moderate-intensity aerobic exercise program for women with gestational diabetes. Obstet Gynecol 1997; 89: 10–15
62 Dye TD, Knox KL, Artal R, Aubry RH, Wojtowycz MA. Physical activity, obesity, and diabetes in pregnancy. Am J Epidemiol 1997; 146: 961–965
63 Dempsey JC, Butler CL, Sorensen TK *et al*. A case-control study of maternal recreational physical activity and risk of gestational diabetes mellitus. Diabetes Res Clin Pract 2004; 66: 203–215
64 Oken E, Ning Y, Rifas-Shiman SL, Radesky JS, Rich-Edwards JW, Gillman MW. Associations of physical activity and inactivity before and during pregnancy with glucose tolerance. Obstet Gynecol 2006; 108: 1200–1207
65 Meher S, Duley L. Exercise or other physical activity for preventing pre-eclampsia and its complications. Cochrane Database Syst Rev 2006; 19: CD005942
66 Sorensen TK, Williams MA, Lee IM, Dashow EE, Thompson ML, Luthy DA. Recreational physical activity during pregnancy and risk of preeclampsia. Hypertension 2003; 41: 1273–1280
67 Marcoux S, Brisson J, Fabia J. The effect of leisure time physical activity on the risk of pre-eclampsia and gestational hypertension. J Epidemiol Community Health 1989; 43: 147–152
68 Spinillo A, Capuzzo E *et al*. The effect of work activity in pregnancy on the risk of severe preeclampsia. Aust NZ J Obstet Gynaecol 1995; 35: 380–385
69 Wolfe LA, Weissgerber TL. Clinical physiology of exercise in pregnancy. A literature review. J Obstet Gynaecol Can 2003; 25: 473–483
70 Hume Jr RF, Bowie JD, McCoy C *et al*. Fetal umbilical artery Doppler response to graded maternal aerobic exercise and subsequent maternal mean arterial blood pressure: predictive value for pregnancy-induced hypertension. Am J Obstet Gynecol 1990; 163: 826–829
71 Watson WJ, Katz VL, Caprice PA, Jones L, Welter SM. Pressor response to cycle ergometry in the midtrimester of pregnancy: can it predict preeclampsia? Am J Perinatol 1995; 12: 265–267
72 Rafla NM. The effect of maternal exercise on umbilical artery blood flow in pregnancy-induced hypertension. J Obstet Gynaecol 2000; 20: 19–23
73 Hackett GA, Cohen-Overbeek T, Campbell S. The effect of exercise on uteroplacental Doppler waveforms in normal and complicated pregnancies. Obstet Gynecol 1992; 79: 919–923
74 Rafla NM. The effect of maternal exercise on umbilical artery velocimetry waveforms in intrauterine growth retardation. J Obstet Gynaecol 1999; 19: 469–473
75 Chaddha V, Simchen MJ, Hornberger LK *et al*. Fetal response to maternal exercise in pregnancies with uteroplacental insufficiency. Am J Obstet Gynecol 2005; 193: 995–999

76 Nabeshima Y, Sasaki J, Mesaki N, Sohda S, Kubo T. Effect of maternal exercise on fetal umbilical artery waveforms: the comparison of IUGR and AFD fetuses. J Obstet Gynaecol Res 1997; 23: 255–259
77 Ertan AK, Schanz S, Tanriverdi HA, Meyberg R, Schmidt W. Doppler examinations of fetal and uteroplacental blood flow in AGA and IUGR fetuses before and after maternal physical exercise with the bicycle ergometer. J Perinat Med 2004; 32: 260–265
78 Heslehurst N, Ells LJ, Simpson H, Batterham A, Wilkinson J, Summerbell CD. Trends in maternal obesity incidence rates, demographic predictors, and health inequalities in 36 821 women over a 15-year period. Br J Obstet Gynaecol 2007; 114; 187–194
79 Yu CK, Teoh TG, Robinson S. Obesity in pregnancy. Br J Obstet Gynaecol 2006; 113: 1117–1125
80 Polley BA, Wing RR, Sims CJ. Randomized controlled trial to prevent excessive weight gain in pregnant women. Int J Obes Relat Metab Disord 2002; 26: 1494–1502
81 Rooney BL, Schauberger CW. Excess pregnancy weight gain and long-term obesity: one decade later. Obstet Gynecol 2002; 100: 245–252
82 Davies GAL, Wolfe LA, Mottola MF, MacKinnon C. Joint SOGC/CSEP clinical practice guideline: exercise in pregnancy and the postpartum period. Can J Appl Physiol 2003; 28: 329–341
83 Camporesi EM. Diving and pregnancy. Semin Perinatol 1996; 20: 292–302
84 Wolfe LA, Davies GAL. Canadian guidelines for exercise in pregnancy. Clin Obstet Gynecol 2003; 46: 488–495
85 Borg GA. Psychophysical bases of perceived exhaustion. Med Sci Sports Exerc 1982; 14: 377–381

Kristi Borowski Jennifer R. Niebyl

Drugs in pregnancy

Each pregnancy carries a risk of major congenital anomaly of 2–3%.[1] The risk increases to 7–10% if minor malformations are included. Drug exposure has been associated with 2–3% of all birth defects. Given the fact that half of pregnancies are unplanned, it is important to minimize exposure to unnecessary medications in reproductive-aged women regardless of their plan for pregnancy.

In addition to prescription medications, many pregnant women also take over-the-counter medications (OTCs). Acetaminophen is the most common OTC with nearly two-thirds of pregnant women taking the medication during pregnancy.[2] Nearly 15% of pregnant women take ibuprofen and pseudoephedrine.[2]

Despite the thought in the early 20th century that the uterus acted as a shield and protected the fetus, it is now known that the placenta allows the transfer of any drug or chemical unless it is of great size, has low lipid solubility, or is destroyed or altered during passage.[3] Heparin and insulin are examples of drugs that do not cross the placenta and this is due to their large molecular weight.

There is a marked species specificity in drug teratogenesis.[4] For example, thalidomide was not found to be teratogenic in rats and mice but is a potent human teratogen, with at least 20% of exposed fetuses affected. Thus, extrapolating from animal studies to humans can be hazardous and of limited clinical applicability.

Kristi Borowski MD
Fellow, Division of Maternal-Fetal Medicine, Department of Obstetrics and Gynecology, University of Iowa Hospitals and Clinics, 200 Hawkins Drive, Iowa City, IA 52242, USA
E-mail: kristi-borowski@uiowa.edu

Jennifer R. Niebyl MD (for correspondence)
Professor and Head, Department of Obstetrics and Gynecology, University of Iowa Hospitals and Clinics, 200 Hawkins Drive, Iowa City, IA 52242, USA
E-mail: jennifer-niebyl@uiowa.edu

Table 1 US Food and Drug Administration categories of labeling for drug use in pregnancy

A	**Controlled studies show no risk** Adequate, well-controlled studies in pregnant women have failed to demonstrate a risk to the fetus in any trimester of pregnancy
B	**No evidence of risk in humans** Adequate, well-controlled studies in pregnant women have not shown increased risk of fetal abnormalities despite adverse findings in animals, or, in the absence of adequate human studies, animal studies show no fetal risk. The chance of fetal harm is remote, but remains a possibility
C	**Risk cannot be ruled out** Adequate, well-controlled human studies are lacking, and animal studies have shown a risk to the fetus or are lacking as well. There is a chance of fetal harm if the drug is administered during pregnancy, but the potential benefits may outweigh the potential risk
D	**Positive evidence of risk** Studies in humans, or investigational or post-marketing data have demonstrated fetal risk. Nevertheless, potential benefits from the use of the drug may outweigh the potential risk. For example, the drug may be acceptable if needed in a life-threatening situation or serious disease for which safer drugs cannot be used or are ineffective
X	**Contra-indicated in pregnancy** Studies in animals or humans or investigational or post-marketing reports have demonstrated positive evidence of fetal abnormalities or risk which clearly outweigh any possible benefit to the patient

The US Food and Drug Administration (FDA) has five categories of labeling for drug use in pregnancy. The rating system weighs the degree to which available information has ruled out risk to the fetus against the drug's potential benefit to the patient. The ratings, and their interpretation, are described in Table 1. It is important to emphasize that these categories were meant for prescribing physicians and not for addressing inadvertent exposure. For example, isotretinoin (Accutane) and oral contraceptives are both category X. Oral contraceptives receive this category due to lack of benefit and not due to significant fetal risk. For a woman who finds out at 12 weeks she is pregnant and has been taking her oral contraceptive pills throughout the first trimester, there is not significant risk to the fetus, but there is no benefit to the patient to continue on the medication at this point. This is a very different situation than a woman who is 12 weeks' pregnant and has been taking Accutane daily and is at risk for miscarriage, fetal malformation as well as risks for mental retardation, blindness and deafness.

The critical period for organogenesis or the classic teratogenic period is from 31–71 days after the last menstrual period in a normal 28-day menstrual cycle. Timing of the exposure is key to the malformation pattern noted at birth. Administration of drugs early in the period of organogenesis will lead to defects in the neural tube or heart which form early (Fig. 1), whereas exposure later in the period may lead to abnormalities such as cleft palate. Exposure to a teratogen prior to day 31 produces an all-or-none effect. This means the

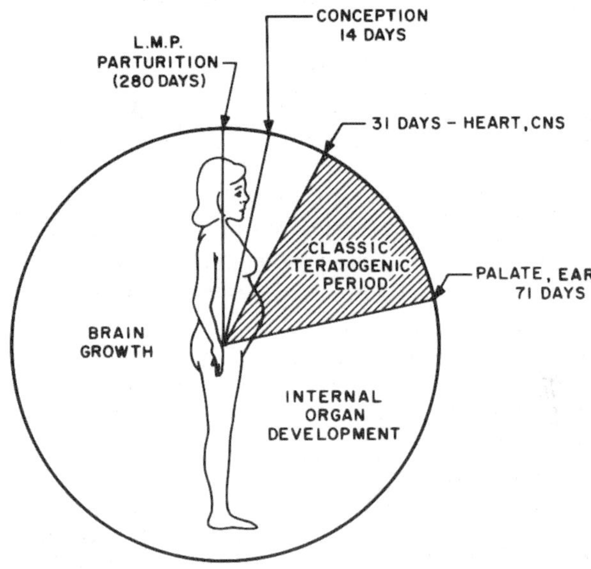

Fig. 1 The classic teratogenic period in the human. *Reproduced with the permission of the copyright owner* © Lippincott, Williams & Wilkins from: Niebyl JR (ed). Drug Use in Pregnancy, 2nd Edn. Philadelphia, PA: Lea & Febiger, 1988; chapter 1, p2.

exposure leads to abortion and the conceptus does not survive, or there is survival without congenital anomalies.

By 10 weeks after the last menstrual period, all of the major organ systems have formed. Continued development and refinement of many systems continues into the second and third trimester of pregnancy and, for some organs like the brain, into the first year of life. Use of medications and drugs in the second and third trimester are not without risk. Fetal alcohol syndrome may develop due to alcohol exposure in the latter parts of pregnancy. Coumadin can lead to fetal intracranial bleeding that results in brain damage near the end of pregnancy or in labor.

Wilson's six general principles of teratogenesis demonstrate the important factors leading from exposure to malformation.[5] The principles are as follows: (i) genotype and interaction with environmental factors; (ii) timing of exposure; (iii) mechanisms of teratogenesis; (iv) manifestation; (v) agent; and (vi) dose effect. The idea that the genotype of the fetus plays a role in susceptibility to malformation is becoming increasingly more obvious with the information from the Human Genome Project. There is evidence in humans that a specific genotype may confer a risk for teratogenesis.

The principle of timing of exposure suggests that susceptibility varies with the developmental stage of the fetus. Exposure during the critical time in organogenesis from 2–8 weeks after conception is more likely to be associated with a structural defect than exposure in the third trimester. For each organ system, most believe there is a critical window after which abnormal embryogenesis cannot be initiated. A specific example of this is neural tube defects which result from failure of the neural tube to close. Closure of the neural tube occurs between 22–28 days after conception, so medications would not show an effect on the neural tube after this time period.

The principle of mechanism of teratogenesis suggests that susceptibility and pattern of malformation is due to the mechanism of action of the specific medication. The final manifestation of exposure is ultimately death, malformation, growth restriction or functional disorder. The manifestation is often determined by the timing of the exposure. Exposure prior to organogenesis may lead to pregnancy loss or no manifestation, while exposure during the critical period of embryogenesis may lead to malformation. This same exposure in the fetal period may lead to growth restriction or functional disorder.

The fifth principle is the agent, which must have access to the fetus to have an effect on it. When discussing medications in pregnancy, the drugs must cross the placenta to have an effect on the fetus. This concept also involves maternal metabolism of drugs. The idea that maternal genotype in the drug metabolism pathway plays a role in disease has been shown with relation of smoking to low birth weight and alcohol to neurobehavioral development in the offspring.[6]

The final principle is dose effect, which implies that increasing effect is noted with dosage increases. The manifestation of exposure may vary with increases in drug dose or duration of exposure.

TERATOGENIC DRUGS

Currently, there are many drugs in use that have not been evaluated in human pregnancy due to the short length of time they have been available. It is possible that some of these are teratogens, and of concern are those in a drug class that has shown to be teratogenic.

Anticonvulsants

Women with epilepsy who take anticonvulsant medication during pregnancy have a risk of fetal malformations that is 2–3 times that of the general population. In the past, it was thought that epileptic women may be at increased risk for a fetus with congenital anomalies regardless of anticonvulsant use, but studies comparing women with epilepsy and medication to those with no medication have not shown this association.[7,8] Valproic acid (Depakene) and carbamazepine (Tegretol) each carry a risk of approximately 1% for neural tube defect.[9] Anti-epileptic drugs in combination have been shown to increase the risk of fetal malformations in multiple studies. Valproic acid has also shown a dose-dependent risk for major congenital anomalies, with increased malformations noted at doses above 800–1000 mg/day.[10]

Carbamazepine, phenytoin (Dilantin) and Phenobarbital are all folic acid antagonists and have been implicated through this mechanism in neural tube defects, clefting and cardiovascular defects. Although epileptic women on anticonvulsants were not included in the Medical Research Council study, most authorities would recommend folic acid 4–5 mg daily for these women.[11] In addition to the isolated birth defects described previously, phenytoin use in pregnancy has been associated with fetal hydantoin syndrome in up to 10% of offspring.[12] Findings in fetal hydantoin syndrome include: microcephaly, developmental delay, mental retardation, growth deficiency, nail and phalangeal hypoplasia, hypertelorism and nasal bone hypoplasia. Epoxide hydrolase deficiency may indicate susceptibility to fetal hydantoin syndrome.[13]

Lamotrigine (Lamictal) is an inhibitor of dihydrofolate reductase, which decreases embryonic folate levels in animals. An international registry was compiled which noted congenital anomalies in 2.9% of patients on lamotrigine monotherapy, which was similar to both the general population and women in other registries on monotherapy.[14] A small registry has been published showing no increase risk for congenital anomalies in the offspring of women using oxycarbazepine, but further evaluation of this drug is necessary.

Most agree the benefits of anticonvulsant therapy outweigh the risks of discontinuation during pregnancy. There may be patients who have been seizure-free for greater than 2 years, who have a normal electro-encephalogram in whom withdrawal of the drug before pregnancy is beneficial.[15] Reduction to anticonvulsant monotherapy is recommended if possible. Enzyme-inducing anticonvulsants are thought to produce a vitamin K deficiency which is associated with neonatal bleeding. Some authors have suggested maternal vitamin K supplementation for the last month of pregnancy, in addition to neonatal administration, but this practice has not been proven in controlled trials.

Analgesics

There is no evidence of teratogenic effect when aspirin is taken in the first trimester.[16,17] Aspirin inhibits prostaglandin synthesis and decreases platelet aggregation which can lead to an increased risk of bleeding in the peripartum period. No teratogenicity has been reported with non-steroidal anti-inflammatory agents (NSAIDs), but chronic use can lead to oligohydramnios and constriction of the fetal ductus arteriosis and pulmonary hypertension. Acetaminophen (Tylenol), propoxyphene (Darvon) and codeine have not been associated with congenital malformations, but the narcotics have been associated with addiction and withdrawal symptoms in the newborn period. Pain management in pregnancy should be managed initially with acetaminophen.

Anticoagulants

Warfarin (Coumadin) is an oral anticoagulant that crosses the placenta and whose use in pregnancy has been associated with warfarin embryopathy. Warfarin embryopathy occurs in approximately 5% of patients exposed to the medication between 6–9 weeks' gestation.[18] It consists of bone stippling seen on radiological examination, nasal hypoplasia, ophthalmological abnormalities including bilateral optic atrophy and mental retardation. In addition to these findings associated with first trimester use, maternal hemorrhage and fetal intracranial hemorrhage have been reported with use throughout pregnancy.

Both unfractionated heparin (UFH) and low molecular weight heparin (LMWH) are alternatives to coumadin use in pregnancy. Heparin is a large molecule that does not cross the placenta and, because of this, does not have an adverse effect on the fetus. Maternal concerns have been raised due to reports of thrombosed valves, leading to increased maternal morbidity and mortality in women with anticoagulation for mechanical heart valves.[19] This has been attributed to inadequate dosing during pregnancy, but this is an assumption. Risks involved with UFH use also include immune, IgG-mediated thrombocytopenia.[20] Long-term use of UFH has been associated with osteoporosis with vertebral fractures as well as sterile abscesses at the injection site.[21] Some 36% of patients had more than a 10% decrease from baseline bone density to postpartum values.[22]

LMWH has also been associated with valve thrombosis and maternal mortality, although the exact risk is unknown. LMWH has the advantage over UFH of once-daily dosing and possibly decreased risks of thrombocytopenia and osteoporosis. However, in pregnancy, the clearance of LMWH is increased which suggests the need for twice-daily dosing. Cost of LMWH is substantially higher than either UFH or coumadin.

Antihypertensives

Antihypertensive drugs are commonly used in pregnancy for chronic hypertension, diabetes and cardiovascular disease. Alpha-methyldopa (Aldomet) has been used extensively in pregnancy for the treatment of hypertension. No teratogenic effects have been attributed to the drug. The Cochrane Database reviewed antihypertensive drugs in pregnancy and questioned the utility of treatment in mild-to-moderate hypertension. The review also suggested that, in drug comparison trials, there appears to be no specific advantage of one class of antihypertensive drugs to another.[23]

Propranolol (Inderal) is a β-adrenergic blocking agent in wide-spread use, with a variety of indications. No evidence for teratogenicity has been documented. Multiple studies of propranolol in pregnancy have shown an increased risk of intra-uterine growth restriction or skewing to lower birth weights.[24] Studies from Scotland suggest improved outcome with the use of atenolol (Tenormin) to treat chronic hypertension during pregnancy.[25] Ultrasound monitoring for growth abnormalities is recommended.

Angiotensin-converting enzyme inhibitors (ACE inhibitors) (*e.g.* enalapril [Vasotec], captopril [Capoten]) can cause fetal renal tubular dysplasia in the second and third trimesters, leading to oligohydramnios, fetal limb contractures, craniofacial deformities, and hypoplastic lung development.[26] A recent, large cohort study found an increased risk of congenital malformation with isolated first trimester exposure to ACE inhibitors, with a RR of 2.71.[27] Infants exposed *in utero* to ACE inhibitors were at increased risk for cardiovascular and CNS malformations. Angiotensin II receptor antagonists (*e.g.* losartan [Cozaar]) have been shown to have second and third trimester findings consistent with ACE inhibitors and are not recommended in pregnancy.

Thyroid drugs

Propylthiouracil (PTU) and methimazole (Tapazole) are both antithyroid drugs that cross the placenta and can lead to fetal goiter. These drugs are thionamides that inhibit thyroid peroxidase mediated iodination of tyrosine in thyroglobulin and thus lead to decreased thyroid hormone production. Methimizole has been associated with cutis aplasia (scalp defects), choanal atresia, esophageal atresia and increased maternal side effects.[28] Agranulocytosis is a severe complication that occurs in less than 0.5% of all patients receiving a thionamide. Because both medications are equally effective, the drug of choice for hyperthyroidism in pregnancy is propylthiouracil. This drug is not available throughout the world and, therefore, methimazole (or carbimazole) should then be substituted.

Thyroid hormones, triiodothyronine (T_3) and thyroxine (T_4), both cross the placenta poorly and, therefore, do not correct fetal hypothyroidism caused by the antithyroid medication as they do maternal hypothyroidism. To prevent this, it is recommended to use the lowest dose of antithyroid medication to keep maternal free thyroxine at the upper limit of the normal range. By the third trimester, 30% of women no longer require antithyroid medication.

Radioactive iodine (^{131}I or ^{125}I) is the first-line treatment for adults with Grave's disease, but is contra-indicated in pregnancy. Women of reproductive age should have pregnancy testing prior to the procedure to prevent exposure during pregnancy as well as to prevent hypothyroidism in early pregnancy. Iodine is not concentrated by the fetal thyroid until after 12 weeks of pregnancy; therefore, inadvertent exposure prior to that time proves no specific risk to the fetal thyroid from radioactive iodine.[29]

The need for thyroxine increases in many women with primary hypothyroidism during pregnancy. This is demonstrated by an increase in thyroid stimulating hormone (TSH). This increase has been noted to occur by 5 weeks' gestation; therefore, women with hypothyroidism should increase their levothyroxine (Synthroid) by 30% as soon as pregnancy is confirmed (2 extra doses each week) and then have further dosing adjustments based on the maternal TSH levels.[30]

Psychoactive drugs

Lithium (Eskalith, Lithobid) exposure in early pregnancy has been associated with a rare cardiovascular malformation – Ebstein's anomaly. This occurs in only 1 out of 20,000 births in the non-exposed population. In the International Register of Lithium Babies, 217 infants with first trimester exposure were evaluated with 25 (11.5%) being malformed.[31] Of the infants with a birth defect, 18 had cardiovascular anomalies with 6 of them being Ebstein's anomaly. Two other studies showed no difference in major anomalies with lithium exposure in pregnancy.

Complications including goiter and hypothyroidism have been seen in newborns exposed to lithium. Perinatal effects of lithium can include hypotonia, lethargy and poor feeding in the newborn period. Polyhydramnios has been reported in two cases with maternal lithium treatment. Nephrogenic diabetes insipidus has been reported in adults on lithium, and is suspected in the fetus in cases of polyhydramnios. It is usually recommended that drug therapy be changed in pregnant women on lithium to avoid fetal drug exposure. This is complicated by a 70% relapse rate of bipolar disorder with lithium discontinuation in 1 year compared to 20% if the drug is continued.

The management is also complicated by the fact that many of the other mood stabilizers are known teratogens. Finding a drug to switch to in pregnancy is difficult. Should the decision to continue on lithium be made, appropriate prenatal diagnosis should be available with fetal echocardiography. Newer antipsychotic medication such as olanzipine (Zyprexa) and respiridone (Risperdal) have almost no safety data at this point.

Depression in women of child-bearing age is extremely common, with 10–15% affected. Tricyclic antidepressants (imipramine, amitiriptyline) as well as selective serotonin re-uptake inhibitors (SSRIs) are commonly prescribed for these patients. Imipramine has been associated with cardiovascular defects and neonatal withdrawal in one small study.[3] Amitriptyline has been more widely used without associated birth defects. SSRIs (*e.g.* fluoxetine [Prozac], paroxetine [Paxil]) have been associated with neonatal withdrawal in the newborn period after *in utero* exposure.[32] SSRI use in pregnancy has also been associated with an increased risk for pulmonary hypertension of the newborn.[33]

Paroxetine use in the first trimester has been associated with an increase in congenital cardiac malformations in two recent, unpublished, epidemiological studies. This led the FDA to recommend additional warnings in the product labeling and assign the drug to category D (Table 1). In evaluation of over 500 pregnancies with first trimester fluoxetine exposure, no increase in major malformations was noted.[34,35] Researchers have not found that antidepressant use has adversely affected cognition, language or development in children, but that depression itself does.[36]

Antibiotics

Antibiotics are commonly used to treat or prevent infection in pregnancy. Due to maternal and fetal effects, care should be used when determining which antibiotic to use. Pregnant women should also be cautioned regarding risk of yeast infection following antibiotic use.

Penicillin and its derivatives are safe in pregnancy. The Collaborative Perinatal Project evaluated 3546 mothers with first trimester penicillin use and found no increase in birth defects.[16] Clavulanate is added to penicillins to broaden their antimicrobial coverage. No increase in birth defects has been identified with first trimester use. A randomized, control trial in women with preterm premature rupture of membranes found an increase in necrotizing enterocolitis in the amoxicillin/clavulanate group compared to both the control and erythromycin groups.[37] A mechanism of pathogen selection leading to abnormal microbial gastrointestinal colonization and then necrotizing enterocolitis has been suggested. A study of Michigan Medicaid patients found a 25% increase in birth defects with the use of cefaclor, cephalexin and cephradine,[3] but other studies have shown no teratogenicity with the cephalosporins.

No increase in birth defects was noted with the use of erythromycin in 79 pregnant women in the Collaborative Perinatal Project or 6972 in the Michigan Medicaid data.[3,16] Clindamycin has been reviewed as well, and there is no indication of teratogenicity. Studies have failed to show an increase in birth defects with use of metronidazole in early or late pregnancy. Concern regarding its use has been due to carcinogenicity seen with high doses in animals, but this has not been seen in humans.[38] No increase in birth defects with the use of nitrofurantoin in pregnancy has been noted.

Sulfonamides have been studied in human pregnancy and have not been associated with an increase in birth defects.[16] Sulfonamides compete with bilirubin for bindings sites on albumin, raising the level of free bilirubin in the serum and increasing the risk of hyperbilirubinemia in the neonate.[39] The sulfonamides do not cause damage *in utero* because the placenta can clear free-bilirubin. There is a theoretical risk if the drug were present in the blood of the neonate after birth that hyperbilirubinemia could result. Due to this potential risk, sulfonamides are not recommended in the third trimester. Trimethoprim is a competitive inhibitor of dihydrofolate reductase and is often used in combination with a sulfonamide drug to treat urinary tract infections. A recent case control study of 1242 infants with neural tube defects found an increased risk with the use of trimethoprim/sulfonamide during the first 2 months after conception with an OR of 4.8.[40] An increase in cardiovascular defects were also noted with early use of the medication with an OR of 4.2.

Tetracyclines are bound by chelation to calcium in developing bone and teeth. This produces brown discoloration of the deciduous teeth, hypoplasia of the enamel and inhibition of bone growth.[41] While bone incorporation can occur early in pregnancy, the brownish discoloration occurs in the second and third trimesters. Because of these findings, alternative antibiotics are recommended in pregnancy. The fluoroquinolones (*e.g.* ciprofloxacin, norfloxacin, levofloxacin) have an affinity for bone and cartilaginous tissue and are associated with arthralgia in children. Quinolone exposure was studied prospectively in 200 pregnant women who were compared to pregnant control women exposed to non-teratogenic antibiotics during pregnancy. No differences in birth defects or development were noted.[42]

The aminoglycosides(gentamicin, tobramycin) are used in pregnancy in the setting of pyelonephritis and chorioamnionitis. Ototoxicity has been reported with first trimester use of streptomycin with doses as low as 1 g biweekly for 8 weeks.[43] No other known teratogenic effect has been associated with aminoglycosides in the first trimester. Nephrotoxicity may be increased when aminoglycosides are combined with cephalosporins. When combined with curariform drugs, a neuromuscular blockade may result.

Antiretrovirals

Zidovudine (ZDV) should be included as a component in the antiretroviral regimen in pregnant women whenever possible, due to its long history of safety and efficacy. The Pediatric AIDS Clinical Trials Group Protocol 076 prospectively evaluated children exposed to ZDV in the perinatal period through age 4 years. No adverse effects were observed in the exposed children.[44] In 1989, the International Antiretroviral Registry was established to detect any major teratogenic effect of antiretroviral drugs. Over 1000 pregnancies with first trimester exposure to ZDV and lamivudine were ascertained through January 2004, with no increase in teratogenicity reported.[45]

Not all antiretroviral drugs are considered safe in pregnancy. Efavirenz is not recommended during pregnancy due to malformations in monkeys receiving the medication in the first trimester, as well as three case reports of neural tube defects in women taking the medication.[46] Didanosine and stavudine use in pregnancy is not recommended due to case reports of lactic acidosis and an advisory warning from Bristol-Myers Squibb in 2001.[47]

Retinoids

Retinoids are known to be teratogenic in humans. These derivatives of vitamin A are lipid soluble and accumulate in the body, with the exception of isotretinoin (Accutane) which is not detectable in the serum 5 days after discontinuation of the medication. Isotretinoin is a drug marketed for treatment of cystic acne and is contra-indicated in pregnancy (FDA category X). It is one of the most widely used teratogenic drugs in reproductive-aged women in the US.

In an early report of 154 exposed human pregnancies, there were 21 cases of birth defects, 12 spontaneous abortions, 95 elective abortions and 26 normal infants in women who took isotretinoin during early pregnancy.[48] Those infants born with birth defects showed a characteristic pattern or syndrome including central nervous system (CNS), craniofacial, cardiac and thymic abnormalities. The findings included microtia/anotia (small or absent ears), micrognathia, cleft palate, heart defects, thymic defects, retinal or optic nerve anomalies, and CNS findings of hydrocephalus, retinal defects and blindness.[48] This pattern of findings is consistent with retinoic acid embryopathy. The risk of structural defects is estimated at approximately 25%, with an additional 25% with mental retardation.[49]

Given the significant teratogenic effect and the large number of exposed reproductive-aged women, the manufacturer of isotretinoin began a pregnancy prevention program in 1988. The pregnancy prevention program states that before initiating isotretinoin all women of reproductive potential must either abstain from sexual intercourse or use two methods of effective contraception simultaneously, have a negative pregnancy test and then wait until the second or third day of the next period before initiating the medication. Despite these recommendations, exposed pregnancies continue to occur. A survey looking at compliance with the pregnancy prevention program found that 99% of women were told to avoid pregnancy by their doctor during treatment and that, of sexually active women, 99% were using contraceptives.[50] Approximately half of women underwent a pregnancy test prior to starting the medication. Among 124,000 women, 402 pregnancies occurred, which resulted in 32 live births.

Etretinate (Tegison) is a retinoid marketed for psoriasis and has teratogenic risk similar to that of isotretinoin. The medication is stored in the subcutaneous fat and slowly released. The drug has been detected over 2 years after discontinuation, making the exact length of time that pregnancy should be avoided unknown. High doses of vitamin A have been associated with birth defects (25,000 IU/day), but with levels in prenatal vitamins (5000 IU/day) there have been no documented risks. Topical tretinoin (Retin-A) has not been associated with teratogenic risk.

Chemotherapeutics

Methotrexate (amethopterin) is a folic acid antagonist that has been associated with first trimester use and characteristic birth defects. Methotrexate is related to aminopterin and has similar findings with first trimester use. The most consistent findings in infants born to mothers with first trimester exposure include CNS abnormalities, limb defects and craniofacial findings. There is likely both a critical window of exposure and dosage for teratogenic effects. It has been suggested that exposure between 6–8 weeks' gestation is critical, as well as a methotrexate dose of greater than 10 mg/week.[51] It is unknown if exposure during the second or third trimesters results in growth abnormalities.

Cyclophosphamide (Cytoxan) is an alkylating agent used for cancer chemotherapy. Human malformation has resulted after first trimester exposure. Skeletal, palatal and eye malformations have all been described.[52] Low birth-weight may be associated with use in the second and third trimesters, but also may be related to underlying disease state.

There is an increase in the rate of spontaneous abortion and major birth defects when cancer chemotherapy is used during embryogenesis. Use of chemotherapeutic agents in the second and third trimester lead to an increase in the risk of still-birth, intra-uterine growth restriction and myelosuppression in the newborn.[52]

KEY POINTS FOR CLINICAL PRACTICE

- Major congenital anomalies occur in 2–3% of all pregnancies and 2–3% of these are due to drug exposure.
- Three key concepts to drug exposure during pregnancy are the type of medication, the gestational age at exposure, and the drug dosage.
- During pregnancy each mediciation must have the maternal and fetal risks and benefits evaluated to determine if the medication use is indicated.

References

1 Wilson JG, Fraser FC. Handbook of Teratology. New York: Plenum, 1979

2 Werler M, Mitchell A, Hernandez-Diaz S, Honein M. Use of over-the-counter medications during pregnancy. Am J Obstet Gynecol 2005; 193: 771–777

3 Briggs GG, Freeman RK, Jaffe SJ. Drugs in Pregnancy and Lactation, 7th edn. Philadelphia, PA: Lippincott Williams & Wilkins, 2005

4 Blake DA, Niebyl JR. Requirements and limitations in reproductive and teratogenic risk assessment. In: Niebyl JR. (ed) Drug Use in Pregnancy. Philadelphia, PA: Lea & Febiger, 1988

5 Wilson JG. Current status of teratology – general principles and mechanisms derived from animal studies. In: Wilson JG, Fraser FC. (eds) Handbook of Teratology. New York, Plenum, 1977; 47

6. Polifka JE, Friedman JM. Medical genetics: 1. Clinical teratology in the age of genomics. Can Med Assoc J 2002; 167: 265–273

7 Holmes LB, Harvey EA, Coull BA *et al*. The teratogenicity of anticonvulsant drugs. N Engl J Med 2001; 344: 1132–1138
8 Monson RR, Rosenberg L, Hartz SC, Shapiro S, Heinonen OP, Slone D. Diphenylhydantoin and selected congenital malformations. N Engl J Med 1973; 289: 1049–1052
9 Rosa FW. Spina bifida in infants of women treated with carbamazepine during pregnancy. N Engl J Med 1991; 324: 674–677
10 Perucca E. Birth defects after prenatal exposure to antiepileptic drugs. Lancet Neurol 2005; 4: 781–786
11 Dansky LV, Rosenblatt DS, Andermann E. Mechanisms of teratogenesis: folic acid and antiepileptic therapy. Neurology 1992; 42: 32
12 Hanson JW, Smith DW. The fetal hydantoin syndrome. J Pediatr 1975; 87 :285
13 Buehler BA, Delimont D, VanWaes M *et al*: Prenatal prediction of risk of the fetal hydantoin syndrome. N Engl J Med 1990; 322: 1567–1572
14 Cunnington M, Tennis P and the International Lamotrigine Pregnancy Registry Scientific Advisory Committee. Lamotrigine and the risk of malformations in pregnancy. Neurology 2005; 64: 955–960
15 Callaghan N, Garrett A, Goggin T. Withdrawal of anticonvulsant drugs in patients free of seizures for two years. N Engl J Med 1988; 318: 942–946
16 Heinonen OP, Slone S, Shapiro S. Birth Defects and Drugs in Pregnancy. Littleton, MA: Publishing Sciences Group, 1977
17 Werler MM, Mitchell AA, Shapiro S. The relation of aspirin use during the first trimester of pregnancy to congenital cardiac defects. N Engl J Med 1989; 321: 1639–1642
18 Jones KL. Smith's Recognizable Patterns of Human Malformation, 5th edn. Philadelphia, PA: WB Saunders, 1997
19 Ginsberg JS, Chan WS, Bates SM, Kaatz S. Anticoagulation of pregnant women with mechanical heart valves. Arch Intern Med 2003; 163: 694–698
20 Warkentin TE, Levine MN, Hirsh J *et al*. Heparin-induced thrombocytopenia in patients treated with low-molecular-weight heparin or unfractionated heparin. N Engl J Med 1995; 332: 1330–1335
21 Bonow RO, Carabello B, McKay CR *et al*. ACC/AHA guidelines for the management of patients with valvular heart disease. J Am Coll Cardiol 1998; 32: 1486–1588
22 Barbour LA, Kick SD, Steiner JF *et al*. A prospective study of heparin-induced osteoporosis in pregnancy using bone densitometry. Am J Obstet Gynecol 1994; 170: 862
23 Abalos E *et al*. Antihypertensive drug therapy for mild to moderate hypertension during pregnancy. Cochrane Database System Rev 3, 2006
24 Redmond GP. Propranolol and fetal growth retardation. Semin Perinatol 1982; 6: 142
25 Rubin PC, Clark DM, Sumner DJ. Placebo-controlled trial of atenolol in treatment of pregnancy-associated hypertension. Lancet 1983; 1: 431
26 Hanssens M, Keirse MJNC, Vankelecom F *et al*. Fetal and neonatal effects of treatment with angiotensin-converting enzyme inhibitors in pregnancy. Obstet Gynecol 1991; 78: 128
27 Cooper WO, Hernandez-Diaz S, Arbogast PG *et al*. Major congenital malformations after first-trimester exposure to ACE inhibitors. N Engl J Med 2006; 354: 2443–2451
28 Cooper DS: Antithyroid drugs. N Engl J Med 2005; 352: 905–917
29 Burrow GN. Thyroid diseases. In: Burrow GN, Ferris TF. (eds) Medical Complications During Pregnancy. Philadelphia, PA: WB Saunders, 1988; 229
30 Alexander EK, Marqusee E, Lawrence J *et al*. Timing and magnitude of increases in levothyroxine requirements during pregnancy in women with hypothyroidism. N Engl J Med 2004; 351: 241–249
31 Linden S, Rich CL. The use of lithium during pregnancy and lactation. J Clin Psychiatry 1983; 44: 358
32 Moses-Kolko EL, Bogen D, Perel J *et al*. Neonatal signs after late *in utero* exposure to serotonin reuptake inhibitors: literature review and implications for clinical applications. JAMA 2005; 293: 2372–2383
33 Chambers CD, Hernandez-Diaz S, Van Marter LJ *et al*. Selective serotonin-reuptake inhibitors and risk of persistent pulmonary hypertension of the newborn. N Engl J Med 2006; 354: 579–587

34 Pastuszak A, Schick-Boschetto B, Zuber C *et al.* Pregnancy outcome following first-trimester exposure to fluoxetine (Prozac). JAMA 1993; 269: 2446
35 Goldstein DJ, Corbin LA, Sundell KL. Effects of first-trimester fluoxetine exposure on the newborn. Obstet Gynecol 1997; 89: 713
36 Nulman I, Rovert J, Stewart DE *et al.* Neurodevelopment of children exposed *in utero* to antidepressant drugs. N Engl J Med 1997; 336: 258
37 Kenyon S, Boulvain M, Neilson J. Antibiotics for preterm rupture of the membranes: a systematic review. Obstet Gynecol 2001; 104: 1051–1057
38 Beard CM, Noller KL, O'Fallon WM *et al.* Lack of evidence for cancer due to use of metronidazole. N Engl J Med 1979; 301: 519
39 Harris RC, Lucey JF, MacLean JR. Kernicterus in premature infants associated with low concentration of billirubin in the plasma. Pediatrics 1950; 23: 878
40 Hernandez-Diaz S, Werler MM, Walker AM, Mitchell AA. Folic acid antagonists during pregnancy and the risk of birth defects. N Engl J Med 2000; 343: 1608–1614
41 Cohlan SQU, Bevelander G, Tiamsic T. Growth inhibition of prematures receiving tetracycline. Am J Dis Child 1963; 105: 453
42 Loebstein R, Addis A, Ho E *et al.* Pregnancy outcome following gestational exposure to fluoroquinolones: a multicenter prospective controlled study. Antimicrob Agents Chemother 1998; l42: 1336–1339
43 Robinson GC, Cambon KG. Hearing loss in infants of tuberculous mothers treated with streptomycin during pregnancy. N Engl J Med 1964; 271: 949
44 Culnane M, Fowler MG, Lee SS *et al.* Lack of long-term effects of *in utero* exposure to zidovudine among uninfected children born to HIV-infected women. JAMA 1999; 281: 151–157
45 Antiretroviral Pregnancy Registry Steering Committee. Antiretroviral pregnancy Registry International Interim Report for 1 January 1989 through 31 January 2004. Wilmington, NC: Registry Coordinating Center; 2004. Available from <www.apregistry.com>
46 Perinatal HIV Guidelines Working Group. Public Health Service Task Force. Recommendations for use of antiretroviral drugs in pregnant HIV-1-infected women for maternal health and interventions to reduce perinatal HIV-1 transmission in the United States. June 23, 2004, Available from <http://AIDSinfo.nih.gov>
47 Bristol-Myers Squibb. Important drug warning. Available from <http://www.fda.gov/medwatch/safety/2001/zerit&videx_letter.htm>
48 Lammer EJ, Chen DT, Hoar RM *et al.* Retinoic acid embryopathy. N Engl J Med 1985; 313: 837
49 Adams J. High incidence of intellectual deficits in 5 year old children exposed to isotretinoin '*in utero*'. Teratology 1990; 41: 614
50 Mitchell AA, Van Bennekom CM, Louik C. A pregnancy-prevention program in women of childbearing age receiving isotretinoin. N Engl J Med 1995; 333: 101–106
51 Feldkamp M, Carey JC. Clinical teratology counseling and consultation case report: low dose methotrexate exposure in the early weeks of pregnancy. Teratology 1993; 47: 533–539
52 Zemlickis D, Lishner M, Degendorfer P *et al.* Fetal outcome after *in utero* exposure to cancer chemotherapy. Arch Intern Med 1992; 152: 573

Robert L. Brent

Environmental causes of human congenital malformations

When I had completed medical school and graduate school, the scientific world did not even have the correct figure for the number of human chromosomes. Gregg[1] had recently described the teratogenicity of rubella virus infection during pregnancy. The teratogenic risk of the folic acid antagonists was established[2,3] and there were experimental studies indicating that nutritional deficiencies could produce birth defects in animals.[4]

What have we learned and accomplished in the past 50 years? Thousands of previously unknown genetic diseases have been described and many of their genes have been identified since the 1950s.[5,6] The fields of prenatal intrauterine diagnoses, intervention and treatment have been created. Metabolic and biochemical screening have become standard care for pregnant women and newborns. Over 50 teratogenic environmental drugs, chemicals and physical agents have been described[7–10] using modern epidemiological tools and the talents of clinical dysmorphologists.[11–17] The basic science and clinical rules for evaluating teratogenic risks have been established (Table 1).[18] The development of the rubella vaccine and the recognition of the importance of adequate folic acid intake in women of reproductive age are forerunners for the prevention of birth defects from teratogenic infectious agents and nutritional components that are important for normal development. The completion of the first stage of the Human Genome Project in the year 2000 offers the geneticist and teratologist immense opportunities to evaluate the concepts of polygenic and multifactorial etiologies[19,20] of congenital malformations.

Robert L. Brent MD PhD,
Head, Clinical and Environmental Teratology Research Laboratory, Room 308, R/A, Alfred I. duPont Hospital for Children, Box 269, Wilmington, DE 19899, USA.
E-mail: rbrent@nemours.org

Table 1 Evaluation of the allegation that a particular environmental agent causes congenital malformations or is responsible for malformations in an individual patient

Epidemiological studies

Controlled epidemiological studies consistently demonstrate an increased incidence of a particular spectrum of embryonic and/or fetal effects in exposed human populations

Secular trend data

Secular trends demonstrate a positive relationship between the changing exposures to a common environmental agent in human populations and the incidence of a particular embryonic and/or fetal effect

Animal developmental toxicity studies

An animal model can be developed which mimics the human developmental effect at clinically comparable exposures. Since mimicry may not occur in all animal species, animal models are more likely to be developed once there is good evidence for the embryotoxic effects reported in the human. Developmental toxicity studies in animals are indicative of a potential hazard in general rather than the potential for a specific adverse effect on the fetus when there are no human data on which to base the animal experiments

Dose–response relationship (pharmacokinetics and toxicokinetics)

Developmental toxicity in the human increases with dose (exposure) and the developmental toxicity in animal occur at a dose that is pharmacokinetically (quantitatively) equivalent to the human exposure

Biological plausibility

The mechanisms of developmental toxicity are understood and the effects are biologically plausible:

- Mechanisms of action (MOA)
- Receptor studies
- Nature of the malformations
- Teratology principles

Modified from several references.[7,8,18,26,36–38,41]

EMOTIONAL IMPACT OF CONGENITAL MALFORMATIONS

Reproductive problems encompass a multiplicity of diseases including sterility, infertility, abortion (miscarriage), stillbirth, congenital malformations (due to environmental or hereditary etiologies), fetal growth retardation and prematurity.[7–10,13] These clinical problems occur commonly in the general population and, therefore, environmental causes are not always easy to corroborate (Table 2). Severe congenital malformations occur in 3% of births. According to the Centers for Disease Control, severe congenital malformations (including those birth defects that cause death, hospitalization, and mental retardation) necessitate significant or repeated surgical procedures, are disfiguring, or interfere with physical performance. That means that each year in the US, 120,000 newborns are born with severe birth defects. Genetic diseases occur in about 11% of births. Spontaneous mutations account for less than 2–3% of genetic disease. Therefore, mutations induced from preconception exposures of environmental mutagens are difficult end-points to document (Table 2). It may surprise the reader to know that birth defects

Table 2 Background reproductive risks per million pregnancies

Reproductive risk	Frequency
Immunologically and clinically diagnosed spontaneous abortions per million conceptions	**350,000**
Clinically recognized spontaneous abortions per million clinically recognized pregnancies	**150,000**
Genetic diseases per million births	**110,000**
Multifactorial or polygenic genetic environmental interactions (*i.e. neural tube defects, cleft lip, hypospadius, hyperlipidemia, diabetes*)	90,000
Dominantly inherited disease (*i.e. achondroplasia, Huntington's chorea, neurofibromatosis*)	10,000
Autosomal and sex-linked genetic disease (*i.e. cystic fibrosis, hemophilia, sickle-cell disease, thalassemia*)	1200
Cytogenetic (chromosomal abnormalities) *i.e. Down's syndrome (trisomy 21), trisomy 13, trisomy 18, Turner's syndrome, 22q deletion, etc.*	5000
New mutations*	3000
Severe congenital malformations# (*due to all causes of birth defects: genetic, unknown, environmental per million births*)	**30,000**
Prematurity/million births	**40,000**
Fetal growth retardation/million births	**30,000**
Stillbirths (> 20 weeks)/million births	**2000–20,900**
Infertility	**7% of couples**

**The mutation rate for many genetic diseases can be calculated. This can be readily performed with dominantly inherited diseases when offspring are born with a dominant genetic disease and neither parent has the disease.*

#Congenital malformations have multiple etiologies including a significant proportion that are genetic.

account for 440,000 children's deaths each year in the low- and middle-income nations from congenital malformations. That represents 3.7% of the deaths in children. In the high-income countries, congenital malformations are the second highest cause of death in children, accounting for 20% of the deaths.

DISEASES OF AFFLICTION

Along with cancer, psychiatric illness, and hereditary diseases, reproductive problems have been viewed throughout history as diseases of affliction. Inherent in the reactions of most cultures is that these diseases have been viewed as punishments for misdeeds.[21–24] Regardless of the irrationality of this viewpoint, these feelings do exist. Ancient Babylonian writings recount tales of mothers being put to death because they delivered malformed infants. One George Spencer was slain by the Puritans in New Haven in the 17th century, having been convicted of fathering a cyclopean pig, since the Puritans were unable to differentiate between George Spencer's cataract and the malformed pigs cloudy cornea.[21] In modern times, some individuals with reproductive problems reverse the historical perspective, and blame others for the occurrence of their congenital malformations, infertility, abortions and hereditary diseases. They place the responsibility of their illness on environmental agents dispensed by their healthcare provider or utilized by their employer.[21–24]

Reproductive problems alarm the public, the press and some scientists to a greater degree than most other diseases. In fact, severely malformed children are disquieting to healthcare providers, especially if they are not experienced in dealing with these problems. No physician will be comfortable informing a family that their child was born without arms and legs. The objective evaluation of environmental causes of reproductive diseases is clouded by the emotional climate that surrounds these diseases, resulting in the expression of partisan positions that either diminish or magnify the environmental risks. These non-objective opinions can be expressed by scientists, the laity or the press.[23,24] It is the responsibility of every physician to be aware of the emotionally charged situation when a family has a child with a birth defect. The inadvertent comment by the physician, nurse, resident or student in attendance at the time of the child's delivery can have grave consequences for the physician and the family. Comments such as, 'Oh, you had an X-ray during your pregnancy', or 'You did not tell me that you were prescribed tetracycline while you were pregnant', can direct the patient's family to an attorney rather than to a teratology or genetic counselor.

BASIC PRINCIPLES OF TERATOLOGY

Labeling an environmental exposure as teratogenic is inappropriate unless one characterizes the exposure with regard to the dose, route of exposure and the stage of pregnancy when the exposure occurred. Labeling an agent as teratogenic only indicates that it may have the potential for producing congenital malformations. A 50-mg dose of thalidomide administered on the 26th day post-conception has a significant risk of malforming the embryo. That same dose taken during the 10th week of gestation will not result in congenital malformations.[25] One milligram of thalidomide taken at any time during pregnancy will have no effect on the developing embryo. We know that X-irradiation can be teratogenic.[26–30] However, if the dose is too low or the X-ray does not directly expose the embryo, there is no increased risk of congenital malformations (Fig. 1).[7,8,26] So a list of teratogens only indicates teratogenic potential. Evaluation of the dose and time of exposure could indicate that there is no teratogenic risk or that the risk is significant.

When evaluating studies dealing with the reproductive effects of any environmental agent, important principles should guide the analysis of human and animal reproductive studies. Paramount to this evaluation is the application of the basic science principles of teratology and developmental biology.[7,8,26] These principles are as follows:

1. *Exposure to teratogens follows a toxicological dose–response curve. There is a threshold below which no teratogenic effect will be observed; as the dose of the*

teratogen is increased, both the severity and frequency of reproductive effects will increase (Fig. 1; Table 3).

2. *The embryonic stage of exposure is critical in determining what deleterious effects will be produced and whether any of these effects can be produced by a known teratogen. Some teratogenic effects have a broad, and others a very narrow, period of sensitivity. The most sensitive stage for the induction of mental retardation from ionizing radiation is from the 8th to 15th week of pregnancy, a lengthy period. Thalidomide's period of sensitivity is about 2 weeks (Table 4).*[25]
3. *Even the most potent teratogenic agent cannot produce every malformation.*

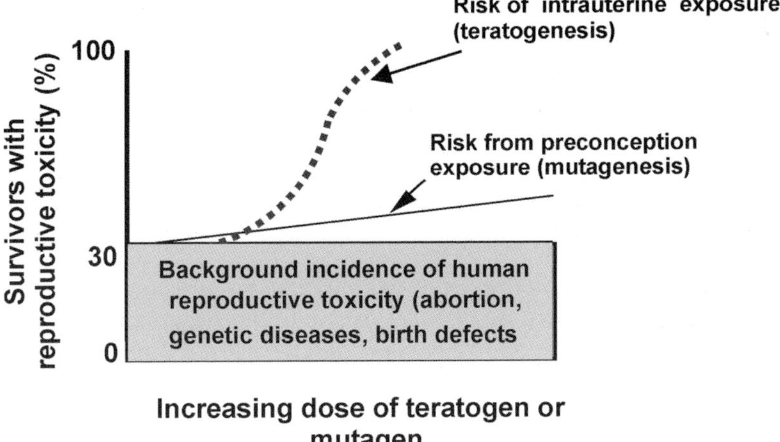

Fig. 1. Dose–response relationship of reproductive toxins comparing preconception and post-conception risks. Reprouced with permission of Wiley-Liss Inc © 1999 from Brent[26]

Table 3 Stochastic and threshold dose–response relationships of diseases produced by environmental agents

Relationship	Stochastic phenomena	Threshold phenomena
Pathology	Damage to a single cell may result in disease	Multicellular injury
Site	DNA	High variation in etiology, affecting many cells and organ processes
Diseases	Cancer, mutation	Malformation, growth retardation, death, chemical toxicity, *etc*.
Risk	Some risk exists at all dosages; at low exposures, the hypothetical risk is below the spontaneous risk	No increased risk below the threshold dose
Effect	The incidence of the disease increases with the dose but the severity and nature of the disease remain the same	Both the severity and incidence of the disease increase with dose

Modified from Brent.[26]

Table 4 Developmental stage sensitivity to thalidomide-induced limb reduction defects in the human

Days from conception for induction of defects	Limb reduction defects
21–26 days	Thumb aplasia
22–23 days	Microtia, deafness
23–34 days	Hip dislocation
24–29 days	Amelia, upper limbs
24–33 days	Phocomelia, upper limbs
25–31 days	Pre-axial aplasia, upper limbs
27–31 days	Amelia, lower limbs
28–33 days	Pre-axial aplasia, lower limbs; phocomelia, lower limbs; femoral hypoplasia; girdle hypoplasia
33–36 days	Triphalangeal thumb

Modified from Brent and Holmes.[24]

4. *Most teratogens have a confined group of congenital malformations that result after exposure during a critical period of embryonic development. This confined group of malformations is referred to as the syndrome that describes the agent's teratogenic effects.*

5. *While a group of malformations may suggest the possibility of certain teratogens, they cannot definitively confirm the causal agent because some teratogenic syndromes mimic genetic syndromes. On the other hand, the presence of certain malformations can eliminate the possibility that a particular teratogenic agent was responsible because those malformations have not been demonstrated to be part of the syndrome or because the production of that malformation is not biologically plausible for that particular alleged teratogen.*

ETIOLOGY OF CONGENITAL MALFORMATIONS

The etiology of congenital malformations can be divided into three categories – unknown, genetic, and environmental (Table 5). The etiology of a majority of human malformations is unknown. A significant proportion of congenital malformations of unknown etiology is likely to have an important genetic component. In fact, newly published findings are describing genetic causes for malformations or syndromes whose etiology were previously listed as unknown. Malformations with an increased recurrent risk, such as cleft lip and palate, anencephaly, spina bifida, certain congenital heart diseases (pyloric stenosis, hypospadias, inguinal hernia, talipes equinovarus, and congenital dislocation of the hip) fit in the category of multifactorial disease as well as in the category of polygenic inherited disease.[19,20] The multifactorial/threshold hypothesis postulates the modulation of a continuum of genetic characteristics by intrinsic and extrinsic (environmental) factors.

Spontaneous errors of development may account for some of the malformations that occur without apparent abnormalities of the genome or

Table 5 Etiology of human congenital malformations observed during the first year of life*

Suspected cause	Percentage of total
Unknown	**65–75**
Polygenic	
Multifactorial (gene-environment interactions)	
Spontaneous errors of development	
Synergistic interactions of teratogens	
Genetic	**15–25**
Autosomal and sex-linked inherited genetic disease	
Cytogenetic (chromosomal abnormalities)	
New mutations	
Environmental	**10**
Maternal conditions: alcoholism, diabetes, endocrinopathies, phenylketonuria, smoking and nicotine, starvation, nutritional deficits	4
Infectious agents: rubella, toxoplasmosis, syphilis, herpes simplex, cytomegalovirus, varicella-zoster, Venezuelan equine encephalitis, parvovirus B19	3
Mechanical problems (deformations): amniotic band constrictions, umbilical cord constraint, disparity in uterine size and uterine contents	1–2
Chemicals, prescription drugs, high-dose ionizing radiation, hyperthermia	<1

*Modified from several references.[7,8,26,36–38,41]

environmental influence. Spontaneous errors of development may indicate that we may never achieve our goal of eliminating all birth defects because a significant percentage of birth defects are due to the statistical probability of errors in the developmental process, similar to the concept of spontaneous mutation. It is estimated that 30–40% of all conceptions are lost before term, many within the first 3 weeks of development. The World Health Organization estimated that 15% of all clinically recognizable pregnancies end in a spontaneous abortion, 50–60% of which are due to chromosomal abnormalities.[31–34] Finally, 3–6% of offspring are malformed, which represents the background risk for human maldevelopment (Table 2).

FACTORS AFFECTING SUSCEPTIBILITY TO DEVELOPMENTAL TOXICANTS

A basic tenet of environmentally produced malformations is that teratogens or a teratogenic milieu have certain characteristics in common and follow certain basic principles. These principles determine the quantitative and qualitative aspects of environmentally produced malformations.

Embryonic stage

The types and risk of malformations caused by teratogenic agents usually results in a spectrum of malformations that varies depending on the stage of exposure and the dose. The developmental period at which an exposure occurs will determine which structures are most susceptible to the deleterious effects of the drug or chemical and to what extent the embryo can repair the damage. This period of sensitivity may be narrow or broad, depending on the environmental agent and the malformation in question. The period of susceptibility to thalidomide-induced limb defects is very narrow (Table 4),[25] while susceptibility period for radiation-induced microcephaly is very broad.[26]

Dose or magnitude of the exposure

The quantitative correlation of the magnitude of the embryopathic effects to the dose of a drug, chemical or other agent is referred to as the dose–response relationship. This is extremely important when comparing effects among different species because the use of mg/kg doses is ,at most, a rough approximation. Dose equivalence among species for drugs and chemicals can only be accomplished by performing pharmacokinetic studies, metabolic studies and dose–response investigations in the human and the species being studied, while ionizing radiation exposures in rads or Sieverts (Sv) are comparable in most mammalian species.[26]

Threshold dose

The threshold dose (no-adverse-effect-level, NOAEL) is the dosage below which the incidence of death, malformation, growth retardation, or functional deficit is not statistically greater than that of controls (Fig. 1; Table 3). The threshold level of exposure is usually from less than one to two orders of magnitude below the teratogenic or embryopathic dose for drugs and chemicals that kill or malform half the embryos. An exogenous teratogenic agent, therefore, has a no-effect dose as compared to mutagens or carcinogens that have a stochastic dose response curve (Fig. 1; Table 3). Stochastic phenomena, namely mutation and oncogenesis, are hypothesized not to have a threshold. Therefore, there is no exposure that does not have a theoretical risk. The severity and incidence of malformations produced by every exogenous teratogenic agent that has been appropriately studied have exhibited threshold phenomena during organogenesis.

Pharmacokinetics and metabolism of the drug or chemical

The physiological alterations in pregnancy and the bioconversion of compounds can significantly influence the teratogenic effects of drugs and chemicals by affecting absorption, body distribution, active form(s) and excretion of the compound.

Physiological alterations in the mother during pregnancy affect the pharmacokinetics of drugs:

1. Decreased gastrointestinal motility and increased intestinal transit time resulting in delayed absorption of drugs absorbed in the small intestine due to increased stomach retention and enhanced absorption of slowly absorbed drugs.

2. Decreased plasma albumin concentration which alters the kinetics of compound normally bound to albumin.
3. Increased plasma and extracellular fluid volumes that affect concentration-dependent transfer of compounds.
4. Renal elimination, which is generally increased but is influenced by body position during late pregnancy.
5. Inhibition of metabolic inactivation in the maternal liver.
6. Variations in uterine blood flow, although little is known about how this affects transfer across the placenta.

The fetus also undergoes physiological alterations that affect the pharmacokinetics of drugs:

1. The amount and distribution of fat varies with development and affects the distribution of lipid-soluble drugs and chemicals.
2. The fetal circulation contains a higher concentration of unbound drug largely because the plasma fetal protein concentrations are lower than in the adult.
3. The functional development of pharmacological receptors is likely to proceed at different rates in the various tissues.
4. Drugs excreted by the fetal kidneys may be recycled via amniotic fluid swallowing by the fetus.

The role the placenta plays in drug pharmacokinetics has been reviewed by Juchau and Rettie[35] and involves: (i) transport; (ii) the presence of receptors sites for a number of endogenous and xenobiotic compounds (β-adrenergic, glucocorticoid, epidermal growth factor, IgG-Fc, insulin, low-density lipoproteins, opiates, somatomedin, testosterone, transcobalamin II, transferrin, folate, retinoid); and (iii) the bioconversion of xenobiotics. Bioconversion of xenobiotics has been shown to be important in the teratogenic activity of several xenobiotics. There is strong evidence that reactive metabolites of cyclophosphamide, 2-acetylaminofluorene, and nitroheterocycles (niridazole) are the proximal teratogens. There is also experimental evidence that suggests that other chemicals undergo conversion to intermediates that have deleterious effects on embryonic development including phenytoin, procarbazine, rifampicin, diethylstilbestrol, some benzhydrylpiperazine antihistamines, adriamycin, testosterone, benzo(a)pyrene, methoxyethanol, caffeine, and paraquat.

The major site of bioconversion of chemicals *in vivo* is likely to be the maternal liver. Placental cytochrome P450-dependent monooxygenation of xenobiotics will occur at low rates unless induced by such compounds as those found in tobacco smoke. However, the rodent embryo and yolk sac have been shown to possess functional cytochrome P450 oxidative isozymes capable of converting pro-teratogens to active metabolites during early organogenesis. In addition, cytochrome P450-independent bioactivation has been suggested: for example, there is strong evidence that the rat embryo can reductively convert niridazole to an embryotoxic metabolite.

As defined by Juchau and Rettie,[35] there are several experimental criteria that would suggest that a suspected metabolite is responsible for the *in vivo* teratogenic effects of a chemical or drug: (i) the chemical must be convertible to the intermediate; (ii) the intermediate must be found in or have access to the tissue(s) affected; (iii) the embryotoxic effect should increase with the concentration of the metabolite; (iv) inhibiting the conversion should reduce the embryotoxic effect of the agent; (v) promoting the conversion should increase the embryotoxicity of the agent; (vi) inhibiting or promoting the conversion should not alter the target tissues; and (vii) inhibition of biochemical inactivation should increase the embryotoxicity of the agent. It is readily apparent why there may exist marked qualitative and quantitative differences in the species' response to a teratogenic agent.

Placental transport

The placenta controls the exchange between the embryo and the maternal organism. The placenta varies in structure and function among species and for each stage of gestation. Thus, differences in placental function and structure may affect our ability to apply teratogenic data developed in one species directly to other species, including the human. Yet, as pharmacokinetic techniques and the actual measurement of metabolic products in the embryo become more sophisticated, the appropriateness of utilizing animal data to project human effects may improve.[35]

While it has been alleged that the placental barrier was protective and, therefore, harmful substances did not reach the embryo, it is now clear that there is no 'placental barrier' *per se*. Yet the package inserts on many drugs state that: 'this drug crosses the placental barrier'.[26] The uninitiated may infer from this statement that this characteristic of a drug is both unusual and hazardous. The fact is that most drugs and chemicals cross the placenta. It will be a rare chemical that will cross the placental barrier in one species and be unable to reach the fetus in another. No such chemical exists except for selected proteins whose actions are species-specific.

Genetic differences

The genetic constitution of an organism is an important factor in the susceptibility of a species to a drug or chemical. More than 30 disorders of increased sensitivity to drug toxicity or effects in the human are due to an inherited trait.

ENVIRONMENTAL AGENT EXPOSURE DURING PREGNANCY RESULTING IN REPRODUCTIVE TOXICITY[7–9]

Table 6 lists environmental agents that have resulted in reproductive toxicity and or congenital malformations in human populations. The list cannot be used in isolation because so many other parameters must be considered in analyzing the risks in individual patients. Many of these agents represent a very small risk while others may represent substantial risk. The risks will vary with the magnitude, timing and length of exposure. More information can be obtained from more extensive reviews or summary articles. Table 7 includes agents that have had concerns raised about their reproductive risks but, after

Table 6 Proven human teratogens or embryotoxins: drugs, chemicals, milieu and physical agents that have resulted in human congenital malformations

REPRODUCTIVE TOXIN AND ALLEGED EFFECTS
Aminopterin, methotrexate – growth retardation, microcephaly, meningomyelocele mental retardation, hydrocephalus, and cleft palate
Androgens – masculinization of the developing fetus can occur from androgens and high doses of some male-derived progestins
Angiotensin converting enzyme (ACE) inhibitors – fetal hypotension syndrome in 2nd and 3rd trimester resulting in fetal kidney hypoperfusion, and anuria, oligohydramnios, pulmonary hypoplasia and cranial bone hypoplasia. No teratogenic effect in the first trimester although a recent publication[54] contests this conclusion
Angiotensin II receptor blocking agents – the effects of this group of drugs is very similar to the ACE inhibitors
Antituberculous therapy – INH, PAS has an increased risk for some CNS abnormalities
Caffeine – moderate caffeine exposure is not associated with birth defects; high exposures are associated with an increased risk of abortion but the data are inconsistent
Chorionic villous sampling (CVS) – vascular disruption malformations, *i.e.* limb reduction defects
Cobalt in hematemic multivitamins – fetal goiter
Cocaine – vascular disruptive type malformations in very low incidence, pregnancy loss. Inconsistent reports of decrease in cognitive function
Corticosteroids – high exposures administered systemically have a low risk for cleft palate in some studies, but the epidemiological studies are not consistent
Coumarin derivatives – early exposure during pregnancy can result in nasal hypoplasia, stippling of secondary epiphysis, intrauterine growth retardation. CNS malformations can occur in late pregnancy exposure due to bleeding
Cyclophosphamide and other chemotherapeutic agents and immunosuppressive agents like cyclosporine or leflunomide – many chemotherapeutic agents used to treat cancer have a theoretical risk for producing malformations in the fetus when administered to pregnant women, especially since most of these drugs are teratogenic in animals, but the clinical data are not consistent. Many of these drugs have not been shown to be teratogenic, but the numbers of cases in the studies are small. Caution is the byword
Diethylstilbestrol – administration during pregnancy produces genital abnormalities, adenosis, clear cell adenocarcinoma of vagina in adolescents. The latter has a risk of 1:1000 to 1:10,000, but the other effects, such as adenosis can be quite high
Ethyl alcohol – fetal alcohol syndrome consists of microcephaly, mental retardation, growth retardation, typical facial dysmorphogenesis, abnormal ears, small palpebral fissures. It is the most common environmental cause of a decrease in intellectual performance
Ionizing radiation – the threshold for major birth defects is greater than 20 rad (0.2 Gy) at the most sensitive stage of embryogenesis (18–35 days post-conception). Radiation can increased the risk for some fetal effects such as micocephaly or growth retardation at mid-gestation, but the threshold for these effects is higher
Insulin shock therapy – this therapeutic modality when administered to pregnant women resulted in microcephaly, mental retardation. This therapy is no longer used
Lithium therapy – continuous exposure during pregnancy for the treatment of manic-depressive illness has an increased risk for Ebstein's anomaly and other malformations, but the risks appear to be very low

Table 6 *(continued)* Proven human teratogens or embryotoxins: drugs, chemicals, milieu and physical agents that have resulted in human congenital malformations

Minoxidil – the effect of the growth promotion of fetal hair was discovered for this drug because administration during pregnancy resulted in hirsutism in newborns

Methimazole – aplasia cutis has been reported to be increased in mothers administered this drug during pregnancy*

Methylene blue intra-amniotic instillation – fetal intestinal atresia, hemolytic anemia and jaundice in neonatal period. This procedure is no longer utilized to identify one twin

Misoprostol – a low incidence of vascular disruptive phenomena, such as limb reduction defects and Mobius syndrome have been reported in pregnancies in which this drug was used to induce an abortion. Autism has also been associated with *in utero* exposure[55]

Penicillamine (D-penicillamine) – this drug results in the physical effects referred to as lathyrism, the results of poisoning by the seeds of the genus Lathyrus. It causes collagen disruption, cutis laxa, and hyperflexibility of joints. The condition appears to be reversible and the risk is low

Progestin therapy – very high doses of androgen hormone derived progestins can produce masculinization. Many drugs with progestational activity do not have masculinizing potential. None of the commonly used progestational drugs have the potential for producing non-genital malformations

Propylthiouracil – this drug and other antithyroid medications administered during pregnancy can result in an infant born with a goiter

Radioactive isotopes – tissue- and organ-specific damage is dependent on the radioisotope element and distribution, *i.e.* high doses of ^{131}I administered to a pregnant woman can cause fetal thyroid hypoplasia after the 8th week of development

Retinoids (Acutane) – systemic retinoic acid, isotretinoin, Etretinate can cause increased risk of central nervous system, cardio-aortic, ear and clefting defects. Microtia, anotia, thymic aplasia and other branchial arch, aortic arch abnormalities and certain congenital heart malformations

Retinoids, topical – topical administration is very unlikely to have teratogenic potential because one cannot attain a teratogenic serum level from topical exposure to retinoids

Streptomycin – streptomycin and a group of ototoxic drugs can affect the eighth nerve and interfere with hearing; it is a relatively low-risk phenomenon. Even children are less sensitive to the ototoxic effects of these drugs when compared to adults

Sulfa drug and vitamin K – these drugs can produce hemolysis in some subpopulations of fetuses

Tetracycline – this drug produces bone and teeth staining, No other malformations are at increased risk

Thalidomide – this drug results in an increased incidence of deafness, anotia, pre-axial limb reduction defects, phocomelia, ventricular septal defects and GI atresias. The susceptible period is from the 22nd to the 36th day post-conception. Autism has also been associated with *in utero* exposure[55]

Trimethorpin – this drug was frequently used to treat urinary tract infections and has been linked to an increased incidence of neural tube defects. The risk is not high, but it is biologically plausible because of the drug's effect on lowering folic acid levels. This has resulted in neurological symptoms in adults taking this drug

Vitamin A – the same malformations that have been reported with the retinoids have been reported with very high doses of vitamin A (retinol). Dosages to produce birth defects would have to be in excess of 25,000–50,000 units per day

Vitamin D* – large doses given in vitamin D prophylaxis are possibly involved in the etiology of supravalvular aortic stenosis, elfin faces, and mental retardation

Table 6 *(continued)* Proven human teratogens or embryotoxins: drugs, chemicals, milieu and physical agents that have resulted in human congenital malformations

Warfarin (Coumarin) – early exposure during pregnancy can result in nasal hypoplasia, stippling of secondary epiphysis, intrauterine growth retardation. CNS malformations can occur in late pregnancy exposure due to bleeding

ANTICONVULSANTS

Diphenylhydantoin – treatment of convulsive disorders increases the risk of the fetal hydantoin syndrome, consisting of facial dysmorphology, cleft palate, VSD, growth and mental retardation

Trimethadione and paramethadione – treatment of convulsive disorders increases the risk of characteristic facial dysmorphology, mental retardation, V-shaped eye brows, low-set ears with anteriorly folded helix, high-arched palate, irregular teeth, CNS anomalies, severe developmental delay

Valproic acid – treatment of convulsive disorders increases the risk of spina bifida, facial dysmorphology and autism.[55] A threshold (NOAEL) has been suggested for exposures below 1000 mg/day and a serum level below 70 μg%

Carbamazepine – treatment of convulsive disorders increases the risk facial dysmorphology

Primidone, phenobarbital, Lamotrigine and other anticonvulsants – anticonvulsants all have real or hypothetical risks for a group of malformations and reduction in cognitive function. The actual risks are difficult to determine, but most authorities are of the opinion that some type of regimen must be utilized to prevent or decrease convulsive episodes during pregnancy. Anticonvulsant polytherapy increases the risk of developmental effects

CHEMICALS

Carbon monoxide poisoning – CNS damage has been reported with very high exposures, but the risk appears to be low*

Lead – very high exposures can cause pregnancy loss; intrauterine teratogenesis is not established at very low exposures below 20 μg% in the serum of pregnant mothers

Gasoline addiction embryopathy – facial dysmorphology, mental retardation

Methyl mercury – Minamata disease consists of cerebral palsy, microcephaly, mental retardation, blindness, cerebellum hypoplasia. Other endemics have occurred from adulteration of wheat with mercury containing chemicals that are used to prevent grain spoilage. Present environmental levels of mercury are unlikely to represent a teratogenic risk, but reducing or limiting the consumption of carnivorous fish has been suggested in order not to exceed the EPA's MPE (maximum permissible exposure), which is far below the toxic effects of mercury

Polychlorinated biphenyls – poisoning has occurred from adulteration of food products (Cola-colored babies, CNS effects, pigmentation of gums, nails, teeth and groin; hypoplastic deformed nails; intrauterine growth retardation; abnormal skull calcification). The threshold exposure has not been determined, but it is unlikely to be teratogenic at the present environmental exposures

Toluene and gasoline addiction – facial dysmorphology, mental retardation

EMBRYONIC AND FETAL INFECTIONS

Cytomegalovirus infection – retinopathy, CNS calcification, microcephaly, mental retardation

Rubella – deafness, congenital heart disease, microcephaly, cataracts, mental retardation

Table 6 *(continued)* Proven human teratogens or embryotoxins: drugs, chemicals, milieu and physical agents that have resulted in human congenital malformations

Herpes simplex – fetal infection, liver disease, death

Human immunodeficiency virus – perinatal HIV infection

Parvovirus infection, B19 – stillbirth, hydrops

Syphilis – maculopapular rash, hepatosplenomegaly, deformed nails, osteochondritis at joints of extremities, congenital neurosyphilis, abnormal epiphyses, chorioretinitis

Toxoplasmosis – hydrocephaly, microphthalmia, chorioretinitis, mental retardation

Varicella Zoster – skin and muscle defects, intrauterine growth retardation, limb reduction defects, CNS damage (very low increase risk)

Venezuelan equine encephalitis – hydranencephaly, microphthalmia, central nervous system destructive lesions, luxation of the hip.

Rubeola (wild-type measles) – the measles virus can infect the placenta and this severe infection can cause pregnancy loss, which is uncommon

Malaria – pregnancy loss by miscarriage or stillbirth. Maternal demise

MATERNAL DISEASE STATES

Corticosteroid secreting endocrinopathy – mothers with Cushing's disease can have infants with hyperadrenocortism, but anatomical malformations do not appear to be increased

Iodine deficiency – can result in embryonic goiter and mental retardation

Intrauterine problems of constraint and vascular disruption – these types of defects are more common in multiple-birth pregnancies, pregnancies with anatomical defects of the uterus, placental emboli, amniotic bands; birth defects such as club feet, limb reduction defects, aplasia cutis, cranial asymmetry, external ear malformations, mid-line closure defects, cleft palate and muscle aplasia, limb reduction defects, cleft lip, omphalocele, encephalocele)

Maternal androgen endocrinopathy (adrenal tumors) – masculinization

Maternal depression and the use of antidepressants – at the present time, there is a controversy as to whether the SSRI exposures during pregnancy represent a risk for congenital malformations. The data are inconsistent and more studies and well-performed animal studies are necessary.[55–62] There is data indicating the presence of fetal growth retardation and postnatal hyperactivity that is transient

Maternal diabetes – caudal and femoral hypoplasia, transposition of great vessels and other malformations

Maternal folic acid in reduced amounts – an increased incidence of neural tube defects (NTDs) and possibly other mid-line malformations

Maternal phenylketonuria – abortion, microcephaly, and mental retardation. Very high risk in untreated patients

Maternal starvation – IUGR, abortion, NTDs

Tobacco smoking – abortion, IUGR, and stillbirth. Question of decrease in cognitive function a possibly and increase in some birth defects, although this is controversial

Zinc deficiency – neural tube defects*

*Controversial.

careful and complete evaluation, the agents were found not to represent an increased reproductive risk.[36–41]

References for the environmental agents can be found in review articles and texts dealing with teratogenesis.[5,6,11,16,34,42–47]

Table 7 Agents erroneously alleged to have caused human malformations

Agent	Allegation
Bendectin	Alleged to cause numerous types of birth defects including limb reduction defects, heart malformations and many other malformations
Diagnostic ultrasonography	No significant hyperthermia, therefore no reproductive effects. Newer ultrasound equipment and lengthy procedures could raise the intrauterine temperature, This can be monitored to make certain that the fetal temperature is not significantly increased
Electromagnetic fields (EMFs)	Alleged to cause abortion, cancer, and birth defects
Progestational drugs	Alleged to cause numerous types of non-genital birth defects, including limb reduction defects, heart malformations and many other malformations)

ROLE OF THE PHYSICIAN IN COUNSELING FAMILIES

The clinician must be cognizant of the fact that many patients believe that most congenital malformations are caused by a drug or medication taken during pregnancy. Counseling patients about reproductive risks requires a significant degree of both knowledge and skill. Physicians must also realize that erroneous counseling by inexperienced health professionals may be a stimulus to non-meritorious litigation.[22]

Unfortunately, some individuals have assumed that if a drug or chemical causes birth defects in an animal model or *in vitro* system at a high dose, then it has the potential for producing birth defects at any dose.[48,49] This may be reinforced by the fact that many teratology studies reported in the literature using several doses do not determine the no-effect dose.

Ignoring the basic tenets of teratology appears to occur most commonly in the evaluation of environmental toxic exposures where the exposure was very low or unknown and the agent has been reported to be teratogenic at a very high dose or a maternally toxic dose in animal models.[48,49] In most instances, but of course not all instances, the actual population exposure is revealed to be orders of magnitude below the threshold dose and the doses that were used in animal studies or toxic exposures in the population. This has occurred with 2,4,5-T, PCBs, Pb, Cd, pesticides, herbicides, veterinary hormones and some industrial exposures.

Unfortunately, we do have examples where environmental disasters have been responsible for birth defects or pregnancy loss in exposed populations (methyl mercury in Japan, PCBs in the Orient, organic mercury in the Middle East, lead poisoning in the 19th and early 20th centuries) and we do have many examples of the introduction of teratogenic drugs (Table 6). Therefore, we can never generalize as to whether a chemical or drug is safe or hazardous unless we know the magnitude of the exposure.

Before their baby is born, parents may be concerned about the risks of various environmental exposures. If the child is born with congenital malformations they may question whether there was a causal relationship with an environmental exposure:

1. *Has the environmental agent been proven to increase the risk of congenital malformations in exposed human populations? In other words, is the agent a proven human teratogen?*
2. *Should a woman of reproductive age or who is pregnant be concerned about increased risks of reproductive effects from exposure to a particular environmental agent?*
3. *If a child is born with congenital malformations and the mother was exposed during her pregnancy to a particular environmental agent, was the agent responsible for the child's birth defects?*
4. *Should a physician report or publish a case of a patient or cluster of patients who were born with congenital malformations and whose mother was exposed to an environmental agent?*[50]

Scholarly evaluation

When a physician responds to a parent's inquiry ('What caused my child's birth defect?'), the physician should respond in the same scholarly manner that would be utilized in performing a differential diagnosis for any clinical problem. Physicians have a protocol for evaluating complex clinical problems; *i.e.* 'fever of unknown origin', 'failure to thrive', 'congestive heart failure', or 'respiratory distress'. If a mother of a malformed infant had some type of exposure during pregnancy, such as a diagnostic radiological examination or medication during pregnancy, the consulting physician should not support or suggest the possibility of a causal relationship before performing a complete evaluation. Likewise, if a pregnant woman who had not yet delivered had some type of exposure during pregnancy, the consulting physician should not support or suggest the possibility that the fetus is at increased risk before performing a complete evaluation. As mentioned previously, only a small percentage of birth defects are due to prescribed drugs, chemicals and physical agents (Table 5).[9,36,51] Even when the drug is listed as a teratogen, it has to have been administered during the sensitive period of development for that drug and above the threshold dose for producing teratogenesis. Furthermore, the malformations in the child should be the malformations that are included in the teratogenic syndrome produced by that drug. It should be emphasized that a recent analysis pointed out that there are no drugs with measurable teratogenic potential in the list of the 200 most prescribed drugs in the US.[51]

After a complete examination of the child and a review of the genetic and teratology medical literature, the clinician must decide on whether the child's malformations are due to a genetic cause or an environmental toxin or agent. The clinician may not be able to conclude, definitively or presumptively, the etiology of the child's birth defects. This information must then be conveyed to the patient in an objective and compassionate manner. A similar situation exists if a pregnant women has been exposed to a drug, chemical or physical agent, since the mother will want to know the risk of that exposure to her unborn child. If one wishes to answer the generic question, 'Is a particular environmental drug, chemical or physical agent a reproductive toxicant?' then a formal approach is recommended that includes a 5-part evaluation as described in Table 1.[18]

Some typical analyses of the risks of reproductive effects for Bendectin, sex steroids, diagnostic ultrasound, and electromagnetic fields demonstrate the usefulness of an organized approach to determine whether an environmental agent has been demonstrated to be a reproductive toxin.[36–41]

There are resources that can assist the physician with the medical literature evaluation and the clinical evaluation of the patient.[5,6,11,16,34,42–47]

Clinical evaluation

There are many articles and books that can assist the physician with the clinical evaluation, although physician training programs do not usually prepare generalists to perform sophisticated genetic counseling or teratology counseling.[11,16] Besides the usual history and physical evaluation, the physician has to obtain information about the nature, magnitude and timing of the exposure. The physical examination should include descriptive and quantitative information about the physical characteristics of the child. While some growth measurements are routine, many measurements utilized by these specialized counselors are not part of the usual physical examination, *i.e.* palpebral fissure size, ear length, intercanthal distances, total height-to-trunk ratio, and many others. Important physical variations in facial, hand and foot structure as well as other anatomical structures may be suggestive of known syndromes, either teratologic or genetic.

Evaluation of the reproductive risk of an environmental exposure that occurred during pregnancy or the cause of a child's malformation in which an exposure occurred during pregnancy

The vast majority of consultations involving pregnancy exposures conclude that the exposure does not change the reproductive risks in that pregnancy. In many instances, the information that is available is so vague that the counselor cannot reach a definitive conclusion about the magnitude of the risk. Information that is necessary for this evaluation is:

1. What was the nature of the exposure?
2. Is the exposure agent identifiable? If the agent is identifiable, has it been definitively identified as a reproductive toxin with a recognized constellation of malformations or other reproductive effects?
3. When did the exposure occur during embryonic and fetal development?
4. If the agent is known to produce reproductive toxic effects, was the exposure above or below the threshold for these effects?
5. Were there other significant environmental exposures or medical problems during the pregnancy?
6. Is this is a wanted pregnancy or is the family ambivalent about carrying this baby to term?
7. What is the medical and reproductive history of this mother with regard to prior pregnancies and the reproductive history of the family lineage?

Evaluation of the reproductive risk of an environmental exposure that occurred during pregnancy

After obtaining all this information, the counselor is in a position to provide the family with an estimate of the reproductive risks of the exposure. Here are some examples of consultations that have been referred to our clinical teratology service:

Patient 1

A 26-year-old pregnant woman was in an automobile accident in her 10th week of pregnancy and sustained a severe concussion. Although she did not convulse post-injury, the treating neurosurgeon prescribed 300 mg of diphenylhydantoin during her first 24 hours in the hospital. Fortunately, she recovered from the injury without any sequelae but her primary physician was concerned that she had received an anticonvulsant associated with a teratogenic syndrome. No other exposure to reproductive toxins occurred in this pregnancy and the family history for congenital malformations was negative, except for an uncle with neurofibromatosis. The primary physician requested a consultation with regard to the teratogenic risk. While diphenylhydantoin administered chronically throughout pregnancy has been associated with a low incidence of characteristic facial dysmorphogenesis, reduced mentation, cleft palate and digital hypoplasia, there are no data to indicate that one day of therapy would cause any of the features of this syndrome. Furthermore, the lip and palate have completed their development by the 10th week. This was a wanted pregnancy and the mother chose to continue her pregnancy. She delivered a normal 3370-g boy at term.

Patient 2

A 25-year-old woman was seen in the emergency service of her local hospital with nausea, vomiting and diarrhea. She had just returned from a cruise on which a number of the passengers became ill on the last day of the trip with similar symptoms. The emergency ward physician ordered a pregnancy test followed by a flat plate of the abdomen because there was evidence of peritoneal irritation. Both of these studies were negative. But 1 week later, she missed her menstrual period and a week later her pregnancy test was positive. Her obstetrician was concerned because she had been exposed to a radiological procedure at a time when she was pregnant. The obstetrician referred the patient for counseling after obtaining an ultrasound that indicated that the embryo was approximately 7 days post-conception at the time of the radiological examination. The patient advised the counselor that she was ambivalent about the pregnancy because of the 'dangers' of the X-rays to her embryo. The estimated exposure to the embryo was less than 500 mrad (0.005 Sv). This exposure is far below the exposure that is known to affect the developing embryo. Just as important is the fact that the embryo was exposed during the first 2 weeks post-conception, a time that is less likely to increase the risk of teratogenesis, even if the exposure was much higher.[26,52] After evaluation of the family history and after she received counseling about the risks of the X-ray, the prospective mother decided to continue the pregnancy. She delivered a 3150-g normal baby.

Evaluation of whether a child born with congenital malformations was caused by an environmental exposure during pregnancy, has a genetic etiology or whose cause cannot be determined

Patient 3

A mother of a 30-year-old man born in the Azores in 1960 with congenital absence of the right leg below the knee had pursued compensation for her son because she was certain that she must have received thalidomide during her pregnancy.[24] The German manufacturer of thalidomide refused compensation claiming that thalidomide had never been distributed in the Azores. The mother fervently believed that thalidomide was responsible for her son's malformations and I received a letter from her asking for my opinion. I requested her son's medical records, X-rays and photographs of the malformations. She sent me the X-ray studies of his hips and legs and his complete evaluation performed at the local hospital in the Azores. He had none of the other stigmata of thalidomide embryopathy (pre-axial limb defects, phocomelia, facial hemangioma, ear malformations, deafness, crocodile tears, ventricular septal defect, intestinal or gall bladder atresia, kidney malformations). Most importantly, his limb malformations were not of the thalidomide type. He had a unilateral congenital amputation, with no digital remnants at the end of the limb. His pelvic girdle was completely normal which would be unusual in a thalidomide malformed limb. Finally, his limb defect involved only one leg; the other leg was completely normal. This would be very unusual in a true thalidomide embryopathy. In this particular case, the young man had a congenital amputation, probably due to vascular disruption, etiology unknown. Known causes of vascular disruptive malformations are cocaine, misoprostol and chorionic villous sampling. It is difficult to determine whether any amount of appropriate counseling will put closure on this problem for this mother.

Patient 4

A family claimed that the anti-nausea medication, Bendectin,[36,37,53] taken by the mother of a malformed boy, was responsible for her son's congenital limb reduction defects. Bendectin was taken during the mother's pregnancy after the period of limb organogenesis, but some limb malformations can be produced by teratogens later in pregnancy. The malformation was unaccompanied by any other dysmorphogenetic effects. The boy's malformations were the classical split-hand, split-foot syndrome, which is dominantly inherited. This malformation has a significant portion of cases that are due to a new mutation. Since neither parent manifested the malformation, the conclusion had to be that a new mutation had occurred in the sex cells of one of the parents. Therefore, the risk of this malformation occurring in the offspring of this boy would be 50%. Obviously, Bendectin was not responsible for this child's malformations. In spite of the obvious genetic etiology of the malformed child's birth defects, a legal suit was filed. A jury decided for the defendant – namely, that Bendectin was not responsible for the child's birth defects.

It should be apparent that determining the reproductive risks of an exposure during pregnancy or the etiology of a child's congenital malformations is not a simple process. It involves a careful analysis of the medical and scientific literature pertaining to the reproductive toxic effects of exogenous agents in humans and animals, as well as an evaluation of the exposure and biological plausibility of an increased risk or a causal connection between the exposure and a child's congenital malformation. It also involves a careful physical examination, a review of the scientific literature pertaining to genetic and environmental causes of the malformations in question. Abridged counseling based on superficial and incomplete analyses is a dis-service to the family.

CONCLUSIONS

There have been significant advances in embryology, teratology, reproductive biology, genetics and epidemiology in the last 50 years that have provided scientists and clinicians with a better perspective on the causes of congenital malformations. We still cannot provide the families of children with malformations a definitive diagnosis and etiology for every malformed child. However, there are numerous environmental drugs, chemicals and physical agents that have been documented to produce congenital malformations and reproductive effects. While this multitude of teratogenic agents (agents that produce congenital malformations from exposures during pregnancy) account for only a small proportion of malformations, it is important to remember that all these environmentally produced birth defects are potentially preventable. The most common known cause of congenital malformations is genetic, but the largest group, unfortunately, is unknown. There are a number of important clinical rules that are important for clinicians to utilize when determining the cause of their patient's congenital malformations.

1. No teratogenic agent should be described qualitatively as a teratogen (an agent that causes birth defects), since a teratogenic exposure includes not only the agent, but also the dose and the time in pregnancy when the exposure occurs.
2. Even agents that have been demonstrated to result in malformations cannot produce every type of malformation. Known teratogens may be presumptively implicated by the spectrum of malformations they produce (the syndrome that describes the clinical manifestations of the teratogenic agent). It is easier to exclude an agent as a cause of birth defects than to definitively conclude that it was responsible for birth defects, because of the existence of genocopies of some teratogenic syndromes.
3. When evaluating the risk of exposures, the dose is a crucial component in determining the risk. Teratogenic agents follow a toxicological dose–response curve. This means that each teratogen has a threshold dose, below which, there is no risk of teratogenesis, no matter when in pregnancy the exposure occurred.
4. The evaluation of a child with congenital malformations cannot be adequately performed unless it is approached with the same scholarship and intensity as the evaluation of any other complicated medical problem.
5. Each physician must recognize the consequences of providing erroneous reproductive risks to pregnant women exposed to drugs and chemicals

during pregnancy or alleging that a child's malformations are due to an environmental agent without performing a complete and scholarly evaluation.

6. Unfortunately, clinical teratology and clinical genetics are not emphasized in medical school and residency education programs. But physicians have a multitude of educational aids to assist them in their evaluations, which include consultations with clinical teratologists and geneticists, the medical literature and the OMIM website.

References

1 Gregg NM. Congenital cataract following German measles in the mother. Trans Ophthalmol Soc Aust 1941; 3: 35–46
2 Thiersch JB. Therapeutic abortions with a folic acid antagonist, 4-aminopteroylglutamic acid (4-amino P.G.A.) administered by the oral route. Am J Obstet Gynecol 1952; 63: 1298–1304
3 Warkany J, Beautry PH, Horstein S. Attempted abortion with aminopterin (4-aminopteroylglutamic acid). Am J Dis Child 1959; 97: 274–281
4 Warkany J, Schraffenberger E. Congenital malformations of the eyes induced in rats by maternal vitamin A deficiency. Proc Soc Exp Biol Med 1944; 57: 49–52
5 McKusick VA. Mendelian inheritance in man: catalogs of autosomal dominant, autosomal recessive, and X-linked phentotypes, 8th edn. Baltimore, MD: Johns Hopkins University Press, 1998
6 OMIM, Online Mendelian Inheritance of Man. <http://www3./ncbi.nlm.nih.gov/omim>
7 Brent RL, Beckman DA. Environmental teratogens. Bull NY Acad Med 1990; 66:123–163
8 Beckman DA, Fawcett LB, Brent RL. Developmental toxicity. In: Massaro EJ. (ed) Handbook of human toxicology. New York: CRC Press, 1997; 1007–1084
9 Brent RL, Beckman DA. Prescribed drugs, therapeutic agents, and fetal teratogenesis. In: Reece EA, Hobbins JC. (eds) Medicine of the fetus and mother, 2nd edn. Philadelphia, PA: Lippincott-Raven, 1999; 289–313
10 Heinonen OP, Slone D, Shapiro S. Birth defects and drugs in pregnancy. Littleton: Publishing Sciences Group, 1977
11 Aase JM. Diagnostic dysmorphology. New York: Plenum, 1990
12 Beckman DA, Brent RL. Fetal effects of prescribed and self-administered drugs during the second and third trimester. In: Avery GB, Fletcher MA, MacDonald MG. (eds) Neonatology: pathophysiology and treatment, 4th edn. Philadelphia, PA: Lippincott, 1994; 197–206
13 Brent RL. What is the relationship between birth defects and pregnancy bleeding? New perspectives provided by the NICHD workshop dealing with the association of chorionic villous sampling and the occurrence of limb reduction defects. Teratology 1993; 48: 93–95
14 Brent RL, Beckman DA. Teratogens: an overview. In: Knobil E, Neill JD. (eds) Encyclopedia of reproduction, vol. 4, 1999; 735–750
15 Graham Jr JM, Jones KL, Brent RL. Contribution of clinical teratologist and geneticists to the evaluation of the etiology of congenital malformations alleged to be caused by environmental agents, ionizing radiation, electromagnetic fields, microwaves, radionuclides, and ultrasound. Teratology 1999; 59: 307–313
16 Jones KL. Smith's recognizable patterns of human malformations, 5th edn. Philadelphia, PA: W.B. Saunders, 1994
17 Brent RL, Beckman DA. Angiotensin-converting enzyme inhibitors, an embryopathic class of drugs with unique properties: information for clinical teratology counselors. Teratology 1991; 43: 543
18 Brent RL. Methods of evaluating the alleged teratogenicity of environmental agents. In: Sever JL, Brent RL. (eds) Teratogen update: environmentally induced birth defect risks. New York: Alan R. Liss, 1986; 199–201

19 Carter CO. Genetics of common single malformations. Br Med Bull 1976; 32: 21–26
20 Fraser FC. The multifactorial/threshold concept-uses and misuses. Teratology 1976; 14: 267–280
21 Brent RL. Medicolegal aspects of teratology. J Pediatr 1967; 71: 288–298
22 Brent RL. Litigation-produced pain, disease and suffering: an experience with congenital malformation lawsuits. Teratology 1977; 16: 1–14
23 Brent RL. The irresponsible expert witness: a failure of biomedical graduate education and professional accountability. Pediatrics 1982; 70: 754–762
24 Brent RL. Drugs and pregnancy: are the insert warnings too dire? Contemp Obstet Gynecol 1982; 20: 42–49
25 Brent RL, Holmes LB. Clinical and basic science lessons from the thalidomide tragedy: what have we learned about the causes of limb defects? Teratology 1988; 38: 241–251
26 Brent RL. Utilization of developmental basic science principles in the evaluation of reproductive risks from pre- and postconception environmental radiation exposures. Teratology 1999; 59: 182–204
27 Brent RL. Effects and risks of medically administered isotopes to the developing embryo. In: Fabro S, Scialli AR. (eds) Drug and chemical action in pregnancy. New York: Marcel Dekker, 1986; 427–439
28 Brent RL. Radiation teratogenesis. Teratology 1980; 21: 281–298
29 Brent RL, Beckman DA. Developmental effects following radiation of embryonic and fetal exposure to X-ray and isotopes: counseling the pregnant and nonpregnant patient about these risks. In: Hendee WK, Edwards FM. (eds) Health effects of low level exposure to ionizing radiation. Bristol & Philadelphia, PA: Institute of Physics Publishing, 1996; 169–213
30 Brent RL. Ionizing radiation. Contemp Obstet Gynecol 1999; 44: 13,14,16,21,25,26
31 Boue J, Boue A, Lazar P. Retrospective and prospective epidemiological studies of 1,500 karyotyped spontaneous abortions. Teratology 1975; 12: 11–26
32 Hertig AT. The overall problem in man. In: Benirschke K. (ed) Comparative aspects of reproductive failure. Berlin: Springer, 1967; 11–41
33 Simpson JL. Genes, chromosomes and reproductive failure. Fertil Steril 1980; 33: 107–116
34 Sever JL. Infections in pregnancy: highlights from the collaborative perinatal project. Teratology 1982; 25: 227–237
35 Juchau MR, Rettie AE. The metabolic role of the placenta. In: Fabro S, Scialli AR. (eds) Drug and chemical action in pregnancy: pharmacologic and toxicologic principle. New York: Marcel Dekker, 1986; 153–169
36 Brent RL. Bendectin: review of the medical literature of a comprehensively studied human non-teratogen and the most prevalent tortogen-litigen. Reprod Toxicol 1995; 9: 337–349
37 Brent RL. Review of the scientific literature pertaining to the reproductive toxicity of Bendectin. In: Faigman DL, Kaye DH, Saks MJ, Sanders J. (eds) Modern scientific evidence: the law and science of expert testimony, vol. 2. St Paul, MN: West Publishing, 1997; 373–393
38 Brent RL, Gordon WE, Bennett WR, Beckman DA. Reproductive and teratologic effects of electromagnetic fields. Reprod Toxicol 1993; 7: 535–580
39 Brent RL, Jensh RP, Beckman DA. Medical sonography: reproductive effects and risks. Teratology 1991; 44: 123–146
40 Wilson JG, Brent RL. Are female sex hormones teratogenic? Am J Obstet Gynecol 1981; 141: 567–580
41 Brent RL. Non-genital malformations following exposure to progestational drugs: The final chapter of an erroneous allegation. Birth Defects Part A 2005; 73: 906–918
42 Friedman JM, Polifka JE. TERIS. The Teratogen Information System. Seattle, WA: University of Washington, 1999
43 Scialli AR, Lione A Padget GKB. (eds) Reproductive effects of chemical, physical and biologic agents; Reprotox. Baltimore, MD: The Johns Hopkins University Press, 1995
44 Sever JL, Brent RL. (eds) Teratogen update: environmentally induced birth defect risks, New York, Alan R. Liss, 1986; 1–248
45 Shepard TH. Catalogue of teratogenic agents, 8th edn, Baltimore, MD: The Johns Hopkins University Press, 1995

46 Schardein JL. Chemically induced birth defects, 3rd edn. New York: Marcel Dekker, 2000
47 Briggs GG, Freeman RK, Yaffe SJ. Drugs in pregnancy and lactation, 3rd edn. Baltimore, MD: Williams and Wilkins, 1990; 502–508
48 Brent RL. Drug testing in animals for teratogenic effects: thalidomide in the pregnant rat. J Pediatr 1964; 64: 762–770
49 Brent RL. Predicting teratogenic and reproductive risks in humans from exposure to various environmental agents using *in vitro* techniques and *in vivo* animal studies. Cong Anom 1988; 28 (Suppl): S41–S55
50 Brent RL. Congenital malformation case reports: the editor's and reviewer's dilemma. Am J Med Gen 1993; 47: 872–874
51 Friedman JM, Little BB, Brent RL,, Cordero JF, Hanson JW, Shepard TH. Potential human teratogenicity of frequently prescribed drugs. Obstet Gynecol 1990; 75: 594–599
52 Wilson JG, Brent RL, Jordan HC. Differentiation as a determinant of the reaction of rat embryos to X-irradiation. Proc Soc Exp Biol Med 1953; 82: 67–70
53 Brent RL. Commentary on Bendectin and birth defects: hopefully, the final chapter. Birth Defects Res 2003; 67: 79–87
54 Cooper WO, Hernandez-Diaz S, Patrick PH *et al*. Major congenital malformations after first-trimester exposure to ace inhibitors. N Engl J Med 2006; 354: 2443–2451
55 Miller MT, Stromland K, Ventura L *et al*. Autism with ophthalmologic malformations: the plot thickens. Trans Am Ophthalmol Soc 2004; 102: 107–122
56 Hendrick V, Smith LM, Suri R *et al*. Birth outcomes after prenatal exposure to antidepressant medication. Am J Obstet Gynecol 2003; 189: 1810–1811
57 Wisner KL, Gelenberg AJ, Leonard H *et al*. Pharmacologic treatment of depression during pregnancy. JAMA 1999; 282: 1264–1269
58 Malm H, Klaukka T, Neuvonen PJ. Risks associated with selective serotonin reuptake inhibitors in pregnancy. Obstet Gynecol 2005; 106: 1289–1296
59 Zeskind PS, Stephens LE. Maternal selective serotonin reuptake inhibitor use during pregnancy and newborn neurobehavior. Pediatrics 2004; 113: 368–375
60 Kallen B, Otterblad-Olausson P. Antidepressant drugs during pregnancy and infant congenital heart defect. Reprod Toxicol 2006; 21: 221–222
61 Ericson A, Kallen B, Wiholm B-E. Delivery outcome after the use of antidepressants in early pregnancy. Eur J Clin Pharmacol 1999; 55: 503–508
62 Diav Citrin O, Schehtman S, Weinbaum D *et al*. Paroxetine and fluoxetine in pregnancy: a multicenter, prospective, controlled study. Reprod Toxicol 2005; 20: 459

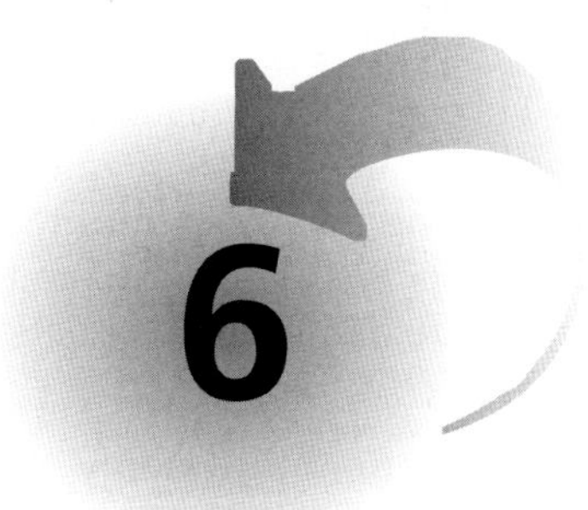

Susan M. White   Lachlan de Crespigny

Counseling for prenatal testing

Counseling for prenatal testing is a challenge for health professionals practising in obstetrics. The process first requires the health professional to perform a risk assessment of each pregnancy and be well-informed of the prenatal testing options for the pregnancy. This information then needs to be conveyed meaningfully to the woman. Finally, the health professional and woman enter a decision-making process with the health professional being mindful of patient autonomy and respecting the woman's right to choose. It is rare for a health professional to possess all of the above skills inherently; hence, the process requires practice, awareness of how women make decisions and self-awareness in order to develop proficiency.

PRINCIPLES OF PRENATAL COUNSELING

Consistent counseling principles should underlie the approach to the three aspects of prenatal testing: (i) choice of tests; (ii) communication of results; and (iii) pregnancy options following communication of results. The term counseling implies a process distinct from simply providing information about a given test. Counseling involves establishing a relationship where the woman's understanding of, and attitude to, prenatal tests, termination of pregnancy and disability are explored. This may include an exploration of the woman's previous experience of disability or termination of pregnancy and an

Susan M. White MBBS FRACP
Clinical Geneticist, Genetic Health Services Victoria, Murdoch Children's Research Institute, Royal Children's Hospital, Parkville, Australia

Lachlan de Crespigny MBBS MD FRCOG FRACOG DDU COGU (for correspondence)
Associate Professor, Department Obstetrics & Gynaecology, University of Melbourne, Honorary Fellow, Murdoch Children's Research Institute, Obstetrician Sonologist, Mercy Hospital for Women and Melbourne Ultrasound for Women, 62 Lygon St Carlton, 3153 Melbourne, Australia
E-mail: lach.dec@symbionhealth.com

understanding of the religious or cultural influences on their attitudes. It is the context of the pregnancy for the woman into which the woman incorporates the scientific information and reaches a decision about a test.[1] Health professionals need to be aware of these factors in order to play a meaningful role in facilitating patient decision-making.

Patient autonomy

A central principle underlying counseling for prenatal testing is respect for patient autonomy. Respect for patient autonomy implies more than simply allowing the patient to reach her own decision: it entails respect for the patient's values, the provision of adequate information about the test, and the implementation of the patient's expressed preferences.[2] Health professionals need to be aware of their own influence on patient decision-making and needs to hold the patient's expressed attitudes towards testing as the key determinant of the decision, not their own judgment of what the patient should do. This underpins the principle of respecting patient autonomy.

Non-directive counseling

A long-held view is that counseling for prenatal testing should be non-directive: in its strictest sense, this implies that the counselor should convey information in a neutral manner without attempting to influence the decision-making of the patient. Proponents for this form of practice argue that attempts to influence patient decision-making amount to paternalism.[3] There is debate as to whether it is truly possible to be non-directive given that all individuals, including health professionals, are shaped by their previous experiences and attitudes. These factors influence the health professional's facial expression, choice of words and demeanor even if they are not consciously wishing to direct the patient toward a particular decision.

Health professionals have reported difficulty with non-directiveness in practice, citing reasons such as that patients request directiveness; that this is different from their usual practitioner–patient relationship, and that they are driven by their own desire to help and support patients in decision-making.[4] Some authors have broadened their description of non-directive counseling to include counseling where a health professional may express a point of view as to how the patient might proceed, with the caveat that this point of view should be formed through listening actively to the cues the patient gives about their motives and experiences. In this definition, non-directive counseling cannot involve direct coercion of the patient, but may include advice giving.[5] Others have argued that directiveness may be acceptable if it is explicitly acknowledged by the health professional, as it may enable clients to consider implications of their decision they had not previously thought about.[6]

Whether or not one believes that it is possible – or desirable – for a health professional to be completely non-directive, it is critical for health professionals to be aware of their own biases and attitudes towards a patient and their situation, and to monitor their own emotional responses to the patient's decision, in an attempt to minimize their influence over the patient. The process of patient decision-making should be grounded in the context of the pregnancy for the patient, and should be owned by the patient, with contributions and facilitation by the health professional.

Language

The language used in prenatal diagnosis counseling can greatly influence the process and outcome. Whether a health professional refers to the fetus as 'baby' or 'fetus' may influence a woman's perception of the viability of the fetus and may convey an attitude on the part of the health professional as to the acceptability of the option of termination of pregnancy. Some authors have argued that the term fetus and pregnant woman are the appropriate terms until the time of completion of prenatal tests.[7] A common clinical practice is to be guided by the terminology used by the couple themselves. Other studies have examined the interpretation of risk in relation to the language used. There is good evidence that the way information is presented can have a significant impact on the decisions couples make. A study of the language used in prenatal diagnosis counseling showed that couples found risks expressed as 1 in X were more worrying than when the same risk was expressed as a percentage.[8] The same study found that couples were particularly worried by genetic jargon and when the following terms were used: rare, abnormal, syndrome, disorder, anomaly and high-risk. The technique of positive framing (*e.g.* presenting a 5% risk of abnormality as 95% chance of no abnormality) is important in putting a risk in context and, in some studies, has influenced take-up of higher-risk options.[9] Thus, it is critical that health professionals are aware of the effects of the language they use. While there are clinical situations when it is appropriate to use terms which increase anxiety, health professionals should use such terms knowing the likely effects on the couple. Terms known to heighten anxiety should be used with special caution when there is a finding of uncertain significance.

THE PRENATAL COUNSELING PROCESS

Pre-test counseling

Having conveyed relevant information, the decision to have a test for fetal abnormality must be reached as an active process between the patient and health professional. Several authors have outlined different models for achieving informed consent about proceeding with or refusing a test, but they have the following principles in common:

1. Provision of adequate information to allow patient decision-making.
2. Respect for patient values and autonomy in the choice they make.[10]

This model of decision-making may result in women making decisions that health professionals do not agree with or are uncomfortable with, but as long as they are informed and deemed capable of such decision-making, then this should be deemed a good outcome of prenatal counseling. A good example of such decisions is the woman of advanced maternal age who decides against screening or diagnostic testing for Down syndrome. This introduces the concept of 'choice to have choice', where patients have the capacity to choose not to have tests if they judge that the information the test provides may not be helpful for them in their decision-making.[11] Such decisions challenge the concept of these tests being routine in pregnancy, and call into question the belief that the knowledge gained by a test is always empowering for a woman. In most circumstances, knowledge and information do enhance patient autonomy. When such information is unwanted, there is the potential to do harm with this information. It may force a couple to make difficult choices about the continuation of the pregnancy causing anxiety and distress for the couple[12] or affect their future relationship with their 'abnormal' child.[11] Unwanted information has the potential to harm seriously the pregnancy experience for couples, particularly if they would not seek pregnancy termination even in the presence of an abnormality.

For these reasons, it is critical that health professionals respect such a decision, even if the health professional deems that the test could provide useful clinical information.

Risk assessment

In terms of the risk of fetal abnormality, each pregnancy can be stratified into high- and low-risk groups on the basis of maternal age, previous obstetric history, family history and previous testing in the pregnancy.

An important component of a risk assessment is the taking of a family history. In particular, specific questions should be asked about any family history of intellectual disability, genetic conditions or children born with any problems. In an ideal setting, a risk assessment would be carried out pre-pregnancy to enable completion of any investigations, and to allow the couple to embark on a pregnancy with a full understanding of the risks involved. In some instances, it may be necessary for relatives affected with possible genetic conditions to be assessed by a geneticist if such an assessment has not recently occurred, as advances in genetic testing mean that there may be new test options in an individual which were not previously available. There are several thousand rare genetic conditions which can cause intellectual disability and congenital abnormalities, some of which may be recognised by the clinical pattern or gestalt, or by specific genetic tests in the affected individual. Male relatives affected with intellectual disability on the maternal side of the family raise the possibility of X-linked mental retardation conditions, the most common of which is Fragile X. Fragile X is screened for antenatally in some countries and carrier testing should be offered to a woman with a family history compatible with X-linked inheritance. A history of consanguinity is important to establish as it means that autosomal recessive conditions are more likely in that family. Racial background determines the most common recessive conditions for which a given couple is at risk. In Caucasian individuals, cystic fibrosis is the most common recessive condition and carrier testing of parents is routinely offered in some countries, while in others testing is only available to those with a family history. In individuals of Mediterranean or Asian background, screening for thalassemia should be offered.

A thorough examination of genetic and obstetric risk factors should generate an assessment of the pregnancy as high risk or low risk. In high-risk or low risk women, pre-test counseling should focus on the potential information to be gained by the test, balanced against the risk of information of uncertain significance. With screening tests, this requires an analysis of the positive predictive value of the test for that population of women.

The application of a risk assessment in some countries determines which tests are offered to a patient, particularly in countries where tests are funded by a public health system. In an ideal setting, the provision of tests would not be determined by risk assessment alone, but would take into account all of the factors influencing a woman's decision-making, such as their life experience, anxiety and need for certainty which may motivate 'low-risk' women to seek diagnostic tests. A woman with a previous child with an intellectual disability of unknown cause may wish to have diagnostic testing for Down syndrome in a subsequent pregnancy despite the fact that her pregnancy is at low-risk for Down syndrome, as she may feel she could not cope with two children with significant disabilities. In other women, screening tests do not provide the reassurance they need in terms of the risks for their pregnancy, and they require the certainty of a diagnostic test. This must be weighed against the risks of more invasive tests; however, if a woman is informed of these risks and still wishes to have the certainty of a diagnostic test, this should be supported.

Provision of test results

While women usually have autonomy in choosing prenatal tests, they commonly do not have autonomy either in receiving results or in pregnancy options following bad news.

Ultrasound results

The communication of ultrasound results is traditionally based on a paternalistic model of the doctor–patient relationship. If an abnormality or marker of aneuploidy is found, the doctor decides what the patient will be told. It is difficult to ask women whether they wish to know about an abnormality once it has been identified. If we are to offer women autonomy over the information they receive, we must ask before the ultrasound examination what information they seek.

Couples are not always aware of what information may be provided by a prenatal diagnostic test;[13] indeed, they may not be aware that a planned test can provide information about the health of their fetus at all. For example, at 'routine' mid-trimester ultrasound examination, at least one in 10 couples may not be aware that they will receive information about the health of their fetus.[14] Most women today appear to have a reasonable understanding that one of the major goals of diagnostic ultrasound and other prenatal tests is to check for fetal abnormality.[15] It might be expected, therefore, that a woman presenting for obstetric ultrasound examination in pregnancy wishes to be told if an abnormality or marker is present. However, not every couple wants all available information and it is not always clear what couples do want to know.

Women can be given more opportunity to participate in setting the goals and outcomes of ultrasound diagnosis. We cannot assume that all couples wish to be told all information about their ultrasound examination. In an unpublished survey of 29 patients, the authors found that although 79%

wished to be told all information following a mid-trimester scan, 21% did not wish to be told about markers. These informed women had given careful thought to testing, had already had testing for aneuploidy and did not want to revisit Down syndrome markers. Although in this survey no women requested not to be told if there was a structural abnormality, occasional women do request general pregnancy information only. A limited scan should be available to such women.

It is unreasonable for a doctor to take a paternalistic approach by telling women what he or she feels is important. Women should be asked before an ultrasound examination to indicate the types of information that they wish to be given, particularly in relation to minor abnormalities and markers of aneuploidy. Those requesting limited information should be informed that minor anomalies may be markers of more serious disorders. Women who would not request abortion if an anomaly is found may not find such information helpful. It is for this reason that doctors do not impose tests such as mid-trimester serum screening on women who do not want the test because they would not consider termination of a pregnancy with Down syndrome. It is anomalous that women can opt in or out of serum screening but have no such options in relation to the breadth of information following ultrasound.

Markers, also called soft-markers, are variations of normal findings that increase the risk of an underlying fetal anomaly, most commonly Down syndrome or some other chromosomal abnormality. Many doctors feel an ethical and legal responsibility to inform the patient of the presence of even a single marker for aneuploidy on a mid-trimester scan.

Being told that such a marker is present causes great distress to the pregnant woman,[16,17] despite the fact that a single marker is a relatively low-risk finding; indeed, some studies suggest that some 'markers' in low-risk women are not associated with any increased risk.

What risk of aneuploidy should be present before we inform the patient of the presence of a marker? To help answer this question, workers have produced likelihood ratios (LRs) to alter the *a priori* background risk.[18,19] Using likelihood ratios, most women with low-risk Down syndrome screening tests, using either first trimester combined or second trimester serum screening testing, remain low risk if a marker of aneuploidy is found at a mid-trimester ultrasound examination.

One group recommended that screening ultrasound should evaluate 8 markers. The authors admit, however, that 'risk adjustment has not been validated in a population with a lower prevalence for fetal aneuploidy owing to first trimester prenatal screening and diagnosis'.[20]

Many would argue that the plethora of poorly documented 'markers' has caused more harm than good for most low-risk women.[21] Indeed Filly *et al.*[21] found that in women at low risk for chromosomal anomalies, neither of two common markers – choroid plexus cysts (particularly if the hands look normal) and echogenic intracardiac foci – increase the risk of aneuploidy.

In summary, different providers manage markers differently, depending in part on other screening test results. Since there are better tests for trisomy 21, we recommend that, in low-risk women, single mid-trimester markers of aneuploidy should not be reported except in centers that run an audited program.

Prenatal testing for chromosomal abnormality

Testing for Down syndrome is usually the major indication for chromosome analysis, but other abnormalities such as sex chromosome abnormalities or normal variants may be discovered incidentally. Women and couples need to be prepared for these possibilities. Couples need the opportunity to limit the information gathered in prenatal chromosome analysis; some couples may opt for a limited chromosome analysis as an alternative to a full karyotype. This would allow for a couple to receive information about the presence or absence of Down syndrome without finding out about chromosome abnormalities of less, or uncertain, significance. A disadvantage of this approach is that a limited chromosome analysis will mean that the test will not detect other rare, but serious, chromosome abnormalities such as chromosome deletions or re-arrangements, which may have a phenotypic effect as serious as Down syndrome. However, an informed couple may still choose this option knowing its limitations.

Combined Down syndrome screening

In prenatal testing, we increasingly ask our patients to understand and respond to relatively complex concepts of risk assessment, including combinations of tests. After a nuchal translucency scan, for example, final results of combined or integrated testing may be delayed. Patients, therefore, press for information, or even a risk figure, based on ultrasound alone. While professional ethics demand that we communicate requested information to patients, acquiescing to such requests may be contrary to the patient's best interests. To provide a series of changing statistics as the sequence of results for ultrasound and serum screening become available is confusing. We would not produce a different risk figure for each analyte of a serum screening test. The woman's best interests are usually best served by explaining why the combined test provides better and less confusing information, and that her interests are served by awaiting full results.

A special problem arises with integrated testing – there may be some weeks to wait for the final serum screen result. Here, the conflict between communicating results and minimizing patient confusion are, in particular, tension. In clinical practice, it would be unethical to withhold information from a couple who had high-risk ultrasound findings simply because an integrated test was planned.

Access to abortion

Philosophy

Perhaps the most controversial area of prenatal diagnosis is abortion. Here, the tension between respecting patient's autonomous choices and the attitudes and judgment of the clinician is especially difficult to disentangle. Patients' autonomous choices regarding abortion are not necessarily supported by health professionals, particularly for women carrying an anomalous fetus.[22,23] The options offered to women have been shown to vary. Surveys have shown that obstetricians, geneticists, ultrasonologists and physicians, in general, vary in their view of which abnormalities are severe enough to offer abortion.[24–27] This variation applies at both 13 and 24 weeks.

The greatest variation is seen in ultrasonologists' attitudes to late-abortion. A mail survey of obstetricians who practice ultrasound had 39 respondents from 82 questionnaires (unpublished study, de Crespigny and Savalescu). Thirty-three carried out interventional procedures, 11 of whom had performed or supervised a trainee to carry out a feticide procedure at 24 weeks or more in the past 3 years. They had carried out a total of 35 procedures. Only one of these conditions might be called 'lethal' (trisomy 18) while less severe abnormalities included transposition of the great vessels (25 weeks) and a suicidal woman with a fetus with probable skeletal dysplasia at 31 weeks.

Of the 39 respondents, 28 would be prepared to carry out a termination at or after 24 weeks for lethal abnormalities, 11 for severe abnormalities, 12 for less severe or minor abnormalities, eight for intellectual handicap, four on maternal psychiatric grounds and four on request by a pregnant woman who is competent, fully informed and not coerced and has had adequate counseling. The response rate (48%) highlights the difficulty in carrying out such surveys.

Central to the debate on allowing women autonomy regarding decisions about abortion is whether the fetus has a recognised legal or moral status. If the fetus is given no legal or moral status until delivery, then women should be given complete autonomy regarding decisions of abortion. This would be consistent with The World Medical Association Declaration on the Rights of the Patient, which states: 'The patient has the right to self-determination, to make free decisions regarding himself/herself'.[28] However, some authors have argued for a limited moral status of the fetus which means that the decision-making of the woman has an impact on another being with some moral status and may be subject to some limits. In practice, this moral status is gestation-dependent which is problematic in its assignation.

McCullough and Chervenak[29] are leaders in promoting discussion of ethical issues in our specialty. Chervenak *et al.*[30] argue that before viability, the only link between the fetus and the pregnant woman is the woman's autonomy. They claim it is up to the pregnant woman to confer moral status before viability.[29] However, after viability, the fetus becomes a patient, to whom doctors have duties. They have been strong advocates of limiting access to late termination of pregnancy except when absence of cognitive developmental capacity is expected.[30]

They argue that third-trimester abortion for such conditions as trisomy 21 or achondroplasia violates professional integrity and social justice concerning fetal patients.[29] They have also argued that the obstetrician's compassionate response to a woman whose pregnancy is affected by such anomalies does not justify terminating such third-trimester pregnancies.[30]

An alternative view is that viability is not pivotal: this would require significant changes to our practice around early abortion and treatment of newborns.[24] Support for this position comes from the fact that late-abortion has been supported by organizations including the UK Royal College of Obstetricians and Gynaecologists.[31]

One of Singer's examples is instructive in illustrating one problem with relating a right to life to viability.[32] Suppose that a woman, 6-months pregnant, was to fly from New York to a New Guinea village and that, once she had arrived in the village, there was no way she could return quickly to a city with modern medical facilities. In New York, the fetus may be viable with intensive medical intervention, but in a New Guinea village, such medical facilities are not available and hence the fetus would not be viable. Are we to say that it would have been wrong for her to have an abortion before she left New York, but now that she is in the village she may go ahead? The trip does not change the nature of the fetus, so why should it remove its claim to life?

Viability may be difficult to determine and may vary according to whether or not fetal abnormality is present. Although a healthy, normally structured fetus may be considered 'viable' at 24 weeks, this might not be the case for a fetus with a major anomaly such as a hypoplastic left heart. Indeed, it may be that few of the anomalous fetuses likely to undergo late abortion would be viable at 24 weeks – to be consistent, those advocating viability as conferring fetal status should also advocate individualizing.

An alternative proposal to limiting abortion to the previable fetus is to claim that all abortion is wrong. While this position is supported by many non-secular ethicists, we question whether it is possible for a person who opposes previable abortion to practice prenatal diagnosis in a way that supports the best interests of patients.

Most legal jurisdictions already accept a 'maternal interests' justification of early abortion and it has been argued that this should be extended to late abortion.[24] This allows late abortion for fetal abnormality but also for some normal pregnancies. This view thus escapes the criticism that can be leveled at current practice around late termination that there is discrimination against fetuses with disability. Discrimination in according a right-to-life depending on the severity of disability would not be considered acceptable after birth and similarly should not be before birth.

Surveys show that, in clinical practice, service providers offer abortion to selected women, depending on the clinician's personal view of the severity of the abnormality – the more severe the abnormality the more obstetricians supported availability of abortion.[24–27] However, in the survey described above, 28% of obstetricians would not facilitate abortion at 24 weeks even for anencephaly. Interestingly, more obstetricians would support access to abortion at 13 weeks for social problems than if there was a cleft lip and palate.

We are unaware of any argument to justify the practice of limiting access to abortion depending on the severity of a fetal abnormality. Either such arguments need to be developed or physicians' practice regarding which patients with a fetal abnormality can access abortion must be reviewed.

Doctors' differing views result in women being offered varying treatments depending on the doctor she sees. Doctors with a conscientious objection to offering a woman legal abortion when it would be available elsewhere should offer her a referral.

Abortion for 'minor' or apparently isolated abnormalities

Abortion in the presence of an apparently isolated 'minor' abnormality, such as cleft lip, is often opposed by both the general public and the medical community. Derogatory terms such as 'designer babies' are used. However, there are several reasons why a couple may consider termination of pregnancy when a minor abnormality is present.

One limitation of ultrasound is that a minor anomaly may be the only detectable sign of an underlying syndrome. We seldom know the risk of such a syndrome, but with some congenital abnormalities it is surprisingly common. One study looked at 22 fetuses with an omphalocele, a normal karyotype and no serious and/or multiple anomalies. The outcome in this subgroup comprised 19/22 (86%) survivors and 3/22 (14%) fetal deaths. Eight infants (36%) from the survivors were healthy, while 11 had various impairments.[33]

Occasionally, an isolated congenital abnormality may occur in both a parent and child, such as cleft lip. For some individuals, living with a cleft lip and the medical and cosmetic consequences can be a traumatic and damaging experience. Some individuals may opt for termination of an affected pregnancy rather than subject the fetus to a similar life experience to themselves. It is important for such a parent to be aware of the improvements in treatment of such abnormalities, and to understand the breadth of experiences that different individuals with congenital abnormalities may have. However, for some couples, their own experience of disability or illness can profoundly influence their own prenatal decisions.

The law

Prenatal diagnosis is a relatively new discipline. It has presented options for pregnant women that were beyond the dreams of our predecessors. Views of both professionals and the general public regarding the goals of prenatal testing and the limits of acceptable practice can lag behind scientific advances. Definition of legal limits of practice often lags even further behind. We usually rely on the law to guide our practice. This leaves a window of time in which professionals may have to act in an uncertain legal environment, leaving them at risk if a colleague or anti-abortionist complains. In those jurisdictions in which legal clarity is absent, practitioners need to support what they believe to be in the patient's best interests while minimizing the legal risk to themselves.

Legal uncertainty can heighten the concern about the activities of anti-abortion groups. This may encourage practitioners not to offer certain procedures. Uncertainty in the law, both criminal and civil, exposes doctors to the risk of legal action, referral to statutory bodies, and being sued by patients not because management is in error or illegal, but because of uncertain legal guidelines. Yet it is often the controversial cases that ultimately establish the laws in our different countries.

Cases proceeding to enquiries, court cases or media coverage lead to complex moral, religious and policy arguments. They can affect prenatal practice or even initiate new laws.[34] They graphically illustrate the legal vulnerability of those in our specialty and how the lives of those in prenatal diagnosis are impacted by local laws, or by the absence of clear laws.

CONCLUSIONS

Health professionals in the field of prenatal diagnosis manage patients who present issues at the cutting edge of much current ethical debate. Consultations in this area require sensitivity, self-awareness and skill in order to ensure an informed, autonomous decision is reached by the woman, facilitated by the health professional. The managing doctor is often the decision maker who determines who can access tests and treatments. It is of concern that current practice often appears to depend primarily on the doctor's subjective assessment of the severity of the abnormality. Providers of prenatal diagnostic services and their patients deserve a clearer ethical framework. They also deserve legal certainty.

We advocate that the physician's role is to support and enhance the autonomy of the pregnant woman not only in choice of prenatal tests, but also in the information she receives, and in management decisions including abortion. Implementation of a principle of respect for autonomy includes both enquiring before an ultrasound examination what information the patient wishes to have communicated and also offering abortion for the full range of abnormalities. Where the physician is limited by law or by personal beliefs in offering abortion, including late abortion, the woman should be offered referral to a center where this is available.

References

1 Lippman A. Embodied knowledge and making sense of prenatal diagnosis. J Genet Couns 1999; 8: 255–274

2 McCullough LB, Chervenak FC. Ethics in Obstetrics and Gynecology. New York: Oxford University Press, 1994

3 De Crespigny L, Savulescu J. Is paternalism alive and well in obstetric ultrasound? Helping couples choose their children. Ultrasound Obstet Gynecol 2002; 20: 213–216

4 Williams C, Alderson P, Farsides B. Is nondirectiveness possible within the context of antenatal screening and testing? Soc Sci Med 2002; 54: 339–347

5 Kessler S. Psychological aspects of genetic counseling. XI. Nondirectiveness revisited. Am J Med Genet 1997; 72: 164–171

6 Clarke A. The process of genetic counselling. In: Harper P, Clarke A. (eds) Genetics, Society and Clinical Practice. London: Routledge, 1997; 179–200

7 de Crespigny L, Chervenak F, McCullough L. Mothers and babies, pregnant women and fetuses. Br J Obstet Gynaecol 1999; 106: 1235–1237

8. Abramsky L, Fletcher O. Interpreting information: what is said, what is heard – a questionnaire study of health professionals and members of the public. Prenat Diagn 2002; 22: 1188–1194

9 Edwards A, Elwyn G, Covey J, Matthews E, Pill R. Presenting risk information – a review of the effects of 'framing' and other manipulations on patient outcomes. J Health Commun 2001; 6: 61–82

10 Marteau TM, Dormandy E. Facilitating informed choice in prenatal testing: how well are we doing? Am J Med Genet 2001; 106: 185–190

11 Boyle RJ, de Crespigny L, Savulescu J. An ethical approach to giving couples information about their fetus. Hum Reprod 2003; 18: 2253–2256

12 Statham H, Solomou W, Chitty L. Prenatal diagnosis of fetal abnormality: psychological effects on women in low-risk pregnancies. Baillière's Clin Obstet Gynaecol 2000; 14: 731–747

13 Marteau TM, Plenicar M, Kidd J. Obstetricians presenting amniocentesis to pregnant women: practice observed. J Reprod Infant Psychol 1993; 11: 3–10

14 Eurenius K, Axelsson O, Gallstedt-Fransson I, Sjoden PO. Perception of information, expectations and experiences among women and their partners attending a second-trimester routine ultrasound scan. Ultrasound Obstet Gynecol 1997; 9: 86–90

15 Whynes DK. Receipt of information and women's attitudes toward ultrasound scanning during pregnancy. Ultrasound Obstet Gynecol 2002; 19: 7–12

16 Filly RA. Obstetrical sonography. The best way to terrify a pregnant woman. J Ultrasound Med 2000; 19: 1–5

17 Baillie G, Heurison J, Mason G. Soft marker screening for aneuploidy: some women's experiences. Br J Obstet Gynaecol 1998; Suppl. 17: 26

18 Nicolaides KH, Snijders RJ, Gosden CM, Berry C, Campbell S. Ultrasonographically detectable markers of fetal chromosomal abnormalities. Lancet 1992; 340: 19

19 Bromley B, Lieberman E, Shipp TD, Benacerraf BR. The genetic sonogram: a method of risk assessment for Down syndrome in the second trimester. J Ultrasound Med 2002; 21: 1087–1096
20 Van den Hof MC , Wilson RD and Diagnostic Imaging Committee, Society of Obstetricians and Gynaecologists of Canada, Genetics Committee, Society of Obstetricians and Gynaecologists of Canada. Fetal soft markers in obstetric ultrasound. J Obstet Gynaecol Can 2005; 27: 592–636
21 Filly RA, Benacerraf BR, Nyberg DA, Hobbins JC. Choroid plexus cyst and echogenic intracardiac focus in women at low risk for chromosomal anomalies. J Ultrasound Med. 2004; 23: 447–449
22 Marteau T, Drake H, Bobrow M. Counselling following the diagnosis of a fetal abnormality: the differing approaches of obstetricians, clinical geneticists, and genetic nurses. J Med Genet 1994; 31: 864–867
23 Wertz DC, Fletcher JC. Ethical problems in prenatal diagnosis: a cross-cultural survey of medical geneticists in 18 nations. Prenat Diagn 1989; 9: 145–157
24 Savulescu J. Is current practice around late termination of pregnancy eugenic and discriminatory? Maternal interests and abortion. J Med Ethics 2001; 27: 165–171
25 Green J. Ethics and late TOP. Lancet 1993; 342: 1179
26 Renaud M, Bouchard L, Kremp O *et al.* Is selective abortion for a genetic disease an issue for the medical profession? A comparative study of Quebec and France. Prenat Diagn 1993; 13: 691–706
27 Norup M. Attitudes towards abortion among physicians working at obstetrical and pediatric departments in Denmark. Prenat Diagn 1998; 18: 273–280
28 World Medical Association Declaration on the Rights of the Patient. <www.wma.net/e/policy/17-h_e.html>
29 Chervenak FA, McCullough LB, Campbell S. Is third trimester abortion justified? Br J Obstet Gynaecol 1995; 102: 434–435
30 Chervenak FA, McCullough LB, Campbell S. Third trimester abortion: is compassion enough? Br J Obstet Gynaecol 1999; 106: 293–296.
31 Royal College of Obstetricians and Gynaecologists. A consideration of the law and ethics in relation to late termination of pregnancy for fetal abnormality. Report of the Royal College of Obstetricians and Gynaecologists Ethics Committee. March 1998
32 Singer P. Writings on an Ethical Life? London: Fourth Estate, 2001: 148
33 Brantberg A, Blaas HGK, Haugen SE, Eik-Nes SH. Characteristics and outcome of 90 cases of fetal omphalocele. Ultrasound Obstet Gynecol 2005; 26: 527–537
34 de Crespigny L, Chervenak F, Coquel PA, Ville Y, McCullough L. Practicing prenatal diagnosis within the law. Ultrasound Obstet Gynecol 2004; 24: 489–494

William Buckett

Obstetric, neonatal, and infant outcomes following assisted reproduction

Assisted reproductive technologies (ARTs) are practised all over the world with clinics offering these services in all developed countries and many parts of the developing world too. Results generated from the European registries by ESHRE, show that over 350,000 ART cycles per year are performed in 28 different countries.[1] With a live birth rate of about 20% across the continent, this accounts for 70,000 deliveries per year. In the US alone, over 120,000 cycles of ART are performed each year resulting in over 35,000 deliveries per year.[2,3] With the incidence of twin pregnancies complicating about 20% of ART pregnancies, about 200,000 babies are born per year as a result of ART and, since the advent of *in vitro* fertilization (IVF), over a million babies have been born.[4]

All this is a far cry from the scepticism and concerns that accompanied the early days of IVF, both in the lay press[5,6] and the medical literature.[7]

However, early studies of pregnancies, deliveries and babies following IVF and gamete intra-fallopian transfer (GIFT),[8–11] and later studies following intra-cytoplasmic sperm injection (ICSI) were re-assuring,[12–14] with the exception of concerns regarding multiple pregnancy.[15] This re-assurance led, in part, to the massive increase in availability and uptake of ART. Nevertheless, even in the early days, it was recognized that large numbers of pregnancies would be needed from ART in order to determine if there really is any risk to the mother or baby.[16]

As the number of pregnancies and babies born following ART has increased, there have been an increasing number of authoritative reports detailing the risks to pregnancy – both singleton and multiple – associated with ART,[17–19] as well as the association of congenital abnormalities and ART.[19–21]

This chapter will discuss those risks associated with ART pertaining to early pregnancy loss, ectopic pregnancy, later miscarriage, congenital abnormality, multiple pregnancy (and their sequelae), and pregnancy outcomes in singleton

William Buckett MD FRCOG
Assistant Professor, Department of Obstetrics and Gynecology, McGill University, Hôpital Royal Victoria, 687 avenue des Pins Ouest, Montréal, Québec H3A 1A1, Canada
E-mail: william.buckett@muhc.mcgill.ca

ART pregnancies. The chapter will also discuss the possible causes associated with these findings, where appropriate.

MISCARRIAGE AND ART

Relatively early in the development of ART, workers became aware of the early pregnancy loss – termed chemical β-human chorionic gonadotropin (β-hCG) abortion or biochemical pregnancy – as opposed to 'later' clinical first trimester miscarriage.[22] Ideally, ART programs should report clinical pregnancy rates where a clinical pregnancy is defined using the WHO/ESHRE definition of ultrasound evidence of an intra-uterine pregnancy. Biochemical pregnancies are, therefore, pregnancies lost before this stage.

Because very early pregnancy losses may occur before an awareness of pregnancy following spontaneous conception, it is impossible to determine the rate of biochemical pregnancy in the population as a whole. However, biochemical pregnancy loss rates following ART are typically around 15–20%,[23,24] although rates from as low as 11% to as high as 35% have been reported.[25–27]

The reasons for biochemical pregnancy loss are unclear. However, maternal age (particularly over 40 years), smoking, and poor embryo quality at transfer have been shown to be associated with an increased risk to biochemical pregnancy following ART.[23]

Clinical miscarriage rates amongst spontaneously conceived pregnancies are reasonably consistent at 10–15% pregnancies.[28–30] However, there are many confounding variables which may affect couples undergoing ART – predominantly maternal age,[30,31] which is higher in women undergoing ART than non-ART pregnancies. Also, the presence of other risks for miscarriage such as polycystic ovary syndrome (PCOS) are over-represented in couples undergoing ART. PCOS is associated with an increased risk of miscarriage, typically reported at about 25%, either following spontaneous conception[32] or following ovulation induction.[33,34]

Following ART, the clinical miscarriage rate is typically around 15%,[1,2,24,35] although it ranges from 10–45% depending on the maternal age.[35] In women with PCOS or in those who are overweight or obese, the clinical miscarriage rate is higher.[36,37]

In conclusion, clinical miscarriage rates seem to be similar following ART compared with spontaneously conceived pregnancies (at around 15%), although the higher maternal age and higher incidence of PCOS seen in women undergoing ART are associated with an increased risk of miscarriage. Biochemical loss is impossible to ascertain following spontaneously conceived pregnancies; however, rates of 15–20% are typical following ART. Overall, therefore, about 30% of women with positive pregnancy tests following ART will lose their pregnancies before the end of the first trimester. This high loss rate highlights the importance of reporting live birth rates following ART, rather than pregnancy rates or clinical pregnancy rates.[38]

ECTOPIC PREGNANCY

Ectopic pregnancy rates have risen over the past decade, although the reasons are unclear; improved and earlier diagnosis certainly has an affect. Currently, estimates are that ectopic pregnancy affects about 2% all pregnancies. Although some earlier case series showed a higher incidence of ectopic pregnancy at about 4% of pregnancies following ART,[39,40] most large prospective studies show a rate of 2.0–2.2% which is similar to that of the general population.[41,42] This change is probably because early in the development of ART, tubal disease was the major indication for ART.

The risk of ectopic pregnancy is dependent on the indication and type of ART. Both GIFT and ZIFT are associated with an increased risk of ectopic pregnancy (3.0–3.6%) compared with IVF-ET as a whole (2.0–2.2%). ICSI, as compared to IVF without ICSI, has a similar ectopic pregnancy rate, whereas oocyte donation (1.5%) and gestational surrogacy (0.9%) have lower rates than IVF or the general population.[42]

Cause of infertility also affects the likelihood of ectopic pregnancy. Tubal disease with hydrosalpinges (4.2%), tubal disease without hydrosalpinges (3.0%), and endometriosis (2.2%) increase the risk. Male factor infertility (1.6%), ovulatory infertility (1.8%), and tubal ligation (1.0%) decrease the risk.[42]

LATE PREGNANCY LOSS

The incidence of late pregnancy loss (after 12 weeks' gestation), either through mid-trimester miscarriage, fetal death, or termination of pregnancy for chromosomal or other abnormality after ART, is typically between 2–4%,[43,44] which is higher than that of spontaneously conceived pregnancies (typically around 1%).[45,46]

One reason for this is advancing maternal age, which is associated with a higher incidence of chromosomal and other abnormalities that may result in mid-trimester termination of pregnancy. However, with the exception of case reports and case series, there is no comparative data for mid-trimester termination of pregnancy following ART. Maternal age is also associated with a higher spontaneous late pregnancy loss rate, both following spontaneous conceptions and following ART.[44]

A further reason for the increased late pregnancy loss is the increased incidence of multiple pregnancy associated with ART (discussed below).

CONGENITAL ABNORMALITY

Initial studies comparing babies born following IVF or ICSI with spontaneously conceived controls suggested no increase in the incidence of congenital abnormalities,[47–49] although the magnitude of these were in the hundreds rather than the thousands or tens of thousands that is needed in order to determine any genuine difference. However, since the start of this century, some two decades after the beginnings of IVF, an increasing number of papers comparing ART babies with spontaneously conceived controls[20,21,50,51] as well as several systemic reviews have been published,[19,52] which show an increase in the risk of congenital abnormality associated with ART.

Current information, therefore, shows that ART is associated with a 1.5-fold increased risk of congenital abnormality when compared with spontaneously conceived controls (Fig. 1).

Subgroup analyses from the major published systemic reviews show a persistent elevated odds ratio when singleton deliveries are compared.

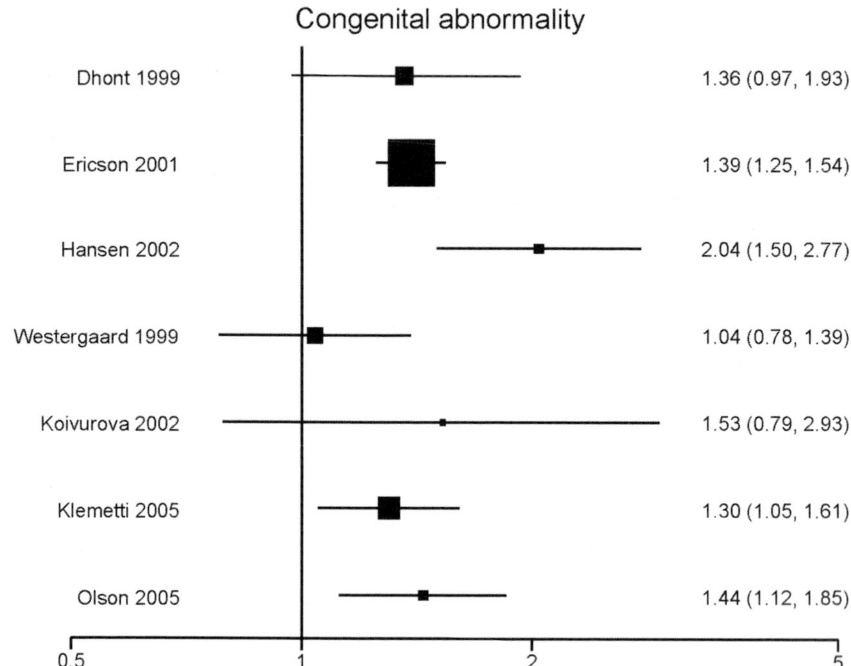

Fig. 1 Odds ratio estimates from major studies comparing major congenital abnormalities in babies born following ART with spontaneously conceived controls.

Similarly, there is no difference when IVF without ICSI is compared with ICSI.[52] Furthermore, a number of studies have compared congenital abnormality risk in babies born following IVF without ICSI and babies born following ICSI and have not found significant differences. Therefore, it would appear that other mechanisms apart from ICSI or multiple pregnancy account for this increase in congenital abnormality.[20,53,54]

Some studies attempted to determine whether any particular abnormalities are associated with ART. Musculoskeletal abnormalities[20,50] and urogenital abnormalities[20,50,55] have been found to be increased in babies born following ART, particularly male babies. Some studies have also found heart malformations to be increased in babies born following ART.[20,21] However, multiple pregnancy is a confounding variable for this, and subgroup analysis of singleton and multiple gestations has not shown any difference.[50]

Chromosomal abnormalities have not been shown to be increased in babies born following ART compared with spontaneously conceived controls. This may, of course, be as a result of mid-trimester termination of pregnancy. As noted above, few data concerning mid-trimester termination of pregnancy for chromosomal or other major abnormalities are available.

It is already well established that chromosomal abnormalities are more frequent in men with severe male factor infertility who are referred for IVF/ICSI.[56] More recently, it has become apparent that chromosomal abnormalities amongst the 'normal' female partners of men who are referred for IVF/ICSI are also increased and indeed is higher with less severe degrees of male factor infertility.[57] These data imply that unexplained female subfertility also confers a higher risk of chromosomal abnormality.

Furthermore, since the association of imprinting disorders and ART,[58,59] more recent evidence has suggested that spontaneous conceptions, with and without ovarian stimulation in the absence of ART, are also associated with imprinting disorders.[60]

In conclusion, there is a genuine, albeit small (1.5-fold), increase in the risk of congenital abnormality amongst children born to couples who conceived following ART. However, it appears that couples with infertility have an *a priori* increased risk for congenital abnormality. Whether any of the myriad features of ART also have a role to increase this risk remains unclear. Research to answer these questions needs careful planning, prospective surveillance, imaginative use of possible control groups, and enough time to generate the data. In the meantime, couples electing to undergo ART should be counseled concerning the small increased risk of congenital abnormality associated with ART although it is unclear whether this is related to their infertility itself or its treatment.

MULTIPLE PREGNANCY

Early in the development of ART, following the advent of ovarian hyperstimulation to produce multiple oocytes and the practice to transfer of multiple embryos in order to improve pregnancy and live birth rates, there was an increase in the rate of multiple pregnancy.[8–11] It is the single most common complication of ART pregnancies and is associated with the huge increase in the multiple pregnancy rate seen over the last two decades (Fig. 2).[61]

A full discussion of the risks of multiple pregnancy (twin pregnancy as well as higher order multiple pregnancy) are beyond the scope of this chapter. Nevertheless, maternal risks include hypertension, pre-eclampsia, preterm labor, anemia and an increased cesarean section rate; fetal or neonatal risks include increased mortality, lower gestational age, lower birthweight, respiratory distress syndrome, necrotizing enterocolitis, sepsis, intracranial hemorrhage, congenital malformations, the twin–twin transfusion syndrome, cerebral palsy and long-term neurological complications. Furthermore, there may be family complications of a psychological, social and financial nature.[62]

Three of the most severe consequences of multiple pregnancy are perinatal death, cerebral palsy, and cost. Perinatal mortality is increased from 4 per 1000 live births in singleton pregnancies to 26 per 1000 live births in twin pregnancies and 63 per 1000 live births in triplet and higher order multiple pregnancies.[63] Cerebral palsy occurs in about 2% children born following a singleton pregnancy, 10% following a twin pregnancy, and over 30% in a triplet or higher order pregnancy.[64] Finally, the cost to the healthcare provider of a twin delivery is about 3–5 times that of a singleton delivery, and a triplet pregnancy at least 10 times this cost.[65,66]

Despite these concerns, over 20% of pregnancies following ART in Europe are twin pregnancies and over 1% are triplet pregnancies.[1] In the US, over 25% of pregnancies following ART are twin pregnancies and about 5% are triplet

Table 1 Randomised trials comparing single embryo transfer with double embryo transfer

		Single embryo transfer		Double embryo transfer	
	No. cycles	Pregnancy rate	Twin rate	Pregnancy rate	Twin rate
Gerris *et al.* (1999)[68]	53	39%	10%	74%	30%
Martikainen *et al.* (2002)[69]	144	32%	4%	47%	18%
Gardner *et al.* (2004)[70]	48	61%	0%	76%	47%
Thurin *et al.* (2004)[71]	661	28%	1%	44%	34%

pregnancies.[2] Therefore, about 50% all babies born following ART belong to a set of multiples. Although it has always been silently accepted that a high proportion of iatrogenic twins and higher order multiple pregnancy was the price to be paid for a reasonable success rate of a treatment that is physically and emotionally demanding and expensive,[62] the need to reduce multiple pregnancy is accepted world-wide.[61]

Single embryo transfer has been seen as a way to reduce twin pregnancy associated with ART;[67] indeed, many prospective randomised trials showed, unsurprisingly, a significant reduction in the incidence of multiple pregnancy while maintaining acceptable live-birth rates.[68–71] However, all these studies showed a lower pregnancy and live-birth rate in the arm where only a single embryo was transferred (Table 1).

Concerns over lower pregnancy and live-birth rates have led to much discussion about the implementation of elective single embryo transfer for all patients,[72,73] and there are marked differences between countries and clinics.[1] Certainly, in unselected patients, elective single embryo transfer significantly decreases the pregnancy and live-birth rate.[74]

Even if single embryo transfer was standard policy for ART, there will always remain a subgroup of patients in whom the transfer of more than one embryo is acceptable. In many countries, the high cost of ART for the patient causes an understandable objection to lower the pregnancy rate. Where female age is above 38 years (or even 40 years), the transfer of more than one embryo is performed more liberally and further clinical research is needed to determine which are the optimal transfer algorithms in this age group. In patients with non-obstructive azoospermia, the recovery by TESE of sperm for ICSI at times is so low that only one or two treatment trials can be performed. Should more than one embryo be obtained in such unfavourable circumstances, the transfer of more than one embryo may be warranted. Similarly, patients undergoing pre-implantation diagnosis because of genetic disease frequently have just one or two unaffected embryos available to them after a long, technically complicated and expensive treatment, perhaps creating a relative contra-indication to limit the number of embryos to one.

Selective fetal reduction or termination has been the safety valve to escape the complications of high-order multiple pregnancy. This secondary prevention is not the best possible solution. Although the clinical outcome of pregnancies reduced to twins is similar to that of naturally conceived twins,[75–77] it offers no solution for the quantitatively much larger problem of twins, which are not as a rule reduced to singletons. There is psychological reluctance in future parents to accept and integrate this procedure in their personal lives. Most patients prefer primary prevention.[78]

PREGNANCY OUTCOME IN SINGLETON PREGNANCIES

Quite reasonably, most earlier descriptive studies presumed that the poorer obstetric outcome associated with ART was as a result of the increased multiple pregnancy rates.[8–12] However, only recently have sufficiently sized and appropriately performed studies and meta-analyses been available to explore the effect of ART in singleton gestations.[17,18,79,80] Although the great majority of singleton ART pregnancies are uncomplicated, there is recent evidence of higher rates of adverse pregnancy outcomes in singleton ART pregnancies compared with spontaneously conceived singleton gestations.

Women with IVF-conceived singletons are at increased risk of pre-eclampsia, gestational diabetes, placenta previa, and perinatal mortality (Table 2). ART singleton pregnancies also have higher relative risks of having induction of labor and both emergency and elective cesarean deliveries.[80]

It is not possible to separate ART-related risks from those secondary to the underlying reproductive pathology at this time. In addition, ART patients are older than average, and age is an independent, contributory risk factor for most of these complications. Although evidence of an effect is convincing, questions remain about whether this is due to treatment effect or to any of the factors related to the underlying infertility.

NEONATAL DEVELOPMENT

ART babies also have increased neonatal morbidity.[50] One study demonstrated an increased frequency of intraventricular hemorrhage following IVF even when controlling for multiple birth, gestational age, and birth weight.[81] Other studies also have suggested an increase in morbidity and mortality but do not sufficiently address the effect of confounders such as birth weight and gestational age.

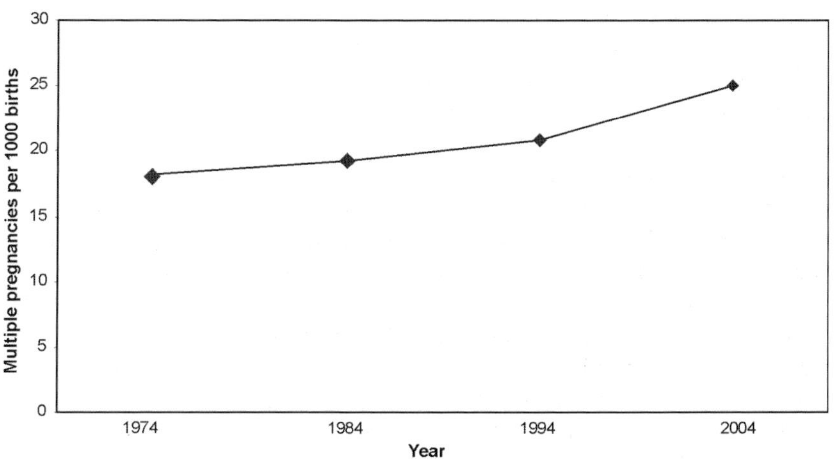

Fig. 2 Multiple pregnancy rates (per 1000 births) in Canada, 1974–2004.

Table 2 Adverse obstetric outcomes in singleton ART pregnancies

	Absolute risk (%)	Odds ratio (95% CI)
Perinatal risks		
Preterm birth	11.5	2.0 (1.7–2.2)
Low birthweight (< 2500 g)	9.5	1.8 (1.4–2.2)
Very low birthweight (< 1500 g)	2.5	2.7 (2.3–3.1)
Small for gestational age	14.6	1.6 (1.3–2.0)
NICU admission	17.8	1.6 (1.3–2.0)
Stillbirth	1.2	2.6 (1.8–3.6)
Neonatal mortality	0.6	2.0 (1.2–3.4)
Cerebral palsy	0.4	2.8 (1.3–5.8)
Maternal risks		
Pre-eclampsia	10.3	1.6 (1.2–2.0)
Placenta praevia	2.4	2.9 (1.5–5.4)
Placental abruption	2.2	2.4 (1.1–5.2)
Gestational diabetes	6.8	2.0 (1.4–3.0)
Cesarean delivery	26.7	2.1 (1.7–2.6)

Modified from Linder *et al.*[81]

A review of the long-term developmental outcomes in children conceived by ART has been re-assuring, demonstrating that the great majority of children are developing normally.[82] However, these evaluations suffer from major methodological limitations, including limited statistical power, selection bias, inadequate or inappropriate comparison groups, and high loss to follow-up. Of concern is a recent study with improved methodology (stratification by gestational age, birthweight, and plurality) that demonstrated an overall increased RR of cerebral palsy (odds ratio 3.7) and suspected developmental delay (odds ratio 4).[83]

The high frequency of twins with concomitant prematurity and low birthweight explained most of the increased risk of neurological problems. However, even singletons had a 2.8-fold increased RR of cerebral palsy compared with controls. Another recent study also showed an increased risk of cerebral palsy for ART children (hazard rate ratio 1.6; 95% confidence interval [CI] 1.1–2.3). However, the risk of cerebral palsy attributed to ART was no longer increased when plurality and preterm delivery were accounted for in the multivariate model, indicating that the increased risk of cerebral palsy for ART children is largely attributable to the increased proportion of IVF children born preterm.[84]

FURTHER RESEARCH

There are three possible groupings of factors responsible for the observed increases in risk of adverse perinatal and neonatal outcomes associated with ART: (i) ART treatment; ii) pharmacological agents, such as those for ovulation induction or pregnancy maintenance; and (iii) underlying infertility.

At this time, it is not possible to evaluate outcomes on the basis of the cause of the infertility or specific infertility treatment because of lack of information, although some studies have shown similar adverse outcomes with non-ART infertility treatments.[50,51]

Identifying and quantifying the perinatal risks for ART-conceived pregnancies is hampered by a myriad of methodological issues. Predominant is the lack of appropriate control groups so that the effects of ART can be differentiated from those of the underlying infertility.

Also, infertility is defined differently across different studies; couples with 1 year of infertility may not be similar to those with 5 years of infertility, and women who become pregnant spontaneously after a period of infertility are likely different from those who never become pregnant spontaneously. The role of the procedure is difficult to study because fertile women cannot be randomly assigned to infertility treatment, and ART has many components.

Nevertheless, future research should concentrate on: (i) infertile women who become pregnant spontaneously compared with infertile treated women; (ii) fertile women who become pregnant with ART compared with fertile women who conceive spontaneously; and (iii) infertile women treated with different types of infertility treatments.

CONCLUSIONS

Although the majority of ART pregnancies and children born following ART are normal, there are concerns about the increased risk for adverse pregnancy outcomes. There is a high pregnancy loss rate, where 25–30% of women with positive pregnancy tests will not deliver a child. Furthermore, over 25% of ART pregnancies are twins or higher-order multiple gestations and more than one half of all ART babies are the products of multiple pregnancy, with its increased prematurity complications. ART singleton pregnancies also demonstrate increased rates of perinatal complications – small for gestational age infants, preterm delivery, congenital abnormality, and perinatal mortality – as well as maternal complications, such as pre-eclampsia, gestational diabetes, placenta previa, placental abruption, and cesarean delivery. Although it is not possible to separate ART-related risks from those secondary to the underlying reproductive pathology, the overall increased frequency of obstetric and neonatal complications should be discussed with the couple.

KEY POINTS FOR CLINICAL PRACTICE

- About 30% of women with a positve pregnancy test following ART will not deliver a child.
- Multiple pregnancy is still the major rusk associated with ART.
- Even in singleton pregnancies there is a slight increase in poor obstetric and neonatal outcomes – mainly as a result of prematurity.
- It is unclear whether these are related to ART or infertility itself.

References

1 Andersen AN, Goosens V, Gianaroli L, Felberbaum R, de Mouzon J, Nygren KG. Assisted reproductive technology in Europe, 2003. Results generated from European registries by ESHRE. Hum Reprod 2007; 22: 1513–1525

2 Society for Assisted Reproductive Technology; American Society for Reproductive Medicine. Assisted reproductive technology in the United States: 2001 results generated from the American Society for Reproductive Medicine/Society for Assisted Reproductive Technology registry. Fertil Steril 2007; 87: 1253–1256
3 Society for Assisted Reproductive Technology. SART national summary 2005 <www.sartcorsonline.com/rpt>
4 International Committee for Monitoring Assisted Reproductive Technology, Adamson GD, de Mouzon J, Lancaster P, Nygren KG, Sullivan E, Zegers-Hochschild F. World collaborative report on *in vitro* fertilization, 2000. Fertil Steril 2006; 85: 1586–1622
5 Auerbach S. Fears aired in test tube baby debate. Washington Post 1974; July 21: A1
6 Wright P. Less risk of test-tube baby being born with brain damage, doctor says. The Times 1974; Sept 7: 4
7 Fitzgerald J. Veto *in vitro*, or turn off the tube. Can Fam Physician 1978; 24: 816
8 Wood C, Trounson A, Leeton JF *et al.* Clinical features of eight pregnancies resulting from *in vitro* fertilization and embryo transfer. Fertil Steril 1982; 38: 22–29
9 Mushin D, Spensley J, Barreda-Hanson M. Children of IVF. Clin Obstet Gynacol 1985; 12: 865–876
10 Beral V, Doyle P, Tan SL, Mason BA, Campbell S. Outcome of pregnancies resulting from assisted conception. Br Med Bull 1990; 46: 753–768
11 Risk B, Doyle P, Tan SL *et al.* Perinatal outcome and congenital malformations in *in-vitro* fertilization babies from the Bourn-Hallam group. Hum Reprod 1991; 6: 1259–1264
12 Palermo G, Joris H, Devroey P, Van Stierteghem AC. Pregnancies after intracytoplasmic injection of single spermatozoon into an oocyte. Lancet 1992; 340: 17–18
13 Bonduelle M, Desmyttere S, Buysse A *et al.* Prospective follow-up study of 55 children born after subzonal insemination and intracytoplasmic sperm injection. Hum Reprod 1994; 9: 1765–1769
14 Wisanto A, Bonduelle M, Camus M *et al.* Obstetric outcome of 904 pregnancies after intracytoplasmic sperm injection. Hum Reprod 1996; (Suppl 4): 121–129
15 MRC Working Party on Children Conceived by *In Vitro* Fertilisation. Births in Great Britain resulting from assisted conception, 1978–87. BMJ 1990; 300: 1229–1233
16 Schlesselman JJ. How does one assess the risk of abnormalities from human *in vitro* fertilization? Am J Obstet Gynecol 1979; 135: 135–148
17 Helmerhorst FM, Perquin DAM, Donker D, Keirse MJNC. Perinatal outcome of singletons and twins after assisted conception: a systematic review of controlled studies. BMJ 2004; 328: 261
18 Jackson RA, Gibson KA, Wu YW, Croughan MS. Perinatal outcomes in singletons following *in vitro* fertilization: a meta-analysis. Obstet Gynecol 2004; 103: 551–563
19 McDonald SD, Murphy K, Beyene J, Ohlsson A. Perinatal outcomes of singleton pregnancies achieved by *in vitro* fertilization: a systematic review and metaanalysis. J Obstet Gynaecol Can 2005; 27: 449–459
20 Hansen M, Kurinczuk JJ, Bower C, Webb S. The risk of major birth defects after intracytoplasmatic sperm injection and *in vitro* fertilization. N Engl J Med 2002; 346: 725–730
21. Koivurova S, Kartikainen AL, Gissler M, Hemminki E, Sovio V, Järvelin MR. Neonatal outcome and congenital malformations in children born after in *in-vitro* fertilization. Hum Reprod 2002; 17: 1391–1398
22 Jones Jr HW, Acosta AA, Andrews MC *et al.* What is a pregnancy? A question for programs of *in vitro* fertilization. Fertil Steril 1983; 40: 728–733
23 Winter E, Wang J, Davies MJ, Norman R. Early pregnancy loss following assisted reproductive technology treatment. Hum Reprod 2002; 17: 3220–3223
24 Buckett WM, Chian RC, Dean NL, Sylvestre C, Holzer H, Tan SL. Pregnancy loss in pregnancies conceived following *in vitro* oocyte maturation (IVM), conventional *in vitro* fertilization (IVF), and intra-cytoplasmic sperm injection (ICSI). Fertil Steril 2007; In press
25 Bellver J, Albert C, Labarta E, Pellicer A. Early pregnancy loss in women stimulated with gonadotropin-releasing hormone antagonist protocols according to oral contraceptive pill pretreatment. Fertil Steril 2007; 87: 1089–1101
26 European Recombinant LH Study Group. Human recombinant luteinizing hormone is as

effective as, but safer than, urinary human chorionic gonadotropin in inducing final follicular maturation and ovulation in *in vitro* fertilization procedures: results of a multicenter double-blind study. J Clin Endocrinol Metab 2001; 86: 2607–2618
27 Barlow P, Lejeune B, Puissant F *et al.* Early pregnancy loss and obstetrical risk after *in-vitro* fertilization and embryo replacement. Hum Reprod 1988; 3: 671–675
28 Miller JF, Williamson E, Glue J *et al.* Fetal loss after implantation: a prospective study. Lancet 1980; ii: 554–556
29 Regan L, Braude P, Trembath PL. Influence of past reproductive performance on risk of spontaneous abortion. BMJ 1989; 299: 541–545
30 Nybo Andersen AM, Wohlfahrt J, Christens P *et al.* Maternal age and fetal loss: population based register linkage. BMJ 2000; 320: 1708–1712
31 Buckett W, Regan L. Sporadic and recurrent miscarriage. In: Shaw RA, Soutter WP, Stanton SL. (eds) Gynaecology, 3rd edn. London: Churchill-Livingston, 2003; 343–360
32 Rotterdam ESHRE/ASRM-sponsored PCOS consensus workshop group. Revised 2003 consensus on diagnostic criteria and long-term health risks related to polycystic ovary syndrome. Fertil Steril 2004; 81: 19–25
33 Homburg R. Pregnancy complications in PCOS. Best Pract Res Clin Endocrinol Metab 2006; 20: 281–292
34 MacGregor AH, Johnson JE, Bunde CA. Further clinical experience with clomiphene citrate. Fertil Steril 1968; 19: 616–622
35 Farr SL, Schieve LA, Jamieson DJ. Pregnancy loss among pregnancies conceived through assisted reproductive technology, United States, 1999–2002. Am J Epidemiol 2007; 165: 1380–1386
36 Wang JX, Davies MJ, Norman RJ. Polycystic ovarian syndrome and the risk of spontaneous abortion following assisted reproductive technology treatment. Hum Reprod 2001; 16: 2606–2609
37 Maheshwari A, Stofberg L, Bhattacharya S. Effect of overweight and obesity on assisted reproductive technology a systematic review. Hum Reprod Update 2007; 13: 433–444
38 Centers for Disease Control and Prevention. Current trends in ectopic pregnancy-United States, 1990–1992. MMWR Surveill Summ 1995; 44: 46–48
39 Ribic-Pucelj M, Tomazevic T, Vogler A, Meden-Vrtovec H. Risk factors for ectopic pregnancy after in vitro fertilization and embryo transfer. J Assist Reprod Genet 1995; 12: 594–598
40 Dubuisson JB, Aubriot FX, Mathieu L, Foulot H, Mandelbrot L, de Joliere JB. Risk factors for ectopic pregnancy in 556 pregnancies after *in vitro* fertilization: implications for preventive management. Fertil Steril 1991; 56: 686–690
41 Verhulst G, Camus M, Bollen N, Van Steirteghem, A, Devroey P. Analysis of the risk factors with regard to the occurrence of ectopic pregnancy after medically assisted procreation. Hum Reprod 1993; 8: 1284–1287
42 Clayton HB, Schieve LA, Peterson HB, Jamieson DJ, Reynolds MA, Wright VC. Ectopic pregnancy risk with assisted reproductive technology procedures. Obstet Gynecol 2006; 107: 595–604
43 Buckett WM, Chian RC, Holzer HEG, Dean N, Usher R, Tan SL. Obstetric outcomes and congenital abnormalities after in vitro maturation, in vitro fertilization, and intracytoplasmic sperm injection. Obstet Gynecol 2007; 110: 885–891
44 Farr SL, Schieve LA, Jamieson DJ. Pregnancy loss among pregnancies conceived through assisted reproductive technology, United States, 1999–2002. Am J Epidemiol 2007; 165: 1380–1388
45 Brigham SA, Conlon C, Farquharson RG. A longitudinal study of pregnancy outcome following idiopathic recurrent miscarriage. Hum Reprod 1999; 14: 2868–2871
46 Confidential Enquiry into Maternal and Child Health. Stillbirth, neonatal and post-neonatal mortality 2000-2003, England, Wales, and Northern Ireland. London: RCOG Press, 2005
47 Morin NC, Wirth FH, Johnson DH *et al.* Congenital malformations and psychosocial development in children conceived by *in vitro* fertilization. J Pediatr 1989; 115: 222–227
48 Sutcliffe AG, D'Souza SW, Cadman J, Richards B, Mckinlay IA, Leiberman B. Minor congenital anomalies, major congenital malformations and development in children conceived from cryopreserved embryos. Hum Reprod 1995; 10: 3332–3337

49 Isaksson R, Gissler M, Tiitinen A. Obstetric outcome among women with unexplained infertility after IVF: a matched case-control study. Hum Reprod 2002; 17: 1755–1761
50 Klemetti R, Gissier M, Sevon T, Koivurova S, Ritvanen A, Hemminki E. Children born after assisted fertilization have an increased rate of major congenital anomalies. Fertil Steril 2005; 84: 1300–1307
51 Olson CK, Keppler-Noreuil KM, Romitti PA *et al*. *In vitro* fertilization is associated with an increase in major birth defects. Fertil Steril 2005; 84: 1308–1315
52 Hansen M, Bower C, Milne E, de Klerk N, Kurinczuk JJ. Assisted reproductive technologies and the risk of birth defects – a systematic review. Hum Reprod 2005; 20: 328–338
53 Bonduelle M, Liebaers I, Deketelaere V *et al*. Neonatal data on a cohort of 2889 infants born after ICSI (1991–1999) and of 2995 infants born after IVF (1983–1999). Hum Reprod 2002; 17: 671–694
54 Place I, Englert Y. A prospective longitudinal study of the physical, psychomotor, and intellectual development of singleton children up to 5 years who were conceived by intracytoplasmic sperm injection compared with children conceived spontaneously and by *in vitro* fertilization. Fertil Steril 2003; 80: 1388–1397
55 Ericson A, Kallen B. Congenital malformations in infants born after IVF: a population-based study. Hum Reprod 2001; 16: 504–509
56 Buckett W, Aird L, Luckas M, Kingsland C, Lewis-Jones I, Howard P. Intracytoplasmic sperm injection. Karyotyping should be done before treatment. BMJ 1996; 313: 1334
57 Gekas J, Thepot F, Turleau C *et al*. Association des Cytogeneticiens de Langue Francaise. Chromosomal factors of infertility in candidate couples for ICSI: an equal risk of constitutional aberrations in women and men. Hum Reprod 2001; 16: 82–90
58 Gosden R, Trasler J, Lucifero D, Faddy M. Rare congenital disorders, imprinted genes, and assisted reproductive technology. Lancet 2003; 361: 1974–1977
59 Chang AS, Moley KH, Wangler M, Feinberg AP, Debaun MR. Association between Beckwith-Wiedemann syndrome and assisted reproductive technology: a case series of 19 patients. Fertil Steril 2005; 83: 349–354
60 Ludwig M, Katalinic A, Gross S, Sutcliffe A, Varon R, Horsthemke B. Increased prevalence of imprinting defects in patients with Angelman syndrome born to subfertile couples. J Med Genet 2005; 42: 289–2891
61 Bissonnette F, Cohen J, Collins J *et al*. Incidence and complications of multiple gestation in Canada: proceedings of an expert meeting. Reprod Biomed Online 2007; 14: 773–790
62 Gerris JM. Single embryo transfer and IVF/ICSI outcome: a balanced appraisal. Reprod Update 2005; 11: 105–121
63 Alexander GR, Wingate MS, Salihu H *et al*. Fetal and neonatal mortality risks of multiple births. Obstet Gynecol Clin North Am 2005; 32: 1–16
64 Pharoah PO. Risk of cerebral palsy in multiple pregnancies. Clin Perinatol 2006; 33: 301–313
65 Ledger WL, Anumba D, Marlow N *et al*. The costs to the NHS of multiple births following IVF treatment in the UK. Int J Obstet Gynecol 2006; 113: 21–25
66 Lukassen HG, Schonbeck Y, Adang EM, Braat ED, Zielhuis GA, Kremer JA. Cost analysis of singleton versus twin pregnancies after *in vitro* fertilization. Fertil Steril 2004; 81: 1240–1246
67 ESHRE Campus Course Report. Prevention of twin pregnancies after IVF/ICSI by single embryo transfer. Hum Reprod 2001; 16: 790–800
68 Gerris J, De Neubourg D, Mangelschots K, Van Royen E, Van de Meerssche M, Valkenburg M. Prevention of twin pregnancy after in-vitro fertilization or intracytoplasmic sperm injection based on strict embryo criteria: a prospective randomized clinical trial. Hum Reprod 1999; 14: 2581–2587
69 Martikainen H, Tiitinen A, Tomas C *et al*. Finnish one versus two embryo transfers after IVF and ICSI: randomized study. Hum Reprod 2002; 16: 1900–1903
70 Gardner DK, Surrey E, Minjarez D, Leitz A, Stevens J, Schoolcraft W. Single blastocyst transfer: a prospective randomized trial. Fertil Steril 2004; 81: 551–555
71 Thurin A, Hausken J, Hillensjo T *et al*. Elective single-embryo transfer versus double-embryo transfer in *in vitro* fertilization. N Engl J Med 2004; 351: 2392–2402
72 Buckett WM, Tan SL. What is the most relevant standard of success in assisted

reproduction? The importance of informed choice. Hum Reprod 2004; 19: 1043–1045
73 Gleicher N, Barad D. The relative myth of elective single embryo transfer. Hum Reprod 2006; 21: 1337–1344
74 Van Montfoort APA, Fiddelers AAA, Janssen M *et al*. In unselected patients, elective single embryo transfer prevents all multiples, but results in significantly lower pregnancy rates compared with double embryo transfer: a randomized controlled trial. Hum Reprod 2006; 21: 338–343
75 Maymon R, Herman A, Shulman A *et al*. First trimester embryo reduction: a medical solution to an iatrogenic problem. Hum Reprod 1995; 10: 668–673
76 Antsaklis AJ, Drakakis P, Vlazakis GP, Michalas S. Reduction of multifetal pregnancies to twins does not increase obstetric or perinatal risks. Hum Reprod 1998; 14: 1338–1340
77 Dodd J, Crowther C. Multifetal pregnancy reduction of triplet and higher-order multiple pregnancies to twins. Fertil Steril 2004; 81: 1420–1422
78 Bergh C, Möller A, Nilsson L, Wikland M. Obstetric outcome and psychological follow-up of pregnancies after embryo reduction. Hum Reprod 1999: 14: 2170–2175
79 McGovern PG, Llorens AJ, Skurnick JH, Weiss G, Goldsmith LT. Increased risk of preterm birth in singleton pregnancies resulting from *in vitro* fertilization-embryo transfer or gamete intrafallopian transfer: a meta-analysis. Fertil Steril 2004; 82: 1514–1520
80 Rimm AA, Katayama AC, Diaz M, Katayama KP. A meta-analysis of controlled studies comparing major malformation rates in IVF and ICSI infants with naturally conceived children. J Assist Reprod Genet 2004; 21: 437–443
81 Linder N, Haskin O, Levit O *et al*. Risk factors for intraventricular hemorrhage in very low birth weight premature infants: a retrospective case-control study. Pediatrics 2003; 111: 590–595
82 Olivennes F, Fanchin R, Ledee N, Righini C, Kadoch IJ, Frydman R. Perinatal outcome and developmental studies on children born after IVF. Hum Reprod Update 2002; 8: 117–128
83 Stromberg B, Dahlquist G, Ericson A, Finnstrom O, Koster M, Stjernqvist K. Neurological sequelae in children born after in-vitro fertilisation: a population-based study. Lancet 2002; 359: 461–465
84 Hvidtjorn D, Grove J, Schendel DE *et al*. Cerebral palsy among children born after in vitro fertilization: the role of preterm delivery – a population-based, cohort study. Pediatrics 2006; 118: 475–482

Isaac Blickstein

Managing multiple pregnancy and birth

The human female is programd by nature to nurture one fetus and to take care of one neonate at a time; hence, the relatively rare birth of twins (about 1:80 to 1:100 births) and the extremely rare occurrence of high-order multiple pregnancies. This ordinary circumstance has not changed since the beginning of mankind until the emergence of effective infertility treatment. Thereafter, it became clear that, within a very small fraction in evolutionary time, all we knew about natural twinning has been profoundly changed by physician-made (iatrogenic) multiple pregnancies.

Undoubtedly, the epidemic dimensions of multiple pregnancies and births have profound perinatal consequences in terms of morbidity and mortality. However, a potential 'advantage' of the increased numbers of multiples is our ability to acquire more experience with these pregnancies and to conduct adequately powered studies. As a result, the amount of information related to these cases increased as well. This chapter discusses a personal selection of several aspects related to the progress in understanding and managing multiple pregnancies and births.

IMPLICATIONS OF CURRENT TRENDS OF MULTIPLE PREGNANCIES

Public health concerns related to the much-increased incidence of higher-order multiples began as early as the late 1980s, when high-order multiples were recognized as a serious side effect of infertility treatment. To overcome the 'epidemic' dimensions of multiple births, two main measures to diminish this problem were implemented: (i) multifetal pregnancy reduction (MFPR); and (ii) decreasing the likelihood of multiple ovulation and number of transferred embryos in assisted conception.[1] Whereas MFPR is considered a 'curative'

Isaac Blickstein MD
Hadassah-Hebrew University School of Medicine, Jerusalem, and Professor, Department of Obstetrics and Gynecology, Kaplan Medical Center, 76100 Rehovot, Israel
E-mail: blick@netvision.net.il

measure that decreases the number of multiple births, the latter is a primary preventive means that may decrease the number of multiple pregnancies. In perspective, both approaches have not been implemented to the same extent and improved MFPR techniques preceded the attempts to improve implantation rates in assisted reproduction techniques (ARTs). Moreover, the pressure to achieve better success rates with infertility treatment disregarded the occurrence of multiple births and the incidence of twins so the number of higher-order multiples continued to escalate in the late 1990s in most developed countries.

The first change in these gloomy trends was reported in the US in the annual vital statistics of 2002.[2] This report showed that twin birth rate had continued its steady increase since 1981, rising 3% for 2002 to 31.1 per 1000 total live births, representing an increased twinning rate of 38% since 1990, and 65% since 1980 (18.9 per 1000 total live births). In contrast, the 2002 rate of triplet and higher-order multiple births decreased slightly (1%), from 185.6 to 184 per 100,000 births, continuing a small (5%), but steady, decline observed since 1999. This welcomed change in trend is strikingly different compared with the average annual increase of 13% (from 37.0 to 193.5 per 100,000 live births; > 400%) between 1980 and 1998.

The change of the trend in the US was even more striking in England and Wales.[3] As in the US, the trend line for twins demonstrated a steady and continuing increase, from 9.95 to 14.66 per 1000 live births during the period 1982 to 2004 (47% increase).[3] Whereas in the US the data seem to represent plateauing of the rates rather than a real decline, the England and Wales data clearly demonstrate a definite turning point in the trend line i n 1998, and the rate of triplet births decreased 52.1% in the following years, from 0.48 to 0.23 per 1000 live births.[4]

The pertinent question, however, is whether the decrease in triplet birth rates with increasing twin rates represents the end of the epidemic of multiple births. Currently, only a few countries have adopted a universal policy of single embryo transfers. Therefore, the more wide-spread policy of double embryo transfers is expected to eliminate the problem of iatrogenic triplets almost entirely, but is not expected to eliminate the excessive rates of twin births following ART, which will still be associated with about 20–30% twin births;[5,6] this is expected to increase the twin birth rate further.[4] In fact, the reduced proportion of higher-order multiples is not expected to change the proportion of multiple births overall, which are dominated by twin maternities.[1]

The increase in twin birth rates and the decrease in triplet birth rates are not entirely independent events. The most plausible cause for the iatrogenic increase in twin births is because twins are the most common multiple birth following ART in centers that do not perform elective single embryo transfers, because ART is increasingly available world-wide, and because many infertility experts hold the view that twins are not to be considered as an adverse outcome. For example, Dickey *et al.*[7] maintain that the essential aim of infertility treatment should be a healthy low order (singleton or twin) birth; therefore, twin as well as singleton births should be counted as ART successes. This argument is further fuelled by as many as 25% of infertile couples undergoing ART that may desire to have an 'instant' family by having twins as the preferred outcome.[7,8]

Whether twins, in general, and the twin rates, in particular, are acceptable or not in terms of morbidity and mortality is currently the center-stage debate among clinicians of both sides of the Atlantic Ocean.[1] Regardless of this controversy, the facts are that 11.9% of twins are born very preterm (< 32 completed weeks), 58.2% are born at < 37 completed weeks, 10.2% weigh < 1500 g (very low birth-weight; VLBW) at birth, and 55.4% weigh less than 2500 g (LBW).[2] These figures represent 7.5-, 5.6-, 9.3-, and 9.1-fold increases compared with the comparative figures in singletons. Given that the total number of twin infants is much higher than the decreased number of triplet infants,[1] there is a definite net increase in preterm and low birth-weight infants. Thus, current trends showing an increase in twin birth rates concomitant with the decrease in triplet birth rates do not herald the end of the 'epidemic' of multiples.

SURVIVAL OF THE EARLY TWIN PREGNANCY

Little is known about the survival of twins during the early stages of spontaneous gestation because ultrasound is not universally performed in the first trimester. It is, therefore, not surprising that data are mostly available for pregnancies following ART. Data from two different studies showed that at least one spontaneous reduction occurred in 35% of twins and 53–59% of triplets.[10,11]

An intriguing finding of a recent comparative study indicates that complete pregnancy loss occurred in 5.1% of the IVF/ICSI twin pregnancies, compared with 21.1% in singletons.[12] This observation was fully supported by La Sala and co-workers in a series of analyses of the Regio Emilia ART database.[10,13–15] This group observed that the lower loss rates of the entire pregnancy in twins occurs irrespective of maternal age, number of transferred embryos, and mode of ART, but seems to be related to the quality of the transferred embryo.[15] All these observations may suggest that the embryological potential for successful development is not the same for twins and singletons and that twin pregnancies after IVF/ICSI have a better survival potential than singletons. It could be speculated that higher implantation rates per transfer (*i.e.* development of more than one live embryo) might represent a better capacity of the uterus for early embryonic development and/or better embryonic quality. Conversely, implantation of one embryo only, despite transfer of many embryos, might represent poor uterine capacity and/or poor embryonic quality, and hence a higher miscarriage rate.

Another aspect refers to the potential outcome of survivors of the so-called 'vanishing' twin syndrome. Recently, Pinborg *et al.*[16] assessed incidence rates of spontaneous reductions in IVF/ICSI twin pregnancies and compared short- and long-term morbidity in survivors of a vanishing co-twin with singletons and born twins. Of all IVF singletons born, 10.4% originated from a twin gestation in early pregnancy. The odds ratio (OR) of LBW was 1.7 (95% CI 1.2–2.2) and 2.1 (95% CI 1.3–3.6) for VLBW in singleton survivors of a vanishing twin versus singletons from single gestations, with corresponding figures for preterm birth. No excess risk of neurological sequelae in survivors of a vanishing co-twin versus the singleton cohort was found, but the OR of cerebral palsy was 1.9 (95% CI 0.7–5.2). In a case-control study comparing outcomes for singleton births that started as either singletons or twins, La Sala and co-workers[17] found a similar frequency of the 'vanishing' twin syndrome (12.2%) but could not confirm the adverse outcomes in terms of birth weight and gestational duration that were found in the Danish cohort.

NUCHAL TRANSLUCENCY THICKNESS IN MULTIPLE PREGNANCY

In a polyzygotic pregnancy, the risk of aneuploidy for each fetus is the same as that for a singleton. However, although a multiple pregnancy does not increase the fetal risk of aneuploidy (which is primarily related to maternal age), the likelihood of the mother having one affected child among her twins is almost doubled (5/3 the risk of a same-age mother). Indeed, a mother of 32 years has a similar risk of an affected twin as does a 35-year-old mother of a singleton.[18] Despite these discouraging figures, there is no indication to perform an invasive procedure merely because the procedure-related risk of pregnancy loss is substantially higher for twins.[19]

Although screening for Down's syndrome using a combination of maternal serum-free β-hCG, pregnancy-associated plasma protein-A (PAPP-A), and fetal nuchal translucency thickness is both theoretically possible and practically achievable,[20] greater reliance is placed on the nuchal translucency thickness risk alone when counselling women about invasive testing.[20,21] Contrary to the observed increase in nuchal translucency in singleton pregnancies from assisted reproduction, the nuchal translucency in dichorionic twins was comparable to the spontaneous ones.[22] Finally, The regression curves of 5th, 50th, and 95th percentiles of nuchal translucency measurements plotted against crown-rump length of triplets and singletons overlapped, supporting the utility of the same cut-off values.[23]

PROPHYLACTIC INTERVENTION TO REDUCE PRETERM LABOR AND LOW BIRTH WEIGHT

Short- and long-term outcomes of multiples are primarily related to the much increased incidence of preterm birth among these pregnancies. As noted above, the ever-increasing multiple birth rates[1] contribute significantly to the continuous increase in preterm births.[24] None of the many prophylactic measures, including cervical cerclage,[25] was effective in reducing the incidence of preterm births in multiple pregnancies. However, during the past decade, nutritional intervention emerged as the only means that consistently improves outcome in multiples.[26] Recently, Luke *et al.*[27] conducted a prospective intervention study of women who participated in a specialized program versus non-participants, which included twice-monthly visits, dietary prescription of 3000–4000 kcal/day, multimineral supplementation, and patient education. The so-called 'program pregnancies' were associated with improved pregnancy outcomes in terms of less pre-eclampsia, preterm premature rupture of membranes, low birth-weight, and significantly longer gestations, higher birth-weights and lower frequencies of neonatal morbidity. These outcomes translated into shorter hospitalization periods and lower cost per twin.[27] It was postulated that adequate weight gain, by yet unclear mechanism(s), increases the efficiency of the uteroplacental unit.[26,27]

Importantly, early weight gain (before 24 weeks' gestation) had a 3–5-fold greater effect on the rate of fetal growth and birth weight than did the weight gained after 24 weeks.[28] In triplets, we found that weight gain was more consequential in terms of fetal growth for underweight and normal-weight than for overweight women.[29]

Although dietary intervention seems appealing, several questions remain to be answered. First, it is unclear how pre-gravid maternal weight (or, more precisely, pre-gravid body mass index [BMI]) alters the effect of weight gain. Studies performed by our group on triplet gestations suggest that whereas pre-gravid BMI is not a good predictor of outcome,[30] the change in maternal BMI (a measure of weight gain corrected for maternal physique) is a good predictor of birth weight in triplets (Levy L *et al.*, Bartfeld Y *et al.*, unpublished observations). Second, the recommended weight gain did not consider its potential effect on future obesity. It might well be that excessive weight gain may work perfectly during the multiple gestation but might turn women with normal pre-gravid BMI into overweight or obese. Finally, it is unclear why not all mothers who gain weight as recommended produce the expected improved effect and, conversely, why not all mothers who failed to meet the recommendation of weight gain have, nonetheless, a favorable outcome. The latter question, perhaps, involves the so-called 'ideal' maternal phenotype to carry multiples. Triplet mothers who were multiparous, older than 35 years, and taller than 165 cm had a significantly better outcome in terms of total triplet birth weight and gestational age at birth compared to younger and shorter nulliparas.[31,32] Indeed, a study that tried to characterize mothers of triplets found that mothers who delivered the heaviest triplets were significantly older, multiparous, taller, heavily built, and gained more weight compared with mothers of average-weight triplets.[30]

MONOZYGOSITY AND MONOCHORIONICITY

All current speculations about the mechanism of zygotic splitting are based on educated deductions.[33] The first theory proposes that every embryo forms an axis along which it develops. According to this theory, monozygotic twining occurs when two axes co-dominate. The second and more popular theory suggests that cells exhibit some genetic differences early in embryonic development that cause them to repel each other. As appealing as they may be, both theories do not explain why monozygotic splitting rates are almost constant in all races, both are unsuitable to explain the formation of monozygotic triplets and quadruplets, and neither is able to explain the invariably increased incidence following all methods of assisted conception. A third pseudomechanical theory suggested that a gap in the zona pellucida is created during the *in vitro* process, leading to herniation of blastomeres through the gap and subsequent division of the cells. This theory is unlikely because it does not explain why ovulation induction alone is associated with a much higher rate of zygotic splitting compared with pregnancies following micromanipulation or assisted hatching, in which the zona pellucida is clearly breached. It follows that any 'new' theory should explain the consistent increase of monozygotic twinning with every method of assisted conception. Data from the East Flanders Prospective Twin Survey – the only population-based series with complete zygosity assessment – show a quasi dose–effect relationship between the method of assisted conception and the incidence of monozygotic twin births.[34] In addition, any 'new' theory to explain zygotic splitting should also explain why embryologists do not observe any physical splitting of the embryo in *in vitro* fertilization (IVF) programs.

Regardless of the unknown mechanism of zygotic splitting, it is clear that monozygotic twinning is one of the most intriguing biological phenomena. However, it is chorionicity, rather than zygosity, that matters. Indeed, most of the perinatal pathology is related to monochorionic (MC) twins, whereas dichorionic monozygotic twins have a similar outcome to dichorionic-dizygotic twins.[33] Most of the specific pathologies – congenital anomalies, twin–twin transfusion syndrome (TTTS), and/or growth restriction – are well known; however, progress in several related issues has been recently made. First and foremost are the significant advances in understanding and treating TTTS. Over the past years, it became clear that TTTS is a manifestation of apparently normal twins, interconnected by transplacental anastomoses. Although all MC placentas have such anastomoses, TTTS occurs as a result of a net shunt of blood via one or more deep arteriovenous anastomoses that are unbalanced by the absence or paucity of compensating anastomoses. It is now also clear that, in addition to this unbalanced shunt, the twins must undergo some adjustment to the on-going hemodynamic change in the form of cardiac, renal, and hormonal adaptation. The severity of maladaptation, and hence of the TTTS, has been categorized by Quintero *et al.*[35] according to its manifestations; these, in turn, enabled a more rational comparison of treatment modalities. Importantly, growth discordance, a previous integral criterion for TTTS, is now considered a consequence of unequal placental sharing and the frequently encountered velamentous cord insertion rather than manifestation of blood shunting.

The advances in understanding and treating TTTS soon translated to a randomized control trial showing a significant advantage of the highly sophisticated fetoscopic laser photocoagulation of the putative anastomoses over the rather simple amnioreduction treatment.[36] In addition, selective reduction of one MC twin by means of cord occlusion techniques was proposed in managing some advanced cases of TTTS,[37] as well as in the case of twin reversed arterial perfusion (TRAP) sequence.[38]

Regardless of the cause, the risks associated with fetal demise in MC twins are also different from those in dichorionic twins. In the past, emboli of a thromboplastin-like material were suspected to cross the inter-twin anastomoses from the dead fetus to the survivor causing end-organ damage. However, in recent years, this theory was discarded and it was established that, following death of one twin, a rapid transfusion from the survivor to the low-resistance (absent) circulation of the dead twin might lead to acute hypovolemia and ischemic end-organ lesions. This, in turn, led to rescue attempts of the survivor by intra-uterine transfusion,[39] although the utility of such heroic measures was questioned.[40]

Because fetal death in MC twins may potentially cause serious damage in the survivor and because this sequence might occur without anomalies or TTTS, the prospective risk of death in MC twins has significant implications for the management of such pregnancies. Recently, Barigye *et al.*[41] analyzed a large cohort of MC twins and found that the subset of 'uncomplicated' MC twins (without signs of TTTS and exhibiting appropriate and concordant growth in each of the structurally normal twins) was at a considerable excess risk (1/23, 4.3%; 95% CI 1/11–1/63) of intra-uterine fetal demise after 32 weeks. With this risk in mind, Cleary-Goldman and D'Alton[42] focused on whether the results of this study seem to suggest that 32 weeks of gestation may be a reasonable date for elective preterm delivery to avoid unexpected intra-uterine fetal death. However, exactly the same study design in the Portuguese population[43] found that the prospective risk of still-birth per pregnancy after 32 weeks of gestation was 1.2% (95% CI 0.3–4.2%). These authors concluded that, under intensive surveillance, the prospective risk of fetal death in MC-diamniotic pregnancies after 32 weeks of gestation does not support a policy of elective preterm delivery.[43]

PROGRESS IN UNDERSTANDING GROWTH ABERRATIONS

Growth discordance is a relatively frequent complication of multiple pregnancies[44–46] implicated in short- and long-term adverse outcomes. At the same time, however, the risk is primarily related to large differences in birth weight, suggesting that lower levels of discordant birth weight might be a result of a normal inter-sibling variation and some form of adaptation of the multiple pregnancy to the limited potential of the uterus to accommodate two large fetuses.[47]

The major progress in recent years in understanding growth discordance is the result of the availability of the 1995–1998 Matched Multiple Birth Dataset from the US National Center for Health Statistics. Analysis showed that mortality was 11 times higher among highly discordant smaller twins (30% or more) compared with concordant smaller twins with risk estimates ranging from 1.08 among 15–19% discordant twins to 2.05 among 30% or more discordant twins. After accounting for the association between fetal growth and discordance, mortality risk was substantially higher among smaller and larger twins who were highly discordant (30% or more).[48] A different analytical approach showed that increased twin birth-weight discordance was associated with increased risk of intra-uterine death and malformation-related neonatal deaths.[49] More recently,[50] severely discordant (> 25%) pairs were classified according to the birth weight of the smaller twin being < 10th, 10–50th, or > 50th percentile, defined as growth-restricted, growth-adapted, and growth-promoted pairs, respectively. Neonatal mortality rate was significantly higher among growth-restricted discordant pairs (OR 2.7; 95% CI 1.3–5.7) and resulted from the higher mortality rates among the smaller, but not among the larger, twins.[50] The results suggest that neonatal mortality is related to absolute growth restriction (*i.e.* < 10th birth-weight percentile) rather than to relative growth restriction (*i.e.* birth-weight discordance > 25%).

Discordant growth in MC twins is of special interest. In contrast to previews views, new data indicate that concordance is more frequent among MC twins that are small for gestational age (SGA).[51] In addition, it was repeatedly observed that growth in MC twins is dependent on the presence of peripheral insertion of the cord and placental territoriality.[52,53] Finally, meticulous analyses of MC placentas identified the existence of arterio-arterial anastomoses from the large to the small twin that occupies a very small (< 10%) placental territory and seems to be entirely dependent on this 'rescue' or 'life-supporting' anastomosis (Lewi L *et al.*, unpublished observations). If such an anastomosis is inadvertently severed during laser therapy for TTTS, fetal death is very likely to follow.

The efficiency of the uteroplacental unit to provide for adequate fetal growth in singletons is usually estimated by defining a given birth weight in relation to other neonates born at the same gestational age, thus leading to the definition of small-, appropriate- and large-for gestational age (SGA, AGA or LGA) infants. Although individual multiples can be similarly defined, such a quantitative measure is not available for the entire multiple pregnancy. Recently, we evaluated US data and defined the entire triplet pregnancy as SGA, AGA or LGA, by calculating the total triplet birth weight as multiples of the median (MoM) birth weight of a singleton infant born at the same gestational age.[54] We showed that an SGA triplet pregnancy (defined as less than 1 SD below the mean MoM) is associated with increased neonatal mortality, as would have been expected for SGA singletons; therefore, this new measure could be a useful proxy for the uteroplacental efficiency in multiple pregnancies.[54]

ANTENATAL CORTICOSTEROIDS IN MULTIPLES

Antenatal corticosteroids (ACSs) are the most effective treatment related to preterm birth. In fact, methods to arrest preterm labor are currently quantified by their ability to postpone birth for at least the 48-h 'window of opportunity' to complete a course of ACSs. Over the years, it was established that only one course should be given, and that this course effectively reduces two of the most significant complications of preterm birth – respiratory distress syndrome (RDS) and intraventricular hemorrhage (IVH). However, this treatment protocol was found to be less effective for twins.[55] It is currently unclear whether the reduced effect of ACSs in twins is a result of inadequate dosing[55] or a result of a different reaction of the multiples to ACS treatment.[56] Recently, our group used an epidemiological approach to evaluate this important clinical question.[57,58] We used the Israel National very low birth weight (< 1500 g) Infant Database to examine the effect of a complete, partial, or no ACS treatment on the frequency of RDS and IVH (grades III and IV) in singletons, twins, and triplets born at < 32 weeks, and weighing < 1500 g at birth. After careful adjustments and rather sophisticated statistics, we found that, irrespective of treatment, the frequency of these adverse outcomes increased with plurality. This finding suggests that the recommended dose of ACSs for singletons seems to be inadequate for multiples, especially in the prevention of RDS. At the same time, however, a complete course of ACS was significantly more effective than a partial course. Interestingly, there was no difference between a partial course and no ACS in relation to RDS whereas it seems that even a partial course has a significant effect on the occurrence of IVH. The latter observation suggests that the dose of ACS might be insufficient for the target tissue related to RDS but seems adequate to reduce the incidence of IVH. Inadequate dosing may be related to the plurality-dependent increase in fetal mass[59] as well as the increased maternal body volume in multiples.

BRAIN DAMAGE AMONG MULTIPLES

Population-based studies from the 1980s and early 1990s show an exponential increase in cerebral palsy (CP) with plurality.[60] Specifically, about a 5-fold and 20-fold increased risk was established for twins and triplets, respectively. Since the diagnosis of CP in usually not made until several years after birth, these frequently cited figures probably do not represent the more recent frequencies of multiple births as a result of the epidemic dimensions of iatrogenic multiples. In addition, these figures do not represent modern perinatal practice whereby twin pregnancies and births are more closely monitored compared to two decades ago.

Little doubt exists that the alarming figures of CP are related to over-representation of multiples among premature and low birth-weight infants. The main question that remains to be answered is related to the contribution of MC twins to the frequency of CP. As discussed above, single fetal demise significantly increases the risk of brain damage in the survivor but, regrettably, no data exist to quantify the proportion of this occurrence among a cohort of multiples. As monozygotic twins comprise about 5% of iatrogenic twins (compared with 1 in 3 of spontaneous twins) and since the proportion of MC twins among monozygotic pairs appears to be unchanged by the mode of conception, it could be assumed that the risk of MC-related CP is decreasing with the increased proportion of iatrogenic multiples.[61] This seemingly encouraging effect of iatrogenic conceptions is offset by the continuous increase in twin births, with a net result of more twins being born preterm and at risk of prematurity-related CP. This effect was estimated using data from the UK related to the frequency of multiples following transfer of three embryos in ART and calculating the risk of CP in the English population.[62] The estimated rates of CP were significantly higher after the transfer of three embryos (16.86 per 1000), transfer of two embryos (8.77 per 1000), or after the transfer of three embryos with a reduction of all triplets to twins (10.31 per 1000) than after spontaneous conception (2.7 per 1000 neonates). Using similar extrapolations, Kiely *et al.*[63] estimated that in the US there might be an 8% increase in the prevalence of CP due solely to the rise in iatrogenic multiple births.

In the absence of chorionicity data among survivors of single fetal death, the best estimate, albeit obviously inadequate, was to examine the frequencies of CP among like- versus unlike-sexed twins. In a series of analyses, Pharoah[64] found an increased risk of CP in the survivors of single fetal death in like-sexed twin sets. Interestingly, the same trend was found among survivors of neonatal death of a co-twin. The latter observation would support the hypothesis that acute intra-uterine bidirectional shunt damaged both twins. This insult, however, caused unequal damage, leading to neonatal death of one twin and CP in its surviving co-twin. Speculations aside, single death in MC twins is seldom observed in real-time and usually is diagnosed some time later, when damage has already occurred. The exception is when impending death is observed following treatment of TTTS.

Finally, several population-based studies reached the same conclusion that whereas the risk of CP is decreasing in singletons born at > 36 weeks and weighing > 2500 g, the risk for twins is increasing 3–4-fold.[60] The main explanation for this epidemiological observation is related to the assumption that post-term occurs earlier in twins than in singletons, in agreement with increased perinatal mortality rates after 38 weeks' gestation.[65]

DELIVERY CONSIDERATIONS

Guidelines regarding the mode of delivery are mainly based on presentation combination and fetal weight. These guidelines have not change over the past decades and national data from the US and UK suggest that about 60% of multiples are delivered by cesarean section. However, some European countries present higher figures, which evidently, cannot be traced to different proportion of malpresentation or low birth weight.[66]

A more plausible explanation is a potentially different approach to the so-called 'premium' pregnancy – a definition that does not exist in obstetric textbooks but, nonetheless, is known to all practicing obstetricians. In such a circumstance, defined in social rather than in medical terms, the abdominal route might be selected for subtle indications rather than an evidence-based decision.[66] From the available guidelines, it appears that most clinicians would consider non-vertex first sets as an indication for a cesarean[67] and all vertex-first twins as candidates for vaginal birth. Controversy exists for vertex-non-vertex pairs[68] and hence the rationale for a randomized multicenter trial for such a combination.[69]

As noted above, there is circumstantial evidence that 'term' occurs earlier in twins and most clinicians who hold this view would consider 38 weeks as the optimal gestational age for delivery.[70] Because nearly 20% of twin pregnancies remain undelivered at 38 weeks, the question of cervical ripening and labor induction may become pertinent for patients eligible for vaginal birth. However, clinicians might be reluctant to use uterotonic means because of the inherent uterine over-distension. Yet, various methods to induce labor, such as oxytocin, prostaglandins, balloons, and, more recently, misoprostol[71] have been described without obvious side-effects. Regardless of the safety of induction, there is insufficient data available to support a practice of elective delivery from 37 weeks' gestation for women with an otherwise uncomplicated twin pregnancy.[72]

EPILOGUE

This chapter covers several issues related to multiple pregnancies and births; however, by no means does it describe the extensive progress in this subject. One of the reasons for this progress is that multiple pregnancies are not that rare anymore and manifestations of twinning are no longer considered as curios of nature. Consequently, more clinical material and experience are available for research with a plethora of publications as a direct effect.

Because the frequencies of multiple births continue to increase, it is expected that adequately powered, and possibly randomized studies, will further increase our understanding of the biology of multiple pregnancy and further improve our management of these high-risk cases.

KEY POINTS FOR CLINICAL PRACTICE

- Current trends showing an increase in twin birth rates concomitant with the decrease in triplet birth rates do not herald the end of the 'epidemic' of multiples.
- Recent data indicate that loss of the entire pregnancy (miscarriage) after ART is lower among twins than among singletons.
- 10% of all IVF singletons are survivors of the vanishing twin syndrome and, hence, have significant perinatal consequences
- Nuchal translucency thickness measurement should be an integral part of first trimester scanning in both mono- and dichorinic twins.
- Early adequate weight gain seems to be the only prophylactic measure that effectively improves outcomes of multiples. However, it is still debatable whether the recommended weight gain is BMI-independent and what its effect on obesity is.
- There is a quasi dose-effect relationship between the method of assisted conception and the incidence of monozygotic twin births. Regardless of the zygotic splitting mechanism, monozygotic twinning is one of the most intriguing biological phenomena, but chorionicity, rather than zygosity, has a clinical relevance.
- It is debatable whether the risk of fetal demise in MC twins indicates an elective preterm birth in uncomplicated cases.
- Severe birth weight discordance *per se,* unless associated with a SGA smaller twin, does not seem to increase perinatal complications.
- Antenatal corticosteroids have a reduced effect in multiples, probably due to increased target tissue mass and increased volume (maternal) of distribution.
- The frequency of CP increases exponentially with plurality: about a 5-fold and 20-fold increased risk for twins and triplets. respectively. These figures are related to over-representation of multiples among premature and low birth-weight infants.

References

1 Blickstein I, Keith LG. The decreased rates of triplet births: temporal trends and biologic speculations. Am J Obstet Gynecol 2005; 193: 327–331

2 Martin JA, Hamilton BE, Sutton PD, Ventura SJ, Menacker F, Munson ML. Births: final data for 2002. Natl Vital Stat Report 2003; 52: 1–113

3 Twins and Multiple Births Association web site. <http://www.tamba.org.uk/html/home.htm> (Accessed May 2006)

4 Simmons R, Doyle P, Maconochie N. Dramatic reduction in triplet and higher order births in England and Wales. Br J Obstet Gynaecol 2004; 111: 856–858

5 Bhattacharya S, Templeton A. What is the most relevant standard of success in assisted

reproduction? Redefining success in the context of elective single embryo transfer: evidence, intuition and financial reality. Hum Reprod 2004; 19: 1939–1942

6 De Sutter P, Van der Elst J, Coetsier T, Dhont M. Single embryo transfer and multiple pregnancy rate reduction in IVF/ICSI: a 5-year appraisal. Reprod Biomed Online 2003; 6: 464–469

7 Dickey RP, Sartor BM, Pyrzak R. What is the most relevant standard of success in assisted reproduction? No single outcome measure is satisfactory when evaluating success in assisted reproduction; both twin births and singleton births should be counted as successes. Hum Reprod 2004; 19: 783–787

8 Ryan GL, Zhang SH, Dokras A, Syrop CH, Van Voorhis BJ. The desire of infertile patients for multiple births. Fertil Steril 2004; 81: 500–504

9 Baor L, Blickstein I. The journey from infertility to parenting multiples: a dream come true? Int J Fertil Womens Med 2005; 50: 129–134

10 La Sala GB, Nucera G, Gallinelli A, Nicoli AN, Villani MT, Blickstein I. Spontaneous embryonic loss following *in vitro* fertilization: incidence and effect on outcomes. Am J Obstet Gynecol 2004; 191: 741–746

11 Dickey RP, Taylor SN, Lu PY *et al*. Spontaneous reduction of multiple pregnancy: incidence and effect on outcome. Am J Obstet Gynecol 2002; 186: 77–83

12 Tummers P, De Sutter P, Dhont M. Risk of spontaneous abortion in singleton and twin pregnancies after IVF/ICSI. Hum Reprod 2003; 18: 1720–1723

13 La Sala GB, Nucera G, Gallinelli A, Nicoli AN, Villani MT, Blickstein I. Spontaneous embryonic loss after in vitro fertilization with and without intracytoplasmic sperm injection. Fertil Steril 2004; 82: 1536–1539

14 La Sala GB, Nucera G, Gallinelli A, Nicoli AN, Villani MT, Blickstein I. Lower embryonic loss rates among twin gestations following assisted reproduction. Assist Reprod Genet 2005; 22: 181–184

15 La Sala GB, Nucera G, Gallinelli A, Nicoli AN, Villani MT, Blickstein I. Spontaneous embryonic loss rates in twin and singleton pregnancies after transfer of top- versus intermediate-quality embryos. Fertil Steril 2005; 84: 1602–1605

16 Pinborg A, Lidegaard O, la Cour Freiesleben N, Andersen AN. Consequences of vanishing twins in IVF/ICSI pregnancies. Hum Reprod 2005; 20: 2821–2829

17 La Sala GB, Villani MT, Nicoli A, Gallinelli A, Nucera G, Blickstein I. Effect of the mode of assisted reproductive technology conception on obstetric outcomes for survivors of the vanishing twin syndrome. Fertil Steril 2006; 86: 247–249

18 Matias A, Montenegro N, Blickstein I. Down syndrome screening in multiple pregnancies. Obstet Gynecol Clin North Am 2005; 32: 81–96

19 Appelman Z, Furman B. Invasive genetic diagnosis in multiple pregnancies. Obstet Gynecol Clin North Am 2005; 32: 97–103

20 Spencer K, Nicolaides KH. Screening for trisomy 21 in twins using first trimester ultrasound and maternal serum biochemistry in a one-stop clinic: a review of three years experience. Br J Obstet Gynaecol 2003; 110: 276–280

21 Maymon R, Neeman O, Shulman A, Rosen H, Herman A. Current concepts of Down syndrome screening tests in assisted reproduction twin pregnancies: another double trouble. Prenat Diagn 2005; 25: 746–750

22 Hui PW, Tang MH, Ng EH, Yeung WS, Ho PC. Nuchal translucency in dichorionic twins conceived after assisted reproduction. Prenat Diagn 2006; 26: 510–513

23 Maslovitz S, Yaron Y, Fait G *et al*. Feasibility of nuchal translucency in triplet pregnancies. J Ultrasound Med 2004; 23: 501–504

24 Martin JA, Hamilton BE, Sutton PD, Ventura SJ, Menacker F, Munson ML. Births: final data for 2003. Natl Vital Stat Report 2005; 54: 1–116

25 Berghella V, Odibo AO, To MS, Rust OA, Althuisius SM. Cerclage for short cervix on ultrasonography: meta-analysis of trials using individual patient-level data. Obstet Gynecol 2005; 106: 181–189

26 Luke B. Improving multiple pregnancy outcomes with nutritional interventions. Clin Obstet Gynecol 2004; 47: 146–162

27 Luke B, Brown MB, Misiunas R *et al*. Specialized prenatal care and maternal and infant outcomes in twin pregnancy. Am J Obstet Gynecol 2003; 189: 934–938

28 Luke B, Nugent C, van de Ven C *et al*. The association between maternal factors and perinatal

outcomes in triplet pregnancies. Am J Obstet Gynecol 2002; 187: 752–757
29 Flidel-Rimon O, Rhea DJ, Keith LG, Shinwell ES, Blickstein I. Early adequate maternal weight gain is associated with fewer small for gestational age triplets. J Perinat Med 2005; 33: 379–382
30 Blickstein I, Rhea DJ, Keith LG. Characteristics of mothers who delivered the heaviest, average-weight, and lightest triplet sets. J Perinat Med 2005; 33: 113–116
31 Blickstein I, Rhea DJ, Keith LG. The likelihood of adverse outcomes in triplet pregnancies estimated by pregravid maternal characteristics. Fertil Steril 2004; 81: 1079–1082
32 Blickstein I, Rhea DJ, Keith LG. Effect of maternal height on gestational age and birth weight in nulliparous mothers of triplets with a normal pregravid body mass index. J Reprod Med 2003; 48: 335–338
33 Blickstein I. Monochorionicity in perspective. Ultrasound Obstet Gynecol 2006; 27: 235–238
34 Derom C, Leroy F, Vlietinck R, Fryns JP, Derom R. High frequency of iatrogenic monozygotic twins with administration of clomiphene citrate and a change in chorionicity. Fertil Steril 2006; 85: 755–757
35 Quintero RA, Morales WJ, Allen MH, Bornick PW, Johnson PK, Kruger M. Staging of twin-twin transfusion syndrome. J Perinatol 1999; 19: 550–555
36 Senat MV, Deprest J, Boulvain M, Paupe A, Winer N, Ville Y. Endoscopic laser surgery versus serial amnioreduction for severe twin-to-twin transfusion syndrome. N Engl J Med 2004; 351: 136–144
37 Nakata M, Chmait RH, Quintero RA. Umbilical cord occlusion of the donor versus recipient fetus in twin-twin transfusion syndrome. Ultrasound Obstet Gynecol 2004; 23: 446–450
38 Weisz B, Peltz R, Chayen B *et al.* Tailored management of twin reversed arterial perfusion (TRAP) sequence. Ultrasound Obstet Gynecol 2004; 23: 451–455
39 Senat MV, Loizeau S, Couderc S, Bernard JP, Ville Y. The value of middle cerebral artery peak systolic velocity in the diagnosis of fetal anemia after intrauterine death of one monochorionic twin. Am J Obstet Gynecol 2003; 189: 1320–1324
40 Blickstein I. Monochorionic pregnancy – where have we been? Where are we going? Am J Obstet Gynecol 2004; 191: 383–384
41 Barigye O, Pasquini L, Galea P, Chambers H, Chappell L, Fisk NM. High risk of unexpected late fetal death in monochorionic twins despite intensive ultrasound surveillance: a cohort study. PLoS Med 2005; 2: e172
42 Cleary-Goldman J, D'Alton ME. Uncomplicated monochorionic diamniotic twins and the timing of delivery. PLoS Med 2005; 2: e180
43 Simoes T, Amaral N, Lerman R, Ribeiro F, Dias E, Blickstein I. Prospective risk of intrauterine death of monochorionic-diamniotic twins. Am J Obstet Gynecol 2006; 195: 134–139
44 Kalish RB, Branum A, Sharma G, Keith LG, Blickstein I. Gestational age-specific distribution of twin birth weight discordance. J Perinat Med 2005; 33: 117–120
45 Blickstein I, Kalish RB. Birthweight discordance in multiple pregnancy. Twin Res 2003; 6: 526–531
46 Blickstein I, Jacques DL, Keith LG. A novel approach to intertriplet birth weight discordance. Am J Obstet Gynecol 2003; 188: 1026–1030
47 Blickstein I, Goldman RD, Mazkereth R. Adaptive growth restriction as a pattern of birth weight discordance in twin gestations. Obstet Gynecol 2000; 96: 986–990
48 Branum AM, Schoendorf KC. The effect of birth weight discordance on twin neonatal mortality. Obstet Gynecol 2003; 101: 570–574
49 Demissie K, Ananth CV, Martin J, Hanley ML, MacDorman MF, Rhoads GG. Fetal and neonatal mortality among twin gestations in the United States: the role of intrapair birth weight discordance. Obstet Gynecol 2002; 100: 474–480
50 Blickstein I, Keith LG. Neonatal mortality rates among growth-discordant twins, classified according to the birth weight of the smaller twin. Am J Obstet Gynecol 2004; 190: 170–174
51 Blickstein I, Mincha S, Goldman R, Machin G, Keith L. The Northwestern twin chorionicity study: testing the 'placental crowding' hypothesis. J Perinat Med 2006; 34: 158–161
52 Loos RJ, Derom C, Derom R, Vlietinck R. Determinants of birthweight and intrauterine growth in liveborn twins. Paediatr Perinat Epidemiol 2005; 19: 15S–22S
53 Quintero RA, Martinez JM, Lopez J *et al.* Individual placental territories after selective laser photocoagulation of communicating vessels in twin-twin transfusion syndrome. Am J Obstet Gynecol 2005; 192: 1112–1118
54 Blickstein I, Salihu HM, Keith LG, Alexander GR. The association between small-for-

gestational age triplet pregnancies and neonatal mortality: a novel approach to growth assessment in multiple gestations. Pediatr Res 2006; 59: 565–569
55 Murphy DJ, Caukwell S, Joels LA, Wardle P. Cohort study of the neonatal outcome of twin pregnancies that were treated with prophylactic or rescue antenatal corticosteroids. Am J Obstet Gynecol 2002; 187: 483–488
56 Jobe AH. Antenatal steroids in twins. Am J Obstet Gynecol 2003; 188: 856
57 Blickstein I, Reichman B, Lusky A, Shinwell ES; Israel Neonatal Network. Plurality-dependent risk of respiratory distress syndrome among very-low-birth-weight infants and antepartum corticosteroid treatment. Am J Obstet Gynecol 2005; 192: 360–364
58 Blickstein I, Reichman B, Lusky A, Shinwell ES; Israel Neonatal Network. Plurality-dependent risk of severe intraventricular hemorrhage among very low birth weight infants and antepartum corticosteroid treatment. Am J Obstet Gynecol 2006; 194: 1329–1333
59 Blickstein I. Is it normal for multiples to be smaller than singletons? Best Pract Res Clin Obstet Gynaecol 2004; 18: 613–623
60 Blickstein I. Do multiple gestations raise the risk of cerebral palsy? Clin Perinatol 2004; 31: 395–408
61 Blickstein I. Estimation of iatrogenic monozygotic twinning rate following assisted reproduction: pitfalls and caveats. Am J Obstet Gynecol 2005; 192: 365–368
62 Blickstein I, Weissman A. Estimating the risk of cerebral palsy after assisted conceptions. N Engl J Med 1999; 341: 1313–1314
63 Kiely JL, Kiely M, Blickstein I. Contribution of the rise in multiple births to a potential increase in cerebral palsy. Pediatr Res 2000: 47: 314A
64 Pharoah PO. Risk of cerebral palsy in multiple pregnancies. Obstet Gynecol Clin North Am 2005; 32: 55–67
65 Minakami H, Sato I. Reestimating date of delivery in multifetal pregnancies. JAMA 1996; 275: 1432–1434
66 Blickstein I. Cesarean section for all twins? J Perinat Med 2000; 28: 169–174
67 Blickstein I, Goldman RD, Kupferminc M. Delivery of breech first twins: a multicenter retrospective study. Obstet Gynecol 2000; 95: 37–42
68 Hogle KL, Hutton EK, McBrien KA, Barrett JF, Hannah ME. Cesarean delivery for twins: a systematic review and meta-analysis. Am J Obstet Gynecol 2003; 188: 220–227
69 Barrett JF. Randomised controlled trial for twin delivery. BMJ 2003; 326: 448
70 Luke B, Brown MB, Alexandre PK *et al.* The cost of twin pregnancy: maternal and neonatal factors. Am J Obstet Gynecol 2005; 192: 909–915
71 Simoes T, Condeco P, Dias E, Ventura P, Matos C, Blickstein I. Induction of labor with oral misoprostol in nulliparous mothers of twins. J Perinat Med 2006; 34: 111–114
72 Dodd JM, Crowther CA. Elective delivery of women with a twin pregnancy from 37 weeks' gestation. Cochrane Database System Rev 2003; CD003582

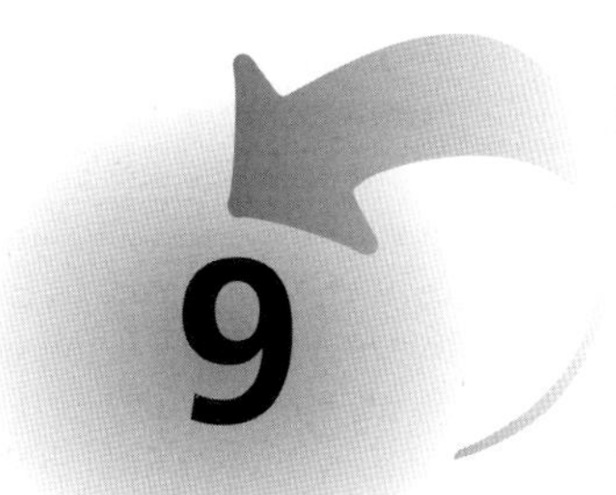

Jean-Claude Veille

Maternal mortality

What sets worlds in motion is the interplay of differences, their attractions and repulsions. Life is plurality, death is uniformity.[1]

The majority of maternal deaths occurring in the world occurs in developing countries (99%). The difference in maternal mortality between rich (mortality risk 1 in 4000–10,000) and poor countries (mortality risk 1 in 15–50) is one of the highest in public health.[2] Post-partum hemorrhage, eclampsia and sepsis are the leading causes for maternal deaths in the developing countries.[2] It is

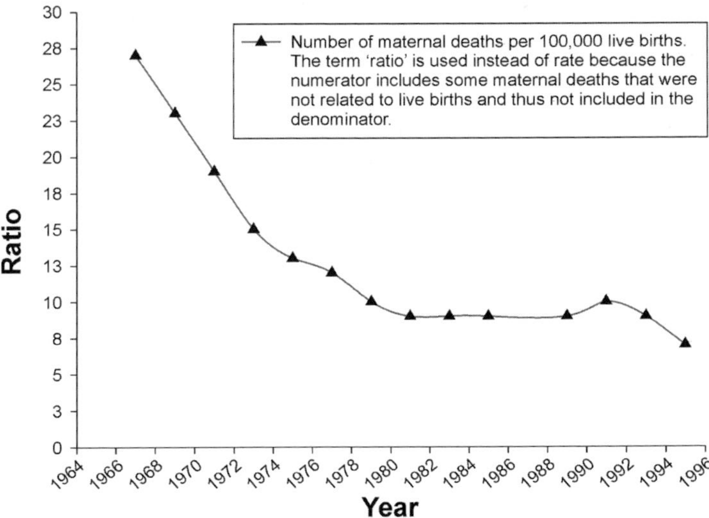

Fig. 1 US maternal mortality ratio by year (1967–1995).

Jean-Claude Veille MD
Former Professor and Chair, Albany Medical Center, Division of Maternal Fetal Medicine, Albany, New York, USA. *Current address*: 5301 F Street, Suite 112, Sacramento, CA 95819, USA
E-mail: vjclaude@comcast.net

estimated that about 500,000 mothers die annually in the world or 1600 maternal deaths per day or about one maternal death per minute. Of these, it is estimated that 100,000–200,000 are related to poorly performed or illegal abortions. Of these, 26% are estimated to be preventable by introducing antenatal, community-based interventions.[3] Access to quality, essential obstetrical care can prevent another 48% of maternal deaths. It is cost-effective to invest in policy markers that reduce maternal mortality in the most efficient manner possible.[4]

It is also noted that death rates rise with parity and maternal age. Maternal and infant death rates in the US are much higher than in many developed countries.[5] One of the six health-related Millennium Development Goals (MDGs) set by the World Health Organization (WHO) is to reduce the maternal mortality ratio (Fig. 1).[6]

MATERNAL MORTALITY – RATIO AND RATE

The US Centers for Disease Control and Prevention (CDC) notes that maternal mortality in the US has declined significantly during the 20th century but little progress has been made during the last 20 years. Figure 2 shows the actual maternal mortality death rates per 100,000 live births with the rapid decline between the years 1900 and 1950. There has been a 'plateau' in the mortality rate since 1960.

An important and impressive decline in maternal mortality occured during the first 50 years of the 20th century (between 1900 and 1950). This decline was observed in all ethnic groups and is attributed to the significant improvement in medical and technological advances including the use of antibiotics.

Data obtained from death certificates compiled by the CDC's National Center for Health Statistics indicate, however, that the annual maternal mortality ratio plateau to approximately 7.5 maternal deaths per 100,000 live births during 1982–1996 (Fig. 2).[7]

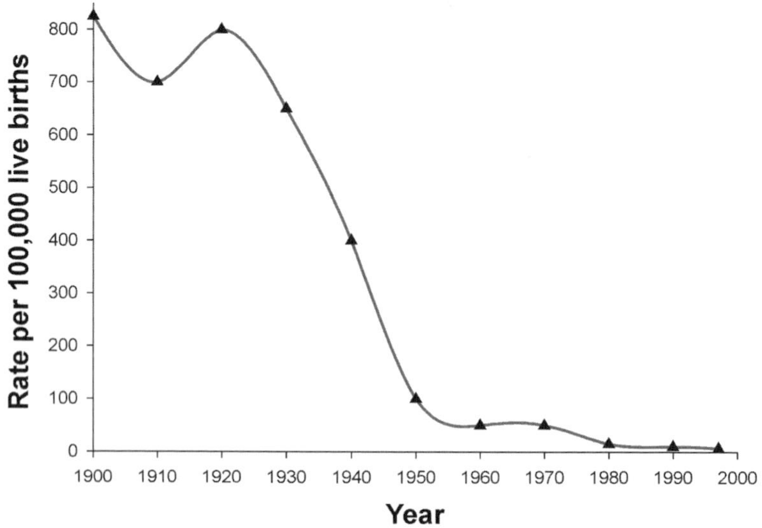

Fig. 2 US maternal mortality rate by year (1900–2000). Adapted from *MMWR* 2004; S2(SS02); 1–8

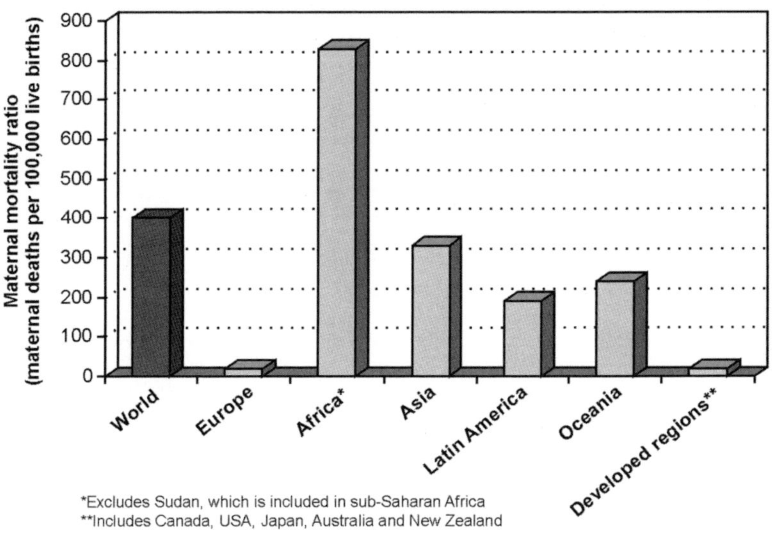

Fig. 3 Maternal mortality estimates by United Nations MDG regions (2000).

Unfortunately, recent estimates published by the United Nations (UN) for the year 2000 show that there is a great disparity in maternal mortality in different parts of the world. The highest rates of maternal mortality are found in Africa, more specifically in sub-Saharan Africa, followed by Asia, Latin America and Oceania (Fig. 3).

During the last 50 years, this overall trend in maternal mortality has also been observed in transitional countries with some achieving a decline of almost 75%. Thailand decreased maternal mortality ratio from 400 deaths per 100,000 live births in 1960 to 50 per 100,000 live births in 1984. Similar declines were observed in Malaysia, Sri Lanka, Matlab, Egypt, Honduras and Bangladesh (Fig. 4).[8]

There are many possible factors, either alone or in combination, responsible for these significant decreases in maternal mortality in these countries. Some

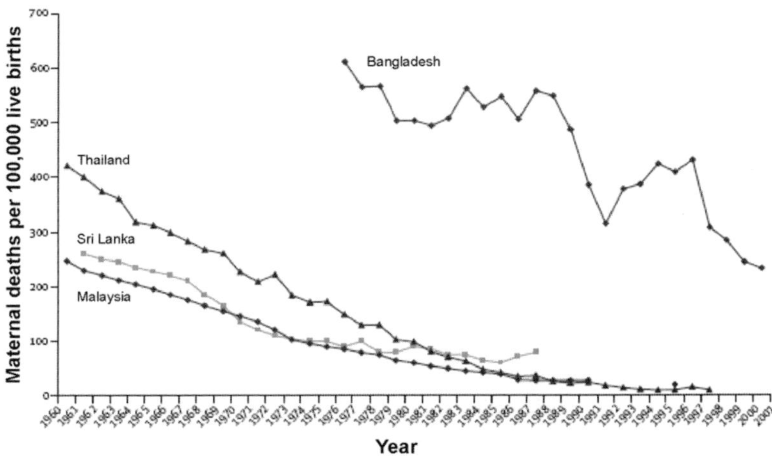

Fig. 4 Maternal death rates per 100,000 live births in Sri Lanka, Thailand, Malaysia, and Bangladesh (1960–2001).

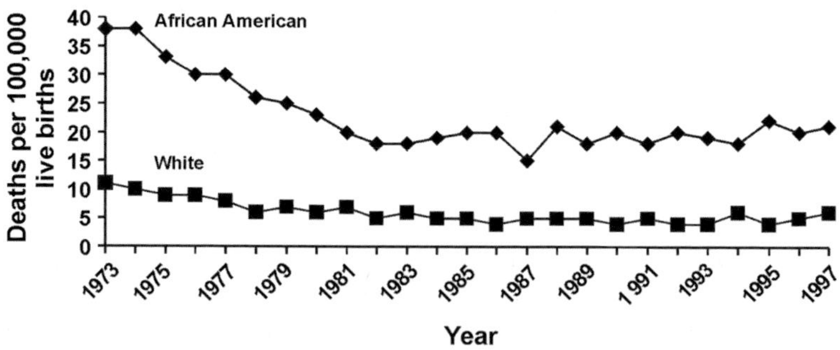

Fig. 5 African American and white women who died of pregnancy complications in the US (1973–1997). Annual number of deaths during pregnancy or within 42 days of delivery per 100,000 live births. Adapted from CDC National Center for Health Statistics.

include a substantial investment in midwifery training, free care, supportive and intense health and family planning services. Implementation of effective systems, international collaboration and policy as well as the introduction of training networks also contribute.

Sri Lanka, for example, achieved an unprecedented decrease from more than 1500 deaths per 100,000 live births to 300 per 100,000 live births in 25 years. This significant decrease in maternal mortality was mostly attributed to the introduction to universal access to midwifery care and to the eradication of malaria.[8]

In the US, the incidence of maternal mortality has not declined substantially over the last 20 years. On average in the US, 2–3 women are dying each day from pregnancy-related complications. Furthermore, the risk of dying if you are African American is increased by 2–4 times over White women (Fig. 5). The race factor differential (Black versus White) was greatest for pregnancies that did not result in a live birth, such as ectopic pregnancy, spontaneous abortion, induced abortion and gestational trophoblastic disease (Fig. 5)

The CDC estimates that half of all deaths from pregnancy could be prevented with better access to prenatal care, quality of care, and life-style habits. Maternal deaths should and need to be a major interest to local, state and federal authorities as rates for maternal mortality are basic health indicators reflecting a nation's health status.

ETIOLOGY

Etiologies for maternal deaths vary from one country to another based on resources. In the US, the leading causes for pregnancy-related deaths are hemorrhage, blood clot, high blood pressure, infection, stroke, amniotic fluid embolism and heart muscle disease such as cardiomyopathy. In a recent survey of maternal mortality in the State of New York, the leading cause for maternal mortality was postpartum hemorrhage.

In 1952, the UK introduced the *Confidential Enquiries of Maternal Deaths in the United Kingdom* (CEMD). This is the longest running example of a national, professional, self-audit in the world. The UK Government requires all maternal deaths be subject to CEMD.[9] During the 'enquiry stage', all relevant hospital professionals involved in a particular case are mandated to participate in the process (CEMD). In a report published in 2000 entitled *Why Mothers Die 1997–1999*, 378 maternal deaths were identified (11.4 deaths per 100,000 live births). Direct causes were responsible for 106 deaths (28%); indirect causes for 136 deaths (36%); co-incidental causes for 29 deaths (8%); and late for 107 deaths (28%).

The majority of direct causes were due to thrombosis and thromboembolism in patients undergoing cesarean delivery. Subsequent to this finding, the committee introduced protocols for the routine use of thromboprophylaxis for surgery. The number of maternal deaths subsequent to this policy fell significantly.

The other causes of direct maternal deaths were hypertensive disorders followed closely by maternal sepsis and ectopic pregnancy. As the result of this on-going task force, new or revised guidelines were established. Besides the use of thromboprophylaxis, the task force recommended the use of routine antibiotics for cesarean deliveries and recommended paying particular attention to women who chronically fail to attend prenatal visits, women who are subject to domestic violence, or women with serious mental illness.

Such prospective and rigorous study underlines the need for accurate and useful information. This accurate information is essential in order to establish effective action and effective corrective actions.

For example, the recent enquiry in New York State resulted in a massive 'information' campaign leading to the publication of large posters on the management of maternal hemorrhage. This combined effort between the New York Department of Health and the American College of Obstetricians and Gynecologists (ACOG) describes the recommended protocols, including the exact medications needed to manage the majority of PPH. The logical next step is to monitor if such standardization in the recognition and the management of PPH will have a significant impact on maternal mortality.

In the US, the CDC is collaborating with state health departments using a Pregnancy Mortality Surveillance System (PMSS). Furthermore, the CDC is collaborating with the Maternal and Child Health Bureau of the Health Resources and Services Administration (HRSA), the ACOG, the Association of Maternal and Child Health Programs, and representatives from nine states to establish guidelines which could be adopted by all States to standardize monitoring and reporting systems. The CDC and the States are also using a Pregnancy Risk Assessment Monitoring System (PRAMS) to analyze women's behavior and experiences before, during and immediately after pregnancy in order to identify women at high risk for health problems.

'Maternal death' is defined by the WHO as: 'death of a woman while pregnant or within 42 days of termination of pregnancy, irrespective of the duration and the site of the pregnancy, from any cause related to or aggravated by the pregnancy or its management, but not from accidental causes'. Others use any maternal deaths within 1 year of being pregnant. Most maternal deaths occur within the first week after delivery and it is 100 times more likely to occur on the first day after birth and in the hospital. It is important to note that this statistic needs to be analyzed further as done by Ronsmans *et al.*[8] There may be some simple reasons for these early maternal deaths occurring in the hospital as summarized in Figure 6.

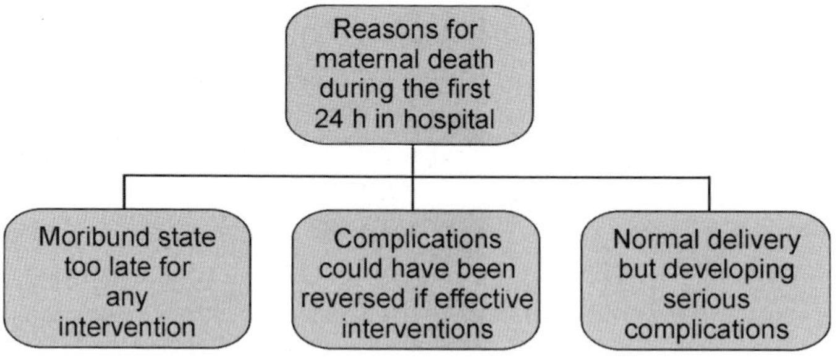

Fig. 6 Proposed reasons for maternal death during the first 24 h in hospital.

The time of death in relation to the pregnancy is illustrated in Figure 7. The vast majority of women die during the first 48 h after birth. Thus, these women are still under the active care of their care providers and, for the most part, still in the hospital where intervention should be readily available.[10]

In Figure 7, maternal mortality rates are calculated based on the number of live births. The figure illustrates the probability of a pregnant women dying of maternal causes.[8] This death may be directly related to the pregnancy (direct) or indirectly related to the pregnancy (indirect) or may occur co-incidentally with the pregnancy or even more than 42 days but less than a year after delivery irrespective of the duration and the site of the pregnancy. Death may also occur from sequelae of direct obstetrical causes.

The *International Classification of Diseases* (10th revision, 1992) assigned specific codes to these respective categories (usually 000-097 codes).[11]

An increasing number of States in the US are currently using a separate item regarding pregnancy status on the death certificate to identify maternal deaths (Table 1).

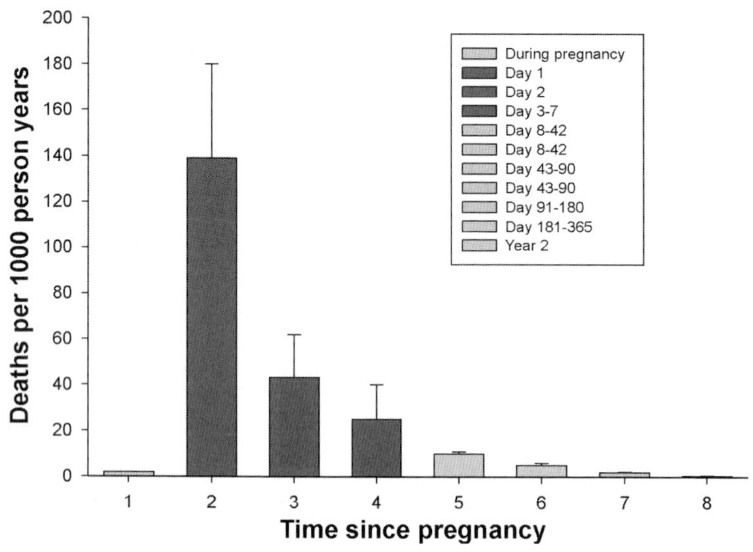

Fig. 7 Maternal mortality rates following pregnancy. Adapted from Ronsmans *et al.*[8]

Table 1 Definitions of maternal deaths

Direct	Due to pre-existing disease aggravated by pregnancy
Indirect	Those in which the cause was unrelated to pregnancy
Co-incidental	Occurring after the internationally defined limit of 6 weeks after delivery
Late	Occurring after 6 weeks but before 1 year from delivery

Table 2 Measures relating to maternal deaths

Maternal mortality ratio	Number of maternal deaths during given time period per 100,000 live births during the same time period
Maternal mortality rate	Number of maternal deaths during given time period per 100,000 women of reproductive age, or women-years of risk exposure, in same time period
Life-time risk of maternal death	Probability of maternal death during a woman's reproductive life, usually expressed in terms of odds
Proportionate mortality ratio	Maternal deaths as proportion of all female deaths of those of reproductive age (usually defined as 15–49 years) in a given time period.

In order to understand the scope of the problem fully, other measures are often reported (Table 2).[12]

Currently, the National Center for Health Statistics is the major source of information for reporting US ratios of maternal mortality. Lack of standardization of death certificates has lead to an under-reporting of maternal death. Furthermore, information from the death certificate may not provide adequate information on all of the events that may have contributed to the death. Closer analysis of maternal death since 1988 indicates that almost half of the cases (48%) had multiple causes-of-death codes covering the series of events leading to death. Thus, information obtained from death certificates is often incomplete or subject to interpretation. As US States revise their death certificates (introducing standard questions or items specifically related to deaths associated with pregnancy, child-birth and the puerperium) exact maternal mortality rates will be difficult to ascertain properly. For example, States which have introduced a separate pregnancy item on the death certificate indicate that maternal mortality is greater than in the States that do not include a separate item on the death certificate. Death certificates are now matched with birth certificates and fetal death to provide a better analysis. In a study done between the years 1995–97 using a 'linking system', there were 35% more maternal deaths identified through surveillance efforts than from the death certificate (Table 3).

Standardization and cross linkage are essential if we are to calculate the number of maternal deaths in a calendar year and relate these to the number of live births registered for the same period of time and presented as rates per 100,000 live births. The number of live births used as the denominator is, however, an approximation of the population of pregnant women who are at risk of a maternal death. This is essential if we are to determine the exact

Table 3 Effect of linking vital records on the identification of pregnancy-related deaths

State	Years	Type of records linked*	Number of deaths		Maternal mortality		Increase (%)
			Without linkage	With linkage	Without linkage	With linkage	
Washington	1977–84	LB & FD	34	57	6.8	10.9	68
West Virginia	1985–89	LB	7	16	5.4	12.4	129
North Carolina	1988–89	LB & FD	19	48	9.5	24	153
Georgia	1990–92	LB	56	73	16.8	21.9	30

*Records linked with death certificates of women of reproductive age: LB, live birth; FD, fetal death.
Adapted from CDC 2001.

causes of maternal deaths in this country and some of the policies needed to implement a decrease in maternal mortality to the goals established by the *Healthy People 2010* which calls for a maternal mortality of 3 per 100,000 live births and for elimination of deaths among certain racial groups.

The UN also adopted the WHO Millennium Development Goals (MDGs) to be achieved by the target date of 2015. For developing countries, according to the 2005 WHO DMG report, the most important goal is to reduce maternal mortality caused by infection and lack of access to antibiotics. For these countries, a good starting point is to concentrate on better reproductive healthcare interventions, sexuality and HIV/AIDS. The UN estimates that there are up to 500 million cases of malaria every year of which 90% occurs in sub-Saharan Africa. Tuberculosis is still very prevalent in many parts of the world and, again, most prevalent in the sub-Saharan area.

The UN is pushing to refinance the Global Fund Against AIDS, Tuberculosis, and Malaria. There is strong evidence that antenatal, antiretroviral treatment decreases perinatal transmission of HIV. Until such funds are renewed, the hope of decreasing maternal mortality in such countries is grim.

Safe motherhood is a vital, cost-effective economic and social investment....
Even one women dying is too many women dying.[13]

Comparison of maternal mortality between countries may be difficult as identification and classification of maternal death is still problematic. Deneux-Tharaux *et al.*[14] compared standardized enhanced methods to identify and classify pregnancy-associated deaths in two states in the US (Massachusetts and North Carolina) and two European countries (Finland and France) between 1999 and 2000. During that period of enhanced monitoring, the authors identified 404 pregnancy-associated deaths. There was great variability in the reporting aspect. Under-reporting varied between 22% (France) to 93% (Massachusetts). This indicates an urgent need to improve the identification and classification of maternal deaths. The causes for deaths varied from one area to another (Fig. 8).

Of the 404 pregnancy-associated deaths, the leading causes for pregnancy-associated maternal death were: France, hemorrhage; Massachusetts, cardiovascular conditions, hemorrhage, pregnancy-induced hypertension;

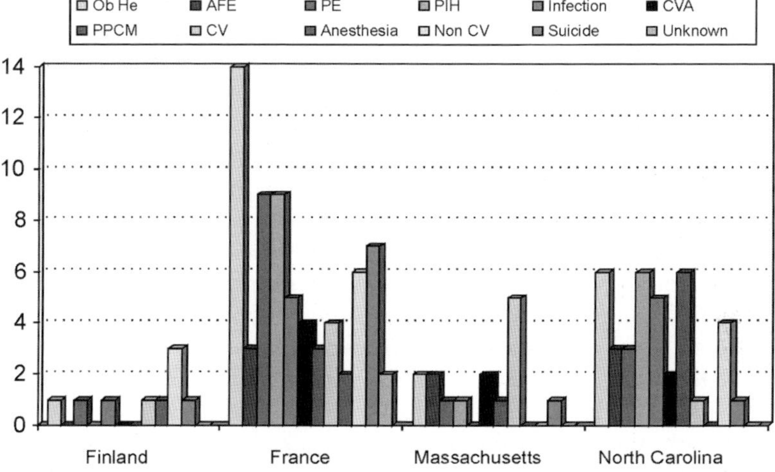

Fig. 8 Pregnancy-associated deaths in Massachusetts, North Carolina, Finland and France. Ob He, obstetrical hemorrhage; AFE, amniotic fluid embolism; PIH, pregnancy-associated-hypertension; CVA, cardiovascular accident; PPCM, peripartum cardiomyopathy; CV, cardiovascular condition other than PPCM; Non-CV, non-cardiovascular medical conditions (hyperemesis, sickle cell, hepatitis, TTP, choriocarcinoma, and melanoma). Adapted from Deneux-Tharaux *et al.*[14]

North Carolina, peripartum cardiomyopathy; and Finland, non-cardiovascular medical conditions.

Figure 9 illustrates the maternal mortality for one decade (1990–2000) for Massachusetts, North Carolina, Finland and France.

Hemorrhage

Researchers in France investigated the reasons why women were dying from post partum hemorrhage. They found that these women had received substandard care. This substandard care occurred in hospitals, in places without a 24-h on-site anesthetist and in places with a low volume of deliveries.[15] These authors have gone on to suggest that mortality due to hemorrhage could be used as an indicator of health quality as it reflects the appropriateness of obstetrical care.[16]

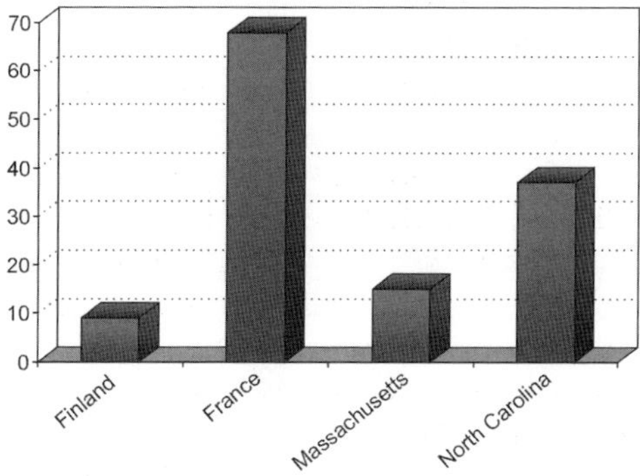

Fig. 9 All causes of maternal mortality for one decade (1990–2000) for Massachusetts, North Carolina, Finland and France. Adapted from Deneux-Tharaux *et al.*[14]

Enhanced methods to identify pregnancy-related deaths are essential; they need to be linked to birth and death certificates and extended for up to 1 year after the end of pregnancy.

Local institutions in the US have established protocols to manage major obstetric hemorrhage. One particular hospital (The New York Hospital Medical Center of Queens), established a multidisciplinary patient safety team which includes individuals from divisions of anesthesia, maternal fetal medicine, neonatology, blood bank, nursing, communication and administration.[17] After forming an obstetric rapid response team (RRT), developing clinical pathways, guidelines and protocols, these authors found that, despite a significant increase in major obstetric hemorrhage cases, there was an improvement in maternal outcomes and fewer maternal deaths. These authors recommend improving hospital systems, creation of hemorrhage drills, and implementing a rapid response team (RRT) that includes a broad spectrum of experts.

Even though much has been done to decrease death from hemorrhage, it remains one of the most frequent causes for maternal mortality is the US and in other developed countries. In countries with fewer resources, it is the single most important causes of maternal death. Hemorrhage is the single most important cause of maternal death world-wide.[3]

Hemorrhage is a comprehensive term that includes multiple etiologies. Hemorrhage can occur with an episiotomy, a vaginal, a vulvar or cervical laceration during spontaneous labor or, more frequently, during operative deliveries such as forceps or vaccum deliveries. Hemorrhage can occur during obstructed labors, with an enlarged fetus, a rupture of the uterus, at the time of a cesarean delivery or at the time of cesarean hysterectomy. Hemorrhage can occur with placenta abnormalities such as abruption placenta, placenta previa, and placenta accrete, percreta or increta, retained placenta, hyditidiform mole, or even there is abnormal implantation such as ectopic pregnancy[18] (Fig. 10).

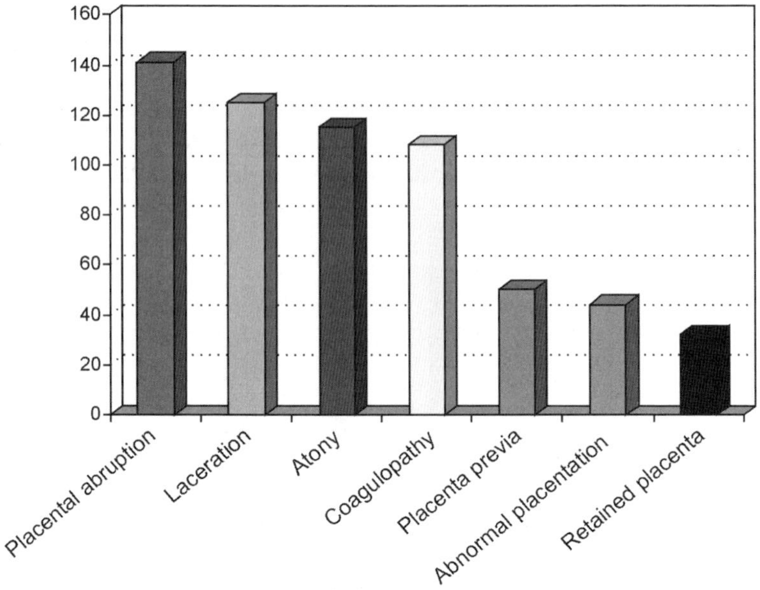

Fig. 10 Causes of hemorrhage in pregnancy (adapted from Chichakli *et al.*[18])

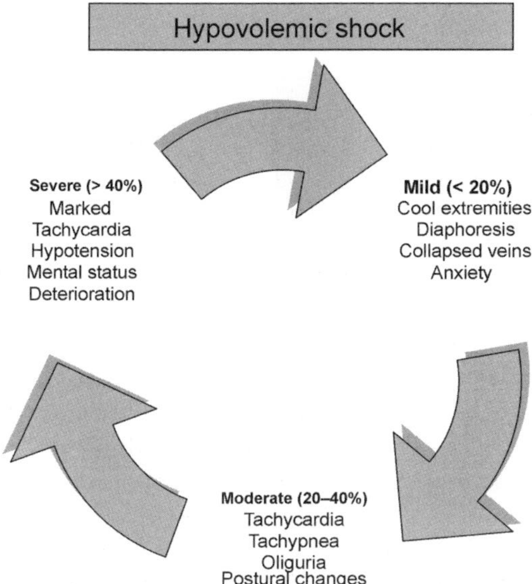

Fig. 11 Hypovolemic shock in pregnancy.

Uterine atony still remains an important contributor to maternal hemorrhage. Atony can occur with an enlarged uterus (such as found in multiple gestations), polyhydramnios, large fetuses, prolonged labors, rapid labor, or chorio-amnionitis. Hemorrhage can also be secondary to coagulation abnormality found in sepsis, amniotic fluid embolism, saline-induced abortions, massive transfusion, severe pregnancy-induced hypertension, congenital or acquired coagulopathies, or patients on anticoagulants. Patients with low blood volume are particularly vulnerable to hemorrhage as they have a decreased ability to compensate for acute blood loss. Small stature women, those with severe pregnancy-induced hypertension or the eclamptic are at greater risks for hypovolemic shock (Fig. 11).

Pregnancy increases total plasma volume, red blood cells and coagulation factors. As such, all normal pregnant patients have a natural tendency to be well prepared for a 'normal' vaginal delivery or a 'normal' cesarean delivery. A blood loss of 500 ml for a vaginal delivery or 1000 ml at the time of delivery is usually well-tolerated by the mother. When blood losses are greater, patients usually are able to adapt well without displaying signs of hypovolemic shock. As the bleeding increases and becomes significant, patients show a progression of symptoms and signs displayed in the non-gravid state. Providers need to be aware of the early signs and symptoms hypovolemic shock. Maternal death results from a failure to recognize and to intervene promptly and efficiently (Fig. 11).

Patients with severe pregnancy-induced hypertension are particularly vulnerable to hypovolemic shock in spite of significant peripheral edema. There is evidence that these patients fail to have the 'physiological' plasma volume expansion when compared to normal patients who do not develop this disorder (Fig. 12).

Khan *et al.*[3] reported a systematic review of the major causes of maternal death in the world as defined previously by the UN. They included all

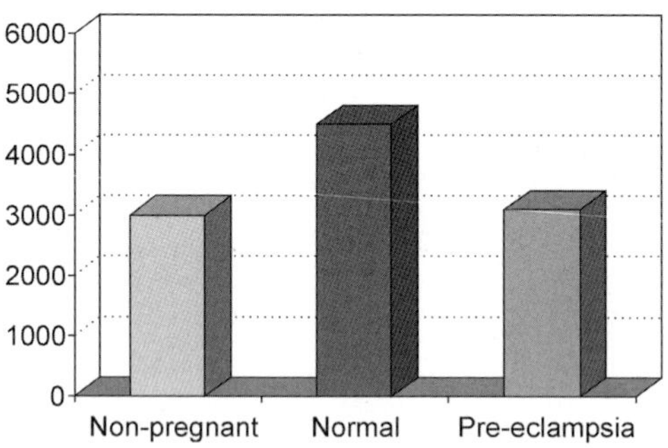

Fig. 12 Plasma volume in the non-pregnant, normal and pre-eclamptic patient.

'reported' maternal deaths occurring either during pregnancy or within 1 year of the end of the pregnancy. The datasets were obtained from 1990 onwards. Personal contacts were also made with country representatives with particular knowledge of the maternal-health field. Using a final count of 34 datasets, they were able to ascertain the causes of maternal death according to geographical region (Fig. 13).

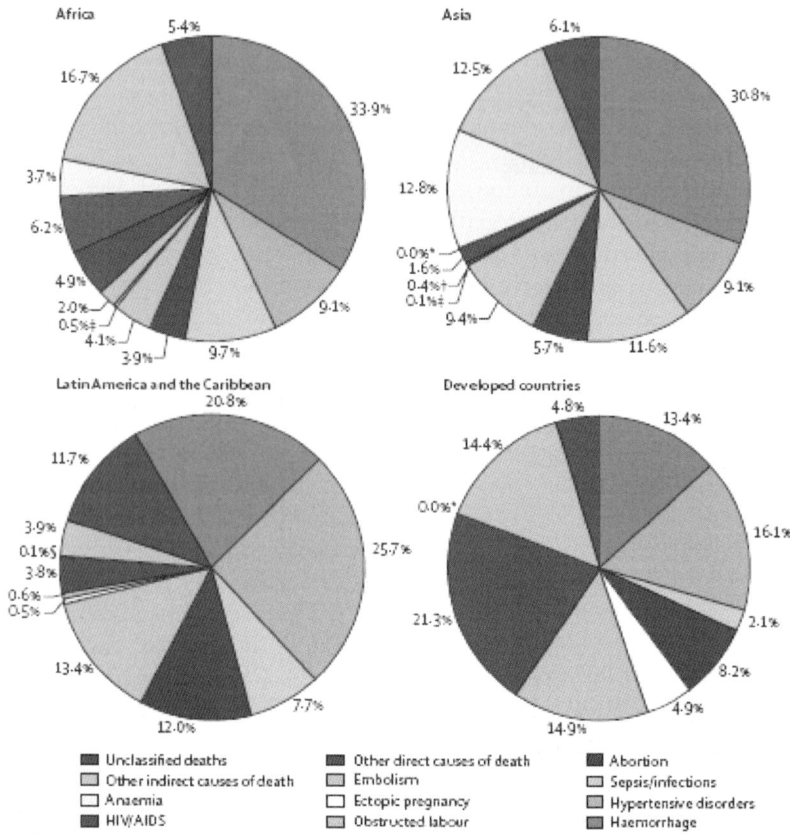

Fig. 13 World-wide causes of maternal death according to geographical region. (Reproduced with the permission of Elsevier © 2006 from Khan *et al.*[3])

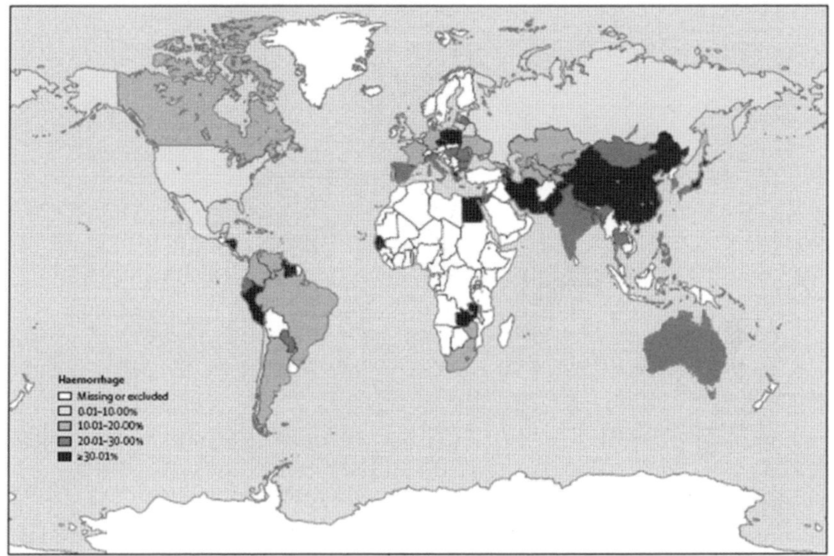

Fig. 14 Geographical distribution of hemorrhage as a cause of maternal death. (Reproduced with the permission of Elsevier © 2006 from Khan *et al.*[3])

Overall, hemorrhage was the leading cause of maternal death in Africa and Asia.[3] Hypertensive disorders represented the highest cause of death in Latin America and in the Caribbean. Within regions, there was also some significant variability. For example, within the South American continent, Peru had the highest incidence of maternal death from hemorrhage whereas in the Asia continent, China, Afghanistan and Iran had the highest incidence. In the African continent, Egypt, Senegal and Zambia were the highest. In Europe, Poland had the highest maternal death rate from hemorrhage. Figure 14 illustrates the geographical distribution of hemorrhage as a cause of maternal death.[3]

Hypertensive disorders

Hypertensive disorders are highest in Latin America and in the Caribbean with regional variations as illustrated in Figure 15. Colombia and Venezuela were found to have the highest reported number of maternal deaths associated with hypertensive disorders. Brazil, Equator, Peru, Chili and Mexico are close second in these regions. North America, Europe, China and Australia follow.[3] There is a large area, especially in the African continent, where data are simply not available; thus, it is difficult to draw solid conclusions regarding the role of hypertensive disorders in maternal deaths. The large 'white' areas have no or missing data, including the entire African continent, the Balkans and the Soviet Union. However, these data demonstrate the need to introduce universal protocols in certain countries to optimize the early recognition and the early management of such disorders.[3]

For example, in the US, magnesium sulfate, either intramuscularly or intravenously, has significantly decreased the number of eclamptic seizures and decreased complications from such disorders. Magnesium sulfate is readily available world-wide and should be considered as part of the preventive plans in countries with a high incidence of hypertensive disorders

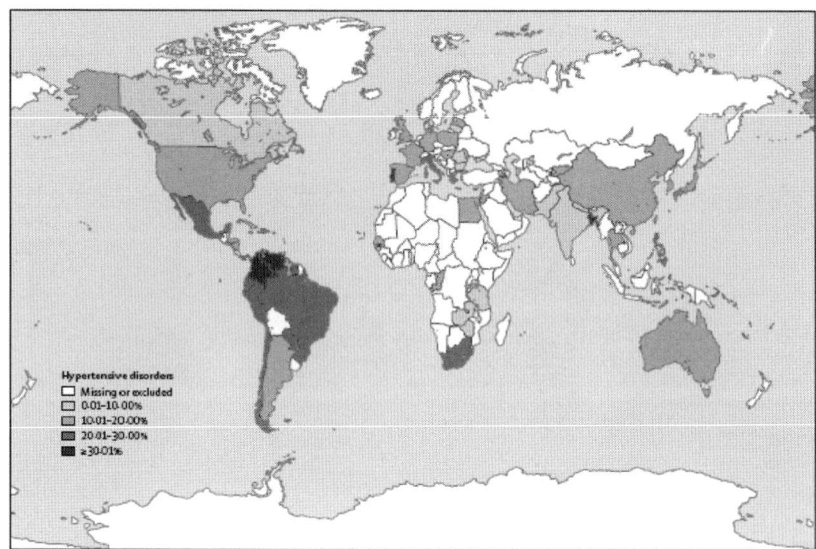

Fig. 15 Geographical distribution of hypertensive disorders as a cause of maternal death. (Reproduced with the permission of Elsevier © 2006 from Khan *et al.*[3])

such as Latin America and the Caribbean. In countries where such treatment is neither accessible nor feasible, other forms of seizure prophylaxis may be instituted prior to transport to the hospital or to other centers providing expertise in such disorders. Each country, county, and state should set standards for the management of the major medical conditions which cause maternal deaths.

Leading the way for decades, the UK has introduced the mandatory *Confidential Enquiries of Maternal Deaths* (CEMD), leading to the recommendation for prevention of thrombo-embolism, infection and standardization for the management of ectopic pregnancies. Areas in the world with increased maternal death rates due to sepsis should develop policies for antibiotic prophylaxis if feasible.

France found that women were dying in hospitals where there was substandard care (such as a lack of a 24-h on-site anesthetist) and in places with a low volume of deliveries.[13]

Abortion

Unsafe abortions remain prevalent in many countries. The WHO estimates that one in eight pregnancy-related deaths results from unsafe abortions.[19] Abortion-related deaths were reported to be the highest in certain parts of Latin America and Eastern Europe (Fig. 16). This increase in maternal deaths may be related to unsafe abortions. In contrast, developed countries have a low risk of complications from abortion procedures and hospitalization is rare.[20]

Table 4 estimates hospitalization rates from induced abortion complications from 13 countries between 1989 and 2003. It is most likely an underestimation as many countries do not support abortions.[21] Table 5 estimates of number of women admitted to hospital for induced abortion complications each year in developing world regions and sub regions in 2005.

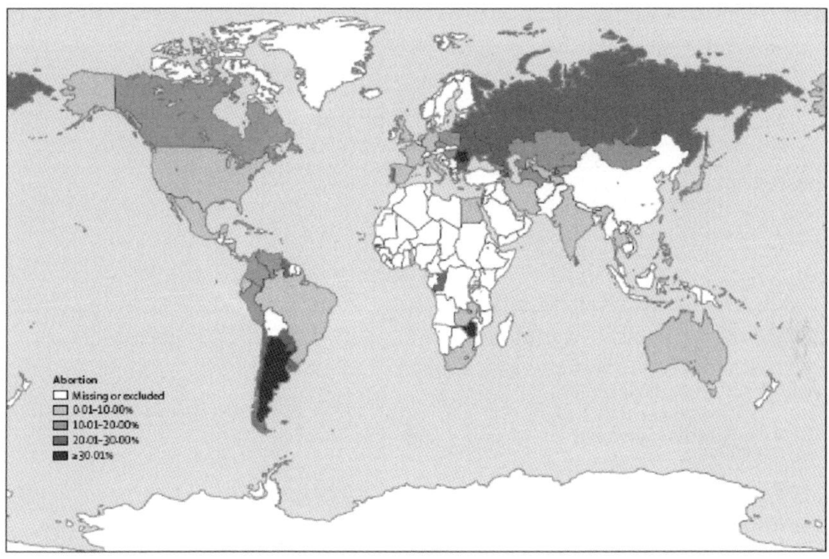

Fig. 16 Geographical distribution of abortions as a cause of maternal death. (Reproduced with the permission of Elsevier © 2006 from Khan *et al.*[3])

It is estimated that 70,000 deaths from unsafe abortions occur annually worldwide. One woman dies every 8 min from unsafe abortion. Many factors are involved. Promotion of increased use of contraception by women, liberalization of abortion laws can be some primary and secondary prevention strategies.[22]

Early and appropriate treatment of post-abortion care for complications will decrease maternal mortality. Another way to prevent maternal death is to make abortion safe, accessible and available. Women living in rural areas with poor

Table 4 Estimated hospitalization rates from induced abortion complications

Continent / Country	Number treated for abortion complications	Annual hospitalization rate for abortion complications/1000 women
Africa		
Egypt (1996)	216,000	15.3
Nigeria (1996)	142,200	6.1
Uganda (2002)	85,000	16.4
Asia		
Bangladesh (1995)	71,800	2.8
Pakistan (2002)	197,000	7.0
Philippines (2000))	78,150	4.4
Latin America		
Brazil (1991)	288,700	8.1
Chile (1990)	31,900	10.0
Columbia (1989)	57,700	7.2
Dominican Republic (1990)	16,500	9.8
Guatemala (2003)	21,600	8.6
Mexico (1990)	106,500	5.4
Peru (1998)	50,200	8.6

Adapted from Singh *et al.* [19]

Table 5 Number of women admitted to hospital for induced abortion complications (2005)

Continent / Country	Estimate of annual rate of hospitalization secondary to induced abortion complications per 1000 women
Africa	
Sub-Saharan Africa	7.4
Eastern Africa	10.0
Central Africa	6.0
Southern Africa	8.0
Western Africa	6.0
Northern Africa	12.0
Total	8.8
Asia (excluding Eastern Asia)	
South-central Asia	4.0
South-east Asia	3.0
Western Asia	8.0
Total	4.1
Latin American & Caribbean	
Caribbean	3.0
Central America	8.0
South America	8.0
Total	7.7
Averaged total	**5.7**

Adapted from Singh *et al.* [19]

access to hospitals are at higher risks. The introduction of misoprostol in parts of Asia, sub-Saharan Africa, Latin America and the Caribbean by well-trained individuals is expected to lower abortion-related morbidity and mortality.[23] Political commitments from healthcare providers and policymakers in these countries will be an important step to reduce the health burden of unwanted pregnancies. Unfortunately, the abortion debate is even more polarized in certain countries. The Pan American Health Organization (PAHO) estimates that more than 4 million abortions are done in Latin America each year.[24] This has become a public-health problem as illegal abortions carry a high rate of death and complications. Emergency contraception, widely available to the public at no or minimal cost, could be a compromise. Even putting the issue of early and safe abortion to a popular referendum, as done in Portugal, may result in a significant decrease in maternal death.[24]

CONCLUSIONS

Maternal mortality is a global problem facing all those involved in women's care. Strong health systems are needed to analyze the cause for these deaths. Women living in rural areas or poor women have the highest risk of dying and carry most of the burden. We need to target specific interventions for specific populations and engage healthcare providers as well as policy makers if we are to meet the challenge set during the meeting of the Fifth Millennium Development Goal (MDG) to reduce maternal mortality by 75% by the year 2015.[25,26] Reducing maternal mortality in each community in each country of the world is a sound medical and economical strategy which would benefit every society at large. The use of the Web has made the world 'flat' and readily accessible. Collection of valid and accurate information is essential to address the reasons why mothers die at an alarming rate world-wide. The creation of an international and even virtual Rapid Deployment Task Force made up of experts in the area should be considered. The task force should review the maternal death rates on a regular basis obtained from accurate data and make practical and measurable recommendations.

Standard, simple, practical epidemiological templates should be made available to low-income countries to increase the ability to collect accurate and relevant data. This should be 'transparent', readily accessible via the Web and regularly updated. Monitoring the impact of these recommendations is essential and should be done regularly and independently by an assigned Monitoring Task Force who would review the impact of these recommendations. In a recent article, Campbell *et al.*[27] looked at strategies for reducing maternal mortality. In particular, they addressed the issue of 'what really works'. Strategies to improve effective intrapartum-care appear to be a primary goal.[22] Safe motherhood has been implemented by the international community for more than 20 years. Since that time, Campbell *et al.*[27] estimated that 10 million women died from pregnancy-related events.

Investing in mother's health is a worthwhile investment for every care provider.

What sets worlds in motion is the interplay of differences, their attractions and repulsions. Life is plurality, death is uniformity.[1]

References

1 Stephens C, Porter J, Nettleton C, Willis R. Disappearing, displaced, and undervalued: a call to action for indigenous health worldwide. Lancet 2006; 367: 2019–2028

2 Potts M. Can family planning reduce maternal mortality? J Obset Gynaecol East Cent Africa 1986; 5: 29–35

3 Khan KS, Woldyla D, Say L, Gulmezoglu AM, Van Look P. WHO systematic review of causes of maternal deaths. Lancet 2006; 367: 1066–1074

4 Jowett M. Safe motherhood interventions in low-income countries: an economic justification and evidence of cost effectiveness. Health Policy 2000; 53: 210–228

5 Puffer RR. Family planning issues relating to maternal and infant mortality in the United States. Bull Pan Am Health Organ 1993; 27: 120–134

6 Hill K, El Arifeen S, Koenig M, Al-Sabir A, Jamil K, Raggers H. How should we measure maternal mortality in the developing world? A comparison of household deaths and sibling history approaches. Bull World Health Organ 2006; 84: 173–180

7. CDC. Weekly MMWR, Sept 2004, 1998/47(34); 705–707

8 Ronsmans C, Graham WJ; on behalf of the Lancet Maternal Survival Series Steering Group. Maternal mortality: who, when, where, and why. Lancet 2006; 368: 1189–1200

9 Confidential Enquiries into Maternal Deaths in the United Kingdom. Why mothers die 1997–1999. London: Stationary Office, 2001

10 Li XF, Forney JA, Kotelchuck M, Glover LH. The postpartum period: the key to maternal mortality. Int J Gynaecol Obstet 1996; 54: 1–10

11 World Health Organization. International Classification of Diseases and Related Health Problems, 10th revision. Geneva: WHO, 1992

12 AbouZahr C, Royston E. Maternal mortality: a global factbook. WHO/MCH/MSM/91.3. Geneva: WHO, 1991

13 Atrash HK, Johnson K, Adams M, Cordero J, Howse J. Preconception care for improving perinatal outcomes: The time to act. Matern Child Health J 2006; 10 (Suppl): 3–11.

14 Deneux-Tharaux C, Berg C, Bouvier-Colle MH *et al*. Underreporting of pregnancy-related mortality in the United States and Europe. Obstet Gynecol 2005; 106: 684–692
15 Bouvier-Colle MH, Ould El Joud D, Varnoux N *et al*. Evaluation of the quality of care for severe obstetrical haemorrhage in three French regions. Br J Obstet Gynaecol 2001; 108: 898–903
16 Wildman K, Bouvier-Colle MH. Maternal mortality as an indicator of obstetrical care in Europe. Br J Obstet Gynaecol 2004; 111: 164–169
17 Skupski DW, Lowenwirt IP, Weinbaum FI, Brodsky D, Danek M, Eglinton GS. Improving hospital system for the care of women with major obstetric hemorrhage. Obstet Gynecol 2006; 107: 977–983
18 Chichakli LO, Atrash HK, Mackay AP, Musani AS, Berg CJ. Pregnancy-related mortality in the United States due to hemorrhage: 1979–1992. Obstet Gynecol 1999; 94: 721–725
19 World Health Organization. The prevention and management of unsafe abortion – report of a Technical Working Group. Geneva: WHO, 1992
20 The Allan Guttmaker Institute. Sharing responsibility: women, society and abortion worldwide. New York: The Allan Guttmaker Institute, 1999 <http://www.guttmaker.org/pubs/sharing.pdf>
21 Singh S. Hospital admission resulting from unsafe abortion: estimates from 13 developing countries. Lancet 2006; 368: 1887–1892
22 World Health Organization. Unsafe abortion: global and regional estimates of the incidence of unsafe abortion and associated mortality in 2000, 4th edn. Geneva: WHO, 2004
23 Okonofua F. Abortion and maternal mortality in the developing world. J Obstet Gynaecol Can 2006; 28: 974–979
24 Replogle J. Abortion debate heats up in Latin America. Lancet 2007; 370: 305–306
25 Sachs JD, McArthur JW. The Millennium Project: a plan for meeting the Millennium Development Goals. Lancet 2005; 365: 347–353
26 World Health Organization. The world health report 2005: make every mother and child count. Geneva: WHO, 2005
27 Campbell OMR, Graham WJ. Strategies for reducing maternal mortality: getting on with what works. Lancet 2006; 368: 1284–1299

Stephen P. Munjanja Franz Majoko
Gunilla Lindmark

Trends in safe motherhood programs in sub-Saharan Africa

The risk of women experiencing serious complications or dying during pregnancy, childbirth or the puerperium continues to be high in sub-Saharan Africa.[1,2] A recent report by the World Health Organization (WHO) highlighted the lack of progress in maternal health in this region, and the concern that most countries will not meet the targets of the Millennium Development Goals (MDGs).[3] The major final causes of maternal mortality and morbidity and the socio-economic factors which raise this risk are well known. Over the past three decades, much information on the interventions which health systems can implement to reduce this risk has become available. Eventually, all these interventions have to be delivered to women through programs, which are packages of routines, tests, procedures, prophylactic regimens and treatments designed to take a woman safely through pregnancy. After the first meeting of the Safe Motherhood Initiative,[4] many countries in sub-Saharan Africa either created safe motherhood programs or strengthened existing ones. This chapter reviews the developments within these programs and examines the major trends. Although fetal and neonatal outcomes are obviously important in maternal health care, in the interests of brevity this chapter will concentrate on the mother.

Stephen P. Munjanja MD(Birm) FRCOG (for correspondence)
Senior Lecturer, Department of Obstetrics and Gynaecology, College of Health Sciences, University of Zimbabwe, Zimbabwe
E-mail: spmunjanja@africaonline.co.zw

Franz Majoko MB ChB PhD(Uppsala) FRCOG
Consultant, Department of Obstetrics and Gynaecology, Singleton Hospital, Sketty Lane, Swansea, UK

Gunilla Lindmark MD(Uppsala) PhD(Uppsala)
Professor, Department of Women's and Children's Health, Section of International Maternal and Child Health, Uppsala University, Uppsala, Sweden

TRENDS IN MATERNAL HEALTH INDICATORS

Maternal mortality

The indicator for maternal mortality, the maternal mortality ratio (MMR), is very difficult to estimate in sub-Saharan Africa because the health information systems are of poor quality. There are major methodological challenges in designing studies or surveys to measure the MMR,[5] and the data are often missing or inadequate.[6,7] In industrialised countries, the estimates are derived from vital registration records of births and deaths, but such databases are underdeveloped in sub-Saharan Africa. Instead, most countries use either the direct or indirect sisterhood methods.[8,9] These are methods which are used during demographic health surveys, and the MMR is calculated from the answers to questions about how many sisters of a respondent have ever lived and how many died during pregnancy. The other methods of estimating the MMR, such as the direct survey, census and the reproductive age mortality study (RAMOS), have rarely been used. In a recent report,[9] only Mauritius had ever conducted a cross-sectional direct survey in sub-Saharan Africa, whilst Cape Verde has conducted a RAMOS; otherwise, all the other countries had used sisterhood methods. Statistical modelling has been used to calculate the MMR when estimates from the reliable methods are not available.[2] However, this method produces estimates with wide confidence intervals, which cannot be used to monitor trends or compare between countries, and there is debate about the most appropriate formula to apply.[10]

Since the methods used to derive MMRs in sub-Saharan Africa are associated with varying degrees of uncertainty, the figures need to be interpreted with caution. The *World Health Report 2005* shows that the MMR in sub-Saharan Africa ranges between 24 (Mauritius) and 2000 (Sierra Leone) per 100,000 live-births.[3] In sub-Saharan Africa, the lowest estimates are for Mauritius, Cape Verde and Botswana whose figures are at 100 per 100,000 live-births or below. At the other extreme are Angola, Niger, Malawi, Sierra Leone and Tanzania which have estimates above 1500 per 100,000 live-births. Table 1 shows the figures for some selected sub-Saharan Africa countries. In the table, the MMRs from 1988 were obtained from country reports,[1] whereas the year 2000 data are from statistical

Table 1 Percentage of women delivered by skilled attendants and maternal mortality ratios in some selected sub-Sahara African countries[1,2]

Country	1988		2000	
	Skilled attendants (%)	MMR[1]	Skilled attendants (%)	MMR[2]
Botswana	78	300	94	100
Ethiopia	10	900	6	850
Ghana	42	700	47	540
Kenya	28	400	42	1000
Mauritius	91	130	99	24
Nigeria	45	750	35	800
Senegal	40	750	58	690
South Africa	–	250	89	230
Tanzania	60	600	36	1500
Zimbabwe	79	330	73	1100

modelling.[2] They are presented not to show any trend but to illustrate the levels of magnitude. The continuing high levels of mortality led to a conclusion in a review[11] that: 'whereas there were grounds for optimism in the trends in maternal mortality in parts of North Africa, Latin America, Asia and the middle East, the situation in sub-Saharan Africa remains disquieting'.

The top five causes of maternal deaths have continued to be hemorrhage, hypertensive disorders/eclampsia, post-abortal sepsis, puerperal sepsis and obstructed labor. This did not change during the 12-year period from 1988 to 2000.[1,12] Malaria and now HIV/AIDS are important indirect causes of death although the proportion attributed to them varies greatly between regions.

There are several reasons behind the lack of improvement, or even deterioration in maternal health in sub-Saharan Africa. Most countries in sub-Saharan Africa have experienced economic difficulties in the past three decades, during which real incomes and standards of living dropped. In addition, there were wars, civil strife, droughts and famine in several countries which compounded the economic decline. Countries then embarked on structural adjustment reforms which decreased social and health security for the most needy by reducing public expenditure.

A second major factor was the growth of the HIV/AIDS epidemic; world-wide, this has affected sub-Saharan Africa the most severely. In this region, women of reproductive age are the most affected as a group, with prevalence figures of 5–24%,[13] with a consequent increase in mortality and morbidity during pregnancy. HIV/AIDS causes 6% of maternal deaths in Africa;[12] since North Africa is a region of lower prevalence, this means that the proportion of deaths caused by HIV/AIDS is much higher than this in sub-Saharan Africa. This is borne out by figures from South Africa, Malawi and Zimbabwe.[14–16] Women with immune suppression from HIV infection are more susceptible to death from direct obstetric causes such as severe anemia, puerperal or post-abortal sepsis and post-surgical infections.[17] They are also more susceptible to malaria, an important indirect cause of maternal death in sub-Saharan Africa.[18] Opportunistic infections such as tuberculosis, *Pneumocystis carnii,* and cryptococcal meningitis are increasingly significant causes of deaths in pregnancy.[17,19]

The last major factor responsible for the failure to improve maternal health was the diversion of resources and effort caused by the HIV/AIDS epidemic, and also by the introduction of the concept of 'reproductive health'. The International Conference on Population and Development (ICPD Cairo) laid out a program of action in reproductive health which was adopted by most members of the United Nations.[20] Reproductive health policies developed in sub-Sahara African countries had very wide scope, which included gender activism, family planning, sexually transmitted diseases, HIV/AIDS, safe abortion, domestic violence and many others. Several of these were vertical programs which competed with safe motherhood for scarce resources. HIV/AIDS was obviously an urgent issue to deal with, but the end result was that maternal healthcare suffered from lack of prioritisation.

Maternal morbidity

A complete picture of the morbidity patterns in sub-Saharan Africa cannot be obtained partly because of the difficulty of definitions,[5] but also because many women still deliver at home without skilled attendants and there is no documentation of complications. Even those who deliver in health facilities frequently do not return for postnatal care.[1] Obviously, the severe morbidities will mirror the main causes of maternal deaths described above. About 15% of pregnancies have complications which require emergency care,[21] but no easily comparable population-based data have been published in sub-Saharan Africa. Two population-based reports on morbidity have been published in West Africa. In one paper, 34.8% of pregnant women developed morbidities but the types were not described.[22] Another paper found that care with a skilled attendant reduced the risk of morbidity.[23] Other reports deal with the continuing morbidity from severe anemia,[24] ruptured uterus,[25] and obstetric fistula.[26]

Severe acute maternal morbidity (SAMM) or near-miss event has been proposed as an additional assessment to maternal death in measuring the risk to mothers and the performance of the obstetric services. Episodes of SAMM are more frequent than maternal death and there is the potential to learn from the survival of the women. Reports of monitoring of SAMM in five African countries show that the leading causes are hemorrhage, hypertension, and sepsis.[27–29]

POLICY TRENDS

Political commitment

Following the UN Conference on Population and Development in Cairo in 1994,[20] countries which had signed up to its agenda for reproductive health were expected to show their commitment by enacting laws to facilitate new policies, and to increase the allocation of resources for reproductive health. National leaders have publicly supported the agenda but very few health budgets have reached the target of 15% of total government expenditure which the leaders of the Organisation of African Unity promised in the Abuja

Table 2 Public health expenditure as percentage of gross domestic product (GDP), general government expenditure on health as percentage of general government expenditure and health expenditure per capita in 1998 and 2002 in selected sub-Sahara African countries.[31,32]

	Public health expenditure (% GDP)		General government expenditure on health (% of total)		Health expenditure per capita (US$)	
Country	1998	2002	1998	2002	1998	2002
Botswana	2.7	3.7	5.6	7.5	133	171
Ethiopia	1.7	2.6	9.4	7.6	4	5
Ghana	1.8	2.3	8.9	8.4	19	117
Kenya	2.2	2.2	8.0	8.4	3	19
Mauritius	1.9	2.2	7.0	8.3	120	113
Nigeria	0.2	1.2	7.1	3.3	9	19
Senegal	2.6	2.3	8.3	11.2	23	27
South Africa	3.2	3.5	11.5	10.7	246	206
Tanzania	1.3	2.7	14.3	14.9	–	13
Zimbabwe	3.3	4.4	12.2	12.2	31	118

Declaration.[30] Table 2 shows the public health expenditure as a percentage of gross domestic product, expenditure on health as a percentage of general government expenditure and health expenditure per capita for selected countries in 1998 and 2002.[31,32] It is very difficult to obtain data regarding national expenditure on reproductive health or maternal healthcare. Both poverty and misallocation of funds are factors which result in very low levels of health expenditure per capita. By contrast, the annual health expenditure per capita in Europe is around US$ 2000.

Safe abortion

After ICPD in 1994, sub-Sahara African countries were expected to reduce the risk of unsafe abortion by reforming abortion laws, and improving access to safe abortion care. Deaths from abortion complications have remained in the list of the top five causes of maternal deaths and the risk from induced abortion remains high.[33] South Africa was the exception and the country introduced reform in several areas of reproductive health.[34] The *Choice on Termination of Pregnancy Act* of 1996 in South Africa, which gave the right to women to have termination on demand up to 12 weeks' pregnancy, is held up as an example of an appropriate reaction to the problem. Early reports on how the Act is working in practice are favorable.[35,36]

Between 1996 and 2003, Burkina Faso, Mali, Niger, Guinea, Chad and Benin changed previously restrictive laws to expand the grounds for legal abortion to include rape, incest and fetal impairment. In 2004, Ethiopia also ratified a new clause which, in addition to the above clauses, allows abortion if the woman is physically disabled or, in the case of a minor, if she is physically or psychologically unprepared to be a mother. These changes, which have been recently reviewed,[37] do not offer much grounds for optimism since countries which already have these clauses continue to suffer high mortality from unsafe abortion. Currently, there are no attempts in other sub-Sahara African countries to introduce significant abortion law reform. However, almost all the sub-Sahara African countries have introduced abortion care interventions at health facility level to reduce complications and mortality. The technique of manual vacuum aspiration is replacing the older procedure of sharp curettage but progress is slow because of regulations which limit its use to doctors in some countries. Mortality from abortion complications has not decreased significantly,[38] suggesting that women at-risk are not gaining access to the safe abortion services and that abortion law reform remains a priority.

Health financing

The structural adjustment economic reforms which many sub-Sahara African countries introduced in the 1980s required them to decrease public expenditure and recover the costs for some services. User fees were introduced in many areas of health. The Bamako Initiative, which was adopted by African health ministers in 1987, had the primary aim of increasing availability and resources for essential drugs,[39] but its recommendations began to be implemented in safe motherhood programs. The aims of introducing user fees were to mobilise revenue, promote efficiency, foster equity, support decentralisation and sustainability, improve the quality of service, and encourage community participation in management. At the community level, some projects encouraged villagers to pool funds that could be loaned to those who needed them for emergency care (transport to hospital, drugs and supplies, treatment).[40] In Nigeria and Sierra Leone, projects run by the Prevention of Maternal Mortality Network (PMMN) reported that this increased the utilisation of emergency obstetric services.[41,42]

However, overall evaluation of the experience of structural adjustment policies and user fees in sub-Saharan Africa has shown that most of the original goals have not been achieved, and that utilisation of the services by those at-risk, who were meant to benefit, had declined.[43–45] User fee revenues have been low, their use seems to have worsened rather than improved equity and there was no improvement in the quality of the service, which was crucial in having the concept accepted by the community. Maternal healthcare is a fundamental human right which cannot be rationed according to ability to pay. It is care which is needed even in the absence of symptoms, which makes user fees particularly harmful. In Europe, maternity care is free or heavily subsidised. To date, most sub-Sahara African countries still have user fees but have exempted primary level facilities and poor people from the scheme. Pregnant women still have to pay when they are transferred with complications to referral institutions and this limits their access to emergency obstetric care.[46,47] Uganda removed all user fees in 2000 and its experience has been considered a success.[48]

Although the introduction of structural adjustment policies and the Bamako Initiative are generally considered to have had a negative effect on maternal health, they stimulated interest in the costs of healthcare,[40] and the cost-effectiveness of certain interventions and strategies.[49–51] The cost of basic and comprehensive obstetric services have been quantified in Uganda.[52] An antenatal visit costs US$ 2.21, a normal vaginal delivery US$ 2.71 and a post-natal visit US$ 2.21. A package of four antenatal visits, a normal delivery and two post-natal visits for a low-risk mother would cost US$ 15.97. Care for complications was more expensive (cesarean section US$ 46.71; managing postpartum hemorrhage US$ 33.44; managing eclampsia US$ 159.66; managing post-abortal complications US$ 12.10; managing puerperal sepsis US$ 8.76). An annual allocation of US$ 2.00 per capita was needed for all women to have required basic and comprehensive obstetric care. The total health expenditure per capita by Uganda for the same year was US$ 14.00.[31]

Both governments and donors have, up to now, funded many projects in reproductive health (including maternal healthcare) in a vertical manner. This causes duplication of certain activities and inefficient use of funds. It is now being suggested that a sector-wide approach to funding and implementation offers maternal health services the opportunity to benefit from other resources within the health system.[53] Uganda has already reported its early experience with this approach.[54]

STRATEGIES FOR MATERNAL HEALTHCARE DELIVERY

There has been a recent evaluation of the strategies that have been used to deliver maternal healthcare.[55] The interest in strategies arises partly from the fact that most sub-Sahara African countries have multiple levels of care for maternal health. In all sub-Sahara African countries, there are at least four and frequently more levels of maternal healthcare, excluding the community level. These levels are: (i) the primary care clinic without maternity beds; (ii) the primary care clinic with maternity beds; (iii) the district hospital; and (iv) the tertiary hospital. Altogether, Tanzania has 6 levels of care,[56] Uganda has 5,[54] and Zimbabwe has 5. The lowest level has little advantage over home deliveries even if there is a skilled worker because there are minimal facilities to cope with emergencies. Planners need to know how to share the resources between the levels in order to obtain the best outcomes in a cost-effective way.

The district model of maternal healthcare delivery

The first reported analysis of strategies examined seven different hypothetical program models of care (conventionally trained traditional birth attendants (TBAs), TBAs with further training, prenatal care for all women, family planning to prevent 20% of pregnancies, health centers, health centers with transport to urban hospital, and health centers with transport to several rural hospitals).[57] The cost-effective analysis showed that investment in health centers and rural hospitals offered the greatest opportunity to save lives per dollar spent. Training of TBAs was the least cost-effective strategy.

In another study in Nigeria, the primary centers and referral hospital were strengthened by re-stocking of equipment and supplies, and giving the midwives communication and life-saving skills. This resulted in an increase in the number of institutional deliveries and a decrease in the prevalence of prolonged labor, postpartum hemorrhage, postpartum sepsis and still-births.[58] This report identified the four major steps that require attention in order to promote survival of the mother and her new-born as: (i) recognition of the problem; (ii) decision making regarding care; (iii) access to care; and (iv) quality of care.

The third analysis of strategy reviewed four models of care described by the organisational characteristics relating to where women give birth and who performs the deliveries. These were: Model 1 – deliveries are conducted at home by a community member who has received brief training; Model 2 – delivery takes place at home but is conducted by a professional; Model 3 – delivery is performed by a professional in a basic essential obstetrical care facility; and Model 4 – all women give birth in a comprehensive essential obstetric care facility with the help of professionals.[59] There was no evidence that Model 1 could reduce the MMR to less than 100 per 100,000 live-births. Models 2–4 in combination had reduced the MMR to 50 or less per 100,000. However, Model 4 did not, on its own, reduce the MMR to less than 100 per 100, 000.

The WHO recommendations for maternal healthcare delivery use the district model. Within the district, only two levels of care are recognised. Previously known as levels 1 and 2,[60] but now described as basic and comprehensive emergency obstetric care, they equate loosely with primary care centers with maternity beds and district hospitals conducting operative deliveries. In a district of 500,000, there must be four facilities offering basic emergency obstetric care (BEmOC) and one facility offering comprehensive emergency obstetric care (CEmOC).[21] The other requirements of district maternity care are discussed under emergency obstetric care below.

The above strategic models and the WHO recommendations suggest that sub-Sahara African countries should offer maternity care on a district basis, and that there should only be two levels of care within the district. Some primary care centers should be upgraded to provide BEmOC and the referral (district) centers should be upgraded to provide CEmOC. There should be good transport links from the community to the BEmOC facilities and an efficient referral mechanism from the latter to the CEmOC facility. The district is small enough to allow local planning, implementation and monitoring of the programs, and, crucially, provides for accountability. In many urban areas of sub-Saharan Africa, where the district as a unit of health delivery is not well developed, accountability in the obstetric services is often missing. One of the features of the decline in maternal mortality in Europe was the growth of professionalism and accountability among those caring for women.[61]

PROGRAM INTERVENTIONS

General health and maternal outcome

The general health of women of reproductive age makes a major contribution towards pregnancy outcome. Poor nutrition, malaria and infestation with intestinal parasites result in anemia and general debilitation, reducing the ability of women to cope with pregnancy. In such a situation, HIV/AIDS increases the risk of unfavorable outcome. Unfortunately, there are no programs addressing this issue in sub-Saharan Africa. The potential of mother and child health (MCH) programs in addressing the general health of women should be utilised more than it is at present.

Antenatal care

In sub-Sahara African countries, the traditional model of antenatal care (ANC) has been provided with varying degrees of compliance by both the patients and staff. Across the sub-continent coverage of antenatal care is 69%,[3] which means that nearly one-third of patients do not receive care. Even among those who do, there are many late bookers. The quality of care women receive is often of poor quality due to non-compliance by the staff and unavailability of supplies.[62,63]

In the past three decades, much has been published on the low effectiveness of ANC in preventing maternal mortality and morbidity,[64,65] the value of individual routines[66,67] and assessments of models of care.[68–70] A systematic review by the WHO showed that effective care could be given to low-risk women with a package of proven interventions taking place over 4–6 planned visits.[71] Following the review, WHO published a recommended model of ANC to be used by low-risk women in developing countries.[72] The evidence-based routines which have been included in this model form the basis of what has been called 'focused antenatal care'.

The routines of focused ANC are goal-oriented and of proven effectiveness. The interventions address the top five causes of maternal deaths, and the top five causes of perinatal deaths (birth asphyxia, prematurity, light for gestational age, neonatal sepsis and neonatal jaundice). A routine which is highly appropriate for sub-Saharan Africa is emergency and birth preparedness which the providers should discuss with the woman from 26 weeks onwards. The pregnant woman should be informed of the danger signs of the main complications likely to occur, and she is also asked to make a birth plan which includes arrangements for transport to the hospital, funds for expenses, and care for any children during her absence. In a randomised, controlled trial in which this counselling was introduced, fewer women delivered at home in the intervention arm than in the control arm.[70]

Table 3 shows the contents of the WHO four-visit model, which should be viewed as a basis on which countries may develop their own programs. Interventions may be added according to the demands of their settings as long as they are evidence-based. The interventions and visits for women with complications will depend on the circumstances.

There are several challenges which programs in sub-Saharan Africa face in implementing the changes but only four will be mentioned here:

1. There should be increased coverage of ANC, and the care must be made more attractive to women who currently do not book, or do so very late. No matter how good or focused an ANC program is, it cannot help those who remain outside it. Any service obstacles, including user fees, should be removed to bring in the 31% who currently do not book.

2. The facilities should have the necessary resources and the staff should have the skills and right attitude to deliver quality care. Studies have shown that the quality of ANC in the screening and treatment for common conditions such as anemia[62] and hypertension[63,73] can be very poor. Programs which have introduced goal-oriented routines should ensure that staff should comply with the protocols.[74]

3. The service should improve the satisfaction of women with care, to increase their compliance with advice and make it more likely that they will deliver at the institution. ANC is sometimes the first or only regular contact women are likely to have with the service for their own health but, so far, the emphasis has been on the routines and not on psychological outcomes. Client satisfaction with antenatal care has received little attention at program level in sub-Saharan Africa but the few reports available show that there is much room for improvement.[75,76] Women spend several hours waiting for a consultation with the midwife which will last 3 minutes. Some health workers exhibit poor communication skills or inappropriate attitudes. These problems have been given by women as reasons for poor utilisation of ANC and programs should start taking them seriously.

4. Antenatal care should provide a realistic pathway for women to receive a higher level of care when complications are detected. Transport is a particular problem and no country has solved this satisfactorily. Simply on the basis of cost and potential, a motorcycle ambulance seems the cheapest way for every BEmOC to have its own transport to the CEmOC. The referral center should have the capacity to admit all the women with complications, such as antepartum hemorrhage, pregnancy hypertension, *etc.*, even if the possibility to undertake sophisticated investigations is

Table 3 WHO antenatal care model (adapted from [72])

	First visit 8–12 weeks	Second visit 26 weeks	Third visit 32 weeks	Fourth visit 38+ weeks
Goals	Assess eligibility for basic ANC	Exclude PIH, multiple pregnancy. Check fetal growth	Assess fetal growth, exclude PIH, anemia, multiple pregnancy	Assess fetal growth, exclude malpresentation, PIH
ACTIVITIES History	Apply classifying form to all women	Assess significant symptoms	Assess significant symptoms	Assess significant symptoms
Examination	Complete general, systemic and obstetrical	Anemia, blood pressure, fetal growth, multiple pregnancy	Anemia, blood pressure, fetal growth, multiple pregnancy	Blood pressure, fetal growth, malpresentation
Investigations	Hemoglobin, syphilis, blood/Rh group HIV, Bacteriuria	± Bacteriuria	Hemoglobin, ± bacteriuria	± Bacteriuria
Treatments	Syphilis and bacteriuria if indicated	Bacteriuria if indicated	Bacteriuria if indicated	Bacteriuria if indicated
Prophylaxis	Tetanus toxoid, iron and folate, ± IPT, ± ARV	Tetanus toxoid, iron and folate, ± IPT, ± ARV	Iron and folate, ± ARV	Iron and folate, ± ARV
Counselling	General pregnancy and nutrition, ± referral	Emergency preparedness, ± referral	Childbirth and emergency preparedness, ± referral	Childbirth and emergency preparedness, ± referral

limited. This may result in the CEmOC booking up to 45% of the deliveries in the district, but those thought to have minor complications can be housed in a maternity waiting home whilst awaiting delivery (see below). This is what already happens in Zimbabwe, where the CEmOC facilities conduct 35–45% of deliveries in the district.

In order to improve the effectiveness of ANC, programs should perform regular audit, starting with process outcomes which are easier to implement. ANC coverage, timing and frequency of visits, quality of care and satisfaction with care can all be monitored using a combination of routinely collected data and periodic surveys.

Maternity waiting homes

The maternity waiting home (MWH) has been proposed as an antenatal intervention to bring women closer to emergency obstetric care. Typically, an MWH is a dormitory to house women in advanced pregnancy next to a CEOC facility. Some of the women are referred there because of problems such as previous cesarean section, but others are admitted because of distance and transport issues. The WHO has reported on the experience of Ethiopia, Nigeria, Malawi, Tanzania and Zimbabwe with MWHs.[77] The effectiveness of MWHs has not been studied rigorously with controlled trials, although some reports have shown favorable effects of stay in a MWH on maternal and perinatal outcomes.[78,79] Within programs, MWHs have not been used consistently, and their construction and administration has often been viewed as a community initiative. The main problem with the MWH is that, unless there is enough capacity to house many women, the referrals will be on the basis of risk, meaning that the majority of women will still face complications away from facilities. In districts where there is only one MWH at the CEmOC facility, its extensive use can cause an unsustainable imbalance in workload as fewer women will deliver at the BEmOC facilities.

The answer to greater use of MWH concept, which is good in principle, may lie in building MWHs at all BEmOC facilities. If in one district there are five MWHs, one each at the four BEmOC and the CEmOC facilities (see below) then perhaps the proportion of women housed in them will approach 100% of the pregnant women in the district. Housing all women from 37 weeks has the potential to prevent two-thirds of the maternal deaths provided the referral mechanisms are functioning. Such MWHs would need to be more attractive to the women than at present, and would need to be built by government to standard physical specifications and not be left to the community.

Skilled attendance

In sub-Saharan Africa, the majority of deaths from direct obstetric causes are preventable and occur because of the absence skilled care during emergencies or childbirth. The availability of trained traditional birth attendants (TBAs) cannot prevent these deaths.[80,81] The WHO and other organisations have defined a skilled attendant as: 'an accredited health professional-such as a midwife, doctor or nurse-who has been educated and trained to proficiency in the skills needed to manage normal (uncomplicated) pregnancies, childbirth, and the immediate postnatal period, and in the identification, management and referral of complications in women and new-borns'.[82] This joint statement was made together with the International Confederation of Midwives (ICM) and the International Federation of Gynaecologists and Obstetricians (FIGO). Since a skilled attendant needs the support of equipment, drugs and other resources to be effective, it was quickly realised that what women needed was skilled attendance which is defined as: 'the presence of a skilled attendant in an enabling environment, providing adequate care during the antenatal period, labor, delivery and the postpartum period'.

Skilled attendance is such an accurate marker of the quality of maternal services that it has been adopted by the UN as an indicator of maternal health for the MDGs. Countries have agreed to scale-up skilled attendance to 100% by the year 2015.[83] Providing an enabling environment if the financial resources are available will be easier than training, employing and retaining the skilled staff. The infrastructural improvements will mainly involve upgrading existing lower level facilities rather than building new ones.

Staffing the facilities with skilled attendants will be more difficult. Until about 20 years ago, most sub-Sahara African countries had enough training capacity to supply their establishment posts, although this was less than what was required. The economic difficulties experienced by most sub-Sahara African countries in the last three decades combined with the structural adjustment policies affected the living standards of health workers, who emigrated in large numbers to work elsewhere.[84,85] Internally, many workers left the public for the private sector, or joined non-governmental organisations working outside the clinical area. The HIV/AIDS epidemic also had a major effect on staff numbers. The mortality from the disease affected workers as their HIV prevalence is the same as that of the general population. The risk of occupational HIV exposure is highest in midwifery and obstetrics amongst the nursing and medical specialities, which reduced the numbers joining these professions. Barrier protection and chemoprophylaxis are not always available. Emigration is sometimes caused by the desire to continue working in the same specialty but in a country with a lower HIV prevalence. As a result of these factors, the number of women delivered by skilled attendants in Zimbabwe, Tanzania and Nigeria actually went down between 1988 and 2000 (Table 1). Botswana, Mauritius and South Africa have the highest figures of skilled attendants at delivery, and they can realistically expect to reach 100% by the year 2015.

Since about 15% of pregnancies have complications which may require operative or intensive care, the right mix of skills is also necessary. The care needed for CEmOC means that skilled attendants alone, as defined above, cannot prevent all deaths.[86] Doctors or other health workers to whom their tasks can be delegated should be available for about 15% of the women. In Tanzania, Burkina Faso, Malawi, the Democratic Republic of Congo and Mozambique, non-medically qualified practitioners have been trained to perform cesarean sections and other obstetric procedures with acceptable results.[87,88] In the short- and medium-term, this may be one solution to the skills' shortage crisis for some countries. However, in other countries, despite the inequalities in access to EmOC between urban and rural areas, and between the public and private sectors in the cities, doctors remain opposed to midwives and other providers gaining essential surgical skills.

Emergency obstetric care

Providing access to emergency obstetric care is now the aim and central activity within programs in sub-Saharan Africa to reduce maternal mortality and morbidity. A strategy which emphasises the importance of EmOC has been adopted by the Africa Union.[89] The barriers to access when complications have arisen led to the model of the 'Three Delays' – delay in deciding to seek care; delay in reaching appropriate care; and delay in receiving care at facilities.[90] This model was used to study the impact of interventions developed to reduce maternal mortality in West Africa by the Prevention of Maternal Mortality Network. Multidisciplinary teams from 12 centers in Nigeria, Ghana and Sierra Leone working with Columbia University, carried out community- and hospital-based interventions over 8 years. Overall, the results showed that: (i) utilisation of the services by the women improved; (ii) more women with complications were seen and treated; (iii) the cesarean section rate went up in most centers; (iv) case fatality rates went down; and (v) in one center, admission-to-treatment intervals became shorter.[91] The network also showed that improving EmOC facilities usually involved upgrading existing centers, and was both feasible and affordable. Community schemes to finance transport to facilities were not as successful as the other interventions and will be difficult to duplicate in other parts of sub-Saharan Africa.

Guidelines for monitoring the use and availability of EmOC have been published by UNICEF/WHO/UNFPA, together with the signal functions of basic and comprehensive EmOC.[21] The variables used for monitoring are now called the 'UN process indicators'. The essential (signal) functions required at a basic EmOC facility are:

- parenteral antibiotics
- parenteral oxytoxics
- parenteral anticonvulsants
- manual removal of placenta
- manual vacuum aspiration of retained products of conception
- assisted vaginal delivery.

The two extra functions in addition to the six above required for comprehensive EmOC are:

- cesarean section
- blood transfusion.

At a district or population level, the UN process indicators which have been recommended to countries are shown in Table 4. Publication of these guidelines has stimulated efforts by countries to evaluate progress in their programs, and to compare with other countries. Table 5 shows the results of reports published from studies in several sub-Sahara African countries.[92–97] The table shows that population coverage for CEmOC is adequate for most countries except Ethiopia and Southern Sudan. Availability of facilities

Table 4 UN process indicators for monitoring the availability and utilisation of obstetric services (adapted from UNICEF guidelines[21]).

Process indicator	Definition	Numerator	Denominator	Recommended level
Availability of EmOC	No. of facilities providing EmOC	No. of facilities providing basic or comprehensive EmOC	500,000 population	1 CEmOC facility per 500,000; 4 BEmOC facilities per 500,000
Proportion of all birth in EmOC facilities	Proportion of all birth in EmOC facilities	No. of births delivered in EmOC facilities in time period	No. of births in are in same time period	> 15%
Met need for obstetric complications	Proportion of women with obstetric complications delivered at EmOC facilities	No. of women with obstetric complications treated in EmOC facilities in time period	No. of women with obstetric complications in same time period	100%
Cesarean sections as proportion of all births	Cesarean sections as proportion of all births	No. of cesarean sections in time period	No. of births in the same time period	5–15%
Case fatality rate	Proportion of women obstetric complications admitted to a facility who die	No. of deaths in a facility due to specific complications during time period	No. of women treated for specific complications in facility in the same time period	< 1%

providing basic EmOC is inadequate in all countries, and the remaining indicators show poor availability and use of EmOC. The cesarean section rates are very low, indicating that although CEmOC coverage is adequate, women with complications are failing to access or utilise it. Overall, these results show the remaining challenges in providing EmOC. Sub-Sahara African countries have many small facilities most of them providing non-basic emergency care. There is quantity but not quality. A process of consolidation is required, in which, based on some characteristics (such as workload, geographical access, communication links, *etc.*), some lower level facilities are upgraded to BEmOC status. It will also be easier to strengthen referral mechanisms between few but effective BEmOC centers and the CEmOC facility than between numerous primary centers and the CEmOC facility.

There are problems with the use of UN process indicators, especially in countries with multiple levels of facilities. The proportion of women with access to EmOC underestimates the proportion being delivered in institutions, because the unavailability of any one signal function, even if the other five are present, disqualifies a facility from BEmOC status. Assisted vaginal delivery seems to be the function that is usually unavailable in non-BEmOC facilities. In countries

Table 5 UN process indicators for EmOC for selected sub-Sahara African countries[92–97]

Country year and population base	Indicators					
	No. of CEmOC per 500,000 population (expected = 1)	No. of BEmOC per 500,000 population (expected = 4)	Proportion of all births in EmOC facilities (expected > 15%)	Met need (expected 100%)	C/s as a proportion of all deliveries (expected 5–15%)	Case fatality rate (expected < 1%)
Ethiopia 2001 (1 district)	0.2	0.4	7.5	8.7	< 0.1	7.2
Kenya 2003 (1 province)	1.6	1.0	8.8	3.0	0.6	5
Malawi 2000 (1 region)	1.7	0.4	30	19.8	1.6	2
Mozambique 2000 (3 districts)	1.3	0.3	12	7.8	1.0	4.7–11.1
Niger 2000 (national)	1	2.4	Not known	19.8	0.5	Not known
Rwanda 2000 (3 districts)	1	Not known	10	30–35	2.0–3.0	2.8–16
Senegal 2001 (national)	1.6	0.26	9.7	11.5	1.1	4.0
Sudan 2003 (1 district)	0.5	0.5	1.5	5	0.1	7.0
Tanzania 2000 (2 districts)	1	Not known	10.3–17.3	14.5–14.9	0.8–1.3	3.3–3.8
Uganda 2003 (national)	1.2	1	5	5	1.0	7.2

where the coverage of assisted deliveries is low, with few obstetric complications seen within the health system, the indicators cannot be used as a tool to monitor the effect of maternal health care programs on maternal mortality.[98]

EMERGING TRENDS

Quality of care

In sub-Saharan Africa, poor quality care limits the benefits which pregnant women can obtain from evidence-based interventions. Apart from the examples of poor quality of ANC in Tanzania and South Africa which have been given above, there are reports of poor quality care in maternal healthcare generally[99] and in the care of obstetric emergencies.[100] In Dar Es Salaam, tests for proteinuria were only available to 33% of women, which meant that antenatal care was not effective in detecting eclampsia, a common complication in that country.[101] In addition to the technical inputs required, programs will need committed health workers who adhere to the clinical guidelines. In rural areas, facilities may not be used because of the perception in the community that the quality of care provided is low.

It has been suggested that maternal death audit is one way to improve quality of care. A recent WHO publication highlighted the important role of maternal death review in reducing maternal mortality.[102] For maternal deaths, the types of review recommended were facility-based audit, confidential enquiries and maternal verbal autopsy. For complications, the publication recommended clinical audit, criterion-based and near-miss audit. In sub-Sahara African countries, some of these approaches were already being used, although not in the formalised and comprehensive manner now envisaged. It is important that programs set aside funds for this important activity in order for it to be integrated into clinical practice rather than remain as a voluntary academic exercise. There are already reports of improved clinical care in West Africa where these interventions have been introduced.[103,104]

SUMMARY

In sub-Sahara African countries, the maternal mortality and morbidity remain high and may be increasing in some areas. There have been very few population-based studies to obtain accurate data and the estimates available depend on methods which have varying degrees of uncertainty. The factors responsible for the lack of improvement include general socio-economic decline, the HIV/AIDS epidemic, and the loss of skilled manpower due to unfavorable conditions of service. The stated political commitments by governments have not resulted in meaningful increases in expenditure on health. Women continue to die from unsafe abortion because legal reform has not taken place in most countries.

Attempts to recover some health costs from patients did not prove a success and the policy of user fees has been amended or withdrawn in several countries. Current strategies for the delivery of maternity care are based on a district model in which several centers equipped and staffed to handle basic obstetric emergencies are linked with a good referral mechanism to a comprehensive emergency obstetric care facility. Programs currently emphasise focused antenatal care, skilled attendance and emergency obstetric care. The quality of care is very variable in programs and this should be addressed if more women are to be persuaded to have deliveries in institutions. Audit of maternal deaths or complications when performed in a formalised and comprehensive manner can improve the quality of maternity care.

The progress made has been in identifying evidence-based interventions and standards of care. It is now up to country programs to deliver them to women in the most cost-effective way. Even within the limited budgets of these countries, there is room for improvement.

KEY POINTS FOR CLINICAL PRACTICE

- The methods used up to now to measure the maternal mortality ratio in SSA are not appropriate for monitoring trends of this indicator.
- Legal reforms and good clinical care for unsafe abortion remain priorities in the region.
- The continuum of clinical care in pregnancy should include focused antenatal care, skilled attendance and emergency obstetric care.
- `User fees' reduce access to EmOC, nd a review should be conducted to justify continuing with such a policy.
- Maternity waiting shelters are an appropriate intervention to increase the proportion of rural women delivering in facilities.
- Quality of care assessments such as maternal death reviews and audits should be integrated into programs.

ACKNOWLEDGEMENTS

S.P. Munjanja and F. Majoko would like to thank the Swedish International Development Cooperation Agency (SIDA) for assistance during the writing of this paper.

References

1 AbouZahr C, Royston E. Maternal mortality. A global factbook. Geneva: World Health Organization, 1991
2 World Health Organization. Maternal mortality in 2000: estimates developed by WHO, UNICEF, UNFPA. Geneva: World Health Organization, 2004
3 World Health Organization. Make every mother and child count. The World Health Report 2005. Geneva: World Health Organization, 2005
4 Starrs A. Preventing the tragedy of maternal deaths. International Safe Motherhood Conference. Nairobi: WHO/UNICEF/UNFPA/World Bank, 1987
5 Campbell O, Graham W. Measuring maternal morbidity and mortality: levels and trends. Research paper no.2. London: Maternal and Child Epidemiology Unit, London School of Hygiene and Tropical Medicine, 1990

6 Campbell O. Measuring progress in safe motherhood programs: uses and limitations of health outcome indicators. In: Berer M, Sundari Ravindran T. (eds) Safe Motherhood Initiatives: Critical Issues. Oxford: Blackwell, 1999
7 Gulmezoglu AM, Say L, Betran AP, Villar J, Piaggio G. WHO systematic review of maternal mortality and morbidity: methodological issues and challenges. BMC Med Res Methodol 2004; 4: 16
8 Graham W, Brass W, Snow RW. Estimating maternal mortality: the sisterhood method. Stud Fam Plan 1989; 20: 125–135
9 Betran AP, Wojdyla D, Posner SF, Gulmezoglu AM. National estimates for maternal mortality: an analysis based on the WHO systematic review of maternal mortality and morbidity. BMC Public Health 2005; 5: 131
10 Hakkert R. Country estimates of maternal mortality: an alternative model. Stat Med 2001; 20: 3505–3524
11 AbouZahr C, Wardlaw T. Maternal mortality at the end of a decade: signs of progress? Bull World Health Organ 2001; 79: 561–568
12 Khan KS, Wojdyla D, Say L, Gulmezoglu AM, Van Look PF. WHO analysis of causes of maternal death: a systematic review. Lancet 2006; 367: 1066–1074
13 UNIAIDS/WHO. Epidemic update – December 2002. UNIAIDS/02.46E. Geneva: UNIAIDS, 2002
14 Majoko F, Chipato T, Iliff V. Trends in maternal mortality for the Greater Harare Maternity Unit: 1976 to 1997. Cent Afr J Med 2001; 47: 199–203
15 Moodley J. Saving mothers: 1999–2001. S Afr Med J 2003; 93: 364–366
16 Bicego G, Boerma JT, Ronsmans C. The effect of AIDS on maternal mortality in Malawi and Zimbabwe. Aids 2002; 16: 1078–1081
17 McIntyre J. Mothers infected with HIV. Br Med Bull 2003; 67: 127–135
18 Brentlinger PE, Behrens CB, Micek MA. Challenges in the concurrent management of malaria and HIV in pregnancy in sub-Saharan Africa. Lancet Infect Dis 2006; 6: 100–111
19 Khan M, Pillay T, Moodley JM, Connolly CA. Maternal mortality associated with tuberculosis-HIV-1 co-infection in Durban, South Africa. Aids 2001; 15: 1857–1863
20 United Nations. Action for the 21st century: reproductive health and rights for all. Program of Action. International Conference for Population and Development. Cairo: United Nations, 1994
21 UNICEF. Guidelines for monitoring the availability and use of obstetric services. New York: UNICEF/WHO/UNFPA, 1997
22 Salihu HM, Adamu YM, Aliyu ZY, Aliyu MH. Pregnancy-associated morbidity in Northern Nigeria. J Obstet Gynaecol 2004; 24: 367–371
23 de Bernis L, Dumont A, Bouillin D, Gueye A, Dompnier JP, Bouvier-Colle MH. Maternal morbidity and mortality in two different populations of Senegal: a prospective study (MOMA survey). Br J Obstet Gynaecol 2000; 107: 68–74
24 Geelhoed D, Agadzi F, Visser L *et al.* Maternal and fetal outcome after severe anemia in pregnancy in rural Ghana. Acta Obstet Gynecol Scand 2006; 85: 49–55
25 Hofmeyr GJ, Say L, Gulmezoglu AM. WHO systematic review of maternal mortality and morbidity: the prevalence of uterine rupture. Br J Obstet Gynaecol 2005; 112: 1221–1228
26 Ezegwui HU, Nwogu-Ikojo EE. Vesico-vaginal fistula in Eastern Nigeria. J Obstet Gynaecol 2005; 25: 589–591
27 Mantel GD, Buchmann E, Rees H, Pattinson RC. Severe acute maternal morbidity: a pilot study of a definition for a near-miss. Br J Obstet Gynaecol 1998; 105: 985–990
28 Kaye D, Mirembe F, Aziga F, Namulema B. Maternal mortality and associated near-misses among emergency intrapartum obstetric referrals in Mulago Hospital, Kampala, Uganda. East Afr Med J 2003; 80: 144–149
29 Filippi V, Ronsmans C, Gohou V *et al.* Maternity wards or emergency obstetric rooms? Incidence of near-miss events in African hospitals. Acta Obstet Gynecol Scand 2005; 84: 11–16
30 Economic Commission of Africa. Abuja Declaration. Abuja, Nigeria: Organisation of African Unity, 2001
31 World Bank. World Development Indicators. Washington, DC: World Bank, 2000
32 World Bank. World Development Indicators. Washington, DC: World Bank, 2005
33 Goyaux N, Alihonou E, Diadhiou F, Leke R, Thonneau PF. Complications of induced

abortion and miscarriage in three African countries: a hospital-based study among WHO collaborating centers. Acta Obstet Gynecol Scand 2001; 80: 568–573
34 Cooper D, Morroni C, Orner P *et al*. Ten years of democracy in South Africa: documenting transformation in reproductive health policy and status. Reprod Health Matters 2004; 12: 70–85
35 Mhlanga RE. Abortion: developments and impact in South Africa. Br Med Bull 2003; 67: 115–126
36 Buchmann EJ, Mensah K, Pillay P. Legal termination of pregnancy among teenagers and older women in Soweto, 1999–2001. S Afr Med J 2002; 92: 729–731
37 Brookman-Amissah E, Moyo JB. Abortion law reform in sub-Saharan Africa: no turning back. Reprod Health Matters 2004; 12 (24 Suppl): 227–234
38 Thonneau PF. Maternal mortality and unsafe abortion: a heavy burden for developing countries. Studies in Health Services Organisation and Policy 2001; 17: 151–174
39 UNICEF. The Bamako Initiative. New York: UNICEF, 1987
40 Borghi J. What is the cost of maternal health care and how can it be financed? Studies in Health Services Organisation and Policy 2001; 17: 247–296
41 Chiwuzie J, Okojie O, Okolocha C *et al*. Emergency loan funds to improve access to obstetric care in Ekpoma, Nigeria. The Benin PMM Team. Int J Gynaecol Obstet 1997; 59 (Suppl 2): S231–S236
42 Fofana P, Samai O, Kebbie A, Sengeh P. Promoting the use of obstetric services through community loan funds, Bo, Sierra Leone. The Bo PMM Team. Int J Gynaecol Obstet 1997; 59 (Suppl 2): S225–S230
43 Gilson L. The lessons of user fee experience in Africa. Health Policy Plan 1997; 12: 273–285
44 Ogunbekun I, Adeyi O, Wouters A, Morrow RH. Costs and financing of improvements in the quality of maternal health services through the Bamako Initiative in Nigeria. Health Policy Plan 1996; 11: 369–384
45 World Bank. World Development Report 2004. Making services work for poor people. Washington, DC: World Bank, 2004
46 Kowalewski M, Mujinja P, Jahn A. Can mothers afford maternal health care costs? User costs of maternity services in rural Tanzania. Afr J Reprod Health 2002; 6: 65–73
47 Sondo B, Testa J, Kone B. [The financial costs of health care: a follow-up survey of women having a high-risk delivery]. Santé 1997; 7: 33–37
48 Health Systems Resource Guide. User fees for health: key issues. 2006 [cited 11/6/2006] <http://www.eldis.org/healthsystems/userfees/>
49 Fox-Rushby JA, Foord F. Costs, effects and cost-effectiveness analysis of a mobile maternal health care service in West Kiang, The Gambia. Health Policy 1996; 35: 123–143
50 Stringer JS, Rouse DJ, Vermund SH, Goldenberg RL, Sinkala M, Stinnett AA. Cost-effective use of nevirapine to prevent vertical HIV transmission in sub-Saharan Africa. J Acquir Immune Defic Syndr 2000; 24: 369–377
51 Adam T, Lim SS, Mehta S *et al*. Cost effectiveness analysis of strategies for maternal and neonatal health in developing countries. BMJ 2005; 331: 1107
52 Weissman E, Sentumbwe-Mugisa O, Mbonye A. Costing Safe Motherhood in Uganda. In: Berer M, Sundari Ravindran T. (eds) Safe Motherhood Initiatives: Critical Issues. Oxford: Blackwell, 1999
53 Goodburn E, Campbell O. Reducing maternal mortality in the developing world: sector-wide approaches may be the key. BMJ 2001; 322: 917–920
54 Orinda V, Kakande H, Kabarangira J, Nanda G, Mbonye AK. A sector-wide approach to emergency obstetric care in Uganda. Int J Gynaecol Obstet 2005; 91: 285–291; discussion 283–284
55 De Brouwere V, Van Lerberghe W. Safe Motherhood Strategies: a review of the evidence. In: Van Lerberghe W, Kegels G, De Brouwere W. (eds) Studies in Health Services Organisation and Policy. Antwerp: European Commission, 2001
56 Urassa DP. Quality aspects of maternal health care in Tanzania. PhD Thesis, Uppsala University, Uppsala, 2004 <urn:nbn:se.uu.diva-4221>
57 Maine D. Safe motherhood programs: options and issues. New York: Centre for Population and Family Health, School of Public Health, Columbia University, 1991
58 Kwast BE. Reduction of maternal and perinatal mortality in rural and peri-urban

settings: what works? Eur J Obstet Gynecol Reprod Biol 1996; 69: 47–53
59 Koblinsky MA, Campbell O, Heichelheim J. Organizing delivery care: what works for safe motherhood? Bull World Health Organ 1999; 77: 399–406
60 World Health Organization. Mother–Baby Package: implementing safe motherhood in countries. Geneva: World Health Organization, 1996
61 Van Lerberghe W, De Brouwere V. Of blind alleys and things that have worked: history's lessons on reducing maternal mortality. Studies in Health Services Organisation and Policy 2001; 17: 7–33
62 Urassa DP, Carlstedt A, Nystrom L, Massawe SN, Lindmark G. Quality assessment of the antenatal program for anaemia in rural Tanzania. Int J Qual Health Care 2002; 14: 441–448
63 le Roux E, Pattinson RC, Tsaku W, Makin JD. Does successful completion of the Perinatal Education Programme result in improved obstetric practice? S Afr Med J 1998; 88 (2 Suppl): 180–182, 184, 187
64 Rooney C. Antenatal care and maternal health: how effective is it? A review of the evidence. Geneva: World Health Organization, 1992
65 Carroli G, Rooney C, Villar J. How effective is antenatal care in preventing maternal mortality and serious morbidity? An overview of the evidence. Paediatr Perinat Epidemiol 2001; 15 (Suppl 1): 1–42
66 Cochrane Library. Pregnancy and Childbirth. Cochrane Database Syst Rev 2005(7)
67 World Health Organization. Reproductive Health Library. Geneva: World Health Organization, 2005
68 Munjanja SP, Lindmark G, Nystrom L. Randomised controlled trial of a reduced-visits programme of antenatal care in Harare, Zimbabwe. Lancet 1996; 348: 364–369
69 Villar J, Ba'aqeel H, Piaggio G *et al.* WHO antenatal care randomised trial for the evaluation of a new model of routine antenatal care. Lancet 2001; 357: 1551–1564
70 Majoko F. Assessing antenatal care in rural Zimbabwe. PhD Thesis, Uppsala University, Uppsala, 2005 <http://urn.kb.se/resolve?urn=urn:nbn:se:uu:diva-6018>
71 Carroli G, Villar J, Piaggio G *et al.* WHO systematic review of randomised controlled trials of routine antenatal care. Lancet 2001; 357: 1565–1570
72 World Health Organization. WHO Antenatal Care Randomised Trial: manual for the implementation of the new model. Geneva: World Health Organization, 2002
73 Urassa DP, Nystrom L, Carlstedt A, Msamanga GI, Lindmark G. Management of hypertension in pregnancy as a quality indicator of antenatal care in rural Tanzania. Afr J Reprod Health 2003; 7: 69–76
74 Majoko F, Nystrom L, Munjanja SP, Lindmark G. Effectiveness of referral system for antenatal and intra-partum problems in Gutu district, Zimbabwe. J Obstet Gynaecol 2005; 25: 656–661
75 Mathole T, Lindmark G, Majoko F, Ahlberg BM. A qualitative study of women's perspectives of antenatal care in a rural area of Zimbabwe. Midwifery 2004; 20: 122–132
76 Mwaniki PK, Kabiru EW, Mbugua GG. Utilisation of antenatal and maternity services by mothers seeking child welfare services in Mbeere District, Eastern Province, Kenya. East Afr Med J 2002; 79: 184–187
77 World Health Organization. Maternity waiting homes. Geneva: World Health Organization, 1996
78 Millard P, Bailey J, Hanson J. Antenatal village stay and pregnancy outcome in rural Zimbabwe. Cent Afr J Med 1991; 37: 1–4
79 Chandramohan D, Cutts F, Chandra R. Effects of a maternity waiting home on adverse maternal outcomes and the validity of antenatal risk screening. Int J Gynaecol Obstet 1994; 46: 279–284
80 World Health Organization. Reduction of maternal mortality: a joint WHO/UNFPA/UNICEF/World Bank statement. Geneva: World Health Organization, 1999
81 Bergstrom S, Goodburn E. The role of traditional birth attendants in the reduction of maternal mortality. Studies in Health Services Organisation and Policy 2001; 17: 77–96
82 World Health Organization. Making pregnancy safer: the critical role of the skilled attendant. A joint statement by WHO, ICM and FIGO. Geneva: World Health Organization, 2004

83 United Nations. Millennium Development Goals. New York: United Nations, 2000
84 World Health Organization. Working together for health. The World Health Report 2006. Geneva: World Health Organization, 2006
85 Chen L, Evans T, Anand S *et al*. Human resources for health: overcoming the crisis. Lancet 2004; 364: 1984–1990
86 Graham W, Bell J, Bullough C. Can skilled attendance at delivery reduce maternal mortality in developing countries? Studies in Health Services Organisation and Policy 2001; 17: 97–130
87 Pereira C, Bugalho A, Bergstrom S, Vaz F, Cotiro M. A comparative study of caesarean deliveries by assistant medical officers and obstetricians in Mozambique. Br J Obstet Gynaecol 1996; 103: 508–512
88 Kowalewski M, Jahn A. Health professionals for maternity services: experience on covering the population with quality maternity care. Studies in Health Services Organisation and Policy 2001; 17: 131–150
89 Africa Regional Committee of WHO. Road map for accelerating the attainment of the millennium development goals relating to maternal and newborn health in Africa. (document AFR/RC54/inf.doc/6). Brazzaville: World Health Organization, Africa Regional Office, 2004
90 Thaddeus S, Maine D. Too far to walk: maternal mortality in context. New York: Centre for Population and Family Health, Columbia University, 1990
91 Prevention of maternal mortality network. Proceedings of the PMM results conference. Accra, June 1996. Int J Gynaecol Obstet 1997; 59 (Suppl. 2): S1–S271
92 Hussein J, Goodburn EA, Damisoni H, Lema V, Graham W. Monitoring obstetric services: putting the 'UN Guidelines' into practice in Malawi: 3 years on. Int J Gynaecol Obstet 2001; 75: 63–73; discussion 74
93 Bailey PE, Paxton A. Program note. Using UN process indicators to assess needs in emergency obstetric services. Int J Gynaecol Obstet 2002; 76: 299–305; discussion 306
94 Lalonde AB, Okong P, Mugasa A, Perron L. The FIGO Save the Mothers Initiative: the Uganda–Canada collaboration. Int J Gynaecol Obstet 2003; 80: 204–212
95 Mekbib T, Kassaye E, Getachew A, Tadesse T, Debebe A. The FIGO Save the Mothers Initiative: the Ethiopia–Sweden collaboration. Int J Gynaecol Obstet 2003; 81: 93–102
96 Program note. Using UN process indicators to assess needs in emergency obstetric services: Niger, Rwanda and Tanzania. Int J Gynaecol Obstet 2003; 83: 112–120
97 Pearson L, Shoo R. Availability and use of emergency obstetric services: Kenya, Rwanda, Southern Sudan, and Uganda. Int J Gynaecol Obstet 2005; 88: 208–215
98 Gottlieb P, Lindmark G. WHO indicators for evaluation of maternal health care services, applicability in least developed countries: a case study from Eritrea. Afr J Reprod Health 2002; 6: 13–22
99 Villar J, Carroli G, Gulmezoglu AM. The gap between evidence and practice in maternal healthcare. Int J Gynaecol Obstet 2001; 75 (Suppl. 1): S47–S54
100 Onah HE, Okaro JM, Umeh U, Chigbu CO. Maternal mortality in health institutions with emergency obstetric care facilities in Enugu State, Nigeria. J Obstet Gynaecol 2005; 25: 569–574
101 Urassa DP, Carlstedt A, Nystrom L, Massawe SN, Lindmark G. Eclampsia in Dar es Salaam, Tanzania – incidence, outcome, and the role of antenatal care. Acta Obstet Gynecol Scand 2006; 85: 571–578
102 World Health Organization. Beyond the numbers: reviewing maternal deaths and complications to make pregnancy safer. Geneva: World Health Organization, 2004
103 Wagaarachchi PT, Graham WJ, Penney GC, McCaw-Binns A, Yeboah Antwi K, Hall MH. Holding up a mirror: changing obstetric practice through criterion-based clinical audit in developing countries. Int J Gynaecol Obstet 2001; 74: 119–30; discussion 131
104 Dumont A, Gaye A, Mahe P, Bouvier-Colle MH. Emergency obstetric care in developing countries: impact of guidelines implementation in a community hospital in Senegal. Br J Obstet Gynaecol 2005; 112: 1264–1269

Laurie Montgomery Irvine

Quality-of-care issues in obstetric services

'Quality of care' is a term used extensively within all areas of the UK National Health Service to try and ensure that the highest standards of practice are maintained. However, what actually constitutes quality of care is not always easy to define, not least because the perception of 'quality' may vary between the different stakeholders. Within obstetric services, obstetricians, midwives and general practitioners provide the core of obstetric care, but defining quality issues must also involve anesthetists, hematologists and pediatricians, and should include the viewpoints of patients and trust managers as well. Within this article, I have tried to establish broader concepts of what may define quality of care in modern obstetric management.

INITIATIVES FOR EVALUATING STANDARDS OF CARE

Assessing quality of healthcare involves three linked, but distinct, groups – the consumers (the patients, and to a certain extent, the media), healthcare providers (obstetrician, midwives and associated professionals), and purchasers (district health authorities and primary care groups).[1] Ideally, the overall judgement of quality of care should take account of all three groups, but the emphasis on what criteria are taken for measurement may differ extensively. The baseline criteria must surely be the delivery of a healthy baby to a healthy mother, but there may be many component parts to this eventual outcome. However, consumers, purchasers and providers all want 'high' quality of care, and care that within an individual unit may be satisfactorily compared against agreed standards of high quality, evidence-based clinical care. The most recent of these is Clinical Governance, defined as: 'a framework

Laurie Montgomery Irvine MD(Lond) FRCOG
Consultant Obstetrician and Gynaecologist, West Hertfordshire Hospitals NHS Trust, Watford General Hospital, Vicarage Road, Watford WD18 0HB, UK
E-mail: laurie.irvine@whht.nhs.uk

through which NHS organisations are accountable for continuously improving the quality of their services and safeguarding high standards of care by creating an environment in which excellence in clinical care will flourish'.[2] The introduction of the National Institute for Health and Clinical Excellence (NICE) and the Commission for Health Improvement (CHI) is designed to facilitate the introduction of clinical governance, but the foundations of these initiatives are based on previously established quality initiatives such as Medical and Clinical Audit, Clinical Guidelines and Clinical Effectiveness.[3–6]

The responsibility for Clinical Governance lies primarily with Trust Chief Executives, including the new Primary Care Trusts (PCTs). However, as standards of care cannot be defined purely on a local level, there is an important role for national bodies in maintaining the components of Clinical Governance. The Royal College of Obstetricians and Gynaecologists has established a Clinical Effectiveness and Standards Board to further the aims of clinical governance, with implementation of standards being maintained by a Clinical Effectiveness Support Unit.[7] The principal components of clinical governance include clinical guidelines, clinical unit, education and training, continuing professional development, clinical risk management, complaints procedures, re-validation of specialist and services accreditation.

ESTABLISHING STANDARDS OF QUALITY OF CARE

Locally set protocols rely on the availability of nationally compiled guidelines. The Royal College of Obstetricians and Gynaecologists produces specific guidelines addressing particular areas of clinical practice. The 'Green-Top' guidelines comprises a series of up-to-date information about subjects such as the management of tubal pregnancies, the use of anti-D immunoglobulin for rhesus prophylaxis and the use of antenatal corticosteroids. These are evidence-based guidelines, and are reviewed on a rolling system.

The NHS has also long established a series of Confidential Enquiries, including those into Maternal Deaths, Perioperative Deaths and Stillbirths and Deaths in Infancy. These are designed to identify cases where substandard practice has resulted in adverse outcome. This should allow the identification of areas of clinical practice where risk management might improve outcome.

METHODS OF EVALUATING QUALITY OF CARE

Clinical audit

Clinical audit relies on the continuing audit cycle aiming to improve standards of care constantly.[8,9] Standards must first be set, using local protocols and national guidelines, together with evidence from randomised controlled trials. Local practice over a set time period is then reviewed, either prospectively or retrospectively, in order to establish whether standards have been achieved, and to make recommendations for changes in clinical practice with the aim of improving standards. These standards are then reviewed again after an agreed time interval, thus establishing a constantly evolving audit cycle.

Risk management

Clinical risk management is an integral part of modern clinical practice. The identification of 'risk events' allows clinical practice involving such events to be monitored, and identify areas for improvement. In obstetric practice, examples might include massive obstetric hemorrhage, shoulder dystocia and neonatal Apgar scores of less than 7 at one minute. Establishment of local protocols for the management of such areas and auditing practice is designed to limit future adverse outcomes from such events. Multidisciplinary training sessions involving mock scenarios have been additionally found to be of benefit in identifying areas of practice needing improvement.

WHAT CONSTITUTES QUALITY OF CARE?

The patient's view

There are several channels in which patients' view points may be expressed. Maternity care in the UK emphasises a woman-focused approach, the aim of *Changing Childbirth* being the establishment of an integrated collaborative service where the views of both practitioner and consumer are acknowledged and applied.[10,11] In addition, *The Patient's Charter* was set up to establish guidelines for overall patient care, in particular, for patients to have clear routes for voicing concerns over their management.[12] Each trust should have a set complaint procedure for dealing with patient concerns. In obstetrics, in common with all other branches of medicine, lack of communication between health professions and patients is continually identified as a main area of concern. One might view the writing of a complaint letter as the ultimate failure of a system that is supposed to foster respect and understanding between a woman and her midwife or doctor. There is evidence to suggest that good communications is valued at a much higher level than mode of delivery or procedures carried out during labor and delivery. In 1989, a study using questionnaires, on 183 postnatal mothers (with healthy infants), 28 midwives and 52 obstetricians, requesting the ranking of 40 different factors.[13] Patients and obstetricians agreed completely about the 'most important' three factors – that the baby was healthy, that the doctors talked in a way that could be understood, and that any questions should be answered by staff. Midwives regarded the explanation of each procedure before it was done as the most important factor. Interestingly, being told the major risks of each procedure before it was carried out was placed much higher by patients (6th), than by midwifes (20th) or obstetricians (17th). This finding could play a part in establishing guidelines for informed consent to surgical or other procedures in obstetric care.

The patients' perception of their quality of care may depend to a certain extent on what the overall outcome has been for them and their baby. A woman who has undergone induction of labor involving prostaglandin administration, artificial rupture of the membranes and Syntocinon augmentation, but with a labor culminating in an emergency cesarean section at full dilatation after an unsuccessful attempt at instrumental vaginal delivery, is bound to have a different view of what constitutes good quality of care than

Table 1 Possible quality of care issues depending on clinical outcome

Clinical scenario	Suggested quality-of-care issues
Spontaneous vaginal delivery, healthy baby	Provision of food and drink Décor and furnishings in labor/postnatal rooms Cost of payphone/car parking
Cesarean section, healthy baby	Incidence of wound infection Need for transfusion Time taken for full mobilisation
Any mode of delivery, with low Apgar score	Need for SCBU admission Need for antibiotics, respiratory support

the woman who has a spontaneous onset of labor resulting in a spontaneous vaginal delivery. A suggested framework of 'quality-of-care issues' governed by clinical outcome is suggested in Table 1. To prioritise quality of care issues based on patient perception is a complex issue, and one which, even if general trends can be established, will always be very individual.

The health professional's view

Medical and midwifery assessments of quality of care tend to involve 'outcome measures', enabling easy statistical analysis, local audit of practice and comparison between units. An example of outcome measures taken from the American College of Obstetrics and Gynecology is listed in Table 2.[14,15] However, hard figures stating the percentage, for instance, of cesarean deliveries, or of epidural rates, within an individual unit compared to other hospitals within the region, is not potentially beneficial to consumers. It does not reflect the variation in case-mix, which may occur between units, particularly with respect to social class, racial and cultural variations. Indeed, with regard to cesarean section rates, there may be wide variations between individual units, regions and even countries.[16] Data collection in a 'binary' form, *i.e.* whether someone has a cesarean section, or not, does not establish why a cesarean delivery was carried out. There cannot be a uniform 'correct' cesarean section rate, as the optimal rate for each unit will be governed by the clinical case-mix, the facilities available, the obstetricians' experience and training, and the mother's wishes.[17] A similar criticism could be made of published epidural rates. A high epidural rate is often regarded as a 'bad' result for an individual unit, but this should not be regarded by itself as a quality-of-care measurement.

A unit dealing with a great deal of high-risk obstetric cases will inevitably be associated with a high epidural rate. The quality of care issue should not solely be about whether someone has an epidural or not, but whether there was a justifiable reason for inserting it, be it a clinical indication or through maternal request. The fact that an outcome measure maybe difficult to obtain should not preclude it from the issues of quality of care.

It is important that there is clear documentation in the obstetric notes of relevant risk factors in the pregnancy. These are often identified antenatally,

Table 2 American College of Obstetricians and Gynecologists obstetric clinical indicators

MATERNAL INDICATORS

- Maternal mortality
- Unplanned re-admission within 14 days
- Cardiopulmonary arrest
- In-hospital initiation of antibiotics 24 h or more after term vaginal delivery
- In-hospital maternal red blood cell transfusion or hematocrit < 22 vol% or hemoglobin of < 7.0 g or decrease in hemoglobin of 3.5 g or more
- Maternal stay more than 5 days after vaginal delivery or more than 7 days after cesarean delivery
- Eclampsia
- Introduction of labor for an indication other than diabetes, premature rupture of membranes, pregnancy-induced hypertension, post-term gestation, intra-uterine growth retardation, cardiac disease, isoimmunization, fetal demise or chorioamnionitis
- Primary cesarean delivery for fetal distress
- Primary cesarean delivery for failure to progress
- Delivery of an infant with a birth weight < 2500 g or respiratory distress syndrome after planned cesarean delivery
- Delivery of an infant with a birth weight < 2500 g or respiratory distress syndrome following induction of labor

NEONATAL INDICATORS

- Delivery of an infant weighing < 1800 g in an institution without a neonatal intensive care unit
- Transfer of a neonate to a neonatal intensive care unit in another institution
- Term infant admitted to a neonatal intensive care unit
- Apgar score of 4 or less at 5 min
- Birth trauma, such as shoulder dystocia, cephalhematoma, Erb's palsy, and clavicular fracture but not caput
- In-born infant with clinically apparent seizures recorded before discharge

Modified from Luthi *et al.*[14] and Loegering *et al.*[15]

although one of the most important notes is on the conduct of labor. When admitted to labor ward in labor, there is a multiplicity of pieces of information that is recorded in the notes. It can be difficult, especially in an emergency situation, to identify that information which enables one to decide on further management of the woman. The partogram is an important part of the labor ward notes and has been widely used in the UK since the early 1970s.[18] On the partogram, a number of important clinical features are recorded, especially the rate of cervical dilatation, position and station and the descent of the presenting part. Also a record of the fetal heart rate.[19] Other important information is the use of Syntocinon to accelerate labor and correct either primary dysfunctional labor or secondary arrest in labor. The benefit of using a partogram is that it represents in a pictorial form on a single page, evidence of progress or lack of progress in labor.

The partogram has become even more important in recent years due to different working patterns on labor ward. With the introduction of shift systems for the registrars, and fixed consultant labor ward sessions, there may be a number of different teams responsible for the woman's labor. The partogram is of benefit in that when different obstetricians take over the management of the case, there is clear evidence of what has occurred before. There is also evidence that using the action and alert line, and with the judicious use of Syntocinon will shorten the length of labor.[20] Other benefits of Syntocinon include the possible reduction in both the operative delivery and cesarean section rate for failure to progress in labor.[21,22]

Clear and accurate documentation in the notes may, at least in part, represent a well-run and organised labor ward. Also, it could imply that the obstetricians and midwives have understood the progress in labor and have acted if there has been delay.

If a woman has had a previous spontaneous vaginal delivery, her chance of subsequent vaginal deliveries is high. A woman who has had one previous cesarean section for whatever reason, has a much higher chance of repeat cesarean section, either as an elective procedure or an emergency. When managing a patient who has had one previous emergency cesarean section, the partogram will give invaluable information on which a decision can be made of mode of delivery in a subsequent pregnancy. As an emergency cesarean section is associated with increased maternal morbidity and mortality, very careful consideration should be given as to whether the woman should be allowed to labor or be delivered by elective repeat cesarean section.[23]

Information contained in the partogram can also be used for audit purposes. For example, the use of Syntocinon to attempt to correct secondary arrest in labor prior to an emergency cesarean section being performed for failure to progress in labor.

The manager's view

Trust executives, together with the accountants, are bound to measure quality of care in terms of financial cost to the trust. This may be broken down into where the unit is saving, and losing, money. The employment of a clinical risk manager and spending of resources on training sessions for staff may involve an initial outlay, but if this means that lengthy in-patient stays of mothers and babies who have complications secondary to poor clinical practice are reduced, substantial savings may be made. In addition, the chance of litigation will be minimised; with obstetrics now comprising an ever-increasing quota of all litigation claims, an initial small outlay could save a trust potentially millions of pounds.

With constant pressure on maternity beds, there is a continual drive to discharge women early from hospital after uncomplicated deliveries. This was critically highlighted in the media in 1998 when Bristol Royal Infirmary established a strict 6-hour discharge policy for 'uncomplicated' vaginal deliveries, in part due to midwifery staffing shortages.[24] Theoretically, if there is a well-established community midwife service, together with family support, this early discharge should not be detrimental to the health of either mother or baby. However, this type of broad policy may have adverse consequences. A recent report in the *British Medical Journal* described one such policy of reduced postnatal in-patient stay resulting in a rise in the re-admission rate of newborn babies from 5.2% to 10.4%, the primary cause being neonatal jaundice.[25,26] Ultimately, trusts may end up spending more money on re-admission, and mothers and babies are left in a situation where the ultimate long-tern establishment of feeding may be compromised. The World Health Organization (WHO) and United Nations Children's Fund (UNICEF) Baby Friendly Initiative emphasised that 'breast is best',[27] but such findings may reflect the deficiencies in current availability of breast-feeding advice and support, not in and outside of hospital. Even well-motivated mothers may find it hard to maintain effective breast-feeding in the face of the physical and psychological upheaval that hospital re-admission may incur.

PROPOSALS FOR ESTABLISHING QUALITY OF CARE

The views of doctors, midwives, patients and managers do not always lie happily together, maybe because of the differing criteria used to set standards of care. Using patient-perceived quality-of-care evaluations can help establish good practice within maternity care. The development of clinical pathways to assess perceived quality of care has been well established within several acute hospital settings,[28] and may help improve efficiency, reduce costs, and improve quality and outcome of care through increased standardisation of practice and improved collaboration and communication between staff.

There are signs that the importance of good communication is being recognised as paramount in the provision of maternity care as well as in medicine in general. At the Birth Centre, run by the leading independent midwife Caroline Flint, all mothers are asked to complete a questionnaire after delivery of their baby. Particular emphasis is placed on the mother's perception of the provision by her midwife of 'good communication, understanding, provision of suitable information, the availability and support of choice'.[29] Within the NHS, the establishment of 'patient partnership' is designed to foster understanding of the important issues facing both medical professionals and patients.[30] However, it remains difficult to establish clear guidelines for what might be termed 'good' quality of care. We would suggest that if an outcome measure is identified, it should not just be how many patients were affected by it, but how they were affected. For example, rather than comparing epidural rates between different obstetric units, a more relevant message might be how many women who stated a preference for epidural analgesia in labor actually received one and how long did they wait before their epidural was sited, from the time of request. With breast-feeding initiatives, identifying which mothers received what they felt to be adequate support with breast-feeding is more important than the overall breast-feeding rate.

When 'informed choice' is now such a part of modern maternity care, how many women who request an induction of labor before 41 weeks, or who request cesarean section for no medical or fetal reason, actually achieve their wish? If they do, are they fully counselled as to the potential risks and benefits of their decision? If they do not, is this because they are simply told 'no' or is it (hopefully) because after discussion with their midwife and obstetrician, they feel better equipped to make a more informed, and perhaps different, decision?

Table 3 Suggested quality-of-care indicators

- Percentage of epidurals inserted within 30 min of request
- Percentage of cesarean section for failed induction of labor
- Percentage of cesarean section for 'fetal distress' without FBS proof
- Percentage of cesarean section for 'fetal distress' within 30 min of decision to deliver
- Percentage of cesarean section or instrumental vaginal delivery where hemoglobin drops by 3 units by day 3
- Percentage of development of wound infection following cesarean section
- Percentage of breech presentations where ECV offered
- Percentage of preterm deliveries receiving antenatal steroid administration
- Percentage of appropriate administration of thromboprophylaxis
- Percentage of mothers breast-feeding who expressed an initial preference to breast feed

A suggested guide to outcome measures is shown in Table 3. Although some of these measures may not be easy to quantify from 'raw' data, this does not mean that they are less worthy of assessment. There may be a general tendency for some to measure what is easily measurable, but we would suggest that this is no guarantee of the quality of what is being measured.

The traditional view that the 'best' outcome of child-birth is a vaginal delivery without medical intervention must be seen as outdated. The most important feature of child-birth must be the safe delivery, by whatever means, of a healthy infant to a healthy mother. If this involves intervention antenatally, in labor or delivery, or in the postnatal period, this should be clearly justifiable, and have a low associated morbidity. Pregnant women should be able to make informed choices with regard to their antenatal, intrapartum and postpartum care, and to receive clear information as to why intervention, may sometimes be indicated. Hard statistical data must be set alongside patient-evaluated outcome measures in order to reach a clear indication of what constitutes good quality of care.

ACKNOWLEDGEMENTS

I should like to thank Julie Spendlove, Research Secretary for her help in the preparation of this manuscript. The views expressed are those of the author, and may not reflect those other members of the department. This paper was, in part, funded by the Watford Gynaecological Research Fund (WGRF).

References

1 Paterson CM, Chapple JC, Beard RW, Joffe M, Steer PJ, Wright CSW. Evaluating the quality of the maternity services – a discussion paper. Br J Obstet Gynaecol 1991; 98: 1073–1078
2 Department of Health. A First Class Service: quality in the new NHS. London: DH, 1998
3 Department of Health. Working for patients. London: Medical Audit, HMSO, 1989

4 Development of Health/NHS Management Executive. Clinical audit: meeting and improving standards in healthcare. London: DH, 1993
5 Mann T. Clinical Guidelines: Using clinical guidelines to improve patient care within the NHS. London: NHS Executive, 1996
6 NHS Executive. Promoting Clinical Effectiveness: a framework for action in and through the NHS. Leeds: NHS, 1996
7 Royal College of Obstetricians and Gynaecologists. Clinical Governance. London: RCOG, 1999
8 NHS Executive. Using clinical audit in the NHS: a position statement. Leeds: NHS, 1996
9 Burnett AC, Winyard G. Clinical audit at the heart of clinical effectiveness. J Qual Clin Practice 1998; 18: 3–19
10 Proctor S. What determines quality in maternity care? Comparing the perceptions of childbearing women and midwives. Birth 1998; 25: 85–93
11 Department of Health. Changing childbirth, Vol 1. London: HMSO, 1993
12 Great Britain, Scottish Office. The Patient's Charter: a charter for health. Edinburgh: Scottish Office, 1991
13 Drew NC, Salmon P, Webb L. Mothers', midwives' and obstetricians' views on the features of obstetric care which influence satisfaction with childbirth. Br J Obstet Gynaecol 1989; 96: 1084–1088
14 Luthi J-C, Dolan MS, Ballard DJ. Evidence-based healthcare quality management in obstetrics and gynecology. Clin Obstet Gynecol 1998; 41: 348–358
15 Loegering L, Reiter RC, Gambone JC. Measuring the quality of health care. Clin Obstet Gynecol 1994; 37: 122–136
16 Stephenson PA, Bakoula C, Hemminki E *et al.* Patterns of use of obstetrical intervention in 12 countries. Paediatr Perinat Epidemiol 1993; 7: 45–46
17 Chamberlain G. What is the correct caesarean section rate? Br J Obstet Gynaecol 1993; 100: 403–104
18 Studd JW, Philpott RH. Partograms and action line of cervical dilatation. Proc R Soc Med 1972; 65: 700
19 Studd JW. Partograms and nomograms in the management of primigravid labour. BMJ 1973; 4: 451–484
20 World Health Organization. Maternal health and safe motherhood programme. World Health Organization partograph in management of labour. Lancet 1994; 343: 1399–1040
21 Phillpott RH, Castle WM. Cervicographs in the management of labour in primigravidae II. The action line and treatment of abnormal labour. J Obstet Gynaecol Br Commonwealth 1972; 79: 599–602
22 Lopez-Zeno JA, Peaceman AM, Adashek JA, Socol ML. A controlled trial of a program for the active management of labor. N Engl J Med 1992; 326: 450–454
23 Hall MH. Confidential enquiry into maternal death. Br J Obstet Gynaecol 1990; 97: 752–753
24 Hospital tells mothers to leave after six hours. Daily Telegraph. 16 September 1998
25 Spurgeon D. Earlier discharge for newborns may increase health risks. BMJ 1993; 319: 469
26 Lock M, Ray JG. Higher neonatal morbidity after routine early hospital discharge. Are we sending newborns home too early? Can Med Assoc J 1999; 161: 249–253
27 Department of Health/UNICEF UK Baby Friendly Initiative. Memorandum of understanding between the National Breastfeeding Working Group and the UNICEF UK Baby Friendly Initiative, London: DH/UNICEF, 1993
28 Chou S-C, Boldy D. Patient perceived quality of care in hospital in the context of clinical pathways: development of an approach. J Qual Clin Practice 1999; 19: 89–93
29 The Birth of Your Baby: Caroline Flint Midwifery Services, 1999
30 NHS Executive. Patient partnership: building a collaborative strategy. Leeds: NHS Executive, 1996

Katherine Shaio Sandhu   Sean Keeler
David E. Seubert

Cervical insufficiency

Preterm birth remains the leading cause of neonatal morbidity and mortality in the world today. Cervical insufficiency is a generous contributor to the pool of preterm births. Accordingly, it is of the utmost importance to gain as much insight as possible into the etiologies of cervical insufficiency and attempt to find treatments which can help decrease the incidence of preterm birth and spontaneous preterm loss. It was estimated that in 2002, approximately 12% of deliveries in the US were premature.[1] Unfortunately, during the last 10 years, the incidence of preterm deliveries and spontaneous preterm losses in the US and Europe has remained unchanged or has even increased. The ideal treatment for cervical insufficiency remains quite controversial. The historical notion that cerclage placement can aid in the prevention of preterm birth caused by the condition of cervical insufficiency is heavily debated.

DEFINITION

The first recognition of 'cervical incompetence' was reported in the literature in 1658 by Cole, Culpetter and Rowland in the *Practice of Physick*.[2] The authors noted that: 'the second fault in women which hindered conception is when the

Katherine Shaio Sandhu MD
Fellow, Division of Urogynecology, Department of Obstetrics and Gynecology, Albert Einstein College of Medicine, Bronx, New York, USA

Sean Keeler MD
Fellow, Division of Maternal Fetal Medicine, Department of Obstetrics and Gynecology, New York University School of Medicine, New York, USA

David E. Seubert MD JD (for correspondence)
Director, Division of Maternal Fetal Medicine and Assistant Professor, Department of Obstetrics and Gynecology, New York University Medical Center, 550 First Avenue, 9N27-BH, New York, NY 10016, USA
E-mail: david.seubert@med.nyu.edu

seed is not retained or the orifice of the womb is so slack that it cannot rightly contract itself to keep in the seed....The fibers of the womb are broken in pieces, one from another and the inner orifice of the womb overmuch slackened.' Despite the description of this condition, a surgical approach for treatment did not emerge until nearly 300 years later.

Traditionally, historical features were used to make the diagnosis of cervical insufficiency. Patients presenting with painless cervical dilation without regular contractions were historically deemed to have cervical incompetence. Harger *et al.*[3] performed an evidence-based analysis of the historical features of cervical insufficiency. The authors listed the following as historical features of cervical insufficiency: (i) history of two or more second-trimester pregnancy losses (excluding those resulting from preterm labor or abruption); (ii) history of losing each pregnancy at an earlier gestational age; (iii) history of painless cervical dilation of up to 4–6 cm; (iv) absence of clinical findings consistent with placental abruption; (v) history of cervical trauma caused by cone biopsy; (vi) intrapartum cervical lacerations; or (vii) excessive forced cervical dilation during pregnancy termination.[3] Other investigators have searched for a more objective means to identify cervical insufficiency. In 1995, a multicentered trial co-ordinated by the National Institute of Child Health and Human Development Maternal Fetal Medicine Unit Network measured cervical lengths transvaginally at 24 and 28 weeks of gestation in singleton pregnancies and then assessed the relation of this measurement to the risk of spontaneous preterm delivery.[4] This study defined the 50 percentile for cervical length as 35 mm, the 10 percentile as 26 mm and the 5 percentile as below 22 mm. The authors concluded that the risk of spontaneous preterm birth increased progressively as the cervical length decreased. At a cervical length less than 26 mm, the relative risk of preterm delivery increased 6-fold.[4] While this study does document a heightened risk of preterm delivery with a shortened cervical length, the positive predictive value was only 17.8% for a cervical length < 25 mm at 24 weeks' gestation.[4] Thus, most patients with a shortened cervix and no historical factors for preterm delivery will not deliver a preterm neonate. Hassan *et al.*[5] performed a retrospective cohort study examining cervical lengths both transabdominally and transvaginally if the cervical length was found to be below 30 mm. The authors concluded that nearly 50% of patients with a cervical length less than or equal to 15 mm had an early spontaneous preterm delivery. However, the authors state that 50% of women with a cervix of 15 mm or less delivered after 32 weeks' gestation.[5,6] The authors further pointed out that only 8% of patients in the series who had a preterm delivery at less than 32 weeks of gestation had a cervical length of 15 mm or less in the midtrimester.[5]

In addition to absolute cervical lengths, cervical effacement can be sonographically visualized. Zilanti *et al.*[7] described an alphabetical progression of cervical effacement which proceeds caudal from the internal cervical os to the external os by the letters 'T', 'Y', 'V' then 'U'. 'T' represents a closed uneffaced cervix. As progressive effacement occurs from the internal os, a 'Y' then 'V' formation occurs. As the cervix opens and the membranes are exposed through the internal os into the vagina, a characteristic 'U' appears. Rust and colleagues[8] reported on a group of patient with a shortened cervix, 82 with a 'T' shaped cervix and no funneling and 82 patients with a 'Y' shaped funnel.

The authors concluded that funneling is a significant risk factor for adverse perinatal outcome including preterm birth, chorioamnionitis, abruption, rupture of the membranes and serious neonatal morbidity.

ROLE OF CERCLAGE

Few topics in the obstetrical literature have generated as much controversy as the dilemma of whether and when to place a cervical cerclage. Proponents and opponents argue around the historical notions versus more objective findings such as cervical length measurements. The advent of dynamic terminology may also aid in the confusion. The historical term of 'cervical incompetence' has been replaced with the term 'cervical insufficiency' to avoid any negative connotations of the word 'incompetence'. 'Prophylactic' or 'elective cerclage' has been replaced with 'history indicated' or primary cerclage. 'Therapeutic' or 'salvage cerclage' has been replaced with 'ultrasound indicated' or 'secondary cerclage'. 'Rescue', 'emergent' or 'urgent' cerclage has been replaced with 'physical exam indicated' or 'tertiary' cerclage.

Cerclage placement was introduced by Prof. V. N. Shirodkar in 1955 at the Grant Medical College in Bombay, India. Shirodkar reported a case series of 30 patients who: 'abort repeatedly between the 4th and 7th month...where one can, by repeated internal examinations...find that the cervix is gradually yielding'.[9] Shirodkar concluded that: 'all these cases can be saved by a simple operation, done during pregnancy when one finds that the cervix is gradually yielding'.[9] Shirodkar's procedures required a strip of fascia lata a "quarter of an inch wide and four and a half inches long" be removed as the material to be used as the suture.[9] An 'anterior colporrhaphy incision and vertical incision through the posterior vaginal wall' was then performed with the fascia lata being attached via an aneurysm needle.[9] These patients were subsequently delivered by cesarean section. Prof. Ian McDonald from the Royal Melbourne Hospital in 1957 published his results of 70 patients with 33 surviving infants.[10] McDonald's diagnosis of cervical incompetence required a combination of 'vaginal discharge', 'lower abdominal discomfort' and a 'lump in the vagina'.[10] McDonald's procedure was a much less invasive procedure than that described by Shirodkar. McDonald used a synthetic suture in a purse-string fashion around the circumference of the cervix. No dissection or colporrhaphy was required. McDonald described a subset of patients not candidates for the procedure: 'it has become apparent that patients in strong labor with the intact membranes bulging beyond the external os are generally not suitable'.[10]

CERCLAGE PLACEMENT

An historic review of randomized controlled trials

Two randomized controlled trials were published in August 1984.[11,12] Lazar and colleagues[11] performed a multicentered controlled trial of cervical cerclage in women at 'moderate risk' for preterm delivery. 'Moderate risk' was defined by a point system; patients falling into this 'moderate risk' group were randomized to cerclage placement versus expectant management. Patients ineligible or in the 'high risk' group included those with previous late spontaneous abortions, a torn or open inner os one finger width or more, an enlarged isthmus greater than 1 cm on hysterogram and those with multiple gestations. The overall preterm delivery rate was only 6% suggesting that perhaps patients with more 'high risk' assessments should have been included. The authors found that the cerclage group had more hospitalizations, received more tocolytic therapies, and had more preterm births than those expectantly managed although this did not reach statistical significance. In the same journal, Rush and colleagues[12] published a randomized controlled trial of cerclage placement in women at 'high risk' for spontaneous preterm delivery. In this group of 194 'high risk' patients, the overall preterm delivery rate was much higher at 33%. Patients were deemed high risk and eligible for study entry if they had 2–4 previous pregnancies that had ended prior to 37 weeks' gestation and at least one previous pregnancy which ended spontaneously between 14–36 weeks' gestation. The authors reported no apparent benefit from cerclage placement including no increase in gestational age in the cerclage group. The authors did report a longer hospitalization and more postpartum fevers in the cerclage group, although this later complication did not reach statistical significance.

The largest randomized controlled trial to date with 1292 patients was published in 1993 by the UK Medical Research Council and the Royal College of Obstetricians and Gynaecologists.[13] This study enrolled patients from 12 countries between 1981 and 1988 if their physician was 'uncertain' about whether cerclage placement was indicated or not. The overall preterm delivery rate in this group was 28%. Of the patients enrolled, 71% had a previous second trimester loss or preterm delivery and 29% had previous cervical surgery. Using the end point of delivery prior to 33 weeks' gestation, the cerclage group (13%) appeared beneficial compared to the no cerclage group (17%) with a $P = 0.03$.[13] Of cerclage patients, 10% had infants weighing less than 1500 g as opposed to the no cerclage group at 13% ($P = 0.05$). After the enrollees were striated into six mutually exclusive cohorts including obstetrical histories and cervical surgeries, only one cohort of patients appeared to have clear benefit from cerclage placement. This group of 107 patients included patients with a history of three or more spontaneous preterm births or preterm deliveries.[13]

In 2001, Althuisius *et al.*[14] published the CIPRACT Trial, an acronym standing for Cervical Incompetence Prevention Randomized Cerclage Trial. The investigators measured cervical lengths in patients with risk factors for cervical incompetence including delivery of a singleton infant prior to 34 weeks' gestation, preterm premature rupture of the membranes prior to 32 weeks' gestation, DES exposure, cold knife conization and uterine anomalies. Patients with a cervical length less than 25 mm were randomized to cerclage placement and bed rest versus bed rest alone. The authors found a significantly higher rate of preterm delivery prior to 34 weeks' gestation in the bed rest group (7/16) versus the cerclage plus bed rest group (0/16; $P = 0.002$).[14] The authors also found that the compound neonatal morbidity, defined as NICU admission or neonatal death was significantly lower in the cerclage plus bed rest group versus the bed rest group.

In 2001, Rust *et al.*[15] conducted the first randomized trial on cerclage where enrollment and randomization was based strictly on sonographic findings. The authors randomized 113 patients with either internal os dilation, membrane prolapse into the endocervical canal involving at least 25% of the cervical length, or a shortened cervix less than 2.5 cm. The authors found that cerclage failed to alter any perinatal outcome variable. The authors proposed a rationale for lack of benefit of cerclage called the 'final common pathway postulate'.[15] Simply stated, if the sonographic findings relate to a structural defect of the cervical stroma, then a reinforcing cerclage should prove beneficial in prolonging gestational age. However, the efficacy of cerclage placement diminishes when a shortened cervix co-exists with preterm contractions, subclinical infection, inflammation, or placental abruption the success diminishes. In 2004, To *et al.*[16] confirmed these findings. in a multicentered trial of 12 hospitals in the UK along with hospitals in five other countries. A total of 47,123 patients were screened and 253 patients with cervical lengths less than 1.5 mm were randomized to cerclage versus expectant management. Preterm delivery rates were 22% in the cerclage group and 26% in the expectantly managed group; thus, cerclage did not show any perinatal improvement. Berghella *et al.*[17] performed transvaginal screening on women with one or more high-risk factors for preterm birth between 14–24 weeks' gestation. Sixty-one patients were randomly assigned to cerclage placement (31 patients) versus bed rest (30 patients). The authors found no difference in any obstetric or neonatal outcomes. A further subanalysis of singleton

Table 1 Summary of seven randomized controlled trials of cerclage placement

Study	Gestational age	Risk category	Type	Results
Lazar & Gueguen (1984)[11]	< 28 weeks	Moderate risk	History indicated	No benefit, possible detriment
Rush *et al.* (1984)[12]	15–21 weeks	High risk	History indicated	No benefit, possible detriment
MRC/RCOG (1993)[13]	14–29 weeks	All categories; 'physician uncertainty'	History indicated	Cerclage beneficial if 3 or more spontaneous losses or preterm deliveries
CIPRACT (2001)[14]	15–27 weeks	High risk	History and ultrasound indicated	Pro-cerclage; cerclage beneficial
Rust *et al.* (2000)[15]	16–24 weeks	High risk – sonographic findings	Ultrasound indicated	No benefit
To *et al.* (2004)[16]	22–24 weeks	Population screening	Ultrasound indicated	No benefit
Berghella *et al.* (2004)[17]	14–24 weeks	High risk	Ultrasound indicated	No benefit

enrollees with a history of preterm births prior to 35 weeks' gestation and a shortened cervix of < 25 mm likewise showed no benefit of cerclage placement.[17]

Table 1 summarizes the seven randomized controlled trials discussed above. The three randomized trials of history-indicated cerclage show no benefit to a possible detrimental effect except in the subset of patients with a history of three prior spontaneous losses or preterm deliveries. The CIPRACT Trial, which used historical factors followed by sonographic findings showed a decrease in the incidence of preterm delivery prior to 34 weeks' gestation and a lower compound neonatal morbidity score with cerclage placement. The ultrasound-indicated randomized controlled trials failed to show a benefit of cerclage placement for any perinatal or neonatal outcome variable.

Berghella *et al.*[18] performed a meta-analysis of four of the above randomized controlled trials.[14–17] The authors reported a significant reduction in preterm birth at less than 35 weeks' gestation in singleton pregnancies from 29.2% in the cerclage group to 34.8% in the expectantly managed or bed-rest group.[18] This reduction of preterm birth also extended to singleton pregnancies with prior preterm births and prior second trimester losses. This reduction was not found in twin gestations. The authors suggested that a 'well-powered trial should be carried out' in the group of patients where benefit was noticed.[18]

PHYSICAL EXAMINATION-INDICATED TERTIARY CERCLAGE

A physical examination or tertiary or emergent cerclage occurs when the cervix is effaced and membranes are exposed in the vagina. Amniocentesis is strongly recommended prior to cerclage placement in these patients since microbial invasion of the amniotic cavity (MIAC) may be as high as 51.5%.[19] Althusius *et al.*[20] conducted a randomized trial of patients meeting physical examination and sonographic evidence of membranes at or beyond a dilated external cervical os before 27 weeks' gestation and randomized 13 patients to receive an emergency cerclage with indomethacin therapy and 10 patients to bed rest only. All patients received antibiotic therapy. The authors found a benefit for cerclage placement with indomethacin therapy in preventing delivery prior to 34 weeks' gestation (7/13 in treated group versus 10/10 in bed rest only group; $P = 0.02$).[20] Terkildsen *et al.*[21] identified 116 patients who underwent emergent cerclage placement between 16–24 weeks' gestation and analyzed factors associated with delivery at or greater than 28 weeks' gestation. The authors identified factors associated with a decreased success rates including nulliparity, presence of membranes prolapsing beyond the external cervical os and gestational age less than 22 weeks at cerclage placement.[21] Daskalakis *et al.*[22] compared 46 patients meeting criteria for emergent cerclage placement including 29 patients actually undergoing the procedure versus 17 patients who declined the procedure and remained on bed rest. All patients received antibiotics and tocolytics. The authors found an enhanced prolongation of gestation (8.8 weeks versus 3.1 weeks), birth weight (2101 g versus 739 g), and live births (25/29 versus 7/17) in the emergent cerclage group versus the bed rest group.[22]

CERVICAL SONOGRAPHIC ASSESSMENT IN MULTIPLE GESTATIONS

The Maternal Fetal Medicine Network of the National Institute of Child Health and Human Development studied 147 sets of twins at 24–28 weeks' gestation.[23]

The investigators found that a cervical length of < 2.5 cm at 24 and 28 weeks' gestation was associated with an increased rate of spontaneous birth prior to 32 weeks' gestation of 26.9% and 13.2%.[23] Guzman *et al.*[24] found an even higher rate of preterm delivery of 50% when the cervical length was below 2.0 cm at 15–24 weeks' gestation and 16.1% between 25–28 weeks' gestation. Guzman found similar results with triplet gestations.[25]

ROLE OF CERCLAGE IN MULTIPLE GESTATIONS

Dor *et al.*[26] randomized twin gestations resulting from induced ovulation to receive a prophylactic cerclage versus expectant management. The investigators followed 22 'sutured' versus 23 'non-sutured' patients. Of the sutured patients, 10 (45.4%) delivered prematurely with a neonatal death rate of 18.2% versus 11/23 (47.8%) delivering prematurely with a neonatal death rate of 15.2% in the non-sutured group.[26] The authors found no support for routine cerclage placement in twin gestations. Newman *et al.*[27] conducted a prospective cohort study of 147 consecutive twin pregnancies over an 8-year period who underwent transvaginal ultrasound cervical length measurement between 18–26 weeks' gestation. Cerclage was offered to patients with cervical lengths less than 2.5 cm. While the authors found that decreasing cervical length was significantly associated with a shorter length of gestation, lower birth weight at delivery, heightened incidence of delivery prior to 34 weeks, PPROM and very low birth weight, midtrimester cerclage placement did not alter these risks.[27] Roman *et al.*[28] studied 3278 triplet gestations of which 248 (7.6%) received a prophylactic cerclage. The investigators found no benefit of prophylactic cerclage placement in triplet gestations in improving pregnancy or neonatal outcomes in triplet pregnancies without a history of cervical insufficiency.

TYPE OF CERCLAGE

To date, no randomized controlled trials exist in the literature comparing the McDonald versus Shirodkar cerclage techniques. A McDonald cerclage is easier to perform and does not require the increased dissection of the Shirodkar procedure. Odibo *et al.*[29] conducted a secondary analysis using data from all published randomized trials including women with a short cervical length and compared preterm birth rates at less than 33 weeks' gestation between patients receiving a McDonald versus a Shirodkar cerclage. The authors found no significant difference in preterm birth prevention between the two groups.

Of even less clarity is the role of transabdominal cerclage. Davis *et al.*[30] conducted a retrospective cohort study of singleton pregnancies in patients who had either a transabdominal or transvaginal prophylactic cerclage. All patients had failed a previous transvaginal cerclage defined as having a preterm delivery at less than 33 weeks despite having a transvaginally placed cerclage. The authors reported a lower incidence of preterm delivery and PPROM in the transabdominal group versus the transvaginal group.[30]

ROLE OF INFLAMMATION

Saki *et al.*[31] recently studied whether the combination of cervical ultrasound and markers of endocervical inflammation can identify a subset of patients who may benefit from cerclage placement and a subset of patients where cerclage may not be beneficial. The investigators enrolled 252 patients with a sonographically short (< 2.5 cm) cervix; cerclage was placed at the 'discretion' of the attending physician (165 patients had cerclage placement and 81 patients did not).[31] The authors had previously reported on the elevated interleukin-8 (IL-8) concentrations in cervical mucus and the risk of preterm delivery.[32] The investigators collected cervical mucus at the time of cervical sonography but did not use the results of the IL-8 concentrations for any management decisions. Overall, cervical cerclage did not reduce the rate of preterm delivery. However, patients with elevated concentrations of IL-8 who had a cerclage had a higher rate of preterm delivery and a shorter procedure to delivery interval than those who did not have a cerclage.[31]

Berghella *et al.*[33] extracted data from all randomized trials including asymptomatic women with a sonographically shortened cervical length below 2.5 cm between 14–27 weeks. These trials randomized the patients to receive cerclage versus no cerclage. Patients who did not receive cerclage were analyzed. The preterm birth rate in women receiving indomethacin before 35 weeks was 29.3% (29/99) versus 42.5% (17/40) who did not receive the medication; the results failed to reach statistical significance. However, preterm birth rates before 24 weeks' gestation were significantly decreased in the group receiving indomethacin therapy at 1.0% (1/99) versus 7.5% (3/40) in the group not receiving the medication.[33] The authors concluded that further research and a randomized trial designed to investigate the role of indomethacin in this subset of patients was warranted.

CONCLUSIONS

Cervical insufficiency is composed of both a functional and structural component. The etiologies of cervical insufficiency are multifactorial in nature. Accordingly, cerclage treatment is not effective for all patients with cervical insufficiency. Ultrasound-indicated cerclage placement in an asymptomatic patient without a history of spontaneous preterm losses or preterm deliveries remains controversial. Currently, there no role for cerclage placement in a low-risk patient with a cervical length less than 2.5 cm. Therefore, routine screening for low-risk patients is not advocated. If the patient has a cervical length less than 2.5 cm and a history of preterm delivery consistent with cervical insufficiency, then there may be a role for cerclage placement. However, the group of patients who would derive benefit from a cerclage procedure has yet to be identified. Physical examination-indicated cerclage may be beneficial but the existing studies lack sufficient power to make appropriate conclusions. If a patient is to undergo a physical examination-indicated cerclage, amniocentesis to rule out MIAC is strongly recommended pre-operatively.

References

1 Martin JA, Hamilton BE, Sutton PD. Births: final data for 2002. Natl Vital Statistics Report 2003; 52.
2 Anonymous. In: Culpepper N, Cole A, Rowland W. (eds) Effective Care in Pregnancy and Childbirth, Vol. 1. New York: Oxford University Press; 1989
3 Harger JH. Cerclage and cervical insufficiency: an evidence-based analysis. Obstet

Gynecol 2002; 100: 1313–1327
4 Iams JD, Goldenberg RL, Meis PJ *et al.*, NICHD HHD MFM Network. The length of the cervix and the risk of spontaneous premature delivery. N Engl J Med 1996; 334: 567–572
5 Hassan SS, Romero R, Berry SM *et al.* Patients with an ultrasonographic cervical length < 15 mm have nearly a 50% risk of early spontaneous preterm delivery. Am J Obstet Gynecol 2000; 182: 1458–1467
6 Romero R, Espinoza J, Erez O, Hassan S. The role of cervical cerclage in obstetric practice: can the patient who could benefit from this procedure be identified? Am J Obstet Gynecol 2006; 194: 1–9
7 Zilianti M, Azuaga A, Calderon F *et al.* Monitoring the effactment of the uterine cervix by transperineal sonography: a new perspective. J Ultrasound Med 1995; 14: 719–724
8 Rust OA, Atlas RO, Kimmel S, Roberts WE, Hess LW. Does the presence of a funnel increase the risk of adverse perinatal outcome in a patient with a short cervix? Am J Obstet Gynecol 2005; 192: 1060–1066
9 Shirodkar VN. A new method of operative treatment for habitual abortions in the second trimester of pregnancy. Antiseptic 1955; 52: 799–800
10 McDonald IA. Suture of the cervix for inevitable miscarriage. J Obstet Gynaecol 1957; 64: 346–350
11 Lazar P, Gueguen S. Multicentred controlled trial of cervical cerclage in women at moderate risk of preterm delivery. Br J Obstet Gynaecol 1984; 91: 731–735
12 Rush RW, Isaacs S, McPherson K, Jones L, Chalmers I, Grant A. A randomized controlled trial of cervical cerclage in women at high risk of spontaneous preterm delivery. Br J Obstet Gynaecol 1984; 91: 724–730
13 MacNaughton MC, Chalmers IG, Dubowitz V *et al.* Final report of the Medical Research Council/Royal College of Obstetricians and Gynaecologists Multicentre Randomised Trial of Cervical Cerclage. Br J Obstet Gynaecol 1993; 100: 516–523
14 Althuisius SM, Dekker GA, Hummel P, Bekedam DJ, van Geijin HP. Final results of the Cervical Incompetence Prevention Randomized Cerclage Trial (CIPRACT): therapeutic cerclage with bed rest versus rest alone. Am J Obstet Gynecol 2001; 185: 1106–1112
15 Rust OA, Atlas RO, Jones KJ, Benham BN, Balducci J. A randomized trial of cerclage versus no cerclage among patients with ultrasonographically detected second trimester preterm dilation of the internal os. Am J Obstet Gynecol 2000; 183: 830–835
16 To MS, Alfirevic Z, Heath VCF *et al.* Cervical cerclage for prevention of preterm delivery in women with short cervix: randomized controlled trial. Lancet 2004; 363: 1849–1853
17 Berghella V, Odibo AO, Tolosa JE. Cerclage for prevention of preterm birth in women with a short cervix found on transvaginal ultrasound examination: a randomized trial. Am J Obstet Gynecol 2004: 191: 1311–1317
18 Berghella V, Odibo AO, To MS, Rust OA, Althuisius SM. Cerclage for short cervix on ultrasonography: Meta-analysis of trials using individual patient-level data. Obstet Gynecol 2005; 106: 181–189
19 Romero R, Gonzalez R, Sepulveda W *et al.* Infection and labor. VIII. Microbial invasion of the amniotic cavity in patients with suspected cervical incompetence: prevalence and clinical significance. Am J Obstet Gynecol 1992; 167: 1086–1091
20. Althuisius SM, Dekker GA, Hummel P, van Geijin HP. Cervical incompetence prevention randomized cerclage trial: emergency cerclage with bed rest versus bed rest alone. Am J Obstet Gynecol 2003: 189: 907–910
21 Terkildsen MFC, Parilla BV, Mumar P, Grobman WA. Factors associated with success of emergent second-trimester cerclage. Obstet Gynecol 2003; 101: 565–569
22 Daskalakis G, Papantoniou N, Mesogitis S, Antsaklis A. Management of cervical insufficiency and bulging fetal membranes. Obstet Gynecol 2006; **107**: 221–226
23 Goldenberg RL, Iams JD, Miodovnik M *et al.* The Preterm Prediction Study: risk factors in twin gestation. National Institute of Child Health and Human Development Maternal-Fetal Medicine Units Network. Am J Obstet Gynecol 1996; 175: 1047–1055
24 Guzman ER, Walters C, O'Reilly-Green C *et al.* Use of cervical ultrasound in prediction of spontaneous preterm birth in twin gestations. Am J Obstet Gynecol 2000; 183: 1103–1107
25 Guzman ER, Walters C, O'Reilly-Green C *et al.* Use of cervical ultrasonography in prediction of spontaneous preterm birth in triplet gestations. Am J Obstet Gynecol 2000; 183: 1108–1113

26 Dor J, Shalev J, Blankstein J, Serr DM. Elective cervical suture of twin pregnancies diagnosed ultrasonically in the first trimester following induced ovulation. Gynecol Obstet Invest 1982; 13: 55–60
27 Newman RB, Kromback S, Myers MC, McGree DL. Effect of cerclage on obstetrical outcome in twin gestations with a shortened cervical length. Am J Obstet Gynecol 2002; 186: 634–640
28 Roman AS, Rebarber A, Pereira L, Sfakianaki AK, Mulholland J, Berghella V. The efficacy of sonographically indicated cerclage in multiple gestations. J Ultrasound Med 2005; 24: 763–768
29 Odibo A, To M, Berghella C, Rust O, Althuisius. Shirodkar versus McDonald cerclage for the prevention of preterm birth (PTB) in women with short cervical length. Am J Perinatol 2006; ahead of print.
30 Davis G, Berghella V, Talucci M, Wapner RJ. Patients with a prior failed transvaginal cerclage: a comparison of obstetric outcomes with either transabdominal or transvaginal cerclage. Am J Obstet Gynecol 2000; 193: 836–839
31 Sakai M, Shiozaki A, Tabata M *et al*. Evaluation of effectiveness of prophylactic cerclage of a short cervix according to interleukin-8 in cervical mucus. Am J Obstet Gynecol 2006; 194: 14–19
32 Sakai M, Ishiyama A, Tabata M *et al*. Relationship between cervical mucus interleukin-8 concentration and vaginal bacteria in pregnancy. Am J Reprod Immunol 2004; 52: 106–112
33 Berghella V, Rust OA, Althuisius SM. Short cervix on ultrasound: does indomethacin prevent preterm birth? Am J Obstet Gynecol 2006; 195: 809–813

Celia Burrell Boon H. Lim

Transvaginal ultrasound – obstetric applications in the second and third trimesters of pregnancy

Transvaginal ultrasound is increasingly being used in the second and third trimesters of pregnancy. It provides high resolution, as the probe can be placed closer to the area being examined. Advantages include: (i) avoiding the discomfort of a full bladder; (ii) reduced problem with acoustic shadowing from the symphysis pubis and the fetal head; (iii) fewer problems with the attenuation of sound waves in obese patients; and (iv) generally not too uncomfortable. Disadvantages include: (i) it is an invasive procedure and may not be acceptable by all patients; and (ii) there is a small possibility of introducing infection in cases of rupture of membrane and a theoretical risk of provoking bleeding in placenta previa.[1]

PLACENTA PREVIA AND PLACENTA ACCRETA

Comparison between transvaginal and transabdominal ultrasound

Transvaginal ultrasound is superior to transabdominal ultrasound in diagnosing placenta previa and placenta accreta.[2] The incidence of placenta previa is about 1:200 but, with a rising cesarean section rate combined with increasing maternal age, the diagnosis of placenta previa and placenta accreta is expected to increase.[2] The National Cesarean Section Audit showed that the rate of cesarean section in England, Wales and Northern Ireland were 21.3%,

Celia Burrell MRCOG (for correspondence)
Senior Specialist Registrar, Department of Obstetrics and Gynaecology, Hinchingbrooke Hospital, Huntingdon, Cambridgeshire PE29 6NT, UK
E-mail: burrellcelia@yahoo.co.uk

Boon H. Lim FRCOG FRANZCOG
Consultant Obstetrician and Gynaecologist, Department of Obstetrics and Gynaecology, Hinchingbrooke Hospital, Huntingdon, Cambridgeshire PE29 6NT, UK
E-mail: boon.lim@hinchingbrooke.nhs.uk

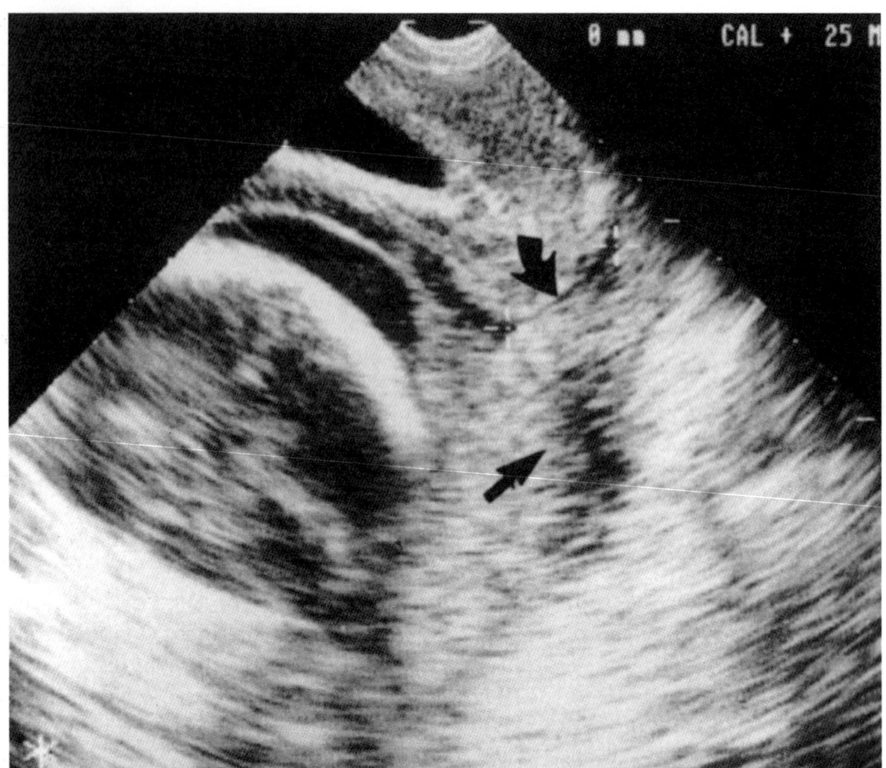

Fig. 1 Transvaginal ultrasound showing diagnostic features of placenta previa. A posterior placenta completely covering the internal cervical os. The cursor (+) shows the cervix to be 25 mm long with the curved arrow identifying the endocervical canal. The straight arrow shows the placenta.

24.2% and 23.9%, respectively.[3] Accurate diagnosis of placenta previa (Fig. 1) and placenta accreta is important in planning subsequent management. A Cochrane Database Review reported only one randomised, controlled trial by Sherman *et al.*[4] consisting of 38 women, that compared the accuracy of transvaginal and transabdominal in diagnosing placenta previa. It showed that transvaginal ultrasound has a good safety profile and produces superior views, especially in cases of posteriorly situated placentas and with the additional benefit of reduced scanning time. Other studies have shown that 26–60% of low-lying placenta diagnosed by transabdominal ultrasound were reclassified by transvaginal ultrasound,[5,6] while, in the third trimester, transvaginal ultrasound changed the transabdominal diagnosis of placenta previa in 12.5%.[7] Leerentveld *et al.*[8] showed the high levels of accuracy of transvaginal ultrasound in predicting placenta previa in the second and third trimester with a sensitivity of 87.5%, specificity of 98.8%, positive predictive value of 93.3%, negative predictive value of 97.6% and false positive rate of 2.33%.

Comstock *et al.*[9] looked at the accuracy of transvaginal ultrasound in diagnosing placenta accreta in high-risk patients – women who had a previous cesarean section and who had an anterior placenta in the current pregnancy. Of 2002 women, 14 had a confirmed diagnosis of placenta accreta, diagnosed between 15–20 weeks' gestation. There were 18 false-positive cases, most of which were due to the lack of visualisation of the echolucent area below the placenta and the myometrium (obliteration of the 'clear space' in the third trimester). They concluded that the presence of multiple, linear, irregular, vascular spaces within the placenta (placental lacunae) was the diagnostic sign with the highest positive predictive value for placenta accreta.[9]

Comparison between magnetic resonance imaging and transvaginal ultrasound

Studies have compared the accuracy of magnetic resonance imaging (MRI), abdominal ultrasound and transvaginal ultrasound in detecting placenta previa. MRI has been proven to be superior to transabdominal ultrasound in detecting placenta previa, especially posterior placentas. It has the advantage of being an objective test – removing inter- and intra-operator dependent errors – and it does not require a full bladder. A Cochrane Database Review showed that there is no randomised, control trial comparing transvaginal ultrasound and MRI in diagnosing placenta previa. The Royal College of Obstetricians and Gynaecologists, therefore, recommends that MRI should only be used in a research context.[2] Uterine scarring from cesarean section increases the incidence of placenta previa from 0.26% with an unscarred uterus to 0.65% after one cesarean section, to as much as 10% after four cesarean sections.[10] Abnormalities in the placentation may result in the attachment of the placenta beyond the endometrium (placenta accreta), extension deeper into the myometrium (placenta increta) and invasion through the serosal layer; this may involve the bladder and surrounding structures (placenta percreta). These conditions can occur in about 5% of patients with placenta previa.[10]

The grey-scale ultrasound findings diagnostic of placenta accreta include: (i) the loss of the normal hypo-echoic retroplacental myometrium zone; (ii) thinning or disruption of the hyperechoic uterine serosa–bladder interface; (iii) the presence of focal exophytic masses; and (iv) lacunar flow within the placentas.[11]

Doppler ultrasound increases the accuracy in diagnosing placenta accreta because it highlights areas of increased vascularity with dilated blood vessels that cross the placenta and the uterine wall.[12] This demonstrates a transition between the retroplacental hypo-echoic zone with normal Doppler signal and the myometrial zone.[13] Levine *et al.*[14] compared MRI, transabdominal and transvaginal ultrasound using grey-scale Doppler, color Doppler and power Doppler in diagnosing placenta accreta. Nineteen patients in the third trimester of pregnancy who were at increased risk for placenta accreta had transvaginal and transabdominal color Doppler and power Doppler, and 18 patients had MRI. Six patients had placenta accreta, confirmed on histology. Transvaginal ultrasound using power Doppler diagnosed five cases with confidence. Transabdominal ultrasound was suspicious or indeterminate in all five cases. In one patient with a posterior placenta and previous myomectomy, the diagnosis of placenta accreta was made after MRI. Levine *et al.*[14] concluded that transvaginal ultrasound with power Doppler had a 86% sensitivity and 92% specificity in diagnosing placenta accreta (see *Key points for clinical practice* at the end of this chapter).

CERVICAL ASSESSMENT

Preterm delivery remains a major cause of perinatal morbidity and mortality and accounts for about 8–10% of all births.[15] Predicting preterm labor and planning subsequent patient management remains a challenge. Research continues to try to assess prediction, intervention and prevention of preterm labor. Changes in the anatomy of the cervix–endocervical shortening, dilation, and herniation of the membranes (funnelling) are considered as changes along a continuum in the early stages of preterm labor. This cervical remodelling can be viewed on ultrasound imaging. Iams *et al.*[16] postulated a multifactorial model of spontaneous preterm labor involving the interaction of pathophysiological processes, including: (i) infection (clinical or subclinical); (ii) uterine activity; (iii) immunological inflammation; (iv) abruption; and (v) abnormal implantation. They suggested that one or more of these factors may act on an otherwise competent cervix to convert it into a distensible conduit through which preterm birth can take place.[16]

Biochemical markers and cervical length measurement in predicting preterm labor

Physiological and hormonal changes in the early stages of preterm labor produce several biochemical markers including cervical fibronectin, α-fetoproteins, alkaline phosphatase, human chorionic gonadotrophin, progesterone, C-reactive protein, cytokines (*e.g.* tumor necrosis factor-α [TNF-α], interleukin [IL]-1, IL-6), collagenases, corticotrophin releasing hormone, salivary estriol, granulocyte colony stimulating factor and metalloproteinase.[17] The US National Institute of Child Health and Human Development Network of Maternal–Fetal Medicine Units (NICHD MFM Network) study showed that α-fetoprotein, alkaline phosphatase and granulocyte-colony stimulating factor were the most promising biochemical markers.[18]

Transvaginal cervical measurement has been assessed independently and as a part of a multimarker in predicting preterm labor. The multifactorial nature of preterm labor makes it unlikely that a single test can be a reliable and accurate predictor. While there is still no major effective tool for predicting the onset of preterm labor in the unselected population, transvaginal ultrasound has shown great potential for the high-risk population. Cervical length > 30 mm or a negative fibronectin test in a patient with possible preterm labor can avoid over-diagnosis and unnecessary intervention.[19] Fetal fibronectin is a basement membrane protein produced by trophoblasts. It acts as a 'glue' holding the placental membrane and the decidua together. Levels > 50 ng/ml between 22–30 weeks' gestation have been associated with preterm labor.[17] It can be argued that there is no role for routine use of either cervical sonography or fibronectin to screen low-risk, pregnant women for preterm labor, but women thought to be at an increased risk may be reassured by a negative test result.[19] The American College of Obstetricians and Gynecologists suggests that cervical length and fetal fibronectin testing are useful in predicting the risk of preterm labor in high-risk women, but most important is their clinical usefulness in providing good negative predictive values.[20]

Fetal fibronectin was found to be independent of cervical length measurements between 21–31 mm. The selective application of fetal fibronectin testing results in a two-step test with performance of 86%, 90%, 63% and 97% for sensitivity, specificity, positive and negative predictive values, respectively.[21] The fetal fibronectin test (fFN) is more accurate in predicting spontaneous preterm birth within 7–10 days of testing among women with symptoms of threatened preterm labor before advanced cervical dilation. With a positive fFN result at 31 weeks', 17 symptomatic women would be needed to be treated with antenatal steroids to prevent one case of respiratory distress syndrome (RDS). If steroids were given to all symptomatic women at 31 weeks without fFN testing, 109 women would need to be treated to prevent one case of RDS.[22]

Rozenberg *et al.*[23] did a prospective, double-blind study comparing fetal fibronectin and transvaginal ultrasonographic cervical assessment to evaluate the risk of preterm labor. Tests were done on 76 patients who were hospitalised with symptoms of preterm labor between 24–34 weeks' gestation. The predictive values of fetal fibronectin and cervical length of ≤ 26 mm considered separately, were approximately equal. In the presence of positive fibronectin and a short cervix, the negative predictive value increased to 94.4%.[23] The presence of fetal fibronectin, a short cervix (≤ 25 mm) and a history of previous preterm delivery are the three strongest predictors for delivery before 32 weeks' gestation. The rate of preterm delivery progressively increases from 0.5% for women with none of these factors to 50% if all three risk factors are present at 22–24 weeks' gestation. It has always been postulated that several pathways can trigger preterm labor; thus, a combination of markers increases the accuracy in predicting preterm delivery.[24]

Cervical assessment using transabdominal, transvaginal and translabial ultrasound

Transvaginal ultrasound is recommended in assessing the cervix as it is more reliable than the transabdominal route.[25] With the abdominal route, bladder overdistension can compress the walls of the lower uterine segment and cervix, creating a deceivingly normal appearance in women with cervical effacement, shortening and dilatation. Furthermore, an underdistended bladder may preclude adequate visualisation of the cervix due to: (i) acoustic shadowing from the symphysis pubis; (ii) refractive shadowing from the bladder/uterine interface; and (iii) loss of the acoustic window provided by the urinary bladder and/or amniotic fluid – or an inability to elevate the fetal head or presenting part. The cervical length is accurately determined as the distance between the internal and external os. The internal os is normally at the level where the cervical canal meets the amniotic sac. The external os is more difficult to define because of acoustic shadowing from rectal gas. This problem can be reduced by scanning with the patient in the lateral decubitus position or elevating the hips with a pillow.[26] Cicero *et al.*[27] showed that patient acceptability was equal for transvaginal, translabial and transperineal sonography. Their study showed that at 22–24 weeks' gestation, the cervix can be visualised adequately by translabial sonography in about 80% of patients. The cervical lengths measured were very similar to those obtained with

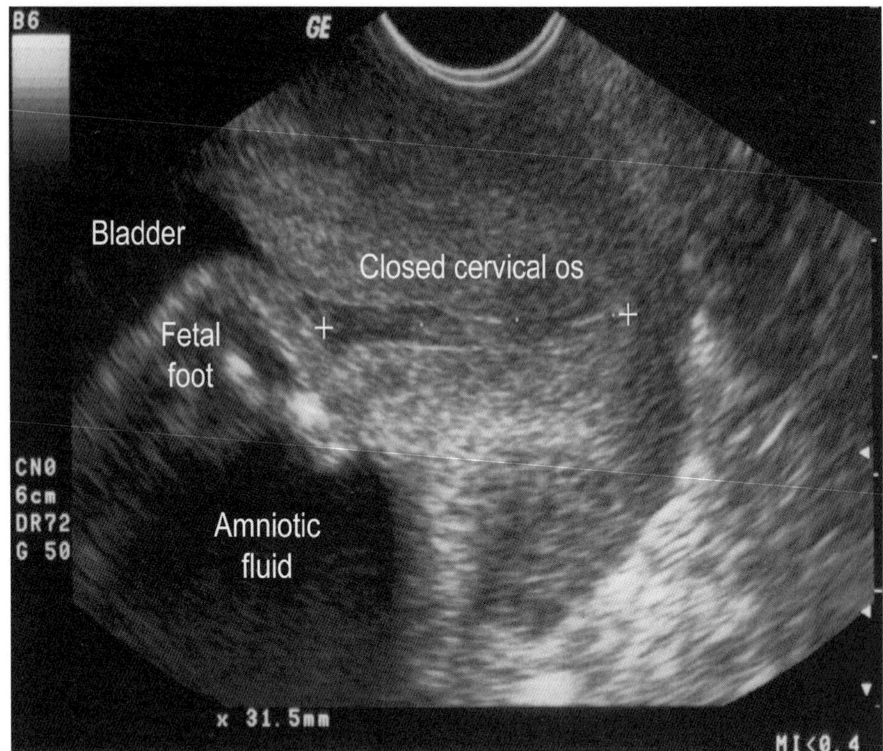

Fig. 2 Transvaginal ultrasound image showing closed cervical os (cervical length 31.5 mm).

transvaginal ultrasound. Carr *et al.*,[28] however, concluded that transvaginal and translabial techniques should not be used interchangeably to measure cervical length because the measurements differed by > 0.5 cm. Rozenberg *et al.*[29] compared two-dimensional assessment of the cervical length and three-dimensional assessment of cervical volume in predicting preterm delivery. They concluded that the cervical volume probably increases the positive predictive value of preterm delivery, but screening high-risk women is best achieved with cervical length.[29]

Cervical changes – funnelling, shortened cervix and dilated cervical os

Several studies have looked at the significance of cervical changes in predicting preterm labor, including: (i) dilated endocervical os (Fig. 2); (ii) shortened cervix; (iii) the presence or absence of funnelling – funnel length and width, percentage funnelling (funnel length/[funnel length plus cervical length] x 100); and (iv) cervical index (1 + funnel length/cervical length). There are many studies looking at the significance of these cervical changes both independently and in combination to predict preterm labor. These studies, however, are heterogeneous with variations in the patient population – low-risk and high-risk, the gestational age at the time of measurement, the frequency of measurements, and the cervical length cut-off used to evaluate predictive ability. Dilatation of the internal cervical os after 25 weeks' gestation

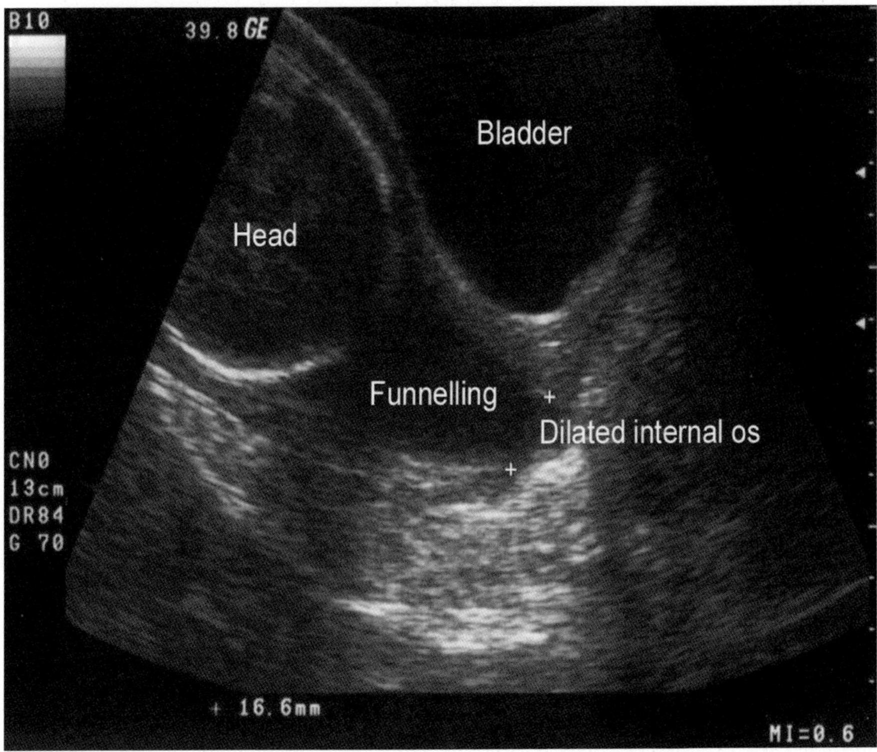

Fig. 3 Ultrasound image showing endocervical canal dilatation and funnelling.

is considered to be the single most significant risk factor for preterm labor, with an adjusted relative risk of 2.4 and 3.4 for examinations done at 25–28 weeks and 32–34 weeks, respectively.[30] Berghella *et al.*[31] showed that funnelling or dilatation of the internal cervical os > 5 mm is associated with a positive predictive value of 33–40% for preterm labor versus 11.3% for a short cervix (Fig. 3). A study by Rust *et al.*[32] showed that patients with cervical funnelling were affected by additional morbidity other than preterm delivery. The study included 82 singleton pregnancies with short cervix (≤ 25 mm) and cervical funnelling and 82 women with matched controls without funnelling at 16–24 weeks' gestation. The group with no funnelling had significantly less morbidity and fewer re-admissions for preterm labor (43.2% versus 67.1%; P = 0.004), chorioamnionitis (2.4% versus 23.2%; P = 0.0002), preterm rupture of membranes (6.1% versus 23.4%; P = 0.002) and abruption (1.2% versus 13.4%; P = 0.007). The mean gestational age at delivery was 36.2 ± 4.6 weeks and 33.8 ± 5.4 weeks (P = 0.003) in the no-funnel and funnel groups, respectively. The presence or absence of funnelling predicted perinatal morbidity rather than the width and depth of the funnelling.[32]

Cervical length is normally distributed and remains relatively constant until about the beginning of the third trimester.[33] In the unselected population, the mean cervical length was found to be 38 mm at 23 weeks,[34] 35 mm at 24 weeks, and 34 mm at 28 weeks (Table 1).[35] After 20 weeks' gestation, the cervix appears to shorten with increasing gestation, with median values falling from 35–40 mm at

Table 1 Cervical length and spontaneous preterm birth in the general obstetric population

Study	Subjects (*n*)	Gestational age (weeks)	Cervix length (mm)	Preterm birth (%)	Sensitivity (%)	Specificity (%)	PPV (%)	NPV (%)
Iams *et al.* (1996)[35]	2915	24	≤ 25	4.3	37	92	18	97
Heath *et al.* (1998)[48]	2567	23	≤ 15	1.5	58		52	
Taipale *et al.* (1998)[49]	3694	18–22	≤ 25	0.8	7	100	15	
Hassan *et al.* (2000)[50]	6877	14–24	≤ 15	3.6	8	99	48	97

Table reproduced with permisson of the publisher Cambridge University Press © 2005 from: *The Prediction of Preterm Labour*. In: Norman J, Greer I. (eds) *Preterm Labour Managing Risk in Clinical Practice*. Cambridge: Cambridge University Press, 2005.[51]

24–28 weeks to 30–35 mm after 32 weeks. At 24 weeks, the cervical length amongst singleton pregnancies has a normal distribution, with the 50th centile at 35 mm and the 10th and 90th at 25 mm and 45 mm, respectively.[34] Crane *et al.*[36] postulated that, of all the cervical changes, transcervical length measurement is the best predictor for preterm delivery (Tables 2 and 3). However, Lueng *et al.*[37] showed

Table 2 Cervical length and spontaneous preterm birth in women with preterm labor

Study	Subjects (*n*)	Gestational age (weeks)	Cervix length (mm)	Preterm birth (%)	Sensitivity (%)	Specificity (%)	PPV (%)	NPV (%)
Iams *et al.* (1994)[52]	60	31 (24–35)	< 30	40	100	44	55	100
Gomez *et al.* (1994)[53]	59	30 (20–35)	< 18	37	73	78	67	83
Timor-Tritsch *et al.* (1996)[54]	70	29 (20–35)	Funnel	27	100	74	60	100
Crane *et al.* (1997)[55]	162	29 (23–33)	< 30	10	88	56	19	97
Rozenberg *et al.* (1997)[23]	76	31	≤ 26	26	75	73	50	89
Rizzo *et al.* (1996)[56]	108	30	≤ 20	43	68	79	71	76
Hincz *et al.* (2002)[57]	82	30.5	≤ 20	17	57	93	62	91

Table reproduced with permisson of the publisher Cambridge University Press © 2005 from: *The Prediction of Preterm Labour*. In: Norman J, Greer I. (eds) *Preterm Labour Managing Risk in Clinical Practice*. Cambridge: Cambridge University Press, 2005.[51]

Table 3 Cervical length and spontaneous preterm birth in high-risk women

Study	Subjects (*n*)	Gestational age (weeks)	Cervix length (mm)	Preterm birth (%)	Sensitivity (%)	Specificity (%)	PPV (%)	NPV (%)
Berghella *et al.* (1997)[58]	102	14–30	< 25	18	59	85	45	91
Owen *et al.* (2001)[59]	183	16–19	< 25	26	19	98	75	
Guzman *et al.* (2001)[60]	469	15–24	≤ 25	6	83	67	15	98

that both a short cervix and funnelling were independent predictors for preterm delivery < 34 weeks. Guzman *et al.*[38] recommended serial ultrasound cervical length assessment from 15 weeks' gestation of at least weekly intervals (or more frequent if necessary), for women with a past history or symptomatic of preterm labor. Transvaginal ultrasound has also been used in assisting intra-operative application of cervical cerclage suture.[39]

The role of cervical cerclage in the management of preterm labor remains controversial. Repeated studies have shown that cervical cerclage does not alter the perinatal outcome in singleton pregnancies.[40–44] A randomised, controlled trial showed that, although transvaginal cervical measurement identified a subgroup of about 1% of the population who are at a high risk of early preterm delivery, subsequent insertion of a cerclage does not reduce the incidence of preterm delivery, neonatal morbidity or mortality.[45] Similarly, tocolysis has no benefit in reducing perinatal death (OR 1.22; 95% CI 0.84–1.78) or decreasing respiratory distress syndrome (OR 0.82; 95% CI 0.64–1.07) or intraventricular hemorrhage (OR 0.73; 95% CI 0.46–1.15).[46] Rozenburg *et al.*[47] used ultrasound to measure cervical length after tocolysis and found that this did not improve the predictive value of preterm delivery (OR 0.97; 95% CI 0.90–1.03; $P = 0.27$).

Multiple pregnancies

Over one million babies have been conceived world-wide using assisted reproduction.[61] In the UK, assisted conception accounts for 1–1.5% of all births.[62] This has resulted in an increase in the incidence of twin pregnancies, and subsequent increase risk of preterm labor (Table 4). A study by Soriano *et al.*[63] looked at risk factors for preterm birth in primigravida with twin gestation ($n = 54$) and the role of transvaginal cervical assessment. The mean cervical length of patients who delivered at < 34 weeks (30.1 ± 6.1 mm) was significantly shorter than that of women who delivered at ≥ 34 weeks (42.2 ± 6.2 mm). Transvaginal cervical measurement > 35 mm at 18–24 weeks in twin gestation can identify patients at low risk for preterm delivery < 34 weeks.[63] Yang *et al.*[64] showed that both cervical length ≤ 30 mm and cervical funnelling in twin pregnancies < 26 weeks' gestation were independent factors strongly

Table 4 Cervical length and spontaneous preterm birth in women with multiple pregnancies

Study	Subj. (*n*)	Gest. age (wks)	Preg.	Cervix length (mm)	Preterm birth (%)	Sensitivity (%)	Specificity (%)	PPV (%)	NPV (%)
Skentou *et al.* (2001)[65]	434	23	Twins	≤ 20	7.8	26.5	97	41	94
Guzman *et al.* (2000)[66]	131	21–24	Twins	≤ 20	9.2	42	85	22	94
To *et al.* (2000)[67]	38	23	Triplets	≤ 25	16	50	91	50	91
Guzman *et al.* (2000)[68]	51	21–24	Triplets	≤ 25	32	60	84	64	82

Table reproduced with permisson of the publisher Cambridge University Press © 2005 from: *The Prediction of Preterm Labour.* In: Norman J, Greer I. (eds) *Preterm Labour Managing Risk in Clinical Practice*. Cambridge: Cambridge University Press, 2005.[51]

Gestational = Gest.
Pregnancy = Preg.
Subjects = Subj.

associated with a high risk for preterm labor. A long cervix > 35 mm is associated with a very low risk of about 4% for preterm labor.[64]

The role of routine cervical assessment at the 20–23 week anomaly scan

The RCOG Working Party Report on *Ultrasound Screening for Fetal Abnormalities* does not recommend that cervical assessment should be done routinely at the 20–23 week anomaly scan;[69] however, several studies looked at the role of routine cervical assessment at the anomaly scan. The Society of Obstetrician and Gynecologists of Canada Obstetric Ultrasound Guideline recommended that cervical assessment should be done routinely at the 16–20 week anomaly scan. They recommended that cervical assessment should be reported as: (i) normal; (ii) abnormal; or (iii) not viewed with explanation.[70] Taipale and Hiilesmaa[49] did transvaginal cervical assessment on 3694 women with singleton pregnancies who came for a routine anomaly scan at 18–22 weeks' gestation. They found that either a short cervix (≤ 29 mm) or cervical os dilatation (≤ 5 mm) was present in 3.6% of the population. They concluded that routine transvaginal cervical assessment at the time of the anomaly scan helps to identify many patients who are at risk for premature delivery; however, the low sensitivity and low positive predictive value limits its usefulness in screening low-risk women.[49] Heath *et al.*[71] measured the cervical length in 2702 women with singleton pregnancies who had routine anomaly scan at 23 weeks' gestation. They showed that 1.6% of the population had cervical length of ≤ 15 mm. Cervical length was significantly shorter in Afro-Caribbean women. Women who had a cervical length of ≤ 15 mm at 23 weeks have a more than 50% chance of spontaneous delivery at < 32 weeks' gestation.[48,71] About

4% of the population had cervical funnelling at routine ultrasound at 23 weeks.[72] The American College of Obstetricians and Gynecologists recommends that, if a short cervix is identified at or after 20 weeks' gestation, this should prompt assessment of: (i) the fetus for anomalies; (ii) uterine activity to rule out preterm labor; and (iii) maternal factors to rule out chorioamnionitis.[73]

Comparison between digital and transvaginal cervical assessment in predicting preterm labor

Digital examination of the cervix remains the oldest method of assessing the risk of preterm labor. However, it can be subjected to inter- and intra-observer variation. Inaccuracy is due to the anatomical configuration of the cervix, because the portion that lies above the anterior fornix or above the bladder base is hidden from the examiner's finger. Several studies have compared digital and transvaginal cervical assessment in various groups of patients – Lim *et al.*[74] looked at low-risk, singleton pregnancies; Berghella *et al.*[75] studied high-risk, singleton pregnancies; Chandra *et al.*[76] assessed post date singleton pregnancies; and Vayssiere *et al.*[77] looked at predicting preterm delivery in twin pregnancies. Lim *et al.*[74] showed that digital assessment tended to overestimate cervical dilatation and underestimate cervical length. The Berghella *et al.*[75] study concluded that ultrasound cervical length measurement was more accurate than digital assessment especially if done at 16–20 weeks. Chandra *et al.*[76] showed that none of the ultrasound characteristics (cervical length, dilatation and funnelling) predicted the primary outcome (rate of vaginal delivery) or secondary outcomes (rate of active labor in 12 h, vaginal delivery in 12–24 h, the mean duration of latent phase and induction to vaginal delivery interval). The Research Group in Obstetrics and Gynaecology (GROG) study[77] showed that transvaginal ultrasound predicted spontaneous delivery at < 34 weeks better than digital examination at 27 weeks but not before 22 weeks. The Society of Obstetricians and Gynecologists of Canada Guideline recommends transvaginal cervical instead of digital assessment[25] (see *Key points for clinical practice* at the end of this chapter).

OTHER USES OF TRANSVAGINAL ULTRASOUND – FETAL ASSESSMENT

Transvaginal ultrasound, as a result of the superior images obtained, is increasingly being used in assessing fetal abnormalities in the second and third trimester. A study by Mashiach *et al.*[78] looked at congenital eye abnormality. Transvaginal ultrasound anomaly scan at 14–16 weeks' gestation diagnosed one cataract (part of a multiple pterygium syndrome) and bilateral anophthalmia anomalies in five high-risk cases in which at least one previous child had congenital eye abnormality.[78] Transvaginal sonography enables better imaging of the fetal heart in various planes and directions in the second trimester, and it enables detection of fetal vascular rings.[79] Bronshtein *et al.*[80] did transvaginal sonographic examination in 36,323 consecutive fetuses at 14–16 weeks in both high- and low-risk pregnancies. Cardiac anomalies were detected in 173 fetuses. Ten fetuses had a cardiac anomaly that differed from the ultrasound diagnosis.[80] With advanced technology available in fetal cardiac surgery, antenatal diagnosis of cardiac abnormality will result in better management planning, counselling, and subsequent improvement in outcome. Transvaginal ultrasound has also been used in assessing the fetal cerebellar vermis.[81,82] Ultrasound has proven to be superior to MRI in detecting fetal cardiac defects, neural tube defects, encephalocele and arachnoid cysts. MRI is less effective in evaluating fetal cardiac abnormalities because MRI scans are not gated for fetal cardiac motion. Small encephalocele and arachnoid cysts are difficult to visualise with MRI due to partial volume averaging of the thin walled structure surrounded by cerebrospinal or amniotic fluid[83] (see *Key points for clinical practice* at the end of this chapter).

CONCLUSIONS

Transvaginal ultrasound provides superior views compared to trans-abdominal scanning. With a rising cesarean section rate and advancing maternal age, the incidence of placenta previa and placenta accreta will continue to increase. Transvaginal ultrasound with power Doppler is very effective in diagnosing placenta previa and placenta accreta, especially in cases of posterior placenta. Cervical assessment is integral, both independently and as a part of a multimarker testing to predict and treat preterm labor. The management of preterm labor remains a challenge. Transvaginal ultrasound has increasingly been used effectively in diagnosing fetal anomalies, in some cases it is more effective than MRI.

KEY POINTS FOR CLINICAL PRACTICE

Transvaginal ultrasound – placenta previa and placenta accreta

- Transvaginal ultrasound provides greater resolution, better image quality and thus is superior to transabdominal ultrasound in diagnosing placenta previa and accreta, especially for posterior placentas.
- Transvaginal ultrasound with power Doppler increases the accuracy in diagnosing placenta accreta.
- With delay in childbirth, increased maternal age combined with rising cesarean section rate, there will be increased abnormal placental location (placenta previa) and abnormal placental attachment (placenta accreta, increta and percreta).
- Antenatal diagnosis of placenta previa and accreta enables better counseling and surgical planning, resulting in reducing fetal and maternal morbidity and mortality.
- Ultrasound findings diagnostic of placenta accreta include: (i) loss of the normal hypo-echoic retroplacental myometrial zone; (ii) thinning/disruption of the hyperechoic uterine serosa–bladder interface; (iii) the presence of focal exophytic masses; and (iv) lacunar flow within the placenta.

KEY POINTS FOR CLINICAL PRACTICE *(Continued)*

Summary of the Royal College of Obstetricians and Gynaecologists Guideline No. 27 – Placenta previa and placenta accreta: diagnosis and management[2]

- Placenta previa major and minor replaced the previous staging of placenta previa Grades I–IV.
- All women should be offered an anomaly scan at 20–24 weeks. Check placental site; if low, offer follow-up: (i) with asymptomatic suspected placenta previa minor, follow-up scan at 36 weeks; or (ii) with asymptomatic suspected placenta previa major, follow-up scan at 32 weeks. If the patient bleeds, treat on individual basis.
- Ultrasound should include color Doppler in cases of placenta previa and suspected placenta accreta.
- Women with placenta previa major, in case of an episode of bleeding, should be offered in-patient management from 34 weeks. Asymptomatic women should be treated on an individual basis.
- All women with placenta previa, major and minor, should be offered counseling before delivery. This should include a discussion about the risks of major hemorrhage, blood transfusion and hysterectomy.
- The mode and timing of delivery depends on clinical judgement and ultrasound findings. If the placental edge is ≤ 2 cm from cervical os, delivery should be by cesarean section. Delivery should involve the most experienced obstetric, anesthetic and hematology staff. All hospitals should have guidelines for the management of massive hemorrhage.

Transvaginal ultrasound – cervical assessment

- Transvaginal cervical measurement, when assessed independently and as a part of a multimarker, shows great potential in predicting preterm labor in the high-risk population.
- The cervical changes seen on ultrasound (endocervical os dilatation, shortening and funnelling) are independent factors that predict preterm labor.
- Transvaginal cervical measurement identifies about 1% of the population who are high risk for preterm delivery, but cervical cerclage does not reduce preterm delivery, neonatal morbidity and neonatal mortality.
- Serial transvaginal cervical length assessment from mid-second trimester for at least weekly intervals is recommended for high-risk women.
- Transvaginal cervical assessment is more reliable, and reproducible compared to digital assessment in predicting preterm labor.

KEY POINTS FOR CLINICAL PRACTICE *(Continued)*

Transvaginal ultrasound – practical hints and techniques[1]

- Ensure that the procedure is clearly explained to the patient and that her privacy is respected at all times.
- Lay the patient comfortably on an examination couch, with the wedge underneath her back or on her side to prevent aortocaval compression. With the pillow placed just below her buttocks, this provides greater comfort, accessibility and manoeuvrability of the probe.
- The probe is placed inside a probe cover and gently inserted in the vagina.
- Insert the probe in the sagittal plane to improve orientation, then transverse plane.
- Watch the advance of the probe to ensure it is not inserted too far.
- Always ensure that the patient is comfortable.
- Systematically examine the lower segment of the uterus, the internal and external os, the endocervical canal, the presence of a fetus and placental site.

References

1 Lim BH. Transvaginal ultrasound – applications in the second and third trimesters of pregnancy. BMUS Bull 2000; 8: 22–25
2 Royal College of Obstetricians and Gynaecologists. Placenta Praevia and Placenta Accreta: Diagnosis and Management. Royal College of Obstetricians and Gynaecologists Guideline no. 27. London: RCOG, 2005.
3 Thomas J, Paranjothy S. The Royal College of Obstetricians and Gynaecologists Clinical Effectiveness Support Unit. National Sentinel Caesarean Section Audit Report. London: RCOG, 2001
4 Sherman SJ, Carlson DE, Platt LD, Mediaris AL. Transvaginal ultrasound: does it help in the diagnosis of placenta praevia? Ultrasound Obstet Gynaecol 1992; 2: 256–260
5 Smith RS, Laurie MR, Comstock CH, Treadwell MC, Kirk JS, Lee W. Transvaginal ultrasound for all placenta that appear to be low lying or over the internal cervical os. Ultrasound Obstet Gynaecol 1997; 9: 22–24
6 Laurie MR, Smith RS, Treadwell MC, Comstock CH, Kirk JS, Lee W. The use of second trimester transvaginal sonography to predict placenta praevia. Ultrasound Obstet Gynaecol 1996; 8: 337–340
7 Oyelese KO, Holden D, Awadh A, Coates S, Campbell S. Placenta praevia: the case for transvaginal sonography. Cont Rev Obstet Gynaecol 1999; 11: 257–261
8 Leerentveld RA, Gilberts EC, Arnold MJ, Wladimiroff JW. Accuracy and safety of transvaginal sonographic placental localization. Obstet Gynecol 1990; 76: 759–762
9 Comstock CH, Love JJ, Bronsteen RA *et al*. Sonograhic detection of placenta accreta in the second and third trimesters of pregnancy. Am J Obstet Gynecol 2004; 190: 1135–1140
10 Clarke SL, Koonings PP, Phelan JP. Placenta previa/accrete and prior caesarean section. Obstet Gynecol 1985; 66: 89–92

11 Finberg H, Williams J. Placenta accrete: prospective sonographic diagnosis in patients with placenta praevia and prior caesarean section. J Ultrasound Med 1992; 11: 333–343
12 Lerner J, Deane S, Timor-Tritsch IE. Characterization of placenta accreta using transvaginal sonography and colour Doppler imaging. Ultrasound Obstet Gynaecol 1995; 5: 198–201
13 Hoffman-Tretin J, Koenigsberg M, Rabin A, Anyaegbunam A. Placenta accreta: additional sonographic observations. J Ultrasound Med 1992; 11: 29–34
14 Levine D, Hulka C, Ludmir J, Li W, Edelman R. Placenta accreta: evaluation with colour Doppler ultrasound, power Doppler ultrasound and MRI. Radiology 1997; 205: 773–776.
15 Andrews WW, Goldenberg RL, Hauth JC. Preterm labour: emerging role of genital tract infections. Infect Agents Dis 1995; 4: 196–211
16 Iams JD, Johnson FF, Sonek J, Sachs L, Gebauer C, Samuels P. Cervical competence as a continuum: a study of ultrasonographic cervical length and obstetric performance. Am J Obstet Gynecol 1995; 172: 1097–1103
17 Obibo AO, Ural SH, Macones G. The prospects for multiple marker screening for preterm delivery: does transvaginal ultrasound of the cervix have a central role? Ultrasound Obstet Gynaecol 2002; 19: 429–435
18 Goldenberg RL, Iams JD, Mercer BM *et al.* for the NICHD MFMU Network. The preterm prediction study: Toward a multiple marker test for spontaneous preterm birth. Am J Obstet Gynecol 2001; 185: 643–651
19 Iams J. Prediction and early detection of preterm labor. Obstet Gynecol 2003; 101: 402–412
20 American College of Obstetricians and Gynecologists. Assessment of Risk Factors for Preterm Birth. Clinical Management Guidelines for Obstetricians & Gynaecologists No 31. ACOG, 2005
21 Hincz P, Wilczynski J, Kozarzewski M, Szaflik K. Two-step test: the combined use of fibronectin and sonographic examination of the uterine cervix for prediction of preterm delivery in symptomatic patients. Acta Obstet Gynaecol Scand 2002; 81: 58–63
22 Honest H, Bachmann L, Gupta J, Kleijnen J, Khan K. Accuracy of cervicovaginal fetal fibronectin test in predicting risk of spontaneous preterm birth. BMJ 2002; 325: 301–304
23 Rozenberg P, Goffinet F, Malagrida L *et al.* Evaluating the risk of preterm delivery: a comparison of fetal fibronectin and transvaginal ultrasonographic measurement of cervical length. Am J Obstet Gynecol 1997; 176: 196–199
24 Goldenberg R, Iams J, Mercer B *et al.* The Preterm Prediction Study: the value of new vs. standard risk factors in predicting early and all spontaneous preterm births. NICHD MFMU Network. Am J Obstet Gynecol 1998; 88: 233–238
25 The Society of Obstetricians and Gynecologists of Canada Guideline No 102 – Ultrasound Cervical Assessment in Predicting Preterm Birth. J Soc Obstet Gynecol Can 2001; 23: 418–421
26 American College of Radiology. Appropriateness Criteria – Premature Cervical Dilatation Guideline. ACR, 2005
27 Cicero S, Skentou C, Souka A, To M, Nicolaides K. Cervical length at 22–24 weeks of gestation: comparison of transvaginal and transperineal-translabial ultrasonography. Ultrasound Obstet Gynaecol 2001; 17: 335–340
28 Carr D, Smith K, Parsons L, Chansky K, Shields L. Ultrasonography for cervical length measurement: agreement between transvaginal and translabial techniques. Obstet Gynecol 2000; 96: 554–558
29 Rozenberg P, Rafii A, Senat M, Dujardin A, Rapon J, Ville Y. Predictive value of two-dimensional and three-dimensional multiplanar ultrasound evaluation of the cervix in preterm labour. J Matern Fetal Neonat Med 2003; 13: 237–241
30 Okitsu O, Mimura T, Nakayama T, Aono T. Early prediction of preterm delivery by transvaginal ultrasound. Ultrasound Obstet Gynaecol 1992; 2: 402–409
31 Berghella V, Kuhlman K, Weiner S, Texeira L, Wapner RJ. Cervical funnelling: sonographic criteria predictive of preterm delivery. Ultrasound Obstet Gynaecol 1997; 10: 161–166
32 Rust OA, Atlas R, Kimmel S, Roberts W, Hess W. Does the presence of a funnel increase the risk of adverse perinatal outcome in a patient with a short cervix? Am J Obstet Gynecol 2005; 192: 1060–1066

33 Tongsang T, Kamprapanth P, Pitaksakorn J. Cervical length in normal pregnancy as measured by transvaginal sonography. Int J Gynaecol Obstet 1997; 58: 313–315
34 Heath V, Southall T, Souka A, Elisseou A, Nicolaides K. Cervical length at 23 weeks of gestation: prediction of spontaneous preterm delivery. Ultrasound Obstet Gynaecol 1998; 12: 312–317
35 Iams J, Goldenberg R, Meis P *et al.* The length of the cervix and the risk of spontaneous preterm delivery. N Engl J Med 1996; 334: 567–572
36 Crane J, Van den Hof M, Armson B, Liston R. Transvaginal ultrasound in the prediction of preterm delivery: singleton and twin gestations. Obstet Gynecol 1997; 90: 357–363
37 Leung TN, Pang MW, Leung TY, Poon CF, Wong SM, Lau TK. Cervical length at 18–22 weeks of gestation for prediction of spontaneous preterm delivery in Hong Kong Chinese women. Ultrasound Obstet Gynaecol 2005; 26: 713–717
38 Guzman ER, Mellon C, Vintzileous AM, Ananth CV, Walters C, Gipson K. Longitudinal assessment of endocervical canal length between 15 and 24 weeks gestation in women at risk for pregnancy loss or preterm birth. Obstet Gynecol 1998; 92: 31–37
39 Quinn MJ. Vaginal ultrasound and cervical cerclage: a prospective study. Ultrasound Obstet Gynaecol 1992; 2: 410–416
40 Berghella V, Odibo A, Tolosa J. Cerclage for prevention of preterm birth in women with a short cervix found on transvaginal ultrasound examination: a randomised trial. Am J Obstet Gynecol 2004; 191: 1311–1317
41 Rust OA, Atlas R, Reed J, van Gaalen J, Balducci J. Revisiting the short cervix detected by transvaginal ultrasound in the second trimester: why cerclage may not help. Am J Obstet Gynecol 2001; 185: 1098–1105
42 Rust OA, Atlas RO, Jones KJ, Benham BN, Balducci J. A randomised trial of cerclage versus no cerclage among patients with ultrasonographically detected second trimester preterm dilatation of the internal os. Am J Obstet Gynecol 2000; 183: 830–835
43 Roman A, Rebarber A, Pereira L, Sfakianaki A, Mulholland J, Berghella V. The efficacy of sonographically indicated cerclage in multiple gestations. J Ultrasound Med 2005; 24: 763–768
44 Palaniappan V, Skentou C, Gibb D, Nicolaides KH. Elective cerclage vs. ultrasound indicated cerclage in high risk pregnancies. Ultrasound Obstet Gynaecol 2002; 19: 475–477
45 To MS, Alfirevic Z, Heath V *et al.* Cervical cerclage for prevention of preterm delivery in women with short cervix: randomised control trial. Lancet 2004; 363: 1849–1853
46 Royal College of Obstetricians and Gynaecologists. Tocolytic drugs for women in preterm labour. Clinical Guideline No. 1(B). London: RCOG, 2002
47 Rozenburg P, Rudant J, Chevret P, Boulogne A. Repeat measurement of cervical length after successful tocolysis. Obstet Gynecol 2004; 104: 995–999
48 Heath VC, Souka AP, Erasmus I, Gibb DM, Nicolaides KH. Cervical length at 23 weeks of gestation: the value of Shirodkar suture for the short cervix. Ultrasound Obstet Gynaecol 1998; 12: 301–303
49 Taipale P, Hiilesmaa V. Sonographic measurement of uterine cervix at 18–22 weeks gestation and the risk of preterm delivery. Obstet Gynecol 1998; 92: 902–907
50 Hassan S, Romero R, Berry S *et al.* Patients with an ultrasonographic cervical length = 15 mm have nearly a 50% risk of early spontaneous preterm delivery. Am J Obstet Gynecol 2000; 182: 1458–1467
51 Norman J, Greer I. (eds) The Prediction of Preterm Labour. In: Preterm Labour Managing Risk in Clinical Practice. Cambridge: Cambridge University Press 2005
52 Iams J, Paraskos J, Landon M, Teteris J, Johnson F. Cervical sonography in preterm labour. Obstet Gynecol 1994; 84: 40–46
53 Gomez R, Galasso M, Romero R *et al.* Ultrasonographic examination of the uterine cervix is better than digital examination as a predictor of the likelihood of premature delivery in patients with preterm labour and intact membranes. Am J Obstet Gynecol 1994; 171: 956–964
54 Timor-Tritsch I, Boozarjomehri F, Masakowski Y, Monteagudo A, Chao C. Can a ‘snapshot’ sagittal view of the cervix by transvaginal ultrasonography predict active preterm labour? Am J Obstet Gynecol 1996; 174: 990–995
55 Crane J, Van Den Hof M, Armson B, Liston R. Transvaginal ultrasound in the prediction

of preterm delivery: singleton and twin gestations. Obstet Gynecol 1997; 90: 357–363
56 Rizzo G, Capponi A, Arduini D, Lorido C, Romanini C. The value of fetal fibronectin in cervical and vaginal secretions and ultrasonographic examination of the uterine cervix in predicting premature delivery for patients with preterm labour and intact membranes. Am J Obstet Gynecol 1996; 175: 1146–1151
57 Hincz P, Wilczynski J, Kozarzewski M, Szaflik K. Two-step: the combined use of fetal fibronectin and sonographic examination of the uterine cervix for prediction of preterm delivery in symptomatic patients. Acta Obstet Gynaecol Scand 2002; 81: 58–63
58 Berghella V, Tolosa J, Kuhlman K *et al.* Cervical ultrasonography compared with manual examination as a predictor of preterm delivery. Am J Obstet Gynecol 1997; 177: 723–730
59 Owen J, Yost N, Berghella V *et al.* National Institute of Child Health and Human Development, Maternal-Fetal Medicine Units Network. Mid-trimester endovaginal sonography in women at high risk for spontaneous preterm birth. JAMA 2001; 286: 1340–1348
60 Guzman E, Walters C, Ananth C *et al.* A comparison of sonographic cervical parameters in predicting spontaneous preterm birth in high risk singleton pregnancies. Ultrasound Obstet Gynaecol 2001; 18: 204–210
61 Cooke I. ART babies: a time bomb in the making. Obstet Gynecol 2005; 7: 177–182
62 Human Fertilization and Embryo Authority. 11th Annual Report and Accounts 2002. London: HFEA, 2002
63 Soriano D, Weisz B, Seidman D *et al.* The role of sonographic assessment of cervical length in the prediction of preterm birth in primigravidae with twin gestation after infertility treatment. Acta Obstet Gynaecol Scand 2002; 81: 39–43
64 Yang J, Kuhlman K, Daly S, Berghella V. Prediction of preterm birth by second trimester cervical sonography in twin pregnancies. Ultrasound Obstet Gynaecol 2000; 15: 288–291
65 Skentou C, Souka A, To M, Liao A, Nicolaides K. Prediction of preterm delivery in twins by cervical assessment at 23 weeks. Ultrasound Obstet Gynaecol 2001; 17: 7–10
66 Guzman E, Walters C, O'Reilly-Green C *et al.* Use of cervical ultrasonography in prediction of spontaneous preterm birth in twin gestations. Am J Obstet Gynecol 2000; 183: 1103–1107
67 To M, Skentou C, Cicero S, Liao A, Nicolaides KH. Cervical length at 23 weeks in triplets: prediction of spontaneous preterm delivery. Ultrasound Obstet Gynaecol 2000; 16: 515–518
68 Guzman E, Walters C, O'Reilly-Green C *et al.* Use of cervical ultrasonography in prediction of spontaneous preterm birth in triplet gestation. Am J Obstet Gynecol 2000; 183: 1108–1113
69 The Royal College of Obstetricians and Gynaecologists Working Party. Report on Ultrasound Screening – Supplement to Ultrasound Screening for Fetal Abnormalities. London: RCOG, 2000
70 The Society of Obstetricians and Gynecologists of Canada Guideline – Content of a Complete Obstetrical Ultrasound Report. J Soc Obstet Gynecol Can 2001; 23: 427–428
71 Heath VC, Southall TR, Souka AP, Novakov A, Nicolaides KH. Cervical length at 23 weeks of gestation: relation to demographic characteristics and previous obstetric history. Ultrasound Obstet Gynaecol 1998; 12: 304–311
72 To M, Skentou C, Liao A, Cacho A, Nicolaides K. Cervical length and funnelling at 23 weeks of gestation in the prediction of spontaneous early preterm delivery. Ultrasound Obstet Gynaecol 2001; 18: 200–203
73 American College of Obstetricians and Gynaecologists. Cervical Insufficiency – American College of Obstetricians and Gynaecologists Clinical Management Guidelines No 48. ACOG, 2003
74 Lim BH, Mahmood TA, Smith NC, Beat I. A prospective comparative study of transvaginal ultrasonography and digital examination for cervical assessment in the third trimester of pregnancy. J Clin Ultrasound 1992; 599–603
75 Berghella V, Tolosa J, Kuhlman K, Weiner S, Bolognese R, Wapner R. Cervical ultrasonography compared with manual examination as a predictor of preterm delivery. Am J Obstet Gynecol 1997; 177: 723–730
76 Chandra S, Crane J, Hutchens D, Young D. Transvaginal ultrasound and digital examination in predicting successful labor induction. Obstet Gynecol 2001; 98: 2–6

77 Vayssiere C, Favre R, Audibert F *et al*. Cervical assessment at 22 and 27 weeks for the prediction of spontaneous birth before 34 weeks in twin pregnancies: is transvaginal sonography more accurate than digital examination? Ultrasound Obstet Gynaecol 2005; 26: 707–712
78 Mashiach R, Vardimon D, Kaplan B, Shalev J. Early sonographic detection of recurrent fetal eye anomalies. Ultrasound Obstet Gynaecol 2004; 6: 640–643
79 Bronshtein M, Lorber A, Berant M, Auslander R, Zimmer E. Sonographic diagnosis of fetal vascular rings in early pregnancy. J Am Cardiol 1998; 81: 101–103
80 Bronshtein M, Zimmer E. The sonographic approach to the detection of fetal cardiac abnormalities in early pregnancy. Ultrasound Obstet Gynaecol 2002; 19: 360–365
81 Ben-Ami M, Perlitz Y, Peleg D. Transvaginal sonographic appearance of the cerebellar vermis at 14–16 weeks gestation. Ultrasound Obstet Gynaecol 2002; 19: 208–209
82 Malinger G, Ginath S, Lerman-Sagie T, Watemberg N, Lev D, Glezerman M. The fetal cerebellar vermis: normal development as shown by transvaginal ultrasound. Prenat Diagn 2001; 21: 687–692
83 Levine D. Ultrasound versus magnetic resonance imaging in fetal evaluation. Topics Magnetic Resonance Imaging 2001; 12: 25–38

Jesus R. Alvarez Joseph J. Apuzzio

Controversies in the management of preterm premature rupture of membranes

Premature rupture of membranes (PROM) is defined as rupture of the fetal membranes occurring prior to the onset of labor. Its management is one of the most controversial topics in obstetrics. Intact fetal membranes with normal amniotic fluid are necessary for normal fetal growth and development. The membranes also serve as a barrier that separates the sterile fetal environment from the bacteria colonized vagina. The incidence of PROM has remained constant through the years and has been reported to be between 3–18.5%.[1] This wide variation in incidence may be secondary to different populations reporting the event, with the highest reported from inner city populations.

Preterm premature rupture of membranes (PPROM) refers to occurrence of this event prior to 37 weeks' gestation and accounts for about one-fourth all cases of ruptured membranes. PPROM is responsible for close to 40% of the cases of preterm births.[2] Because PPROM is the leading cause of preterm birth and perinatal morbidity, it has a tremendous socio-economic impact in society. In the US, preterm birth accounts for 12% of all births, 75% of all neonatal mortality and 50% of long-term neurological impairments in children, 33% of healthcare spending on infants and 10% of spending for children.

PATHOPHYSIOLOGY

PPROM is a complex and multifactorial entity. The fetal membranes are composed of the amnion and the chorion bound together by different layers

Jesus R. Alvarez MD
Third Year Maternal-Fetal Medicine Fellow, Department of Obstetrics, Gynecology and Women's Health, UMDNJ–New Jersey Medical School, 185 South Orange Avenue, E-506, Newark, NJ 07103, USA
E-mail: susomd@yahoo.com

Joseph J. Apuzzio MD (for correspondence)
Professor of Obstetrics, Gynecology and Radiology; Director, Division of Maternal-Fetal Medicine, Department of Obstetrics, Gynecology and Women's Health, UMDNJ–New Jersey Medical School, 185 South Orange Avenue, E-506, Newark, NJ 07103, USA
E-mail: apuzzijj@umdnj.edu

composed of extracellular matrix. This matrix is the key factor for the elasticity and tensile strength of the fetal membranes. The tensile strength guarantees the role of the membranes as a physical and functional boundary for the fetus during human pregnancy.[3] If the extracellular matrix is intact, the fetal membrane's elasticity and tensile strength is at its maximum; hence any process that weakens the matrix causes a release of enzymes, such as matrix metalloproteinases (MMPs), increasing the risk of PPROM.

Risk factors for PPROM are previous pregnancy with PPROM, which carries a recurrence rate of 21%, antepartum hemorrhage, multiple gestation, polyhydramnios (excessive membrane distention), smoking and illicit drug abuse such as heroin and cocaine, cervical insufficiency, and infection. These risk factors are similar to those for preterm birth since they share the same or similar pathways. Nevertheless, the greatest risk factor in PPROM is infection. It has been demonstrated that bacterial proteases decreased the strength and elasticity of the chorioamniotic membranes.[4] Women who are infected with gonorrhea, trichomonas, or chlamydia, and those colonized with Group B β-hemolytic *Streptococcus* spp. (GBS) or *Gardenella vaginalis*, also have an increased risk of PPROM.[5–8] Bacteria which colonize the genital tract have the capability of producing phospholipases which stimulate the release of prostaglandins from the breakdown of arachidonic acid, leading to preterm contractions. Infection also causes a host immune response, releasing pro-inflammatory cytokines and mediators which cause weakening of the fetal membranes by disrupting its extracellular matrix and releasing MMPs.

MMPs are a family of enzymes with varied substrate specificities that decrease membrane strength by increasing collagen degradation. The activation of MMP-9, a 92-kDa type IV collagenase, as an essential mediator of tissue damage is under investigation.

The local physiological signal by amniochorion cells to induce MMP-9 expression is not known, but bacterial products and/or the pro-inflammatory cytokines, IL-1β and TNF-α, as paracrine or autocrine signals may trigger these processes in pregnancies complicated with intra-amniotic infection.[3] In 2003, Romero *et al.*[9] described MMP-3 as a physiological constituent of amniotic fluid that may play a role in the mechanisms of human parturition and in the regulation of the host response to intra-uterine infection. Microbial invasion of the amniotic cavity in preterm gestations has also been associated with a significant increase in amniotic fluid concentration of MMP-7 playing a role in the host defense mechanism.[10] Marked elevations of mid-trimester amniotic fluid MMP-8 have also been found to be associated with subsequent preterm premature rupture of membranes, suggesting that the pathophysiological processes that contribute to preterm premature rupture of membranes may begin early in pregnancy.[11]

Genetic susceptibility may be a risk factor for PPROM. In 2002, the MMP-9 gene promoter activity and its association with PPROM were described. It was concluded that there are cell host-dependent differences in the MMP-9 promoter activity. In African-American neonates born from pregnancies complicated with PPROM, the allele associated with the increase in the MMP-9 promoter activity expression was found to be present, compared to those neonates who delivered at term without PPROM.[12] African-American females who are carriers for the SERPINH1 gene T-allele are also at high risk for premature delivery. This T allele reduces the promoter activity in amnion fibroblasts that deposit fibrillar collagen which gives the tensile strength to the amnion.[13]

RISK FACTORS

Conditions similar to those described above increase the risk of preterm birth and rupture of the fetal membranes. These risk factors are the same for spontaneous mid-trimester PPROM, PPROM, and rupture of membranes at term. Also, cervical insufficiency with cervical dilatation in the second trimester is a continuum to labor at this gestational age. Cervical dilatation exposes the fetal membranes to the vaginal microbial flora, causing weakening of the fetal membranes leading to the release of uterotonic agents and rupture of the membranes. Therefore, infection plays an important role for the occurrence of this entity.

Rupture of the fetal membranes can be caused secondary to an iatrogenic process. Fluid leakage can complicate a pregnancy after amniocentesis or fetoscopies. Fluid leakage has been described in 1% of genetic amniocentesis and 3–5% of diagnostic fetoscopies.[14,15]

EVALUATION OF PPROM

A patient with symptoms suggestive of PPROM should have a prompt evaluation. Patient history has a sensitivity of 90% for the diagnosis of PPROM.[15] It should be determined if the cause of mid-trimester PPROM was spontaneous or secondary to an iatrogenic process since the management may differ.

A patient who complains of leakage of fluid should have a speculum examination to evaluate for gross pooling of amniotic fluid in the vagina. If no fluid is seen on the speculum examination, the patient should be instructed to perform a valsalva maneuver such as coughing to evaluate if any leakage is visualized from the cervical os. A digital examination should be avoided since this increases the risk of infection and little information is obtained from this examination.[16]

Several tests have been utilized to assist in the diagnosis of PPROM if rupture of membranes cannot be determined by a speculum examination alone. The nitrazine paper test and the fern test may be performed. The combination of the patient's history, speculum examination, the nitrazine test, and the fern test for the evaluation of a patient with symptoms suggestive of PPROM yields a sensitivity of 93.1%.[15]

The normal pH of the vagina during pregnancy is between 4.5 and 5.0. When rupture of the membranes occurs and the vaginal mucosa is bathed in amniotic fluid whose pH is close to 7.3, the pH increases above 6.0, causing the nitrazine paper to turn from yellow to blue in color. However, the nitrazine test may give false-positive results if contaminated with semen, blood, some lubricants or if a vaginal infection is present.

The fern test has been described since the 1960s.[17] This test is performed by placing a swab in the posterior fornix of the vagina to obtain vaginal fluid and then performing a smear on a glass slide which should be allowed to dry for

10 min. The microscopic appearance of the smear as arborization or fern pattern is a positive test. The reported specificity of the fern test has been reported to be 84–100%.[18]

Patients with leakage of fluid from the vagina may also have a sonographic evaluation of amniotic fluid volume performed. It is also important to confirm a fetal heart rate, assess the gestational age of the pregnancy, and the position of the fetus. A finding of oligohydramnios may be useful in confirming rupture of the fetal membranes along with the above tests. The cervix can also be assessed by measuring the dilatation of the cervical os, the cervical length, and to determine if funneling is present.

Another test that may can be useful to assess leakage of fluid fetal fibronectin (FFN). This test can be performed after 18 weeks' gestation. A negative test indicates that the membranes are intact since its negative predictive value is 98–99%. Nevertheless, it has a poor positive predictive value due to its high false-positive rate and may not be needed or cost-effective.

If the diagnosis of rupture of the fetal membranes cannot be made with the above tests, an ultrasound-guided invasive test can be performed. A 22-gauge needle is inserted under ultrasound guidance into the amniotic cavity. Amniotic fluid can be obtained and evaluated for glucose, white blood cells, Gram stain, and be sent for culture of the amniotic fluid. Indigo carmine, or Evans blue (1 ml) can be instilled. A tampon is placed in the vagina prior to instillation of dye and kept in place for 30–60 min; when removed, a blue-tinged tampon will be seen if the patient has ruptured membranes.

NEONATAL COMPLICATIONS OF PPROM

Infection

Antenatal infection is the major complication of mid-trimester PPROM. The neonatal mortality for mid-trimester PPROM is approximately 35–40%; in the majority of cases, this occurs secondary to infection.[19–35] Infection decreases the latency period resulting in deliveries at a premature gestational age. Some studies have compared the neonatal mortality of those delivered after mid-trimester PPROM and controls delivered without PPROM having the same gestational age. There was no difference in mortality rate between the groups, indicating that the main factor for neonatal mortality is extreme prematurity secondary to a decrease in latency period.[36,37]

The risk of neonatal mortality has been correlated with the residual amount of amniotic fluid in mid-trimester PPROM (< 26 weeks' gestation). A study by Hadi *et al.*[27] showed that, in pregnancies with PPROM between 20–25 weeks' gestation, the group with a residual amniotic fluid pocket ≥ 2 cm had a greater neonatal survival rate compare to those with a largest pocket of fluid of < 2m (98% versus 31%) for neonates delivered matched for gestational age. They also described that the risk of chorioamnionitis is affected by the residual amniotic fluid volume after mid-trimester PPROM. Hadi *et al.*[27] also showed that, in the group of patients with severe oligohydramnios, a residual largest pocket of fluid < 2 cm, the incidence of chorioamnionitis was 69%.

There is a direct correlation between infection and the severe complications of prematurity. Studies done in 1982 by Garite and Freeman[38] and in 1987 by

Morales[39] have shown that the incidence of severe respiratory distress syndrome and neonatal sepsis or serious infections was inversely proportional to chorio-amnionitis. In 1990, a meta-analysis study showed an association between chorioamnionitis and perventricular leukomalacia (relative risk 3.0) and cerebral palsy (relative risk 1.9). In 1999, Yoon *et al.*[40] described a condition known as fetal inflammatory response syndrome (FIRS), defined as elevated IL-6 in fetal plasma obtained by cordocentesis. Fetuses of mothers with PPROM and FIRS have an impending onset of preterm labor irrespective of the inflammatory state of the amniotic cavity, showing that the fetus has a role in the initiation of labor in this patient population.[40] Furthermore, they showed an association of periventricular white matter lesions secondary to the cytokines released from the intense response of fetuses with FIRS. A follow-up for these fetuses was done for 3 years, and an association between fetuses with FIRS and cerebral palsy was noted.

Intra-uterine fetal demise

The incidence of intra-uterine fetal demise after mid-trimester PPROM varies, but the risk has been reported to be about 9.8%.[19–35] The rate is proportional to the gestational age when PPROM occurs, decreasing as gestational age increases.[24,31] There is also an association between intra-uterine fetal demise and < 2 cm pocket of residual amniotic fluid volume.[30] The majority of cases of intra-uterine fetal demise are attributable to placental abruption, cord prolapse, cord compression, and fetal infection.

Placental abruption is a major risk occurring in up to 50% if PPROM occurs prior to 20 weeks' gestation.[29,31] The highest risk factor is vaginal bleeding prior to the onset of PPROM at an early gestational age.[27,29,31] The risk of placental abruption with PROM at term is 0.4–1.3%.[41] Hence, the greatest risk factor for placental abruption is mid-trimester PPROM. Cord prolapse is not common, but it has grave complications. The incidence has been reported to be 1.9%. The main risk factor for cord prolapse is an unstable lie of the fetus such as transverse lie with the fetal back up.

Musculoskeletal morbidities secondary to PPROM

The majority of fetal limb growth occurs in the second and third trimester of pregnancy. If chronic oligohydramnios is present after mid-trimester PPROM, fetal growth and movements are restricted, and the intra-uterine pressure becomes asymmetric leading to limb position deformities, pulmonary hypoplasia, and craniofascial defects.

In mid-trimester PPROM, the reported incidence for these deformities varies between 3.5–50% for cases with severe oligohydramnios.[19–35] The risk increases when the duration of PPROM is greater than 14 days.[33]

Pulmonary hypoplasia

Pulmonary hypoplasia is associated with PPROM occurring prior to 26 weeks of gestation. The incidence of pulmonary hypoplasia if PPROM occurs after 26 weeks is low (1.4%).[29,31,32,42,43] The incidence of pulmonary hypoplasia as a complication of mid-trimester PPROM varies depending on the gestational age of the pregnancy. Rotschild *et al.*[32] reported an incidence of pulmonary hypoplasia when PPROM occurred at 19 weeks of 50% and at 25 weeks of 10%. In 1994, Vergani *et al.*[44] described an association of severe oligohydramnios and pulmonary hypoplasia. In this study, all fetuses that had pulmonary hypoplasia were born to mothers with a median amniotic fluid of less than 2 cm. It is thought that when PPROM occurs, the pressure gradient between the amniotic cavity and the alveoli is altered leading to a loss of fetal lung fluid to the amniotic cavity, leading to this complication.

MATERNAL COMPLICATIONS OF PPROM

Infection is the most important maternal complication of PPROM. The risk of infection is inversely proportional to the duration of the latency period.[20] chorioamnionitis is a complication for both fetus and mother. Non-reassuring fetal heart occurs more commonly in pregnancies complicated by PPROM. Cord compression due to oligohydramnios and a fetal cardiac response to infection are examples of why the incidence of non-reassuring fetal status increases with PPROM. Also, the incidence of fetal malpresentation increases with PPROM. Because of these factors, the cesarean delivery rates for pregnancies complicated by PPROM increases.

Postpartum endometritis is the most common maternal complication of mid-trimester PPROM. The incidence has been reported to be between 15–40%. Nevertheless, the incidence of postpartum maternal sepsis has been reported to be between 0–3%.[19,30,37]

USE OF TOCOLYTICS IN PPROM

Since PPROM is a major cause of preterm deliveries and perinatal morbidity, the use of tocolytics may be appealing to the obstetrician. However, tocolytic use in a case scenario of PPROM is controversial. Several randomized studies have been done looking at oral tocolytics in PPROM, intravenous tocolytics, and short-term and long-term tocolysis.[45–50] All of these studies failed to show a decrease in perinatal morbidity or improvement in neonatal outcome. Also, the use of tocolytics may be of concern since the incidence of perinatal infection is high and prolongation of these pregnancies may not be desired. Thus, the medical evidence does not justify the use of tocolytics in PPROM.

ANTENATAL CORTICOSTEROID THERAPY IN PPROM

In patients with intact membranes and at risk of preterm labor, studies have shown that the use of a corticosteroid course significantly benefits the preterm infant. A decrease has been shown in the incidence of severe respiratory distress syndrome (RDS), necrotizing enterocolitis (NEC), and intraventricular hemorrhage (IVH).

The use of antenatal corticosteroids is controversial in a pregnancy complicated by PPROM. Prospective, randomized, control studies have not shown a decrease in the rate or severity of RDS in patients receiving antenatal corticosteroids.[51,52] These studies also showed a small increase in postpartum endometritis and neonatal infections.

In 1994, the *National Institute of Health Consensus Conference* recommended the use of antenatal corticosteroids for those patients that were ≤ 32 weeks' gestation.[53] This recommendation was made because there was a decrease in the incidence of IVH and cerebral palsy. Since 1998, the American College of Obstetricians and Gynecologists (ACOG) recommends the use of corticosteroids to gravidas with PPROM before 32 weeks' gestation without evidence of chorioamnionitis to decrease the incidence of RDS, IVH, NEC, and neonatal death.[54] This decision was prompted by a study by Lewis *et al.*[55] where 18% (corticosteroid treated) to 44% (untreated) of infants had respiratory distress with no obvious increased risk for infection (5% to 3%).[55]

Although corticosteroids may potentially increase the risk of perinatal infection, they should be administered to patients with PPROM of less than 32 weeks' gestation, since the neonatal benefits may outweigh the risks.

ANTIBIOTIC PROPHYLAXIS

The purpose of prophylactic antibiotics for patients with PPROM is to decrease the risk of perinatal infections and to increase the latency period. A few randomized control studies have shown a prolongation of the latency period of 5–7 days, and a decrease in the incidence of postpartum endometritis and neonatal sepsis.[56,57] The largest randomized control studies are the NIH Maternal Fetal Medicine Collaborative Group and the Oracle 1 Randomized Trial.[58,59] In both studies, the incidence of severe RDS, severe IVH, neonatal sepsis, pneumonia, and NEC were reduced with the use of ampicillin or erythromycin. However, they reported an increased incidence of NEC in fetuses whose mothers were treated with ampicillin/clavulanic acid, so its use is not recommended. However, prolonged treatment with antibiotics may generate drug-resistant micro-organisms. In 1993, Mcduffie *et al.*[60] reported the development of resistant Enterobacteriaceae after prophylactic ampicillin or amoxicillin were used.

If prescribed, there is no uniformity in how long antimicrobials should be given after the onset of PPROM. The potential benefits of antimicrobials are well described, but there is no consensus on the duration of therapy.

Patients with PPROM should have genital tract cultures obtained for GBS, since these are the most common micro-organisms causing neonatal pneumonia, meningitis, and sepsis. Penicillin G should be started after cultures are obtained with a loading dose of 5×10^6 units intravenously followed by a maintenance dose of 2.5×10^6 units every 4 h. If penicillin G is not available, a 2-g loading dose of intravenous ampicillin should be started followed by 1 g every 4 h. The purpose of this management is to decrease the vertical transmission of GBS and the severe neonatal morbidity that may occur.

A recent study done at University Hospital, Newark, New Jersey showed that after 3 days of intravenous penicillin G therapy, GBS was eradicated from the genital tract in women with PPROM. In this study, daily genital tract GBS cultures were obtained from all patients with PPROM from the time of admission to the end of the latency period. A total of 220 patients were included in the study, 46 tested positive for GBS on admission. For all 46 patients, genital cultures were negative for GBS by day 3. Therefore, it was proposed that 3 days of antimicrobial prophylaxis for GBS should be given.[61]

MID-TRIMESTER PPROM (16–26 WEEKS' GESTATION)

The definition of mid-trimester PPROM as rupture of the fetal membranes occurring between 16–26 weeks' gestation varies among investigators. It can occur secondary to an iatrogenic factor such as amniocentesis. Mid-trimester PPROM affects 0.7% of all pregnancies.[62] In a pregnancy complicated by PPROM, less than 50% of patients will remain pregnant after 1 week of the event and 75–88% will be delivered by 28 days.[42]

Iatrogenic mid-trimester PPROM

Fluid leakage can complicate 1% of genetic amniocentesis, 3–5% of diagnostic fetoscopies, and up to 10% of all operative fetoscopies.[63,64] The outcome of iatrogenic mid-trimester PPROM is different to that of spontaneous mid-trimester PPROM with the exception of PPROM iatrogenically caused after placement of a cervical cerclage. Iatrogenic mid-trimester PPROM is not only a different entity etiologically, it is also different than spontaneous PPROM in its clinical behavior and response to therapeutic measures so it should no longer be viewed as a devastating complication of pregnancy.[65] In 2000, a study by Borgida *et al.*[66] reported the outcome of pregnancies complicated by iatrogenic rupture of membranes compared to those having spontaneous PPROM. In this study, women with PPROM after amniocentesis experience a significantly longer latency period (124 versus 28 days) and delivered at more advanced gestational ages (34.2 versus 21.6). The perinatal survival in the iatrogenically caused PPROM was 91% compared to 9% in the control group of spontaneous PPROM.[66] Hence, the counseling for a patient with iatrogenic mid-trimester PPROM is unique and different to that of spontaneous mid-trimester PPROM, or to the counseling given after PPROM occurs during or after placement of a cervical cerclage.

There are several options for a patient with iatrogenic mid-trimester PPROM if they desire to maintain the pregnancy. Patients with mid-trimester PPROM should be offered a termination of pregnancy irrespective of whether the cause of PPROM was iatrogenic or spontaneous. In some series, neonatal survival when PPROM occurred prior to 24 weeks was 12.5%; if it occurs after 24 weeks, the neonatal survival was 65%.[27] This should be part of the counseling given to these patients.

A patient may be given the option of expectant management since iatrogenic PPROM may be associated with a good perinatal outcome. In a study by Gold *et al.*,[63] 603 patients underwent a genetic amniocentesis during a 32-month period and 7 patients experienced leakage of fluid. Cessation of amniotic fluid leakage and re-accumulation occurred in all cases within 7 days.[63]

Another controversial option that can be offered to a patient with iatrogenic PPROM in which membranes have not 'resealed' after a week of expectant management is serial saline amnio-infusions. In selected cases, amnio-infusion appears to be a technique with low fetal and maternal risk that improves the fetal intra-uterine environment and survival.[68] Studies have shown that, in selected cases, serial amnio-infusions decrease the incidence of pulmonary hypoplasia, increase significantly the latency phase, and without increasing the incidence of perinatal infection.[67–72] The majority of women lose amniotic fluid after amnio-infusion but it is retained in up to 25%. Patients who retain saline fluid after amnio-infusion have the best outcomes and should be the patients selected for serial amnio-infusion therapy. Those who continued to leak the infused fluid and have persistent oligohydramnios are not good candidates for this therapy.

Several experimental therapies for 'resealing' the fetal membranes after mid-trimester PPROM have been tried. Different materials have been used to create the sealer or 'amniopatch', varying from gelatin sponge, fibrin and thrombin, to the most recent use of cryoprecipitate with platelets.[73–75] This experimental approach may be used to reseal the fetal membranes after iatrogenic PPROM. In a case of spontaneous PPROM, this therapy may not be effective since the area of rupture appears to be larger and at the level of the internal os.[76]

Spontaneous mid-trimester PPROM

Spontaneous mid-trimester PPROM risk factors are the same as those for preterm labor (*e.g.* smoking, intra-amniotic infection, cervical insufficiency) with the most important factor being infection. The recurrence rate has been reported to be 13.5–32%.[77–80]

The counseling of a patient with spontaneous PPROM differs from that of an iatrogenic cause, since it carries a poorer outcome. When this event occurs prior to 22 weeks, the best management option is termination of the pregnancy with a diagnosis of inevitable abortion. The mean latency for mid-trimester PPROM is 17 days; therefore, if the patient has no signs or symptoms of infection, it is more likely that the fetus may have a better chance of survival than if PPROM occurred prior to 22 weeks.[22,24,27,30,81,82] However, the chance of having an extremely premature infant are very high, and the long-term complications of extreme prematurity can occur which include cerebral palsy, blindness, and bronchopulmonary dysplasia amongst others.

If PPROM occurs at a gestational age where the fetus is potentially viable (24 weeks' gestation), infection should ruled out and the patient should have cultures obtained from the genital tract and prescribed antimicrobials that are effective for GBS. Expectant management for mid-trimester PPROM is the treatment option of choice since the complications of prematurity outweigh early delivery. As discussed above, tocolytics should probably not be administered and an antenatal steroid course should be given to decrease the incidence of IVH. Those patients that are candidates for serial amnio-infusions may have this therapeutic option.

PPROM OCCURRING AFTER 26 WEEKS' GESTATION

PPROM after 26 weeks' gestation is the most common obstetrical complication that leads to preterm deliveries. The major risks for the fetus are those of prematurity; therefore, therapy for PPROM is aimed at prolonging labor to decrease the risks of prematurity. However, the timing of delivery is still controversial. Patients with PPROM should be delivered if expectant management will not result in a significant prolongation of the pregnancy or if the risks of expectant management outweigh the neonatal risks associated with a preterm delivery.

After 34 weeks of gestation, expectant management is of little benefit, so most studies recommend delivery. If PPROM occurs prior to 32 weeks, one may collect amniotic fluid for fetal lung maturity testing and expectant management with intravenous antimicrobials. If the fetal lung maturity test is positive, delivery of the fetus is then recommended. The controversial area is in the management of PPROM that occurs between 32–34 weeks' gestation. This dilemma will be discussed later.

When counseling a patient, the neonatal survival rate and the risks of prematurity at the gestational age in which the PPROM occurred should be addressed. The risk of pulmonary hypoplasia decreases dramatically after 26 weeks, so serial amnio-infusions may be of minimal benefit after this gestational age.

Maternal surveillance for infection should be employed on every patient. Amniocentesis can be used to assess intra-amniotic infection and clinical parameters should be followed for any signs of chorioamnionitis.

Fetal surveillance with non-stress testing and biophysical profile testing may be employed. The interpretation of fetal heart rate changes that can occur after PPROM on the non-stress test are often difficult to interpret. For example, fetal heart rate changes may be due to an immature fetal neurological development because of prematurity, or secondary to cord compression if oligohydramnios is present, or secondary to intra-amniotic infection. This is an explanation for the many false-positive readings. A biophysical profile may also be performed on patients with PPROM. The absence of fetal breathing and fetal tone are predictive of fetal infection. Positive fetal breathing has a 95% negative predictive value for intra-amniotic infection.[83,84]

CONTROVERSIAL MANAGEMENT OF PATIENTS WITH PPROM

When to deliver?

PPROM prior to 32 weeks' gestation

The evidence suggests that PPROM prior to 32 weeks' gestation should be managed expectantly. In the absence of complications like infections, abruption, active preterm labor, or a non-reassuring fetus, expectant management with antimicrobials and antenatal corticosteroids may help decrease the severe complications of prematurity. Even though neonatal survival has improved dramatically over the years, there is little information about the long-term complications of these preterm infants.

There is some evidence that, for extreme low birth weight (ELBW) premature neonates (< 1000 g), there may be poor neurological development. A study done in 2005 showed the 5-year neurodevelopment outcome for ELBW born in 1996–1997. Only one-fourth of these babies developed normally by age 5 years.[85] In pregnancies complicated by preterm delivery, the incidence for ELBW of cerebral palsy was 9–26%; blindness 1–15%; deafness 9%; and up to 42% had cognitive disabilities.[86] Studies have also shown an association between a poor outcome in the ELBW population and infection.[87]

Because of complications of prematurity and the severe complications of the extreme low birth weight infants, we recommend expectant management with the use of antimicrobials and antenatal steroids until 32 weeks of gestation unless infection is present or the status of the fetus or the mother are not re-assuring.

PPROM occurring after 34 weeks' gestation

Patients that present with PPROM ≥ 34 weeks' gestation should have genital cultures done, prescribed appropriate antimicrobials that covers GBS, and be delivered. Most authorities recommend delivering patients presenting with PPROM ≥ 34 weeks' gestation since there is usually little benefit obtained from expectant management.

PPROM occurring between 32–34 weeks' gestation

The management for patients presenting with PPROM occurring between 32–34 weeks of gestation is unclear. Some authors recommend collection of amniotic fluid for fetal lung maturity testing and expectant management until 34 weeks' gestation unless the fetal lung maturity test is positive. Others recommend the same management as that of PPROM occurring after 34 weeks' gestation. A study done by Cox and Leveno[88] randomly assigned 68 women with PPROM at 30–34 weeks of gestation to expectant management and 61 similar women to immediate delivery. The mean gestational age at delivery was similar for each group (32.0 weeks and 31.7 weeks, respectively) and there was no improvement in pregnancy outcome (*e.g.* birth weight, intraventricular hemorrhage, necrotizing enterocolitis, sepsis, respiratory distress syndrome, or perinatal death) with either management strategy. However, the incidence of chorioamnionitis and antepartum hospitalization was higher in women managed expectantly.[88]

Many obstetricians collect amniotic fluid to evaluate for fetal lung maturity and, if positive, they would proceed to deliver the fetus. However, a study by Refuerzo *et al.*[89] reported no difference in the incidence of major neonatal morbidities including need for mechanical ventilation, grade 2 or 3 necrotizing enterocolitis, grade 3 or 4 intraventricular hemorrhage, or seizures, between the group with positive indices for fetal lung maturity and those with negative indices between the gestational ages of 32–34 weeks (41 patients positive indices and 37 patients negative indices).

However, there is an association between severe RDS and early peri/intraventricular hemorrhages and pro-inflammatory cytokines (IL-8, IL-6) and malondialdehyde (measures lipid peroxidation) was made by Krediet *et al.*[90] in 2006. This association may support a more aggressive approach if PPROM occurs at ≥ 32 weeks' gestation since the risk of infection increases with expectant management. But there are few studies comparing the long-term outcome for those infants electively delivered after PPROM occurred after 32 weeks' gestation and after 34 weeks' gestation. One study looked at the long-term lung effects and preterm deliveries. A reduced risk of RDS in infants born at ≥ 32 weeks' gestational age (conferred possibly by intra-uterine stress leading to accelerated lung maturation) appeared to be of transient effect and was counterbalanced by adverse effects of poor intra-uterine growth on long-term pulmonary outcomes such as chronic lung disease.[91]

The management of PPROM between 32–34 weeks will remain controversial until studies are performed comparing the long-term outcome of those infants delivered electively during this gestational age.

Amniocentesis and ultrasound-guided procedures in PPROM

Amniocentesis and ultrasound-guided procedures may be useful but are controversial tools in the management of patients with PPROM. They can be used as a diagnostic or as a therapeutic tool depending on the gestational age in which the event of PPROM occurs.

As previously described, an ultrasound-guided needle can be introduced into the amniotic cavity for the infusion of 1 ml of indigo carmine or Evans blue for the confirmation or diagnosis of PPROM.

Amniocentesis may be used for the diagnosis of intra-amniotic infection after PPROM occurs. The sample of amniotic fluid obtained can be sent for analysis of glucose, white blood cell count, Gram stain, IL-6, and genital cultures. The most sensitive test is IL-6, reported to be 86–100%. Its specificity is reported to be 79%.[92–94] Nevertheless, this test is not commercially available. The sensitivity of a Gram stain varies between 28–80%, but it is the most specific test, reported to be as high as 98%. Glucose has a reported sensitivity of 81.8% and specificity of 81.6%; white cell count has a reported sensitivity of 57–64% and high specificity (as high as 94%). The frequency of positive cultures obtained by transabdominal amniocentesis at the time of presentation with PPROM in the absence of labor is 25–40%.[95] Promising studies are being done evaluating the association of intra-amniotic MMPs and intra-amniotic infection or inflammatory response. In 2006, a study was done to assess the value of a rapid MMP-8 test from amniotic fluid. It reported a sensitivity of 83%, specificity of 94%, and a negative predictive value of 99% for intra-amniotic infection.[96]

Experimental ultrasound-guided procedures have been reported to be successful in the management of PPROM. We have previously described serial amnio-infusions where, in selected cases, it has been noted to be a relatively safe procedure that can decrease the morbidities associated with severe oligohydramnios and preterm birth.

Another experimental modality that has been used is the use of intra-amniotic surfactant prior to delivery to decrease the incidence of severe RDS. A case control study was done in China were 15 women received intra-amniotic surfactant several hours prior to delivery after an initial dose of theophilline was administered to the mother to induce fetal swallowing. Another 30 women served as controls and did not receive intra-amniotic surfactant prior to delivery. The only statistically significant difference between the groups was a decrease of neonatal RDS and incidence of fetal lung maturity (56.3% to 13.3%, respectively) and the length of hospital stay (32.4 days to 42 days, respectively).[97] Another case series have described similar results of decreased incidence of neonatal RDS, hospital stay, and postpartum surfactant use.[98] There are limited cases reported, so this modality is still experimental and should be viewed as such.

PPROM with a cervical cerclage in place: to remove or not to remove?

The placement of a cervical cerclage is controversial; hence, the management of a patient in which PPROM occurs after placement of a cervical cerclage has caused confusion. If PPROM occurs prior to 24 weeks' gestation, most agree on removing the cerclage and counseling the patient about termination of the pregnancy. Even though it is caused by an iatrogenic process, rupture of membranes after a cervical cerclage should be managed as if it was a spontaneous PPROM.

The controversy is in the management of those cases with PPROM and a cervical cerclage in place after viability is reached. In the US, viability is usually considered to be after 24 weeks of gestation.

The dilemma of whether or not to remove the cervical cerclage encompasses two questions – will maintaining the cerclage increase the incidence of perinatal infection and would it increase the latency period? Several studies have tried to answer these questions.[99–101] A case control study was done by Yeast and Garite[99] showing no statistical difference in the incidence of chorioamnionitis, latency period, and neonatal outcome. Similar results were obtained by a study done by McElrath *et al.*[102] Another study by Moore-Goldman *et al.*[101] showed a decreased latency period for those patients with retained cerclage after PPROM. In this study, there were no differences in incidence of chorioamnionitis and neonatal outcome. Based on the results of all the studies available, there appears to be no benefit in retaining the cervical cerclage. The neonatal outcome is similar and the latency period appears to be similar.

Twin pregnancies and PPROM

It has been reported that PPROM occurs more frequently in twin than singleton gestations (7.4% versus 3.7%).[103] The reported mean gestational age at which PPROM occurs in multifetal gestations is 30 weeks. When compared to a singleton pregnancy with PPROM matched for gestational age, the event occuring in multifetal pregnancies has a shorter latency period.[104,105]

When PPROM occurs in a twin pregnancy, the ruptured sac can be from the presenting fetus, from the sac of the non-presenting fetus, or from the interamniotic membrane. When PPROM occurs from the sac of the presenting fetus, the non-presenting fetus has an increased incidence of RDS as well as prolonged oxygen therapy.[104] There are few cases reported on the management of PPROM when occurring from the non-presenting twin. Nevertheless, some authors have reported success with conservative expectant management and antibiotics with leakage stoppage after a period of several weeks if the event occurs at an early gestational age.

If PPROM occurs early in the second trimester, termination of the pregnancy should be offered, since the risk of continuing the pregnancy outweighs the benefit of expectant management. Nevertheless, some authors have reported four successful cases using selective fetal reduction of the fetus with PPROM in the absence of infection. After this technique is applied, leakage of fluid stops and the second fetus has successfully continued the course of the pregnancy with normal fetal growth.[106,107]

Delayed interval delivery of the presenting twin after PPROM may be an option in selected cases. Contra-indications to offer this option to a patient are suspected placental abruption, intra-amniotic infection, and non-reassuring fetal status of the remaining fetus. A monochorionic placenta is a possible contra-indication but is controversial. The management of a delayed interval delivery is ligation of the umbilical cord with an absorbable suture after vaginal delivery, followed by tocolytics and antimicrobials. The placement of a cerclage is controversial since it may increase the incidence of infection.

Studies in delayed interval twin deliveries are of a small number of subjects and sometimes contradictory in their results. Arias *et al.*[108] reported a case series of 10 patients who underwent this management and reported success in 6 of 10 patients with a mean latency period of 49 days. This study also states that the factor for the failure in the four patients was intra-uterine infection. In 2005, a population-based study was done with 200 pregnancies with delayed delivery, the mean gestational age at first delivery was 23 weeks and the median duration of delay was 6 days. One week of delay in delivery was associated with an increase in infant birth weight of 131 g on average. Survival was 56% for the delayed second twins by 1 year of age, whereas only 24% of the non-delayed second twins survived to 1 year of age.[109]

The timing of when to offer this management is also controversial. The largest study to date, reporting the best time to offer delayed interval in twins, states that when a first twin was delivered at 22–23 weeks, delayed delivery of the second twin was associated with reduced perinatal and infant mortality of the second twin if the interval was less than 3 weeks. Delayed delivery of the second twin when the first was delivered at ≥ 24 weeks had no benefit on mortality.[110]

Herpes genitalis and PPROM

Congenital herpes is a major perinatal infection with possible fatal disease occurring in the neonate. It may be acquired from an infected lower genital tract; hence, if a mother has PPROM with active genital lesions, concerns about perinatal transmission become apparent.

Few studies have looked at the risk of perinatal transmission after PPROM occurs when expectant management is implemented. Major *et al.*[111] identified 29 patients that met the criteria of mothers with PPROM and active genital lesions. No cases of neonatal herpes developed in the delivered newborn infants and all neonatal cultures were negative. This study suggest that expectant management of PPROM with active recurrent genital herpes is warranted.[111] Although there is no good data, some would prescribe antivirals as well in this setting.

PPROM in patients who are HIV positive

In the US, perinatally acquired HIV accounts for 0.6% of all cases of HIV with an estimated range of 144–236 cases a year in 2002.[112] A major risk factor for vertical transmission of HIV is the duration of ruptured membranes prior to delivery. In 1995, Minkoff *et al.*[113] described a significant increase in vertical transmission rate if the duration of rupture of membranes was greater than 4 h in patients with low $CD4^+$ levels. Other studies confirmed that among HIV-infected pregnant women, ruptured membranes greater than 4 h prior to delivery significantly increased the rate of vertical transmission from 25% as compared to 14% among mothers with a shorter length of ruptured membranes less than 4 h prior to delivery.[114]

We performed a retrospective study at our institution where we identified

18 HIV-positive mothers having PPROM. All 18 patients delivered by cesarean section. The mother-to-child transmission rate (MTCT) was 11.1%. Of the 18 patients in the study, 10 mothers had antenatal antiretrovirals (ARVs) and 8 other mothers had no prenatal care and received nevirapine (NVP) and intravenous zidovudine (AZT) at the time of delivery. None of the 10 patients prescribed antenatal ARVs had an infected child. Of those 8 non-clinic patients not receiving antenatal ARVs, the MTCT was 25% (2 of 8). These results occurred irrespective of the maternal viral load and CD4 count. There was no difference in neonatal outcome when the fetuses were delivered after 30 weeks. Our limited study suggests that expectant management after 30 weeks may be offered to patients with antenatal ARVs, but for those patients without antenatal ARVs, this management strategy may be of no benefit.[115]

KEY POINTS FOR CLINICAL PRACTICE

- Patients at 34 or more weeks' gestation with PPROM should be delivered.
- Patients less than 32 weeks gestation with PPROM should be managed conservatively with corticosteriod and antimicrobial prophylaxis unless there is an indication for delivery.
- The management of patients with PPROM between 32 and 34 weeks' gestation is controversial.
- Patients with PPROM and either HIV or genital HSV require individual evaluation and treatment.

References

1 Gunn CS, Mishell DR, Morton DG. Premature rupture of the fetal membranes. Am J Obstet Gynecol 1970; 106: 469

2 Parry S, Strauss 3rd JF. Premature rupture of the fetal membranes. N Engl J Med 1998; 338: 663–670

3 Vadillo-Ortega F, Estrada-Gutierrez G. Role of matrix metalloproteinases in preterm labour. Br J Obstet Gynaecol 2005; 112 (Suppl 1): 19–22

4 McGregor JA, French JI, Lawellin D *et al*. Bacterial protease-induced reduction of chorioamniotic membrane strength and elasticity. Obstet Gynecol 1987; 69: 167–174

5 Edwards LE, Barrada MI, Hamman AA *et al*. Gonorrhea in pregnancy. Obstet Gynecol 1978; 132: 637–641

6 Regan TA, Chao S, James LS. Premature rupture of membranes, preterm delivery, and group B streptoccocal colonization of mothers. Am J Obstet Gynecol 1981 141: 184–186

7. Martin DH, Koutsky L, Eschenbach DA *et al*. Prematurity and perinatal mortality in pregnancies complicated by maternal *Chlamydia trachomatis* infections. JAMA 1982; 247: 1585–1588

8 Minkoff H, Grunebaum AN, Schwarz RH *et al*. Risk factors for prematurity and premature rupture of membranes: a prospective study of the vaginal flora in pregnancy. Am J Obstet Gynecol 1984; 150: 965–972

9 Park KH, Chaiworapongsa T, Kim YM *et al*. Matrix metalloproteinase 3 in parturition, premature rupture of the membranes, and microbial invasion of the amniotic cavity. J Perinat Med 2003; 31: 12–22

10 Maymon E, Romero R, Pacora P *et al*. Matrilysin (matrix metalloproteinase 7) in parturition, premature rupture of membranes, and intrauterine infection. Am J Obstet Gynecol 2000; 182: 1545–1553
11 Biggio Jr JR, Ramsey PS, Cliver SP *et al*. Midtrimester amniotic fluid matrix metalloproteinase-8 (MMP-8) levels above the 90th percentile are a marker for subsequent preterm premature rupture of membranes. Am J Obstet Gynecol 2005; 192: 109–113
12 Ferrand PE, Parry S, Sammel M *et al*. A polymorphism in the matrix metalloproteinase-9 promoter is associated with increased risk of preterm premature rupture of membranes in African Americans. *Mol Hum Reprod* 2002; 8: 494–501
13 Wang H, Parry S, Macones G *et al*. A functional SNP in the promoter of the SERPINH1 gene increases risk of preterm premature rupture of membranes in African Americans. Proc Natl Acad Sci USA 2006; 103: 13463–13467
14 Gold RB, Goyert N, Schwartz DB *et al*. Conservative management of second-trimester post-amniocentesis fluid leakage. Obstet Gynecol 1989; 74: 745–747
15 Rodeck CH. Fetoscopy guided by real-time ultrasound for pure fetal blood samples, fetal skin samples, and examination of the fetus *in utero*. Br J Obstet Gynaecol 1980; 87: 449–456
16 Friedman ML, McElin TW. Diagnosis of ruptured fetal membranes. Am J Obstet Gynecol 1969; 104: 554–550
17 Wagner MV, Chin VP, Peters CJ *et al*. A comparison of early and delayed induction of labor with spontaneous rupture of membranes at term. Obstet Gynecol 1989; 74: 93–97
18 Bennett SL, Cullen JB, Shere DM *et al*. The ferning and nitrazine tests of amniotic fluid between 12 and 41 weeks gestation. Am J Perinatol 1993; 10: 101–104
19 Moretti M, Sibai BM. Maternal and neonatal outcome of expected management of premature rupture of membranes in the midtrimester. Am J Obstet Gynecol 1988; 159: 390–396
20 Taylor J, Garite TJ. Premature rupture of membranes before fetal viability. Obstet Gynecol 1984; 64: 615–620
21 Beydoun SN, Yasin SY. Premature rupture of the membranes before 28 weeks: conservative management. Am J Obstet Gynecol 1986; 155: 471–479
22 Dowd J, Permezel M. Pregnancy outcome following preterm premature rupture of the membranes at less than 26 weeks' gestation. Aust NZ J Obstet Gynaecol 1992; 32: 120–124
23 Bengtson JM, VanMarter LJ, Barss VA *et al*. Pregnancy outcome after premature rupture of the membranes at or before 26 weeks' gestation. Obstet Gynecol 1989; 73: 921–927
24 Major CA, Kitzmiller JL. Perinatal survival with expectant management of midtrimester rupture of membranes. Am J Obstet Gynecol 1990; 163: 838–844
25 Rib DM, Sherer DM, Woods Jr JR. Maternal and neonatal outcome associated with prolonged premature rupture of membranes below 26 weeks' gestation. Am J Perinatol 1993; 10: 369–373
26 Hibbard JU, Hibbard MC, Ismail M, Arendt E. Pregnancy outcome after expectant management of premature rupture of the membranes in the second trimester. J Reprod Med 1993; 38: 945
27 Hadi HA, Hodson CA, Strickland D. Premature rupture of the membranes between 20 and 25 weeks' gestation: role of amniotic fluid volume in perinatal outcome. Am J Obstet Gynecol 1994; 170: 1139–1144
28 Fortunato SJ, Welt SI, Eggleston Jr MK, Bryant EC. Active expectant management in very early gestations complicated by premature rupture of the fetal membranes. J Reprod Med 1994; 39: 13–16
29 Farooqi A, Holmgren PA, Engberg S, Serenius F. Survival and 2-year outcome with expectant management of second-trimester rupture of membranes. Obstet Gynecol 1998; 92: 895–901
30 Shumway JB, Al-Malt A, Amon E *et al*. Impact of oligohydramnios on maternal and perinatal outcomes of spontaneous premature rupture of the membranes at 18–28 weeks. J Matern Fetal Med 1999; 8: 20–23
31 Blott M, Greenough A. Neonatal outcome after prolonged rupture of the membranes starting in the second trimester. Arch Dis Child 1988; 63: 1146–1150

32 Rotschild A, Ling EW, Puterman ML, Farquharson D. Neonatal outcome after prolonged preterm rupture of the membranes. Am J Obstet Gynecol 1990; 162: 46–52
33 Kilbride HW, Yeast J, Thibeault DW. Defining limits of survival: lethal pulmonary hypoplasia after midtrimester premature rupture of membranes. Am J Obstet Gynecol 1996; 175: 675–681
34 Hoekstra JH, de Boer R. Very early prolonged premature rupture of membranes and survival. Eur J Pediatr 1990; 149: 585–586
35 Dinsmoor MJ, Bachman R, Haney EI *et al*. Outcomes after expectant management of extremely preterm premature rupture of the membranes. Am J Obstet Gynecol 2004; 190: 183–187
36 Kurkinen-Räty M, Koivisto M, Jouppila P. Perinatal and neonatal outcome and late pulmonary sequelae in infants born after preterm premature rupture of membranes. Obstet Gynecol 1998; 92: 408–415
37 Morales WJ, Talley T. Premature rupture of membranes at < 25 weeks: a management dilemma. Am J Obstet Gynecol 1993; 168: 503–507
38 Garite TJ, Freeman RK. Chorioamnionitis in the preterm gestation. Obstet Gynecol 1982; 69: 539
39 Morales WJ. The effect of chorioamnionitis on developmental outcome of preterm infants at one year. Obstet Gynecol 1987; 70: 183–186
40 Yoon BH, Romero R, Kim KS *et al*. A systemic fetal inflammatory response and the development of bronchopulmonary dysplasia. Am J Obstet Gynecol 1999; 181: 773–779
41 Knab DR. Abruptio placentae: an assessment of the time and method of delivery. Obstet Gynecol 1978; 52: 625–629
42 Falk SJ, Campbell LJ, Lee-Parritz A *et al*. Expectant management in spontaneous preterm premature rupture of membranes between 14 and 24 weeks gestation. J Perinatol 2004; 24: 611–616
43 Nimrod C, Varela-Gittings F, Machin G *et al*. The effect of very prolonged rupture membranes on fetal development. Am J Obstet Gynecol 1984; 148: 540–543
44 Vergani P, Ghidini A, Locatelli A *et al*. Risk factors for pulmonary hypoplasia in second trimester premature rupture of membranes. Am J Obstet Gynecol 1994; 170: 1359–1364
45 Matsuda Y, Ikenoue T, Hokanishi H. Premature rupture of membranes. Aggressive versus conservative approach: effect of tocolysis and antibiotic therapy. Gynecol Obstet Invest 1993; 36: 102–107
46 Levy DL, Warsof SL. Oral Ritrodrine and preterm premature rupture of membranes. Obstet Gynecol 1985; 66: 621–623
47 Dunlop PDM, Crowley PA, Lamont RF *et al*. Preterm ruptured membranes, no contractions. J Obstet Gynaecol 1986; 7: 92
48 Christensen KK, Ingemarsson I, Liedman T *et al*. Effect of Ritrodrine on labor after premature rupture of the membranes. Obstet Gynecol 1980; 55: 187–190
49 Weiner CP, Renk K, Klugman M. The therapeutic efficacy and cost effectiveness of aggressive tocolysis for premature labor associated with premature rupture of the membranes. Am J Obstet Gynecol 1988; 159: 216–222
50 Garite TJ, Keegan KA, Freeman RK *et al*. A randomized trial of Ritrodrine tocolysis versus expectant management in patients with premature rupture of membranes at 25 to 30 weeks of gestation. Am J Obstet Gynecol 1987; 157: 388–393
51 Morales W, Angel J, O'Brien W *et al*. Use of ampicillin and corticosteroids on PROM: a randomized study. Obstet Gynecol 1989; 73: 721–726
52 Block MF, Kling OR, Crosby WM. Antenatal glucocorticoid therapy for the prevention of respiratory distress syndrome in the premature infant. Obstet Gynecol 1977; 50: 186–190
53 National Institutes of Health. National Institute of Health Consensus Development Conference Statement: Effect of corticosteroids for fetal maturation on perinatal outcomes (NIH Publication No. 95-3784). Bethesda, MD: National Institute of Health, 1994
54 ACOG Practice Bulletin. Clinical Management guidelines for Obstetrician-Gynecologists. Number 1, June 1998
55 Lewis DF, Brody K, Edwards MS *et al*. Preterm premature rupture of membranes: a randomized trial of steroids after treatment with antibiotics. Obstet Gynecol 1996; 88:

801–805
56 Amon E, Lewis SV, Sibai B *et al.* Antibiotic prophylaxis in preterm PROM: a prospective randomized study. Am J Obstet Gynecol 1988; 159: 539
57 Lovett SM, Weiss JD, Diogo MJ *et al.* A prospective double-blind, randomized, controlled clinical trial of ampicillin-sulbactam for preterm premature rupture of membranes in women receiving antenatal corticosteroid therapy. Am J Obstet Gynecol 1997; 176: 1030–1038
58 Mercer BM, Miodovnik M, Thurnau GR *et al.* Antibiotic therapy for reduction of infant morbidity after preterm premature rupture of membranes: a randomized controlled trial. JAMA 1997; 278: 989–995
59 Kenyon SL, Taylor DJ, Tarnow-Mordi W. Broad-spectrum antibiotics for preterm, prelabour rupture of membranes: the Oracle 1 randomized trial. Lancet 2001; 356: 979–988
60 Mcduffie R, McGregor J, Gibbs R. Adverse perinatal outcome and resistant Enterobacteriaceae after antibiotic usage for premature rupture of the membranes and group B streptococcus carriage. Obstet Gynecol 1993; 82: 487–489
61 Alvarez J, Williams S, Apuzzio J. Duration of antimicrobial prophylaxis for Group B *Streptococcus* in patients with PPROM. Presentation at the Society of Maternal Fetal Medicine Annual Meeting February 2007, San Francisco
62 Shucker JL, Mercer BM. Midtrimester premature rupture of the membranes. Perinatology 1996; 20: 389–400
63 Gold RB, Goyert GL, Schwarz DB *et al.* Conservative management of second-trimester post-amniocentesis fluid leakage. Obstet Gynecol 1989; 74: 745–747
64 Quintero RA, Morales WJ, Allen M *et al.* Treatment of iatrogenic previable premature rupture of membranes with intra-amniotic injection of platelets and cryoprecipitate (amniopatch): preliminary experience. Am J Obstet Gynecol 1999; 181: 744–749
65 Quintero RA. Treatment of previable premature ruptured membranes. Perinatology 2003; 30: 573–589
66 Borgida AF, Mills AA, Feldman DM *et al.* Outcome of pregnancies complicated by ruptured membranes after genetic amniocentesis. Am J Obstet Gynecol 2000; 183: 937–939
67 De Santis M, Scavo M, Noia G *et al.* Transabdominal amnioinfusion treatment of severe oligohydramnios in preterm premature rupture of membranes at less than 26 gestational weeks. Fetal Diagn Ther 2003; 18: 412–417
68 Locatelli A, Vergani P, Di Pirro G *et al.* Role of amnioinfusion in the management of premature rupture of the membranes at < 26 weeks' gestation. Am J Obstet Gynecol 2000; 183: 878–882
69 Tan LK, Kumar S, Jolly M *et al.* Test amnioinfusion to determine suitability for serial therapeutic amnioinfusion in midtrimester premature rupture of membranes. Diagn Ther 2003; 18: 183–189
70 Ogunyemi D, Thompson W. A case controlled study of serial transabdominal amnioinfusions in the management of second trimester oligohydramnios due to premature rupture of membranes. Eur J Obstet Gynecol Reprod Biol 2002; 102: 167–172
71 Tranquilli AL, Giannubilo SR, Bezzeccheri V *et al.* Transabdominal amnioinfusion in preterm premature rupture of membranes: a randomised controlled trial. Br J Obstet Gynaecol 2005; 112: 759–763
72 Vergani P, Locatelli A, Strobelt N *et al.* Amnioinfusion for prevention of pulmonary hypoplasia in second-trimester rupture of membranes. Am J Perinatol 1997; 14: 325–329
73 O'Brien JM, Mercer BM, Barton JR *et al.* An *in vitro* model and case report that used gelatin sponge to restore amniotic fluid volume after spontaneous premature rupture of the membranes. Am J Obstet Gynecol 2001; 185: 1094–1097
74 Reddy UM, Shah SS, Nemiroff RL *et al.* *In vitro* sealing of punctured fetal membranes: potential treatment for midtrimester premature rupture of membranes. Am J Obstet Gynecol 2001; 185: 1090–1093
75 Quintero RA, Morales WJ, Bornick PW *et al.* Surgical treatment of spontaneous rupture of membranes: the amniograft – first experience. Am J Obstet Gynecol 2002; 186: 155–157
76 Quintero RA, Morales WJ, Kalter CS *et al.* Transabdominal intra-amniotic endoscopic

assessment of previable premature rupture of membranes. Am J Obstet Gynecol 1998; 179: 71–76

77 Mercer BM, Goldenberg RL, Moawad AH *et al*. The preterm prediction study: effect of gestational age and cause of preterm birth on subsequent obstetric outcome. National Institute of Child Health and Human Development Maternal-Fetal Medicine Units Network. Am J Obstet Gynecol 1999; 181: 1216–1221

78 Naeye RL. Factors that predispose to premature rupture of the fetal membranes. Gynecology 1982; 60: 93–98

79 Asrat T, Lewis DF, Garite TJ *et al*. Rate of recurrence of preterm premature rupture of membranes in consecutive pregnancies. Am J Obstet Gynecol 1991; 165: 1111–1115

80 Lee T, Carpenter MW, Heber WW *et al*. Preterm premature rupture of membranes: risks of recurrent complications in the next pregnancy among a population-based sample of gravid women. Am J Obstet Gynecol 2003; 188: 209–213

81 Shenker L, Reed KL, Anderson CF *et al*. Significance of oligohydramnios complicating pregnancy. Am J Obstet Gynecol 1991; 164: 1597–1599

82 McElrath TF, Robinson JN, Ecker JL *et al*. Neonatal outcome of infants born at 23 weeks' gestation. Obstet Gynecol 2001; 97: 49–53

83 Vintzileos AM, Campbel WM, Nochimson DJ *et al*. Fetal breathing as a predictor of infection in premature rupture of the membranes. Obstet Gynecol 1986; 67: 813–817

84 Roberts AB, Goldstein I, Romero R *et al*. Comparison of total fetal activity measurement with the biophysical profile in predicting intra-amniotic infection in preterm premature rupture of membranes. Ultrasound Obstet Gynecol 1991; 1: 36–39

85 Mikkola K, Ritari N, Tommiska V *et al*. Neurodevelopmental outcome at 5 years of age of a national cohort of extremely low birth weight infants who were born in 1996–1997. Pediatrics 2005; 116: 1391–1400

86 Msall ME, Tremont MR. Measuring functional outcomes after prematurity: developmental impact of very low birth weight and extremely low birth weight status on childhood disability. Ment Retard Dev Disabil Res Rev 2002; 8: 258–272

87 Tarnow-Mordi W, Isaacs D, Smart DH *et al*. Neurodevelopmental impairment and neonatal infections. JAMA 2005; 293: 932

88 Cox SM, Leveno KJ. Intentional delivery versus expectant management with preterm ruptured membranes at 30–34 weeks' gestation. Obstet Gynecol 1995; 86: 875–879

89 Refuerzo JS, Blackwell SC, Wolfe HM *et al*. Relationship between fetal pulmonary maturity assessment and neonatal outcome in premature rupture of the membranes at 32-34 weeks' gestation. Am J Perinatol 2001; 18: 451–458

90 Krediet TG, Kavelaars A, Vreman HJ *et al*. Respiratory distress syndrome-associated inflammation is related to early but not late peri/intraventricular hemorrhage in preterm infants. J Pediatr 2006; 148: 740–746

91 Sharma P, McKay K, Rosenkrantz TS *et al*. Comparisons of mortality and pre-discharge respiratory outcomes in small-for-gestational-age and appropriate-for-gestational-age premature infants. BMC Pediatr 2004; 4: 9

92 Romero R, Yoon BH, Mazor M *et al*. The diagnostic and prognostic value of amniotic fluid white blood cell count, glucose, interleukin-6, and gram stain in patients with preterm labor and intact membranes. Am J Obstet Gynecol 1993; 169: 805–816

93 Gomez R, Romero R, Galasso M *et al*. The value of amniotic fluid interleukin-6, white blood cell count, and gram stain in the diagnosis of microbial invasion of the amniotic cavity in patients at term. Am J Reprod Immunol 1994; 32: 200–210

94 Hussay MJ, Levy ES, Pombar X *et al*. Evaluating rapid diagnostic tests of intra-amniotic infection: Gram stain, amniotic fluid glucose level, and amniotic fluid to serum glucose level ratio. Am J Obstet Gynecol 1998; 179: 650–656

95 Simhan HN, Canavan TP. Preterm premature rupture of membranes: diagnosis, evaluation and management strategies. Br J Obstet Gynaecol 2005; 112 (Suppl 1): 32–37

96 Nien JK, Yoon BH, Espinoza J *et al*. A rapid MMP-8 bedside test for the detection of intra-amniotic inflammation identifies patients at risk for imminent preterm delivery. Am J Obstet Gynecol 2006; 195: 1025–1030

97 Zhang JP, Wang YL, Wang YH *et al*. Prophylaxis of neonatal respiratory distress syndrome by intra-amniotic administration of pulmonary surfactant. Chin Med J (Engl) 2004; 117: 120–124

98 Lisawa J, Pietrasik D, Zwolinski J *et al.* Intraamniotic surfactant supply as RDS prevention. Med Wieku Rozwoj 2003; 7 (Suppl 1): 255–260
99 Yeast JD, Garite TR. The role of cervical cerclage in the management of preterm premature rupture of membranes. Am J Obstet Gynecol 1988; 158: 106–110
100 Blickstein I, Katz Z, Lancet M *et al.* The outcome of pregnancies complicated by preterm premature rupture of membranes with cervical cerclage in place. Int J Gynaecol Obstet 1989; 28: 237–242
101 Moore-Goldman J, Greene MF, Harlow BL *et al.* Outcome of expectant management in preterm premature rupture of membranes with cervical cerclage in place. Abstract presented at the Society of Perinatal Obstetricians Jan 23–27, 1990, Houston, TX
102 McElrath TF, Norwitz ER, Lieberman ES *et al.* Perinatal outcome after preterm premature rupture of membranes with *in situ* cervical cerclage. Am J Obstet Gynecol 2002; 187: 1147–1152
103 Mercer BM, Crocker LG, Pierce WF *et al.* Clinical characteristics and outcome of twin gestation complicated by preterm premature rupture of the membranes. Am J Obstet Gynecol 1993; 168: 1467–1473
104 Bianco AT, Stone J, Lapinski R *et al.* The clinical outcome of preterm premature rupture of membranes in twin versus singleton pregnancies. Am J Perinatol 1996; 13: 135–138
105 Jacquemyn Y, Noelmans L, Mahieu L *et al.* Twin versus singleton pregnancy and preterm prelabour rupture of the membranes. Clin Exp Obstet Gynecol 2003; 30: 99–102
106 De Catte L, Laubach M, Bougatef A *et al.* Selective feticide in twin pregnancies with very early preterm premature rupture of membranes. Am J Perinatol 1998; 15: 149–153
107 Dorfman SA, Robins RM, Jewell WH *et al.* Second trimester selective termination of a twin with ruptured membranes: elimination of fluid leakage and preservation of pregnancy. Fetal Diagn Ther 1995; 10: 186–188
108 Arias F. Delayed delivery of multifetal pregnancies with premature rupture of membranes in the second trimester. Am J Obstet Gynecol 1994; 170: 1233–1237
109 Zhang J, Hamilton B, Martin J *et al.* Delayed interval delivery and infant survival: a population-based study. Am J Obstet Gynecol 2004; 191: 470–476
110 Oyelese Y, Ananth CV, Smulian JC *et al.* Delayed interval delivery in twin pregnancies in the United States: impact on perinatal mortality and morbidity. Am J Obstet Gynecol 2005; 192: 439–444
111 Major CA, Towers CV, Lewis DF *et al.* Expectant management of preterm premature rupture of membranes complicated by active recurrent genital herpes. Am J Obstet Gynecol 2003; 188: 1551–1554
112 Centers for Disese Control. Reduction in perinatal transmission of human immunodeficiency virus – United States, 1985–2006. MMWR 2006; 21: 592–597
113 Minkoff H, Burns DN, Landesman S *et al.* The relationship of the duration of ruptured membranes to vertical transmission of human immunodeficiency virus. Am J Obstet Gynecol 1995; 173: 585–589
114 Landesman SH, Kalisha LA, Burns DN *et al.* Obstetrical factors and the transmission of human immunodeficiency virus type 1 from mother to child. The Women and Infants Transmission Study. N Engl J Med 1996; 334: 1617–1623
115 Alvarez J, Garcia J, Bardeguez A, Apuzzio J. Preterm premature rupture of membranes before 34 weeks in HIV positive patients. When to deliver and what is the vertical transmission rate? Presented at the National Meeting of Infectious Disease in Obstetrics and Gynecology, Monterey, California, August 2006

Richard Brown

Abnormalities of amniotic fluid

Variations in the quantity of amniotic fluid around a fetus may arise from a multitude of causes; however, these differences can provide crucial clues to the health and well-being of the fetus and also influence its continuing development. Assessment of the volume of amniotic fluid is, therefore, an integral and essential component of any obstetric ultrasound evaluation. In this chapter, the physiological aspects of amniotic fluid regulation are touched upon and some of the factors resulting in either an excess accumulation of fluid (polyhydramnios), or a reduction in the fluid volume (oligohydramnios and anhydramnios) are discussed.

AMNIOTIC FLUID PHYSIOLOGY

The maintenance of amniotic fluid is a dynamic process throughout pregnancy but with differing origins for the amniotic fluid at advancing gestational ages. In the first trimester, it is believed that the amniotic fluid is, in the main, a transudate of plasma whose origin is most likely both maternal and fetal with fluid transudation occurring across the maternal surface of the uterine decidua, the placental surface and directly from the fetus through its skin. In the second half of the pregnancy, the increased creatinine and urea concentrations of amniotic fluid indicate a shift towards fetal urine production being the main contributor. However, in addition to fetal urine, there is an additional fetal component in later gestation that is often overlooked but which is of significant importance – the production of fetal lung secretions.

The volume of amniotic fluid in early pregnancy clearly is increasing with the increasing size of the amniotic sac; however, this is not maintained

Richard Brown MBBS DFFP FRCOG
Director of Ultrasound and Assistant Professor of Obstetrics and Gynaecology, Department of Obstetrics & Gynaecology & Division of Maternal and Fetal Medicine, McGill University, Montréal, Québec H3A 1A1, Canada
E-mail: richard.brown@muhc.mcgill.ca

throughout gestation with a plateau at a mean volume of around 770–800 ml between 24–37 weeks of gestation.[1] By 40 weeks, the total fluid volume has declined to less than 600 ml and by 41 weeks of gestation to around 500 ml.

The amniotic fluid space is not a static collection of fluid but rather one whose volume is maintained by a circulatory process with fetal urine and lung fluid production being balanced by fetal swallowing and absorption of fluid through the gastrointestinal tract as well as absorption directly across the amnion and into the fetal circulation. Fetal urine production has been estimated from the rate of fetal bladder filling to be in the region of 25% of the estimated fetal weight per 24 h.[2] In animal models, the production of fetal lung fluid has been estimated at around 100 ml/kg every 24 h. Although the rate of fetal lung fluid production in humans has not been measured, this is now relied upon in therapeutic fetal interventions such as in the fetal therapies for congenital diaphragmatic hernia where tracheal occlusion using either an endotracheal balloon or tracheal clip results in fetal lung fluid being wholly retained within the lower respiratory tract. The result is that, as the lungs expand in volume due to fluid accumulation, the diaphragmatic hernia is gradually reduced.

ASSESSMENT OF AMNIOTIC FLUID VOLUME (AFV)

In current practice, the volume of amniotic fluid is determined non-invasively by ultrasound. Alternate methods used prior to the wide-spread use of ultrasound or in research have relied on the principle of dye dilution; in these techniques, a pre-determined volume of dye is introduced into the amniotic cavity and, after allowing for suitable distribution and mixing within the amniotic fluid, an aliquot of fluid is retrieved and the concentration of dye allows the AFV to be calculated quantitatively.

A variety of ultrasound tools to determine the volume of amniotic fluid have been used. The mainstays of practice are the maximum single deepest pocket and the four-quadrant assessment. The latter involves the estimation of the maximum depth of the amniotic fluid pocket in each uterine quadrant with the uterus being divided into quadrants by the midline being bisected by a horizontal meridian drawn either through the umbilicus or at a point representing half of the height of the uterine fundus.[3,4] This four-quadrant assessment is more commonly referred to as the amniotic fluid index, AFI. Measurement of the fluid volume using the 'bladder scanner', a device used predominantly to calculate post micturition bladder residual volumes, has also been reported as have 3-dimensional volumetric calculations using quantitative 3-dimensional volume acquisition performed by ultrasound.

Normal ranges for the AFI have been calculated and measurements can, therefore, be plotted on such charts and the centiles determined with values lying outside of the normal 5th to 95th percentile range being considered reduced or increased with moderate oligohydramnios and polyhydramnios lying beyond the 2.5th and 97.5th percentiles, respectively. For the single pocket technique, < 3 cm and < 2 cm are considered mild and moderate oligohydramnios and > 8 cm and > 15 cm refer to polyhydramnios. Phelan *et al.*[4] introduced a cut-off of 5 cm based on the four-quadrant assessment as a definition of oligohydramnios.

Of the existing tools, AFI has advantages over the single pocket assessment in that it correlates more closely with direct measurements of amniotic fluid volume and is considered more reliable in the assessment of both increased and reduced amniotic fluid volumes. Moore[5] demonstrated that the correlation coefficient between AFI and a single maximum vertical pocket measurement was only 0.51 (R^2 = 24%) and whilst the correlation was improved in cases of polyhydramnios (r = 0.79), in 58% of cases with oligohydramnios, as defined by an AFI measurement, the single deepest pocket measurement was within normal limits. The fetal position may, for example, result in all the amniotic fluid being sited in a single area producing a normal single pocket measurement whilst the overall volume is in fact reduced.

OLIGOHYDRAMNIOS

A reduction in the AFV is due either to the loss of fluid from the amniotic sac or to a reduction in the production of fluid although, in a proportion of cases, the cause may remain undefined.

Etiology

The single commonest cause of oligohydramnios, accounting for around 25% of cases, is pre-labor rupture of the membranes (PROM).[6] This is particularly likely in those cases approaching term. It should, of course, also be remembered that not in all cases of PROM will the AFV be less than normal. However, in all cases where there is no clear presenting history of PROM but oligohydramnios is found, the possibility should be considered and a more detailed patient history should be taken and a vaginal examination to assess the cervix, the presence of pooling of amniotic fluid and ferning should be performed.

It is those cases in which PROM has been excluded that this chapter will focus. A reduction in the production of amniotic fluid in the second and third trimesters is mediated primarily through a reduced or absent fetal urine output. This, in turn, may be the consequence of an abnormality of the fetal urinary tract or of an alteration in fetal renal function in response to the intra-uterine milieu. Although fetal lung fluid contributes to overall fluid volume, the role of this in oligohydramnios is minor. Obstruction of the respiratory tract as seen, for example, in congenital high airway obstruction syndrome (CHAOS), generally inhibits the recirculation of amniotic fluid to a greater degree than the contribution made to overall fluid volume with polyhydramnios resulting. Pulmonary hypoplasia itself is more often a consequence of diminished amniotic fluid or of a structural defect (*e.g.* congenital diaphragmatic hernia) and, therefore, does not contribute significantly to the development of oligohydramnios.

Placental insufficiency

Intra-uterine growth restriction and placental insufficiency may result in a reduced AFV mediated through a reduction in the fetal urine output. In a hypoxic state, redistribution of blood flow is observed in the fetus with fetal cerebral perfusion being maintained at the expense of visceral, including renal, perfusion.

With reduced renal perfusion and reduced renal plasma flow, there is a reduction in the fetal urine output with consequent oligohydramnios. This is supported by examination of the fetal arterial circulation using Doppler ultrasound with which reduced vascular resistance is seen in the fetal middle cerebral artery whereas there is an increase in the resistance to flow in the renal arteries.[7] These changes in blood flow are mediated through a variety of mechanisms including chemo- and baro-receptors, the influence of the renin–angiotensin system and the release of vasopressin.

Renal tract abnormalities

Oligohydramnios may arise as a consequence of a variety of fetal abnormalities. Renal and urinary tract pathologies directly affecting fetal urine production are the first to be considered. Renal reserve in the fetus, as in the adult, is such that only one functioning kidney is required to maintain normal renal function and adequate urine production. Therefore, in general, only in conditions where both kidneys are affected would one expect to observe abnormalities in the AFV.

In bilateral renal agenesis, the AFV may be normal even until 20 weeks due to the other sources of fluid production discussed above. Once fetal urine production has become the predominant source of amniotic fluid, the AFV will diminish. With this, a number of dysmorphic characteristics evolve over the remaining weeks of the pregnancy; these are referred to as Potter's facies and this condition was previously referred to as Potter syndrome.[8] However, the term Potter syndrome has now been expanded and subdivided to refer to a variety of renal pathologies. Potter syndrome as originally defined is now usually referred to as bilateral renal agenesis (BRA) and three sub-groupings of Potter syndrome are now recognised: Type I now refers to autosomal recessive polycystic kidney disease, Type II to renal dysplasia and Type III to autosomal dominant polycystic kidney disease.

In addition to Potter's facies, the other fetal consequences of severe oligohydramnios include limb deformities, generalized growth retardation and, most importantly, pulmonary hypoplasia. The development of this set of factors is now often referred to as the oligohydramnios sequence.

Bilateral renal agenesis may not be recognized in the first trimester unless the renal tract is carefully imaged, as the AFV will be normal. By the mid second trimester, once fetal urine production has become the predominant source of amniotic fluid, the AFV will begin to diminish. Although the fetal lungs produce fluid, an adequate volume of amniotic fluid is itself required in order to allow normal fetal lung development to occur. In the case of bilateral renal agenesis, the severe oligohydramnios results in marked pulmonary hypoplasia. With the ensuing diminution or absence of lung secretions, anhydramnios may develop. Inability to visualize the fetal kidneys and bladder confirms the diagnosis although expansion of the adrenal glands into the renal fossa may confound the diagnosis as the adrenals may be mistaken for the kidneys. Visualization of the fetal renal arteries with color Doppler may help to determine whether the organs identified are indeed the kidneys. Diagnostic amnio-infusion, the instillation of saline into the amniotic cavity, to facilitate ultrasound visualization may sometimes be of value in confirming the diagnosis.[9]

Bilateral renal dysplasia, polycystic kidney disease (both autosomal dominant and recessive), bilateral multicystic dysplastic kidney disease and renal tubular dysgenesis result in interstitial renal dysfunction and failure resulting in oligohydramnios and, possibly, anhydramnios. The prognosis for these fetuses, if resulting in severe oligohydramnios in the mid-trimester, is essentially similar to that of bilateral renal agenesis with the severity of pulmonary hypoplasia being associated with the degree, gestation at onset and duration of the oligohydramnios and contributing together with the renal failure to early neonatal demise. Severe oligohydramnios for whatever etiology (most commonly preterm pre-labor membrane rupture) in the period up to 26 weeks, the end of the canalicular phase of fetal lung development, is likely to be associated with severe pulmonary hypoplasia.

Urinary tract obstruction will also, if it affects the drainage of urine from both kidneys, result in diminished amniotic fluid. The conditions that may give rise to such a situation include urethral obstruction as seen with, for example, posterior urethral valves, ureteroceles, urogenital septum malformations and bilateral uterovesical junction or pelvi-ureteric junction obstruction. At the worst end of the spectrum, cases of lower urinary tract obstruction (LUTO) are associated with bladder over-distension (megacystis) with back-pressure upon the kidneys resulting in progressive renal damage and renal failure or in bladder rupture leading to urinary ascites and the prune belly syndrome.

As well as isolated renal defects, a variety of genetic conditions may also be associated with renal abnormalities, renal dysfunction and consequent oligohydramnios. For example, in the Smith Lemli Opitz syndrome, the kidneys may be hypoplastic with small cortical cysts or, in some cases, may even be absent. In addition, there may also be other urinary tract abnormalities including ectopic kidney, hydronephrosis, hypoplastic ureter, and hydro-ureter.[10]

The Meckel syndrome (Meckel-Gruber syndrome) is a lethal autosomal recessive disorder characterized by anomalies of the central nervous system (encephalocele), enlarged kidneys demonstrating cystic dysplasia, and malformations of the hands and feet.

Miscellaneous conditions

Gastrointestinal conditions, including gastroschisis and megacystis-microcolon, may also be associated with a reduced AFV as are a variety of aneuploidies and chromosome aberrations, genetic syndromes, structural defects and metabolic conditions (for example, hypothyroidism).

Indomethacin, which is many institutions is commonly used as a tocolytic, is known to be associated with the development of oligohydramnios, especially when used for prolonged periods, due to a reduction in fetal urine production.

Management

The obstetric management of pregnancies complicated by membrane rupture will not be discussed here. In the majority of cases of renal abnormality, no intervention is possible and management will depend on whether the condition is expected to be lethal either *in utero* or to the neonate, or whether survival is anticipated. In the latter cases, the timing of delivery will depend upon many factors including the fetal growth, the severity of oligohydramnios, the rate and degree of damage to the kidneys, and the deterioration in renal function in, for example, cases of urinary tract obstruction.

In some cases of lower urinary tract obstruction, fetal intervention might be considered. In bladder outflow obstruction, the placement of a vesico-amniotic shunt will allow the obstruction to be relieved and limit renal damage. More invasive approaches including open fetal surgery, fetal cystoscopy, electrocautery of posterior urethral valves and puncture/septostomy of ureterocele septae have been undertaken. The detailed discussion of these techniques lies beyond the scope of this chapter. In general, attempts at surgical intervention have been marred by a high intra-uterine loss rate and a high rate of severe renal dysfunction and incidence of renal transplantation in surviving neonates; they are, therefore, only applicable in limited cases.[11]

Pulmonary development has been demonstrated to be improved with the therapeutic instillation of fluid into the amniotic cavity in animal studies; however, in human studies, the data are more limited. A number of recent investigations have addressed the use of amnio-infusion in cases of early membrane rupture (before 26 weeks). Such studies have demonstrated a benefit of the procedure to neonatal outcomes with relatively few maternal and fetal risks despite the fact that, in many cases, the procedure needs to be undertaken serially due to continued fluid leakage. Attempts to minimise the continued leakage by means of plugging the cervix (*e.g.* with gelatin sponges) have also reported some success but these interventions require more extensive evaluation before becoming routine practice.[12–14]

POLYHYDRAMNIOS

Polyhydramnios occurs in around 1–3.5% of pregnancies and is severe in only 5% of these. The principal factors associated with polyhydramnios include maternal diabetes, fetal abnormalities and multiple gestations. Although the majority of cases of polyhydramnios overall are idiopathic (an abnormality will be found in around 20%), in cases of severe polyhydramnios an underlying cause will be identified in the majority (80%). Even in cases where sonographic evaluation is normal, the likelihood of a fetal abnormality is not insignificant and is associated with the degree of hydramnios being 1%, 2% and 11%, respectively, in cases of mild, moderate and severe polyhydramnios.[15,16]

Fetal abnormality and polyhydramnios

A key mechanism in a number of the fetal abnormalities associated with polyhydramnios is abnormal or interrupted turnover of amniotic fluid. Inability to swallow and absorb fluid interrupts the normal turnover of amniotic fluid resulting in an imbalance and net accumulation of fluid. The ability of the fetus to swallow amniotic fluid may be interrupted for various reasons: (i) conditions associated with structural abnormalities of the upper gastrointestinal tract (*e.g.* intrinsic bowel obstruction); (ii) conditions where there is physical obstruction of an otherwise normal upper gastrointestinal tract (extrinsic compression of the bowel); and (iii) neurological conditions that interfere with the neurological control of the swallowing process.

In the obstructive group are conditions such as esophageal atresia and bowel obstructions including pyloric stenosis and duodenal atresia. Duodenal atresia may be suspected sonographically due to the visualization of the characteristic 'double bubble' in the upper abdomen; esophageal atresia is usually suspected due to failure to visualize the fetal stomach or recognise normal filling of the stomach, in conjunction with polyhydramnios. It should, however, be remembered that the stomach may appear normal or be visible in cases of esophageal atresia: firstly, because gastric secretions may fill the stomach at least partially; and secondly, because of the possibility of a co-existent tracheo-esophageal fistula. In these conditions, although the mechanics of the swallowing process are normal, amniotic fluid cannot progress beyond the upper gastrointestinal tract and, therefore, is not absorbed and recycled. The continuing production of fetal urine with the fluid turnover disrupted results in an accumulation of excess amniotic fluid.

Large head and neck masses may also result in polyhydramnios by physically obstructing the oropharynx or upper esophagus, again disrupting the turnover of amniotic fluid. In congenital high airway obstruction syndrome (CHAOS; Fig. 1), lung secretions are trapped within the pulmonary tree and the resulting distension and mediastinal, venous and cardiac compression may give rise to both ascites and polyhydramnios.

Intrathoracic masses may also, through external compression of the upper gastrointestinal tract, result in disturbance to the turnover of amniotic fluid and consequently polyhydramnios. Such conditions include diaphragmatic hernia, cystic adenomatoid malformation, bronchogenic cysts and bronchopulmonary sequestration. A comparable outcome results from situations where the chest itself is compressed restricting its contents. Examples of this include the skeletal dysplasias such as thanatophoric dysplasia or Jeune's asphyxiating thoracic dystrophy.

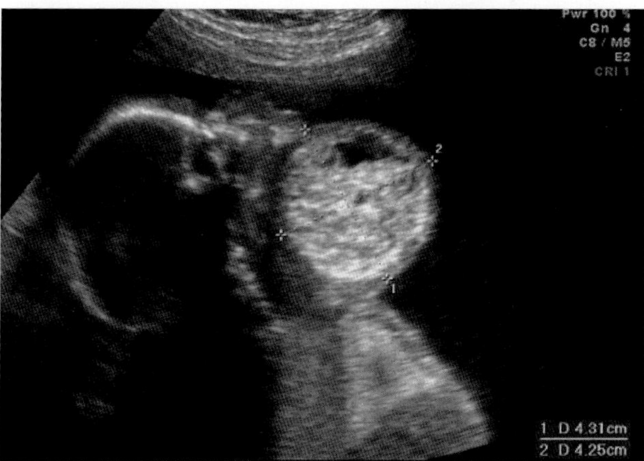

Fig. 1 A large neck tumor causing esophageal obstruction and hence polyhydramnios as well as tracheal obstruction (CHAOS), note the hyperechogenic fetal lung.

The neurological disruption of swallowing encompasses a broad range of conditions including myotonic dystrophy, anencephaly and those presenting with progressive fetal paralysis (*e.g.* arthrogryposis). A variety of genetic conditions may be associated with the presence of polyhydramnios. For example, over one-third of fetuses with Beckwith-Wiedemann syndrome have an increased AFV. In some of these cases, the macroglossia associated with this condition may interfere with fetal swallowing and, hence, the normal turnover of amniotic fluid.[17,18]

Polyhydramnios is often noted in conjunction with fetal hydrops of both immune and non-immune origin. Around half of fetuses found to have hydrops have associated polyhydramnios. The etiology is, in the main, dependent on the etiology of the hydrops itself; for example, fetuses developing high-output cardiac failure due to the presence of arteriovenous anastamoses (*e.g.* sacrococcygeal teratoma) most likely develop polyuria by virtue of increased renal perfusion and an increased glomerular filtration rate.

Diabetes mellitus and diabetes insipidus

In pregnancies complicated by maternal diabetes, polyhydramnios may arise when there is sub-optimal glycemic control. Maternal hyperglycemia leads, in turn, to fetal hyperglycemia and fetal hyperinsulinemia. Hyperglycemia, in part through an osmotic action, results in polyuria; this occurs in the fetus as well as in the child or adult and in this situation this leads to the development of polyhydramnios. Poor glycemic control is also associated with fetal macrosomia and these factors are, therefore, correlated.[19] With improved glycemic control in pregnancy, the incidence of polyhydramnios has fallen; it is now associated with the more severe cases, but its evaluation is very useful in the clinical management. The resulting increase in uterine volume, which is also related to accelerated fetal growth in cases where the maternal glycemic control is poor, is a potential cause of premature delivery, a more significant complication considering the delay in fetal lung maturation also observed with fetal hyperinsulinemia. Although some studies have suggested that the increased incidence of polyhydramnios is confined to those mothers with pre-existing diabetes rather than those who develop gestational diabetes,[20] this is not a consistent finding; however, in cases of gestational diabetes complicated by polyhydramnios, there is no increase in perinatal morbidity.[21]

Fetal diabetes insipdus has also been reported. It is essentially a diagnosis of exclusion and may be suspected when fetal polyuria, as indicated by an increased rate of bladder filling on ultrasound, is observed in the absence of another underlying cause[18] or in the presence of maternal lithium therapy. Lithium is associated with adult nephrogenic diabetes insipidus and is also associated with polyhydramnios which is suspected to be due to the same etiology in the fetus.[22,23]

Multiple gestations

In multichorionic gestations, the causes of polyhydramnios and oligo-hydramnios are similar to those in singleton gestations; however, in the monochorionic gestations, the possibility of feto–fetal transfusion must also be considered.[24] If there is an inequality of exchange across the vascular anastamoses linking the placentas of a monochorionic gestation, then the

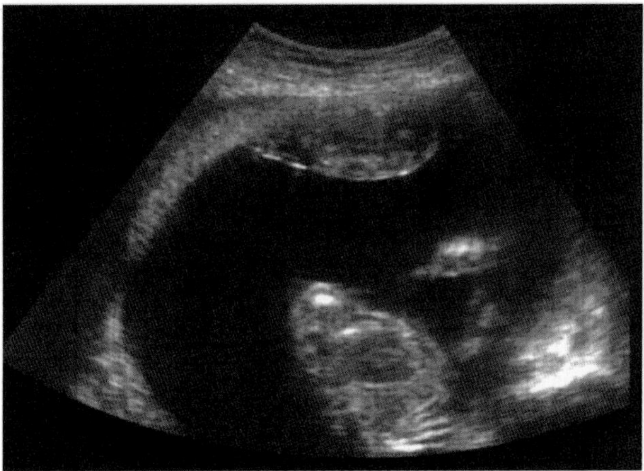

Fig. 2 Polyhydramnios in the larger recipient twin's amniotic sac whilst the smaller donor twin is 'stuck' to the anterior uterine wall.

recipient twin develops polyuria in response to the fluid overload with the consequence of polyhydramnios. The donor twin develops oligohydramnios secondary to hypovolemia and, in the case of the 'stuck' twin (Fig. 2), anhydramnios as its renal perfusion is reduced to preserve the intravascular volume with activation and up-regulation of the renin/angiotensin system in the donor whilst the renin system is down-regulated in the recipient.

Placental abnormalities

Placental chorioangiomas, sonographically well-circumscribed placental tumours that are essentially hemangiomas, have been observed to be associated with an increased incidence of polyhydramnios in approximately 30% of cases.[25,26] Although oligohydramnios has also been observed, this is more typically associated with those cases where there is fetal growth restriction. In approximately 10% of these cases, fetal hydrops will also develop. Cases of chorioangioma have been successfully managed either by direct injection of alcohol into the tumor to cause tumor necrosis or laser photocoagulation of the tumor.[26,27]

Management of polyhydramnios

Clearly, once polyhydramnios is discovered, the search for an underlying etiology is commenced. A detailed sonographic survey is essential with referral to a fetal medicine unit in cases of severe polyhydramnios being advisable. Detailed examination of the brain, upper gastrointestinal tract, head and neck and chest are essential. Evaluation of the long bones and thorax will determine the presence of a skeletal dysplasia and, as congenital cardiac disease is also a common finding, a targeted fetal cardiac echo is recommended. Assessment of fetal movement and tone as well as examination of the joints (ankle, knee, wrist and elbow) and movements at these is key to the diagnosis of neuromuscular abnormalities such as arthrogryposis.

As aneuploidies are common (5–20%), karyotyping is suggested. In cases of severe polyhydramnios, especially if there is co-existent uterine irritability or threatened preterm labor, therapeutic amni-drainage can be combined with diagnostic amniotic fluid sampling. Again, in severe cases, an assessment of the risk of preterm labor by means of assessment of the cervical length by endovaginal ultrasound might be of value.

Concurrently, the mother should be assessed for diabetes and also evaluated for causes of hydrops – maternal antibody status with regard to immune hydrops and virology testing with regard to the infective causes of non-immune hydrops. Cordocentesis and fetal hemoglobin estimation may be of value in both situations with fetal transfusion and correction of an underlying anemia resulting in resolution of hydrops and the associated polyhydramnios in cases of rhesus iso-immunisation or parvovirus-induced fetal red cell aplasia.

Specific fetal abnormalities are managed accordingly if this is feasible. For example, mediastinal shift due increased lung volume in cases of macrocystic congenital adenomatoid malformation might respond to needle puncture and drainage of the cystic lesions. Similarly. the drainage or shunting of pleural effusions may relieve mediastinal shift and intrathoracic cardiac and venous compression. Cases of congenital diaphragmatic hernia with a predicted poor postnatal prognosis may be managed by intra-uterine fetal therapy; fetal endotracheal balloon occlusion being less invasive than either fetal tracheal clipping or open fetal surgery. In cases of severe twin–twin transfusion syndrome (Quintero stage II, III or IV),[28] management is usually by fetoscopic photocoagulation of the vascular anastamoses identified on the placental surface[29] or, in some centers, by serial amnioreduction or amnion septostomy.

Amnio-reduction or amni-drainage have been mentioned in passing and may be of value in the reduction of both maternal symptoms and in the reduction of the risk of preterm labor. There remains some controversy as to the value of the procedure from a therapeutic standpoint given the high likelihood of recurrence of polyhydramnios; however, aggressive and, if necessary, repeated amnio-reduction has resulted in prolongation of pregnancy. In cases of severe polyhydramnios, there are concerns that removing too large a volume of amniotic fluid in one instance might increase the risk of abruptio placentae due to sudden uterine decompression. However, the risk of such complications with the removal of significant volumes of amniotic fluid appears small at around 1.5% when assessed in both singleton and monochorionic twin gestations.[16,30]

As previously mentioned, indomethacin, often used during pregnancy as a tocolytic, is known to be associated with the development of oligohydramnios, due to a reduction in fetal urine production. Postnataly, prostaglandin synthase inhibitors are also used therapeutically to close a persistently patent ductus arteriosus; this may also happen during pregnancy if such agents are used. Therefore, in pregnancy, the use of indomethacin is generally restricted to gestations of 32 weeks or less where the risk of premature closure of the ductus *in utero* appears small. This potential side effect of reduced fetal urine production is used to advantage in the treatment of polyhydramnios. Administration of indomethacin has been demonstrated to reduce the amniotic fluid volume in cases of idiopathic polyhydramnios as well as in cases where underlying pathology is evident.[31–33] The amniotic fluid volume may increase rapidly after discontinuation of the indomethacin;[31–34] therefore, some authors have advocated more prolonged treatment with regular ultrasound monitoring and discontinuation of therapy if oligohydramnios develops. The use of indomethacin therapy may also be combined with amnio-drainage to achieve a longer lasting effect on normalizing the amniotic fluid volume.[35] However, there remain a number of concerns associated with the use of indomethacin. Not only is there the risk of ductal closure,[36] but other neonatal complications may arise. Indomethacin therapy has been associated with increased risks for both necrotizing enterocolitis and intraventricular hemorrhage in particular and there are both theoretical and observed concerns regarding the longer term impact of indomethacin on the fetal kidney; there have been reports of renal dysgenesis and chronic renal failure suspected to be caused, at least in part, by ante-natal indomethacin therapy.[37–40] Treatment with indomethacin should be used with caution and, in the first instance, perhaps limited to a shorter duration. Fetal echocardiography may be of value to assess whether there is any evidence of ductal constriction with the dose being reduced or treatment discontinued if this is observed.[33]

KEY POINTS FOR CLINICAL PRACTICE

- Abnormalities of amniotic fluid can provide crucial information as to the health and well-being of a pregnancy.
- Of existing techniques, the utrasonographic four-quadrant measurement of amniotic fluid index is the most useful assessment.

Oligohydramnios

- The single commonest cause is pre-labor membrane rupture.
- Placental insufficiency can result in both fetal growth restriction and due to fetal adaptive mechanisms, oligohydramnios.
- Renal abnormalities of varying types can contribute to a reduced fetal urine production. Some of these abnormalities that would be associated with a poor perinatal outcome if untreated may be amenable to intra-uterine interventions.

Polyhydramnios

- Occurs in around 1–3.5% of pregnancies and is severe in 5% of these.
- The principal factors associated with polyhydramnios include maternal diabetes, fetal abnormalities and multiple gestations.
- Although the majority of cases of polyhydramnios overall are idiopathic (an abnormality will be found in around 20%), in cases of severe polyhydramnios there is an underlying cause in around 80%.
- Depending on the etiology, the treatment may include procedures such as amnio-drainage or pharmacological management with indomethacin.

References

1 Brace RA. Physiology of amniotic fluid volume regulation. Clin Obstet Gynecol 1997; 40: 280–289

2 Rabinowitz R, Peters MT, Vyas S, Campbell S, Nicolaides KH. Measurement of fetal urine production in normal pregnancy by real-time ultrasonography. Am J Obstet Gynecol 1989; 161: 1264–1266

3 Phelan JP, Ahn MO, Smith CV, Rutherford SE, Anderson E. Amniotic fluid index measurements during pregnancy. J Reprod Med 1987; 32: 601–604

4 Phelan JP, Smith CV, Broussard P, Small M. Amniotic fluid volume assessment with the four-quadrant technique at 36–42 weeks' gestation. J Reprod Med 1987; 32: 540–542

5 Moore TR. Superiority of the four-quadrant sum over the single-deepest-pocket technique in ultrasonographic identification of abnormal amniotic fluid volumes. Am J Obstet Gynecol 1990; 163: 762–767

6 Mercer LJ, Brown LG, Petres RE, Messer RH. A survey of pregnancies complicated by decreased amniotic fluid. Am J Obstet Gynecol 1984; 149: 355–361

7 Arduini D, Rizzo G. Fetal renal artery velocity waveforms and amniotic fluid volume in growth-retarded and post-term fetuses. Obstet Gynecol 1991; 77: 370–373

8 Potter EL. Facial characteristics of infants with bilateral renal agenesis. Am J Obstet Gynecol 1946; 51: 885–888

9 Gembruch U, Hansmann M. Artificial instillation of amniotic fluid as a new technique for the diagnostic evaluation of cases of oligohydramnios. Prenat Diagn 1988; 8: 33–45

10 Lowry RB, Opitz JM. Variability in the Smith-Lemli-Opitz syndrome: overlap with the Meckel syndrome. Am J Med Genet 2005; 14: 429–433

11 Holmes N, Harrison MR, Baskin LS. Fetal surgery for posterior urethral valves: long-term postnatal outcomes. Pediatrics 2001; 108: E7

12 De Santis M, Scavo M, Noia G *et al.* Transabdominal amnioinfusion treatment of severe oligohydramnios in preterm premature rupture of membranes at less than 26 gestational weeks. Fetal Diagn Ther 2003; 18: 412–417

13 O'Brien JM, Barton JR, Milligan DA. An aggressive interventional protocol for early midtrimester premature rupture of the membranes using gelatin sponge for cervical plugging. Am J Obstet Gynecol 2002; 187: 1143–1146

14 Vergani P, Locatelli A, Verderio M, Assi F. Premature rupture of the membranes at < 26 weeks' gestation: role of amnioinfusion in the management of oligohydramnios. Acta Biomed 2004; 75 (Suppl 1): 62–66

15 Dashe JS, McIntire DD, Ramus RM, Santos-Ramos R, Twickler DM. Hydramnios: anomaly prevalence and sonographic detection. Obstet Gynecol 2002; 100: 134–139

16 Hara K, Kikuchi A, Miyachi K, Sunagawa S, Takagi K. Clinical features of polyhydramnios associated with fetal anomalies. Congenit Anom (Kyoto) 2006; 46: 177–179

17 Elliott M, Bayly R, Cole T, Temple IK, Maher ER. Clinical features and natural history of Beckwith-Wiedemann syndrome: presentation of 74 new cases. Clin Genet 1994; 46: 168–174

18 Kirshon B. Fetal urine output in hydramnios. Obstet Gynecol 1989; 73: 240–242

19 Vink JY, Poggi SH, Ghidini A, Spong CY. Amniotic fluid index and birth weight: is there a relationship in diabetics with poor glycemic control? Am J Obstet Gynecol 2006; 195: 848–850

20 Goldman M, Kitzmiller JL, Abrams B, Cowan RM, Laros Jr RK. Obstetric complications with GDM. Effects of maternal weight. Diabetes 1991; 40 (Suppl 2): 79–82

21 Shoham I, Wiznitzer A, Silberstein T *et al.* Gestational diabetes complicated by hydramnios was not associated with increased risk of perinatal morbidity and mortality. Eur J Obstet Gynecol Reprod Biol 2001; 100: 46–49

22 Ang MS, Thorp JA, Parisi VM. Maternal lithium therapy and polyhydramnios. Obstet Gynecol 1990; 76: 517–519

23 Krause S, Ebbesen F, Lange AP. Polyhydramnios with maternal lithium treatment. Obstet Gynecol 1990; 75: 504–506

24 Denbow ML, Fisk NM. The consequences of monochorionic placentation. Baillières Clin Obstet Gynaecol 1998; 12: 37–51

25 Jauniaux E, Ogle R. Color Doppler imaging in the diagnosis and management of chorioangiomas. Ultrasound Obstet Gynecol 2000; 15: 463–467

26 Sepulveda W, Alcalde JL, Schnapp C, Bravo M. Perinatal outcome after prenatal diagnosis of placental chorioangioma. Obstet Gynecol 2003; 102: 1028–1033
27 Quarello E, Bernard JP, Leroy B, Ville Y. Prenatal laser treatment of a placental chorioangioma. Ultrasound Obstet Gynecol 2005; 25: 299–301
28 Quintero RA, Morales WJ, Allen MH, Bornick PW, Johnson PK, Kruger M. Staging of twin-twin transfusion syndrome. J Perinatol 1999; 19: 550–555
29 Ville Y, Hecher K, Ogg D, Warren R, Nicolaides K. Successful outcome after Nd:YAG laser separation of chorioangiopagus-twins under sonoendoscopic control. Ultrasound Obstet Gynecol 1992; 2: 429–431
30 Elliott JP, Sawyer AT, Radin TG, Strong RE. Large-volume therapeutic amniocentesis in the treatment of hydramnios. Obstet Gynecol 1994; 84: 1025–1027
31 Cabrol D, Landesman R, Muller J, Uzan M, Sureau C, Saxena BB. Treatment of polyhydramnios with prostaglandin synthetase inhibitor (indomethacin). Am J Obstet Gynecol 1987; 157: 422–426
32 Carmona F, Martinez-Roman S, Mortera C, Puerto B, Cararach V, Iglesias X. Efficacy and safety of indomethacin therapy for polyhydramnios. Eur J Obstet Gynecol Reprod Biol 1993; 52: 175–180
33 Moise Jr KJ. Indomethacin therapy in the treatment of symptomatic polyhydramnios. Clin Obstet Gynecol 1991; 34: 310–318
34 Sandruck JC, Grobman WA, Gerber SE. The effect of short-term indomethacin therapy on amniotic fluid volume. Am J Obstet Gynecol 2005; 192: 1443–1445
35 Kirshon B, Mari G, Moise Jr KJ. Indomethacin therapy in the treatment of symptomatic polyhydramnios. Obstet Gynecol 1990; 75: 202–205
36 Savage AH, Anderson BL, Simhan HN. The safety of prolonged indomethacin therapy. Am J Perinatol 2007; 24: 207–213
37 Buderus S, Thomas B, Fahnenstich H, Kowalewski S. Renal failure in two preterm infants: toxic effect of prenatal maternal indomethacin treatment? Br J Obstet Gynaecol 1993; 100: 97–98
38 Gloor JM, Muchant DG, Norling LL. Prenatal maternal indomethacin use resulting in prolonged neonatal renal insufficiency. J Perinatol 1993; 13: 425–427
39 Pomeranz A, Korzets Z, Dolfin Z, Eliakim A, Bernheim J, Wolach B. Acute renal failure in the neonate induced by the administration of indomethacin as a tocolytic agent. Nephrol Dial Transplant 1996; 11: 1139–1141
40 Robin YM, Reynaud P, Orliaguet T, Lemery D, Vanlieferingen P, Dechelotte P. Renal tubular dysgenesis-like lesions and hypocalvaria. Report of two cases involving indomethacin. Pathol Res Pract 2000; 196: 791–794

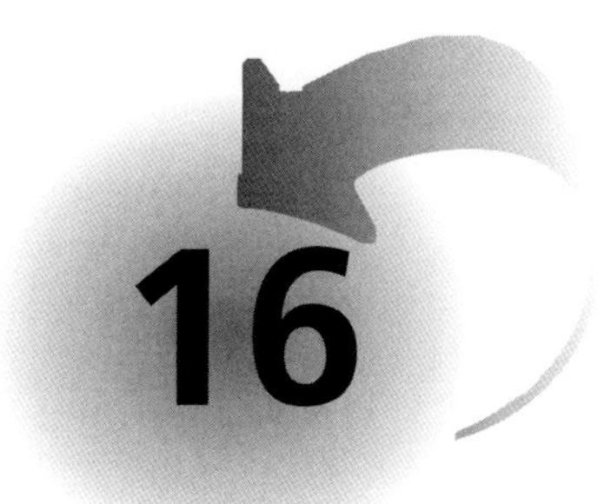

Olanrewaju Sorinola

Urinary tract injuries at cesarean section

Iatrogenic injury to the urinary tract may occur during pelvic surgery due to its close anatomical proximity to the reproductive organs. The bladder and distal ureters are the most commonly involved organs. Though cesarean sections have been associated with lower rates of urological complications than other pelvic surgeries, awareness of possible complications is important to prevent maternal morbidity.

The term 'cesarean section' is derived from two Latin words, *caedere* means to cut and *sectio* means an act of cutting or subdivision. There are other explanations for the origin of this word. Numa Pompolis, king of Rome, in 715 BC, brought in a law which forbade the burial of a pregnant woman unless her child had been removed and buried separately. This practice was called *Lex Caesarea* in 200 BC when the kings became *Caesars*. At this time, the operation was only performed post-mortem. The first recorded successful section was done by Jacob Nufe, a swinegelder, in 1588. His wife had a prolonged and obstructed labor. He used his swine gelding instruments to cut the baby out. His wife survived and had subsequent pregnancies.[1] James Barlow was the first physician to perform cesarean section on a live patient and she survived.[2]

The evolution of cesarean section during the 20th century as a relatively safe procedure has revolutionised obstetric practice. Repeat section has been a major contributor to the increased incidence of cesarean sections. The increase in the frequency of iatrogenic urological injuries was noted ever since the classical vertical incision through the body of the uterus was replaced by the incision in the lower uterine segment.[3]

INCIDENCE

A Medline search from 1951 to date, using the keywords urinary tract, cesarean section and injury, generated 104 articles dealing with urinary tract injuries at

Olanrewaju Sorinola MRCOG MMedSc
Consultant Obstetrician and Gynaecologist, Warwick Hospital, Lakin Road, Warwick CV34 5BW, UK
E-mail: olanrewaju.sorinola@swh.nhs.uk

Table 1 Anatomical changes in the urinary tract during pregnancy

• The kidneys enlarge by 1 cm during pregnancy because the renal vasculature volume and interstitial space are increased but true hypertrophy probably does not occur
• The renal collecting system (calyces, renal pelvis and ureters) undergo dilatation and develop decreased peristaltic activity, with accompanying hypertrophy of smooth muscle and hyperplasia of connective tissue
• The bladder is displaced anteriorly and superiorly as the uterus enlarges due to the intimate anatomical relationship between the bladder, the cervix and the lower uterine segment. Therefore, the bladder becomes more of an abdominal organ as pregnancy advances. As term approaches, with the descent of the presenting fetal part, the base of the bladder broadens
• The anatomical changes in the urethra are relatively minor. The upward displacement of bladder results in an elongation of the urethra

cesarean section. On limiting to English language and human, 76 articles were obtained. The reported incidence of bladder injury at the time of cesarean section ranges from 0.14–0.56%.[4,5] Phipps *et al.*[4] reported an overall incidence of 0.28%. Incidence in repeat cesarean section was 0.56% and in primary cesarean deliveries was 0.14%. Eisenkop *et al.*[6] reported an overall incidence of 0.31% (0.6% in repeat sections and 0.19% in primary sections) and 0.09% incidence of ureteric injury. Rajasekar and Hall[7] reported fewer incidences (0.14% bladder injuries overall and 0.027% ureteric injuries in 11,284 cesarean deliveries). No cases of urethral injuries were found in the Medline search.

ANATOMICAL CHANGES DURING PREGNANCY

Table 1 details the anatomical changes in the urinary tract during pregnancy.

RISK FACTORS

The main risk factors for urinary tract injuries during cesarean section are classified as follows.

Obstetric factors

Prolonged labor before section, cesarean section at full cervical dilatation, emergency section for failed instrumental delivery, concurrent uterine rupture and cesarean hysterectomy.

Surgical factors

Haste in performing the section, repeat section, surgical skill and experience of the operator. Rajasekar and Hall[7] reported that all the incidents of urinary tract injuries in their series happened during the early hours of the morning when the junior doctor is often without direct supervision. Dense adhesions, vaginal wall tears, massive intra-operative hemorrhage and attempts to control bleeding especially during repeat sections are also predisposing factors.

Anatomical factors

Anomalies of the ureter (*e.g.* duplication or mega-ureter) may be associated with uterine anomalies, distortion of pelvic anatomy by masses or adhesions, and abnormal course of the ureter due to pelvic kidney are also to be noted.[8]

TYPES/MECHANISMS OF INJURY

Bladder injury

Most injuries occur in the dome of the bladder and rarely involve the trigone.[4] Bladder injuries occur due to:[3,6,9]

1. Surgical difficulty encountered while developing the bladder flap over the lower uterine segment. The difficulty is caused usually by scar tissue from previous surgery.
2. Inadvertent cystostomy during the uterine incision is the next common cause.
3. Extension of the uterine incision into the bladder may occur along with the extension of incision into the cervix or vagina.
4. Bladder injury due to incision into the vagina rather than the lower uterine segment. With an effaced and dilated cervix, vagina can be mistaken for the lower uterine segment and it becomes difficult to separate bladder from the vagina.
5. Bisection of the bladder during cesarean section and delivery through bladder has also been reported.

Ureteric injury

Types of injuries include ureteric angulation or occlusion by improperly placed sutures, direct ureteric damage from crush/clamp injury, partial or complete transection and ischemia.[10] Many authors suggest that the predisposition of left ureter to injury is due to its anterior location with dextrorotation of the gravid uterus.

The mechanisms of ureteric injury are as follows:[6,11]

1. Transection of the ureter due to extension of uterine incision into the cervix or vagina.
2. In attempts to achieve hemostasis, ureter may be included in blind, mass ligature.
3. Less commonly, the extension of the uterine incision into the broad ligament damages the ureter directly.
4. Ureteric injuries have been reported to occur in association with ruptured bladder causing avulsion of the distal ureters.

Genito-urinary fistulae

Bladder and ureteric injuries, if unrecognised, may give rise to vesico-uterine/vesico-vaginal and uretero-uterine fistulae, respectively. Vesico-vaginal fistulae (Fig.1) and vesico-uterine fistulae (VUF) may develop immediately after

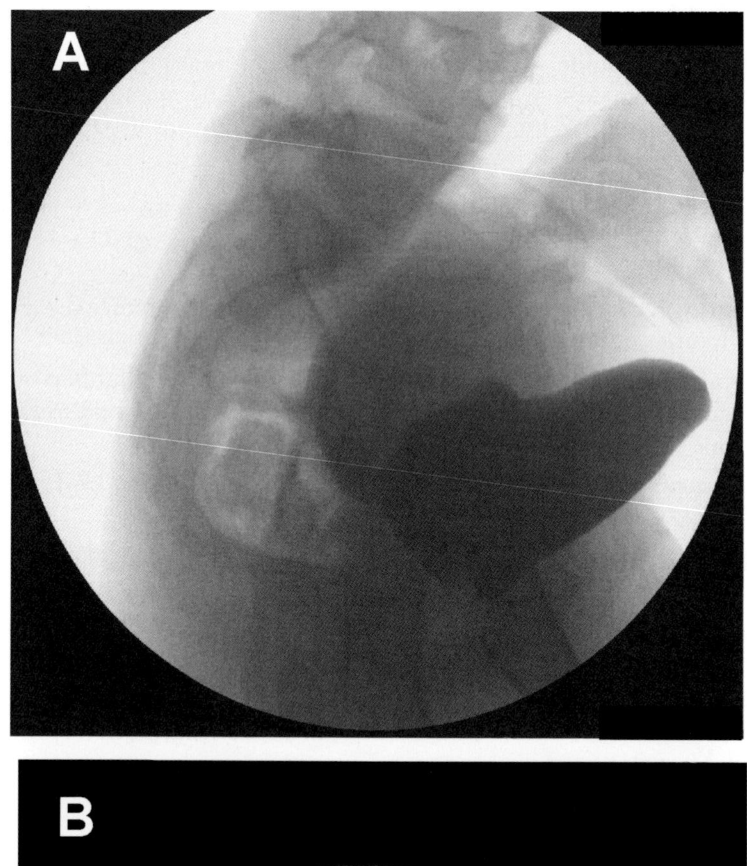

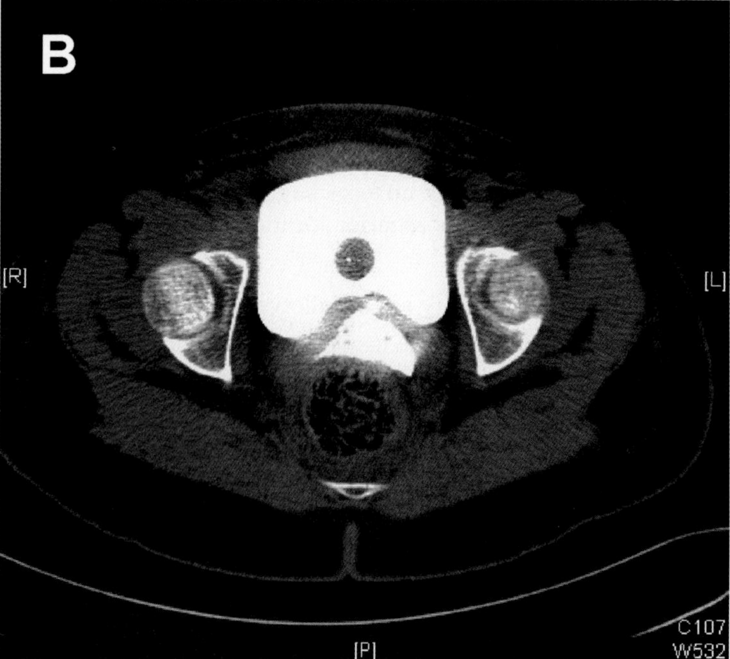

Fig. 1 Vesico-vaginal fistula. (A) The plain film shows a lateral view of a cystogram with leakage of dye into the vagina. (B) The CT cystogram demonstrates the fistulous tract from the left side of the bladder into the vagina.

cesarean section, manifest late in the puerperium, or occur after repeated procedures. The fistulous communication is usually between the posterior supratrigonal part of the bladder and the anterior lower segment of the uterus or, rarely, the cervix. Delayed fistula formation may result from infection, devascularisation, clamping, or hematoma formation in the urinary bladder. Repeat cesarean section may cause progressive devitalisation and scarring of the bladder base injuring its vascular network.[12] Uretero-uterine fistulae have been associated with damage caused by a low transverse uterine incision during cesarean section either due to extension of the incision or in the process of achieving hemostasis. Small necrotic tears in the ureter or uterus along with localised infection can become fistulous.[13]

PREVENTION

Primary prevention

Avoiding injury to the urinary tract is possible by following the points mentioned in Table 2.

Secondary prevention

When injuries do occur, early recognition and repair during the primary surgery, most often result in less morbidity for the patient and a more successful outcome.[10]

MANAGEMENT

Bladder injury

Most bladder injuries are grossly apparent intra-operatively. Red vascular appearances of the muscularis, urine draining through the dome, or the visualisation of the Foley's bulb are all tell-tale signs of bladder wall laceration. If there is suspicion of a bladder perforation, methylene blue, or indigo carmine injected into the urethral catheter with observed leakage of blue dye

Table 2 Prevention of urinary tract injuries during cesarean section

- Bladder should be adequately drained by a Foley's catheter before cesarean section except in the direst circumstances
- The peritoneal cavity should be entered at the most superior aspect of the abdominal incision, especially in patients undergoing repeat cesarean section
- Careful sharp dissection should be employed to mobilise the bladder flap adequately in patients with extensive scarring between bladder and lower uterine segment. This provides better visualisation of the lower uterine segment and drops the ureters out of the field
- The lower uterine scar should be pointing upwards at each end
- While attaining hemostasis, it is best to use compression on the bleeding area rather than blind hemostasis sutures
- The uterus can be exteriorised for better exposure to suture
- If there is any suspicion of ureteric injury, it is best to involve a urologist

into the abdomen confirms lack of integrity of the lower urinary tract. The first step is a thorough evaluation of the extent, size and location of the injury, and a determination of whether the trigone or ureters are involved (Fig. 2). Most injuries are located in the dome of the bladder and do not involve the trigone or ureters.[14]

Bladder dome injury

Simple cystostomy in the dome is closed in two or three layers; the first layer is a simple running closure of the mucosa using 3-0 absorbable suture. The second layer is a running stitch of 2-0 or 3-0 absorbable suture incorporating the submucosa and muscularis. The bladder is filled with methylene blue dye to confirm the integrity of the repair and defects are closed with figure-of-eight stitches. A third running stitch of absorbable suture may be placed in the serosa if the margins can be approximated. Postoperatively, the bladder should be drained for 7 days.

Trigonal or ureteric injury

A minority of injuries extend to the trigone or ureters. Ureteric integrity must be confirmed prior to repair of the cystostomy. This may be done by a variety of methods as described below. If the ureters are not injured, bladder tear can be closed as mentioned above. If ureteric injury is noted, then the management is as described below.

Ureteric injury

The management of ureteric injury during cesarean section depends on the nature and location of the defect as well as the timing of the diagnosis of the injury (Fig. 3). Intra-operative diagnosis of ureteric injury is still very difficult compared with bladder injury.[8] In the presence of suspected or apparent injuries to the ureters during cesarean section, early involvement of the urologist is important as the surgeon may face several difficulties:

1. Obstetric facilities designated for vaginal or abdominal deliveries are often inadequately equipped with the urological tools.
2. The large uterus as well as bleeding from the engorged pelvic blood vessels may render surgical dissection of the bladder and the distal ureters cumbersome.
3. A pfannenstiel incision, which is usually made by obstetricians during cesarean section, may impede proper dissection and exposure of the ureters.

Diagnosis

One or more of the following diagnostic methods may be needed:

1. **Dye test** – injection of 5–10 ml of indigo carmine dye intravenously and directly visualising bilateral spill of blue dye from the ureteric orifices through a cystoscope or cystostomy defect (if bladder also injured). If the spill of the dye is symmetric and no dye is noted in the retroperitoneal space, ureteric injury can usually be excluded. However, given the decreased peristalsis and ureteric dilatation commonly observed in late pregnancy coupled with renal under-

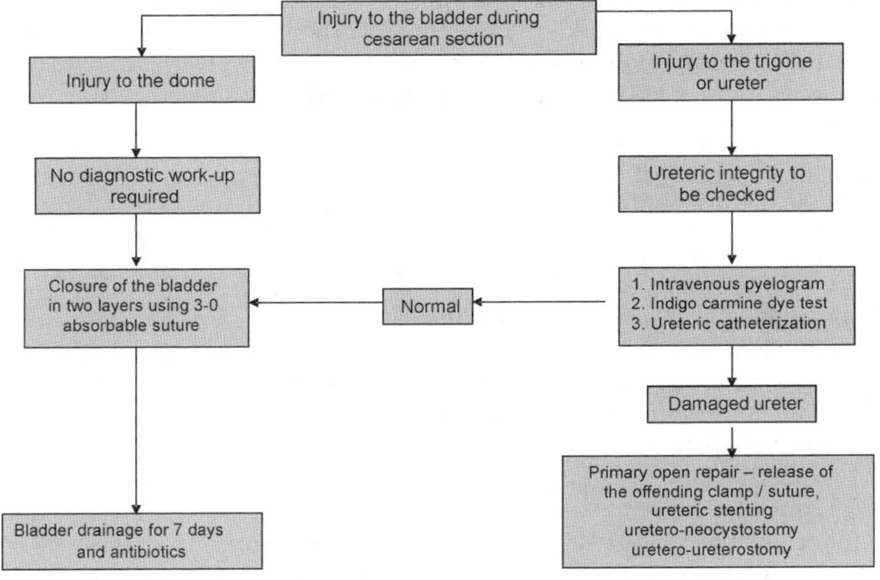

Fig. 2 Schematic flow chart for the management of bladder injuries during cesarean section.

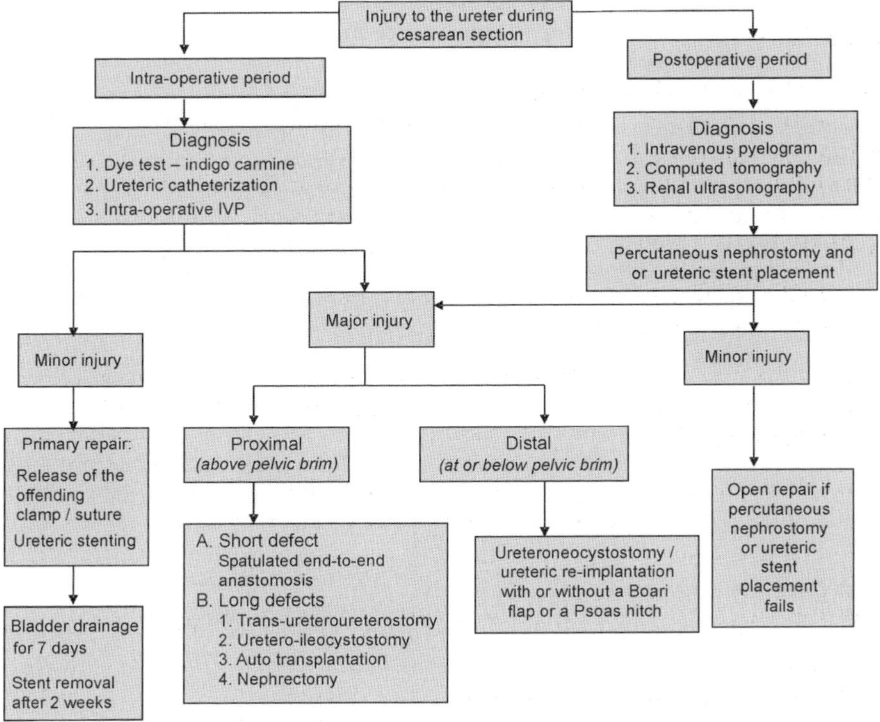

Fig. 3 Schematic flow chart for the management of ureteric injuries during cesarean section.

perfusion in some cases, renal excretion of the contrast medium may be impaired. On the other hand, efflux of urine into a bloody operative field may not be identifiable. Also, some urinary tract anomalies with duplication of the collecting systems may not readily lend themselves to evaluation by this technique.

2. **Imaging** – an intra-operative intravenous pyelogram (IVP) may confirm ureteric integrity if dye can be traced in both ureters to the bladder. This technique also suffers from some of the limitations described above. In addition, operating tables in delivery units may not be designed for intra-operative radiography and may limit the quality of the study.

3. **Ureteric catheterization** – inserting a ureteric catheter in a retrograde manner through the cystoscope or directly into the orifices following a cystostomy (if the bladder is involved or a cystoscope is unavailable) is probably the preferred diagnostic method.[10] The risk of ureteric perforation during insertion and ureteric spasm with transient anuria after removal are potential disadvantages. There is also the possibility of passing a catheter through a partially transected ureter and thus falsely assured. However, failure to advance the catheter easily through the ureter into the renal pelvis indicates ureteric damage. When fluoroscopy is available, retrograde imaging of an intact ureter virtually eliminates the necessity for ureteric catheterization.

Intra-operative period

1. **Minor injury** – kinking or ligation of a ureter by an improperly placed clamp or suture may be treated easily by removal of the offending clamp or suture. If required, after removal of the clamp or suture, a double J, 7-F or 8-F ureteric catheter should be inserted to the level of the renal pelvis and a retroperitoneal drain should there be any leakage of urine. A Foley's catheter is left in place for 7 days, and the ureteric catheter is removed via cystoscopy after 14 days. IVP is not usually required in minor injury.[14]

2. **Major injury** – Management depends on the location and the extent of injury as detailed in Figure 3. Distal ureter injury, such as transection or crush injuries with extensive devascularisation, are best treated with uretero-neocystostomy. Tension on the ureter should be relieved by Boari-flap or Psoas muscle hitch. A suction drain is placed near the anastomosis site to prevent the formation of urinoma. A Foley's catheter is left in place for 7 days. The ureteric catheter is left in place for at least 3 weeks and is removed only after ensuring integrity of the repair with an IVP. Extensive injuries to the proximal ureter during cesarean section are rare. When identified, they should be repaired by end-to-end anastomosis for short defects, or trans-ureteroureterostomy for long defects.

Post-operative period

Unrecognised ureteric injury should be suspected postoperatively if a patient experiences:

- costovertebral angle pain
- oliguria
- unexplained or persistent fever
- persistent abdominal distension with or without ileus
- unexplained hematuria

- watery vaginal discharge
- rise in white cells and serum creatinine.

IVP is able to identify ureteric injury in more than 95% of cases. Renal ultrasonography has limited value due to the physiological dilatation of the upper urinary tract during pregnancy and the early postpartum period.[15] In attempting to establish urinary drainage, the options include percutaneous nephrostomy tube with or without an antegrade stent or a retrograde ureteric stent placement.[15,16] Placement of a percutaneous nephrostomy tube provides rapid and effective urinary tract drainage and is useful in patients with obstruction and urinary tract sepsis. Additionally, this may be the only procedure required in resolving the ureteric injury, particularly if the mechanism has been related to ligation or entrapment with absorbable suture as the obstruction may resolve after resorption of the suture material.[17]

For major injuries, the traditional doctrine is to delay surgical repair of ureteric injuries for several weeks after percutaneous nephrostomy. Pregnancy causes vascular congestion in the pelvis and the gravid uterus could alter the normal anatomical relationships of pelvic organs. Delayed repair affords time for the involution of the tissues, clearance of infection, and the re-establishment of adequate blood supply.[11] However, Davis[14] suggested that immediate repair can be undertaken if the injury is diagnosed within 10–14 days of surgery, if the patient is young and healthy, if infection is not present, and if extensive devascularisation of the ureter is unlikely.

Genito-urinary fistulae

Obstetric genito-urinary fistula tends to present in various ways. Most patients have urinary incontinence or persistent vaginal discharge. If the fistula is very small, leakage may be intermittent, occurring only at maximal bladder capacity or with particular body positions. Other features include: (i) unexplained fever; (ii) hematuria; (iii) recurrent cystitis or pyelonephritis; (iv) vaginal, suprapubic or flank pain; and (v) abnormal urinary stream. The management depends on the type of fistula and its location but there are some key principles that apply to all repairs – accurate diagnosis, timing of repair, appropriate expertise, and detailed postoperative care with follow-up. Examination under anesthesia, dye test (methylene blue), cystoscopy, cystogram and/or intravenous urography are important diagnostic investigations. An IVU is useful where there is suspicion of a ureteric fistula, while the cystogram can diagnose VVF. The timing of repair is critical, more so in the developing world. A 2–3 month wait is common to eradicate infection and for the tissues to become healthier and less friable. However, in the developed world, repairs can usually be done after a few weeks.

Vesico-uterine

VUF deserves special mention as it used to be the least common of all genitourinary fistulae constituting about 5%; however, with a rising cesarean section rate, this may change. There are three common presentations of VUF following Cesarean section: (i) urinary incontinence with cyclical hematuria; (ii) urinary incontinence alone; and (iii) Youssef's syndrome,[18] *i.e.* amenorrhoea and menouria (menstruation through the bladder) in the absence of urinary incontinence. Presentation depends on the level of the fistula. Those arising above the isthmus will present as Youssef's syndrome. The cervical isthmus acts as a sphincter that will only relax if it is distended with menstrual fluid; however, such distension is prevented in the presence of a high fistula as a lower pressure route of exit into the bladder is available. Likewise, the isthmic sphincter prevents urine from entering the vagina; hence, these women are continent. Fistulae arising below the level of the isthmus can present with incontinence alone or with menouria; some menstruation still occurs vaginally.

Conservative management by bladder catheterization for at least 4 weeks is indicated when the fistula is detected just after the delivery since there is good chance for spontaneous closure. Surgical treatment involves ureteric catheterization via cystoscopy followed by an abdominal transperitoneal repair in which the bladder is opened and the fistulous tract excised. The defects in the uterus and bladder are repaired using absorbable sutures and omentum interposed between them. Postoperatively, the bladder is drained via a urethral catheter for 14 days.

Vesicovaginal

Spontaneous healing of small fistulae can occur following continuous free catheter drainage for 3–4 weeks. If this fails, an abdominal or vaginal approach will be chosen according to the practice of the operator and the site of the fistula. Occasionally, a supporting graft, the Martius pedicle graft of fibrofatty tissue is brought down from one labium majus to cover and reinforce the repaired fistula and provide increased vascularity. The postoperative care is the same as in VUF repair.

Ureteric fistulae

Though rare, spontaneous healing can occur, especially where there has been incomplete division of the ureter and where it has been possible to pass a ureteric catheter. Re-implantation of the ureter is usually done via an abdominal transperitoneal approach.

KEY POINTS FOR CLINICAL PRACTICE

- Injury to the urinary tract during cesarean section is not that common but knowledge of the obstetric, surgical and anatomical factors that can predispose to injury is the key to prevention.
- While bladder injury is easily recognised, recognition of ureteric injury is more difficult.
- Early investigation and treatment in ureteric injury can reduce morbidity and save kidney function.
- Genitourinary fistulae are probably under-reported and some go unrecognised especially as spontaneous healing of small fistulae can occur.
- The type and timing of treatment should be individualised.

References

1 Chamberlain G. Caesarean section. In: Chamberlain G, Steer P. (eds) Turnbull's Obstetrics. London: Churchill, 2001; 601–617
2 Yasin SY, Walton DL, O'Sullivan MJ. Problems encountered during caesarean section. In: Plauche W, Morrison J, O'Sullivan MJ. (eds) Surgical Obstetrics. Oxford: Saunders, 1992; 431–445
3 Faricy PO, Augspurger RR, Kaufman JM. Bladder injuries associated with caesarean section. J Urol 1978; 120: 372
4 Phipps MG, Watabe B, Clemons JL, Weitzen S, Myers DL. Risk factors for bladder injury during caesarean section. Am J Obstet Gynecol 2005; 105: 156–160
5 Feeney JK. Injury to the ureter in gynecologic and obstetric operations. Ir J Med Sci 1959; 399: 126
6 Eisenkop SM, Richman R, Platt LD, Paul RH. Urinary tract injury during caesarean section. Obstet Gynecol 1982; 60: 591–596
7 Rajasekar D, Hall M. Urinary tract injuries during obstetric intervention. Br J Obstet Gynaecol 1997; 104: 731–734
8 Sorinola OO, Begum R. Ureteric injuries during gynaecological surgery. In: Studd J. (ed) Progress in Obstetrics and Gynaecology, 16th edn. Edinburgh: Elsevier, Churchill Livingstone 2005; 303–320
9 Franzini M. Delivery through the bladder during cesarean section. J Urol 1981; 125: 422–423
10 Yossepowitch O, Baniel J, Livine PM. Urological injuries during caesarean section: intraoperative diagnosis and management. J Urol 2004; 172: 196–199
11 Onura VC, al Ariyan R, Koko AH, Abdelwahab AS, al Jawini N. Major injuries to the urinary tract in association with childbirth. East Afr Med J 1997; 74: 523–526
12 Porcaro AB, Zicari M, Antiolli SZ *et al*. Vesicouterine fistulas following caesarean section. Int Urol Nephrol 2002; 34: 335–344
13 Saltutti C, Cello VD, Costanzi A *et al*. Ureterouterine fistula as a complication of cesarean section. J Urol 1994; 152: 1199–1200
14 Davis JD. Management of injuries to the urinary and gastrointestinal tract during cesarean section. Obstet Gynecol Clin North Am 1991; 26: 469–480
15 Razvi HA, Denstedt JD. Endoscopic management of ureteral injury after cesarean section. J Endourol 1994; 8: 345–347
16 Dowling RA, Corriere JN, Sandler CM. Iatrogenic ureteral injury. J Urol 1986; 135: 912
17 Harshman MW, Pollack HM, Banner MP, Wein AJ. Conservative management of ureteral obstruction secondary to suture entrapment. J Urol 1982; 127: 121
18 Youssef AF. Menouria following lower segment caesarean section: a syndrome. Am J Obstet Gynecol 1957; 73: 759

Gillian Fowler Nigel Holland

Investigation and management of anal sphincter injury following childbirth

Obstetric trauma following childbirth is the leading cause of fecal incontinence in women. Injury to the anal sphincter complex is common, diagnosed clinically in 0.4–2.5% of vaginal deliveries[1–3] where mediolateral episiotomy is performed and up to 19% with midline episiotomy.[4] Concerns have been expressed that sphincter injuries are missed clinically at time of delivery.[5] Indeed, studies using endo-anal ultrasound have reported occult anal sphincter injury in up to 35% of women after their first delivery.[6]

There has been a steady increase in medicolegal cases associated with anal sphincter. Most causes relate to failure to recognise sphincter injury at time of delivery. The aim of this report, therefore, is to provide a comprehensive review of the diagnosis and evidence for the management of obstetric anal sphincter injury.

ANATOMY AND IMAGING OF THE ANAL SPHINCTER COMPLEX

Anatomy of the sphincter complex

The anal sphincter complex consists of the external anal sphincter (EAS) and internal anal sphincter (IAS) together with the puborectalis part of the levator ani sling. Our anatomical understanding of the anal sphincter and surrounding structures has been greatly enhanced by endo-anal ultrasound.[7–11] The EAS consists of three parts – deep, superficial and subcutaneous (Fig. 1).[7]

Gillian Fowler MRCOG (for correspondence)
Specialist Registrar in Obstetrics and Gynaecology, Warrington District General Hospital, Croft Wing, Lovely Lane, Warrington WA5 1QG, UK
E-mail: fowlergillian@yahoo.co.uk

Nigel Holland MD FRCOG DipVen
Consultant Obstetrician and Gynaecologist, Warrington District General Hospital, Croft Wing, Lovely Lane, Warrington WA5 1QG, UK

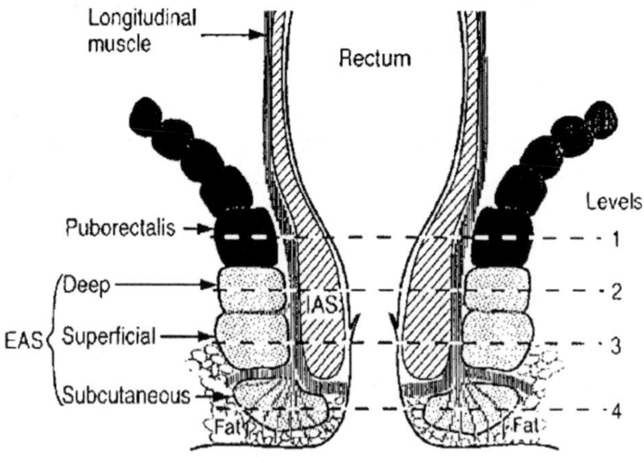

Fig. 1 Cross-section through anal sphincter complex.

The deep part lies at the uppermost aspect of the sphincter complex and is in continuity with the puborectalis which lies above it. The superficial aspect lies caudal to the deep aspect and together they surround the IAS. The subcutaneous part of the EAS lies below the level of the IAS. The IAS itself is a direct continuation of the longitudinal muscle of the rectum. Morphologically, both the EAS and IAS are separate and heterogeneous.

Endo-anal ultrasound

Endo-anal ultrasound is a well-established technique for imaging both the IAS and EAS (Fig. 2).[12] It is used routinely in the investigation of fecal incontinence,

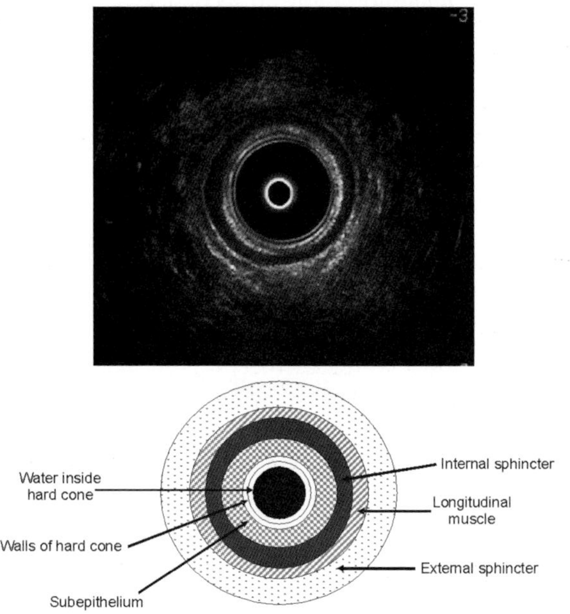

Fig. 2 Endo-anal ultrasound: view of a normal intact IAS and EAS.

providing a high resolution 360° image from within the anal sphincter complex.[12] Studies have proven it to be accurate in the assessment of sphincter defects when compared to histology findings and anorectal physiology testing.[10,11] To obtain images, a specialized ultrasound probe is inserted into the anal canal. Concerns have been expressed that the anal probe may distort the anatomy of the anal sphincter, leading to inappropriate interpretation of ultrasound findings.

Differences between male and female EAS anatomy

Several authors have reported a difference between male and female EAS anatomy based on endo-anal ultrasound findings.[7,8] The EAS muscle fibers appear to slope inferiorly and join anteriorly lower down the anal canal compared with male anatomy. Imaging using end-anal ultrasound just above this point shows an apparent anterior defect.[7] It is the difficulty in interpreting this natural anterior defect that, according to some authors, has resulted in over-reporting of ultrasound diagnosed obstetric anal sphincter defects.[8]

FUNCTION OF THE ANAL SPHINCTERS

A structural and functionally intact anal sphincter complex is essential to maintain continence. Disruption of the anatomy or physiology can lead to anal incontinence. The anus is normally closed by the tonic activity of the IAS. The IAS contributes approximately 70–85% of the resting anal sphincter pressure. This is reduced to 40% after sudden distension of the rectum and 65% during constant rectal distension. Hence, the IAS is responsible for maintaining anal continence at rest.[13]

The EAS is responsible for the majority of the squeeze tone. Like the IAS, it is continually active; however, during rises in the intra-abdominal pressure such as laughing, coughing and sneezing, contraction of the EAS protects against fecal leakage. The peak pressures are found at approximately 2 cm from the anal verge which is the point at which the EAS and IAS overlap.

The anorectal complex receives innervation from sensory, motor and autonomic nerves and by the enteric nervous system. The pudendal nerve arises from sacral nerves (S2, S3, S4) and supplies the EAS providing both sensory and motor function.[14]

Rectal distension is associated with a fall in anal resting pressure known as the recto-anal inhibitory reflex.[15] The EAS initially contracts, followed by a reflex inhibition of the IAS. The amplitude and duration of this relaxation increases with the volume of rectal distension. The bowel contents are periodically 'sampled' by specialized receptors in the upper anal canal by the transient relaxation of the IAS. The 'sampling' process together with the recto-anal inhibitory reflex allows the discharge of flatus but is also associated with a subconscious contractile reflex of the EAS to prevent release of rectal contents if it is not a suitable time for defecation.[16]

EFFECT OF VAGINAL DELIVERY ON ANORECTAL INJURY FUNCTION

During vaginal delivery, the tissues of the genital tract are stretched and distended to enable the passage and delivery of the fetus. This can lead to disruption to anorectal function by either direct muscle trauma in the form of tears in the anal sphincter complex or by injury to the nerve supply to the anorectal region. Disruption of the EAS muscle fibers or impaired function by interruption of the nerve supply to the muscle leads to symptoms of fecal urgency. If the injury also involves the IAS, fecal incontinence symptoms tend to be worse and fecal leakage can occur at rest. Injuries to both EAS and IAS often co-exist.

Anal manometry

The function of the anal sphincter complex can be measured objectively by anal manometry. This technique evaluates the contraction and relaxation of the anal sphincters by inserting a perfusion catheter into the anal canal. Squeeze pressures are principally due to the EAS and resting pressure due to the IAS. Anal manometry cannot distinguish whether the underlying pathology is of mechanical disruption of the anal sphincter muscles or neurological trauma to the pudendal nerve.

Pudendal nerve terminal motor latency (PNTML)

The pudendal nerve can be assessed by the PNTML measurement. This test is undertaken using the St Mark's electrode to stimulate the nerve either transrectally or transvaginally while the evoked response of the external anal sphincter is observed. Prolonged conduction times result from demyelination of the nerve sheath which can occur as a result of direct trauma during passage of the fetal head or stretching of the pudendal nerves during elongation of the birth canal.[17,18]

Neurophysiology tests in women in both the antenatal and postnatal period who have undergone elective cesarean section have shown no change in manometry pressures, no change in bowel function and no sphincter defects on ultrasound.[19–21] Fecal incontinence symptoms and PNTML have, however, been shown following emergency cesarean section.[22,23] These studies conclude that labor can result in changes in the function of the anal sphincter complex as shown by physiological testing although sphincter muscle tears do not occur without vaginal delivery.

Prolonged PNTML has been shown in 33% of primigravid women and 50% of multiparous women within 48 h of delivery in one study.[24] However, when re-assessed at 2 months' postpartum, studies have demonstrated a normal PNTML in 60–80% of these women, indicating that injury to the pudendal nerve conduction is reversible.[24,25] Anal sphincter striated muscle fiber density was also increased 2 months' postpartum, indicating re-innervation of the sphincter muscles occurs following the initial denervation. These neuropathic injuries tend to be asymmetrical.[26]

Anal sensation has been assessed in some studies.[27–29] A combination of antenatal, immediate postpartum (within 72 h) and at 2 months' postpartum were undertaken and either no change or a return to normal measurements postpartum including patients with a known anal sphincter injury. Authors from these studies conclude that anal sensation in isolation plays a minor role in the development of obstetric-related fecal incontinence.

It is important to highlight that, although injuries to the anorectal region occur at childbirth, most patients remain asymptomatic at that time. Many studies have shown a fall in anal sphincter squeeze pressures after the menopause.[30–32] Estrogen receptors have been identified in the anal sphincter and the loss of estrogen at the menopause may explain this associated decline in anorectal function.[32]

RISK FACTORS FOR ANORECTAL INJURY

In order to prevent anorectal injury, it is important to identify risk factors. The majority of research assessing risk factors relates to third degree tears. Based on the overall risk of third degree tears as 1% of vaginal deliveries, a number of risk factors have been identified by retrospective studies. These include induction of labor (up to 2%), epidural analgesia (up to 2%), birthweight over 4 kg (up to 2%), persistent occipito-posterior position (up to 3%), primiparity (up to 4%), second stage longer than 1 h (up to 4%), and forceps delivery (up to 7%).[33–47] These risk factors were confirmed by systematic review of 14 studies.[48] Other risk factors, such as shoulder dystocia, have been suggested but evidence is contradictory.

Parity

Some population-based studies of fecal incontinence have assessed obstetric history. The first vaginal delivery carries the greatest risk of new-onset fecal incontinence[49,50] and each subsequent delivery adds to that risk.[51]

Episiotomy

The evidence in the literature for the role of episiotomy is contradictory. Traditional teaching is that episiotomy protects the perineum from uncontrolled trauma during delivery. Although several authors have demonstrated a protective effect with mediolateral episiotomy,[34,35,43] others have reported the converse.[39,52,53] The type of episiotomy is important. Evidence reports mediolateral episiotomy (favored in the UK and European practice) to have a significantly lower risk of sphincter injury compared with a midline episiotomy (favored in the US), 2% versus 12%.[54,55] The confusion in the evidence may be explained by variations in clinical practice which are not reflected in the studies. There will be differences in the experience of the accoucheur for a normal delivery and the rate of episiotomy also varies. The differences between medical and midwifery staff in conducting a mediolateral episiotomy have been studied, with doctors performing episiotomies which are longer and at a wider angle compared with midwifes.[56,57] Current evidence is unable to support the routine use of episiotomy to prevent anal sphincter injury.

Assisted vaginal delivery

The incidence of anal sphincter damage and fecal incontinence symptoms following instrumental delivery is higher than following normal vaginal delivery.[6,58,59] Over the last few years, vacuum extractor or ventouse has become the favored instrument for assisted vaginal delivery rather than forceps. This is based on the evidence from many studies,[60] including a Cochrane review of 10 trials which showed the use of the vacuum extractor instead of forceps was associated with significantly less maternal trauma (odds ratio [OR], 0.4; 95% confidence interval [CI], 0.3–0.5).[61]

However, compared with forceps delivery, vacuum extraction is significantly more likely to fail with its own implications (OR 1.7; 95% CI 1.3–2.2).[61] In addition, the neonatal risks associated with ventouse delivery are greater, with increased risks of cephalohematoma and retinal hemorrhage.[61,62]

Other risk factors

Studies assessing the risk factors for neuropathy following childbirth have reported injury to be more common in the presence of a prolonged labor particularly the second stage, large size of the fetal head.[2,6,63–66] Many of these factors may result in the need for an assisted vaginal delivery. Further vaginal delivery may result in further pudendal nerve damage.[67]

Many of the risk factors identified are components of normal vaginal delivery and cannot be avoided. The majority of women with these risk factors deliver without anorectal injury. Attempts to develop an antenatal risk scoring system for sphincter injury have so far been unsuccessful.[68] Studies are needed to assess the effect of interventions to prevent sphincter injury.

PROTECTION AGAINST ANAL SPHINCTER INJURY

Increased awareness of the complications of childbirth is fueling requests by women for elective cesarean section in otherwise low-risk pregnancies. Indeed, a survey of female obstetricians in 1996 revealed 31% would themselves request elective cesarean section due to the potential risk of perineal trauma.[69] This view contrasts with the recent UK NICE guidelines which report an increased risk of maternal morbidity with cesarean section compared with vaginal delivery.[70]

Elective cesarean section as opposed to emergency cesarean has been shown to be protective against fecal incontinence.[71] Cesarean section late in the first stage of labor (more than 8 cm dilatation) or in the second stage does not protect the function of the anal sphincter.[72]

CONSEQUENCES OF ANAL SPHINCTER INJURY

Childbirth has a significant impact on the physical and psychological well-being of women, with up to 91% of women reporting at least one new symptom 8 weeks following delivery.[73] Women with recognized anorectal injury have increased morbidity compared with those with first and second degree tears.

Anal incontinence affects 4–6%[74–76] of women up to 12 months following delivery with 40,000 mothers affected each year in the UK.[73,77–79] In women with a clinically recognised anal sphincter injury, however, symptoms are more common with fecal incontinence, fecal urgency, dyspareunia and perineal pain reported in 30–50% of women and symptoms may persist for many years.[2,19,80]

It is recognized that obstetric trauma is the commonest cause of anal incontinence. The International Continence Society defines anal incontinence as the involuntary loss of flatus or feces which becomes a social or hygiene problem. It can be affected by many factors such as stool consistency and volume, colonic transit, compliance of the rectal reservoir and mental function. The most important factor in maintaining continence is an anatomically normal anal sphincter complex and its intact neurological function. It was previously thought neuropathic injury to the pelvic nerves and pudendal nerve was the leading cause of incontinence following childbirth. It has only been since the advent of endo-anal ultrasound that sphincter defects were diagnosed in women who were previously diagnosed with a neurogenic cause for their fecal incontinence.[12]

Anal incontinence has been described as the 'unvoiced symptom' as affected individuals avoid seeking medical advice.[81] Many do not seek medical attention due embarrassment and the taboo nature of the problem. Some women are discouraged from discussing their symptoms because they feel they are a normal consequence of childbirth.[3,80] The true incidence of anal incontinence and impact on women following childbirth are, therefore, unknown.

In addition to anal incontinence the longer term consequences of anorectal injury include perineal pain, dyspareunia and anorectal fistula. Perineal pain can lead to significant morbidity following vaginal delivery. It can interfere with the women's ability to bond with her newborn. If severe, it may lead to problems with voiding of urine and defecation. Perineal pain and dyspareunia have been reported in many studies to affect up to 50% of women following anorectal injury and may persist for many years.[2,80] There is a considerable impact on women's psychosexual health, with many avoiding intercourse for many years.

Abscess formation, wound breakdown and rectovaginal fistula are serious, but fortunately rare, consequences of anorectal injury. It is thought that most rectovaginal fistulas following sphincter repair are caused by failure to recognize the true extent of the initial injury which leads to wound breakdown.[82] Wound breakdown rates of 10% had previously been reported after sphincter repair.[83] However, the recent randomised control trials (RCTs) assessing methods of repair failed to report any cases of wound breakdown.[84–86] This may be a reflection of the routine use of broad-spectrum antibiotics in protocols for sphincter repair.[87]

CLINICAL RECOGNITION OF ANAL SPHINCTER INJURY

Occult anal sphincter injury

In one of the first studies to use endo-anal ultrasound following vaginal delivery, Sultan *et al.*[6] reported anal sphincter injury in up to 35% of women after their first delivery, suggesting that the vast majority of sphincter injuries are not diagnosed clinically at time of delivery. Since this initial work, many studies using endo-anal ultrasound in the postpartum period have reported occult sphincter rates ranging between 6.8–28%.[59,88]

In one study, perineal examination by an experienced person was shown to double the clinical detection rate of sphincter injury.[5] This study went further

Table 1 Classification of perineal trauma

Type of tear	Definition
First degree tear	Injury to perineal skin
Second degree tear	Injury to perineum involving perineal muscles but not involving the anal sphincter
Third degree tear	Injury to perineum involving the anal sphincter complex
3A	Less than 50% of EAS thickness torn
3B	More than 50% of EAS thickness torn
3C	Both EAS and IAS torn
Fourth degree tear	Injury to perineum involving the anal sphincter complex (both EAS and IAS) and anal epithelium

to question whether anal sphincter injuries are truly 'occult' or simply missed clinically at the time of delivery.[5]

There is no question that the addition of postpartum endo-anal ultrasound increases the detection of sphincter injury.[5,89] It is also recognized that symptoms of fecal incontinence following an anal sphincter injury are not commonly reported in the immediate postpartum period and many patients remain asymptomatic for many years. The diagnosis of obstetric anal sphincter damage is, therefore, often delayed for many years and the opportunity for early intervention, either by physiotherapy or surgical repair, is missed. The importance of early diagnosis has been highlighted in a recent paper by Faltin *et al.*[88] Results of this RCT showed a reduction in fecal incontinence symptoms at 12 months in women who had a surgical repair of sphincter injury diagnosed by endo-anal ultrasound at time of delivery compared with no repair.

There is, however, limited availability of endo-anal ultrasound equipment, trained staff and poor patient acceptability of the technique. Consequently, systematic examination of the perineal area by experienced staff following delivery remains the method of detecting sphincter injury in clinical practice and is advocated by both midwifery and obstetric colleges while postpartum endo-anal ultrasound remains, at the moment, a research tool.[5,90]

Third and fourth degree anal sphincter injury

The wide variation in the classification of clinically recognised perineal trauma amongst obstetricians has been highlighted by many authors.[76] Since 2001, the same accepted classification has been used by the UK Royal College of Obstetricians[87] and International Consultation on Incontinence.[91]

A third degree perineal tear is defined as a partial or complete disruption of the anal sphincter muscles, which may involve either or both the EAS and IAS muscles. To standardize classification, third degree tears have, therefore, been sub-classified as 3A, 3B or 3C (Table 1).

A fourth degree tear is defined as a disruption of the anal sphincter muscles with a breach of the rectal mucosa. Obstetric anal sphincter injury encompasses both third and fourth degree perineal tears.

TECHNIQUE AND METHOD OF REPAIR OF OBSTETRIC ANAL SPHINCTER INJURY

The UK Royal College of Obstetrics and Gynaecology (RCOG) produced national guidelines for the management of anal sphincter injury in 2007 based on best available evidence.[92] Together with a recently published Cochrane systematic review on the method of repair of obstetric anal injury,[93] it provides recommendations on each aspect of sphincter repair.

Setting of repair

The RCOG recommends that repair of anal sphincter injury takes place in an operating theatre. This provides aseptic conditions and adequate light. Regional or general anesthesia enables the sphincter muscle to relax, enabling the retracted torn ends to be retrieved and brought together without tension.[94]

Antibiotics

Infection following anal sphincter repair is associated with a high risk of anal incontinence and fistula formation.[94] There is no RCT evidence to support the use of antibiotics; indeed, a recent Cochrane review looking at antibiotic prophylaxis versus placebo or no antibiotics for fourth degree tears did not find any published RCTs. Intra-operative intravenous and postoperative oral broad-spectrum antibiotics have been used in all RCTs assessing different repair techniques. Typical regimens include cefuroxime 1.5 g and metronidazole 500 mg in theatre, followed by a 7-day course of cephalexin 500 mg and metronidazole 500 mg, three times daily.[84–86,94] Metronidazole in particular is used to cover the risk from anaerobic bacteria of fecal origin.

Laxatives

Traditionally, women received constipating agents following sphincter repair. This was based on the experience of colorectal surgeons who were undertaking secondary sphincter repair on patients with fecal incontinence, with the aim to avoid liquid fecal matter contaminating the wound. Primary repair differs from secondary repair as women do not have pre-existing fecal incontinence at time of repair. The use of postoperative laxatives and stool softeners is supported by the opinion that it acts to avoid passing a hard stool which, in turn, could disrupt the repair.[94]

There is only one RCT comparing the outcome of postoperative laxatives versus constipating agents following primary sphincter repair.[95] In the laxative group, patients had a significantly earlier and less painful bowel motion and earlier postnatal discharge. However, there was no difference in the symptomatic or functional outcome of repair between the two regimens.

In the published RCTs, stool softeners (lactulose, 10 ml three times daily), together with a bulking agent (ispaghula husk, Fybogel one sachet twice daily) were used for 10 days following repair.

Technique of repair

The patient is placed in lithotomy for both types of repair which should be performed under full aseptic conditions in theatre under general or regional

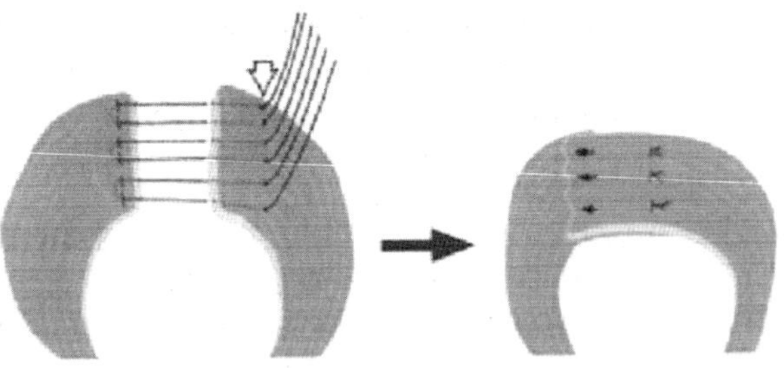

Fig. 3 Overlap technique for repair of the external anal sphincter (with permission from Sultan AH *et al.*[94]).

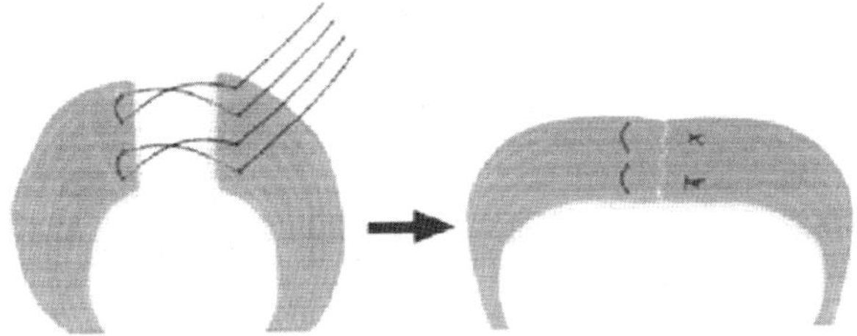

Fig. 4 End-to-end approximation of the external anal sphincter (with permission from Sultan AH *et al.*[94]).

anesthesia. The following repair techniques were first described by Sultan and form the basis for many training workshops throughout the UK and in the published RCTs.[84–86,94,96] The ends of the external anal sphincter are grasped using appropriate forceps. If injury to the anal mucosa or IAS is identified, it should be repaired before the EAS. The anal epithelium is repaired with interrupted 3/0 polyglactin, with knots lying within the anal canal. The IAS is repaired with interrupted 3/0 polydioxanone (PDS).

The overlap technique

The torn ends of the EAS should be mobilised free. For an overlap repair, approximately 2 cm of one end of the EAS should be laid over the other end in a 'double-breasted jacket' fashion (Fig. 3).[94]

The end-to-end repair

The edges of the torn sphincter are identified and repaired in apposition with three or four interrupted mattress sutures (Fig. 4).[94] The vaginal mucosa and perineal muscles should then be repaired using an absorbable material such as vicryl 2/0 in a continuous, non-locking fashion. Finally, the perineal skin is closed with subcuticular using the same suture material.

Which suture material?

There are important differences in suture materials which may affect the outcome of sphincter repair. Monofilament materials such as polydioxanone (PDS) or polypropylene (Prolene) have previously been recommended for sphincter repair as they are less likely to harbor micro-organisms compared with modern braided sutures such as polyglactin (Vicryl).[97] However, Prolene is a non-absorbable suture and shown to be associated with an increased risk of suture sinuses and a 30% suture migration rate in one study.[98]

PDS or Vicryl (polyglactin) are both recommended for sphincter repair. Both suture types are absorbable, with complete absorption in 180 days and 70 days, respectively. Suture materials have only been assessed in one RCT.[84] Braided polyglactin (coated Vicryl 2/0) and monofilament polydioxanone (PDS 3/0) were compared; with no differences found across the two groups in terms of anal incontinence, perineal pain or suture migration at 12 months' follow-up.

The external anal sphincter (EAS)

As described, there are two recognized methods of repairing torn EAS – end-to-end (approximation) method and overlap technique. Traditionally, primary anal sphincter repair involved end-to-end repair of the torn ends of the external anal sphincter. Since the publication of a retrospective study suggested improved outcome using an overlap technique,[94] four RCTs have been completed.[84–86,96]

In each RCT, women were randomised to end-to-end approximation or overlap repair of the EAS. The number of recruited patients varied (range, 41–112) with one study underpowered.[96] Patient follow-up assessed anal continence scores and quality of life, together with a mixed combination of ultrasound and anal manometry findings. The duration of follow-up varied at 3 months[86,96] or 12 months.[84,85]

There were also differences in the degree of sphincter injury in women recruited across the RCTs. Three studies[84,86,96] included all EAS injuries (3A–C) whereas one study[85] only recruited women with disruption greater than 50% (3B and 3C). In this study, patients with 3B tears had the remaining EAS fibers divided to perform an overlap technique. This contrasts with the other studies where overlap was undertaken without division of EAS fibers.

No significant difference was found between the groups in terms of fecal incontinence rates in three of the RCTs.[84,86,96] In one RCT, an improvement in outcome was seen with overlap repair.[85] In addition to the difference in approach to the overlap technique in 3B tears in this study, there was a potential difference in the experience of the clinician undertaking the repair. In contrast to the other studies, sphincter injuries were repaired by three trained clinicians rather one of a larger number of trained clinicians as in the other studies. As such, the benefit of an overlap repair shown in this RCT may not be applicable across other obstetric units.

The internal anal sphincter (IAS)

The original description of the overlap technique includes separate repair of the internal anal sphincter.[94] The IAS has a role in maintaining continence[99] and studies have shown increased anal incontinence in women with both IAS and EAS injury compared with EAS injury alone.[43] It is recognized that identification of the IAS is not always possible in clinical practice; indeed, it was not identified separately from the EAS in all of the RCTs.[84] Whether the IAS should be repaired separately from the EAS is not clear from current evidence but, if identified, it would seem advisable to repair it separately.

WHO SHOULD UNDERTAKE SPHINCTER REPAIR?

Traditionally, anal sphincter injury repair was carried out at the time of injury by trainee obstetricians. It is recognized that inexperienced attempts at anal sphincter repair can contribute to maternal morbidity. As a result, in some units repair would be delayed and repair was undertaken by colorectal surgeons, experienced in secondary sphincter repair.

Deficiencies in the training of both obstetricians and their trainees in the repair of sphincter injury has been highlighted.[100] As a result, many workshops are now available throughout the UK. Attendance at a hands-on training workshop has been shown to increase both awareness of perineal anatomy and recognition of anal sphincter injury.[101]

The RCOG recommends that sphincter repair is performed by appropriately trained obstetricians but do not define what training should involve. There are differences in experience of operators in the RCTs of third degree tear repair. In three of the four published RCTs, large numbers of clinicians were trained in workshops to perform the repairs.[84,86,96] In contrast, another study used three senior operators who undertook the repairs.[85] There is no sub-analysis in these RCTs to assess the effect of operator experience on outcome. Available evidence supports the view of the RCOG that repair by an appropriately trained obstetrician is likely to provide consistent, high-standard repair with better patient outcomes.

OUTCOME OF PRIMARY ANAL SPHINCTER INJURY REPAIR

Endo-anal ultrasound (EAUS) and neurophysiological tests, together with patient symptoms of anal incontinence, have been used to assess the outcome of primary anal sphincter repair. The development of incontinence does not appear to be directly related to neuropathy as shown by EMG and PNTML. Poor outcome instead appears to be related to a persistent sphincter defect as detected on EAUS.[28,36,102]

Primary anal sphincter repair has traditionally been undertaken by trainee obstetricians using an end-to-end approximation of the torn ends of the external anal sphincter. Many prospective and retrospective studies have assessed the outcome in these women, with anal incontinence reported in about 40%.[36,38] Persistent sphincter defects have been reported on EAUS in 54–88%.[2,36,38] The incidence of symptoms are much higher when fecal urgency,[2] anal discomfort, dyspareunia and anal incontinence during sexual intercourse are considered.[38]

A retrospective study by Sultan *et al.*,[103] in 1999, suggested improved outcomes using an overlap technique. The RCTs comparing end-to-end approximation with overlap repair which resulted from this study form the evidence base for primary sphincter repair.[84–86,96] The RCT evidence has shown that 60–80% of women will be asymptomatic at 12 months following primary repair of obstetric anal sphincter injury. Lower rates of persistent defects have also been shown, occurring in 19–36% of women.[84–86,96]

Based on the evidence from the four RCTs published, patients who have an anal sphincter tear repaired using either the end-to-end or overlap technique with a similar intra- and postoperative protocols as described above can be counseled that the outcome of primary repair is likely to be good and the most common symptom experienced is incontinence to flatus.

FOLLOW-UP AFTER OBSTETRIC ANAL SPHINCTER INJURY

Women should be followed up at 6 weeks' postpartum, ideally by a consultant with an interest in anorectal injuries.[87] The delivery details and the anal sphincter injury should be discussed. Direct and specific questioning about symptoms of fecal incontinence, particularly fecal urgency and associated symptoms of dyspareunia and perineal pain, should be made. The use of a validated fecal incontinence questionnaire may be helpful and can be posted to the patient in advance of the appointment.

It is important that women are warned of the possible sequelae of anal sphincter injury. They may not be symptomatic at the time of review but should be advised on how to obtain advice if symptoms develop at a later date. Undertaking EAUS and manometry, where available, will help with the counseling about mode of delivery in future pregnancy.

Symptomatic women should be sent to a specialist center or to a colorectal surgeon. Further management of fecal incontinence symptoms will depend on the results of EAUS and manometry. Symptomatic women with the sphincter defect may be offered a secondary sphincter repair. Any future delivery would be by cesarean section. In women without a sphincter defect or with milder symptoms, benefit has been shown by dietary manipulation to regulate bowel function and advice on avoiding gas-producing foods. Diarrhea or incontinence of loose stool is the common distressing symptom. Medications can firm the stool, *e.g.* constipating agents (such as loperamide or codeine phosphate) or bulking agents.

Many clinicians advocate the involvement of a physiotherapist to teach pelvic floor exercises (PFEs) in the postpartum management of women with anal sphincter injury. The evidence for PFE following anal sphincter injury is sparse. One study reported lower anal incontinence rates at 1 year in women taught PFE by a physiotherapist following third degree tear but lacked a control group.[104]

FUTURE PREGNANCY AND MODE OF DELIVERY

A plan for the management of subsequent pregnancies and the mode of delivery should be part of the follow-up for women sustaining anal sphincter injury. There are no Cochrane reviews or RCTs to suggest the best method of delivery following obstetric anal sphincter injury and, as such, opinions differ between clinicians.

There is limited data regarding the likelihood of sphincter injury if vaginal delivery occurs in a subsequent pregnancy. Attempts to develop an antenatal risk scoring system for sphincter injury have so far been unsuccessful.[68] Studies assessing vaginal delivery following third degree tear have shown worsening fecal incontinence symptoms in 17–24% of women.[20,36,72,105] This is particularly true of women who had transient incontinence after the index delivery.[105]

Review of all women with a previous anal sphincter injury by a senior clinician at booking is essential. The detail of the previous sphincter injury and the follow-up is important to help in planning the mode of delivery. An assessment of symptoms of anal incontinence, namely fecal urgency, incontinence of feces (solid or liquid) and incontinence of flatus should be made. When obtaining a history, it is important to remember that patients with transient incontinence following third degree tear are more likely to have worsening fecal incontinence symptoms.[105] Routine use of one of the validated fecal incontinence questionnaires is useful.

The RCOG guidelines recommend that all women who have sustained an anal sphincter injury in a previous pregnancy should be counseled regarding the risk of developing anal incontinence or worsening symptoms with subsequent vaginal delivery. Women who are symptomatic or who have abnormal endo-anal ultrasound or manometry, should be offered the option of elective cesarean section.[106]. If asymptomatic, there is no clear evidence as to the best mode of delivery.

The patient's own experience of labor or other obstetric-related factors may influence the preference about the mode of delivery. Patients who have had a difficult or traumatic delivery may request elective cesarean section.[107]

CONCLUSIONS

Obstetric anal sphincter injury is the leading cause of fecal incontinence in women. These injuries may be clinically recognized as a third or fourth degree tear or occult, diagnosed using ultrasound. Repair of injuries recognised at delivery by an experienced operator, using a standard protocol and either end-to-end or overlap techniques of the external sphincter has been proven to improve greatly the outcome for women by reducing symptoms of fecal incontinence and the persistence of sphincter defects seen on follow-up ultrasound.

KEY POINTS FOR CLINICAL PRACTICE

- Obstetric anal sphincter injury is the leading cause of fecal incontinence in women.
- Symptoms of fecal incontinence may be delayed for many years.

Repair of sphincter injury

- Trained operators should undertake repair in theatre using a standard intra-operative and postoperative protocol.
- Broad-spectrum intra-operative and postoperative antibiotics are recommended to avoid the risk of infection and wound dehiscence.
- Evidence from randomised controlled trials suggests outcome of overlap and end-to-end techniques for repairing the external anal sphincter are equivalent. Where possible, the internal anal sphincter should be repaired separately from the external anal sphincter.
- There is no difference in the outcome between monofilament sutures (polydioxanone) and braided sutures (such as Vicryl) for sphincter repair.
- Stool softeners and a bulking agent are advised for 10 days following repair.

KEY POINTS FOR CLINICAL PRACTICE *(continued)*

Follow-up and future delivery

- Women should be counseled about the future risk of fecal incontinence.
- Review should occur at 6 weeks following delivery. Endo-anal ultrasonography and manometry should occur where available.
- Symptomatic women should be referred to a colorectal surgeon.
- Women should be reviewed early in future pregnancies. Symptomatic women or those with abnormal endo-anal ultrasonography or neurophysiology tests should be offered delivery by cesarean section.
- There is no evidence to guide the management of asymptomatic women.

References

1 Zetterstrom J, Mellgren A, Jenson LL. Effect of delivery on anal sphincter morphology and function. Dis Colon Rectum 1999; 42: 1253–1260

2 Sultan AH, Kamm MA, Hudson CN, Bartram CI. Third degree obstetric anal sphincter tears: risk factors and outcome of primary repair. BMJ 1994; 308: 887–891

3 Walsh CJ, Mooney EF, Upton GJ, Motson RW. Incidence of third-degree perineal tears in labour and outcome after primary repair. Br J Surg 1996; 83: 218–221

4 Fenner DE, Genberg B, Brahma P, Marek L, DeLancey JOL. Fecal and urinary incontinence after vaginal delivery with anal sphincter disruption in an obstetrics unit in the United States. Am J Obstet Gynecol 2003; 189: 1543–1549

5 Andrews V, Thakar R, Sultan AH. Occult anal sphincter injuries: myth or reality? Br J Obstet Gynaecol 2006; 113: 195–200

6 Sultan AH, Kamm MA, Hudson CN, Thomas JM, Bartram CI. Anal-sphincter disruption during vaginal delivery. N Engl J Med 1993; 329: 1905–1911

7 Sultan AH, Kamm MA, Hudson CN, Nicholls JR, Bartram CI. Endosonography of the anal sphincters: normal anatomy and comparison with manometry. Clin Radiol 1994; 49: 368–374

8 Bollard RC, Gardiner A, Lindow S, Phillips K, Duthie GS. Normal female anal sphincter. Dis Colon Rectum 2002; 45: 171–175

9 Sultan AH, Nicholls RJ, Kamm MA, Hudson CN, Beynon J, Bartram CI. Anal endosonography and correlation with *in vitro* and *in vivo* anatomy. Br J Surg 1993; 80: 508–511

10 Sultan AH, Kamm MA, Talbot IC, Nicholls RJ, Bartram CI. Anal endosonography for identifying external sphincter defects confirmed histologically. Br J Surg 1994; 81: 463–465

11 Law PJ, Kamm MA, Bartram CI. A comparison between electromyography and anal endosonography in mapping external anal sphincter defects. Dis Colon Rectum 1990; 33: 370–373

12 Law PJ, Kamm MA, Bartram CI. Anal endosonography in the investigation of faecal incontinence. Br J Surg 1991; 78: 312–314

13 Gibbons CP, Bannister JJ, Trowbridge EA, Read NW. An analysis of anal sphincter pressure and anal compliance in normal subjects. Int J Colorect Dis 1986; 1: 231–237

14 Duthie HL, Gairns FW. Sensory nerve-endings and sensation in the anal region of man. Br J Surg 1960; 47: 585–595

15 Gaston EA. The physiology of fecal incontinence. Surg Gynecol Obstet 1948; 87: 280–290

16 Miller R, Bartolo DC, Cervero F, Mortensen NJ. Anorectal sampling: a comparison of normal and incontinent patients. Br J Surg 1988; 75: 44–47

17 Neill ME, Swash M. Increased motor unit fibre density in the external anal sphincter muscle in ano-rectal incontinence: a single fibre EMG study. J Neurol Neurosurg Psychiatry 1980; 43: 343–347
18 Kiff ES, Swash M. Slowed conduction in the pudendal nerves in idiopathic (neurogenic) faecal incontinence. Br J Surg 1984; 71: 614–616
19 Crawford L, Quint E, Pearl M, DeLancey J. Incontinence following rupture of the anal sphincter during delivery. Obstet Gynecol 1993; 82: 527–531
20 Tetzschner T, Sorensen M, Lose G, Christiansen J. Anal and urinary incontinence in women with obstetric anal sphincter rupture. Br J Obstet Gynaecol 1996; 103: 1034–1040
21 Nazir M, Stein R, Carlsen E, Jacobsen AF, Nesheim B. Early evaluation of bowel symptoms after primary repair of perineal rupture is misleading – an observational cohort study. Dis Colon Rectum 2003; 46: 1245–1250
22 Haadem K, Dahlstrom JA, Ling L, Ohrlander S. Anal sphincter function after delivery rupture. Obstet Gynecol 1987; 70: 53–56
23 Walsh CJ, Mooney EF, Upton GJ, Motson RW. Incidence of 3 degree perineal tears in labour and outcome after primary repair. Br J Surg 1996; 83: 218–221
24 Snooks SJ, Swash M, Mathers SE, Henry MM. Effect of vaginal delivery on the pelvic floor: a 5-year follow-up. Br J Surg 1990; 77: 1358–1360
25 Allen RE, Hosker GL, Smith AR, Warrell DW. Pelvic floor damage and childbirth: a neurophysiological study. Br J Obstet Gynaecol 1990; 97: 770–779
26 Lubowski DZ, Jones PN, Swash M, Henry MM. Asymmetrical pudendal nerve damage in pelvic floor disorders. Int J Colorect Dis 1988; 3: 158–160
27 Small KA, Wynne JM. Evaluating the pelvic floor in obstetric patients. Aust NZ J Obstet Gynaecol 1990; 30: 41–45
28 Chaliha C, Sultan AH, Bland JM, Monga AK, Stanton SL. Anal function: effect of pregnancy and delivery. Am J Obstet Gynecol 2001; 185: 427–432
29 Cornes H, Bartolo DCC, Stirrat GM. Changes in anal sensation after childbirth. Br J Surg 1991; 78: 74–77
30 McHugh SM, Diamant NE. Effect of age, gender and parity on anal canal pressures. Contribution of impaired anal sphincter function to fecal incontinence. Dig Dis Sci 1987; 32: 726–736
31 Haadem K, Dahlstrom JA, Ling L. Anal sphincter competence in healthy women: clinical implications of age and other factors. Obstet Gynecol 1991; 78: 823–827
32 Haadem K. Estrogen receptors in the external anal sphincter. Am J Obstet Gynecol 1991; 164: 609–610
33 Buekens P, Lagasse R, Dramaix M, Wollast E. Episiotomy and third degree tears. Br J Obstet Gynaecol 1985; 92: 820–823
34 Anthony S, Buitendijk SE, Zondervan KT, van Rijssel EJC, Verkerk PH. Episiotomies and the occurrence of severe perineal lacerations. Br J Obstet Gynaecol 1994; 101: 1064–1067
35 Poen AC, Felt-Bersma RJF, Dekker GA, Deville W, Cuesta MA, Meuwissen SGM. Third degree obstetric perineal tears risk factors and the preventative role of mediolateral episiotomy. Br J Obstet Gynaecol 1999; 104: 563–566
36 Poen AC, Felt-Bersma RJF, Strijers RLM, Dekker GA, Cuesta MA, Meuwissen SGM. Third degree obstetric perineal tear: long-term clinical and functional results after primary repair. Br J Surg 1998; 85: 1433–1438
37 Donnelly V, Fynes M, Campbell D, Johnson H, O'Connell R, O'Herlihy C. Obstetric events leading to anal sphincter damage. Obstet Gynecol 1998; 92: 955–961
38 Gjessing H, Backe B, Sahlin Y. Third degree obstetric tears: outcome after primary repair. Acta Obstet Gynaecol Scand 1998; 77: 736–740
39 Wood J, Amos L, Rieger N. Third degree anal sphincter tears: risk factors and outcome. Aust NZ J Obstet Gynaecol 1998; 38: 417
40 Samuelsson E, Ladfors L, Wennerholm UB, Gareberg B, Nyberg K, Hagberg H. Anal sphincter tears: prospective study of obstetric risk factors. Br J Obstet Gynaecol 2000; 107: 926–931
41 Eason E, Labercque M, Wells G, Feldman P. Preventing perineal trauma during childbirth: a systematic review. Obstet Gynecol 2000; 95: 464–471

42 Janders C, Lyrenas S. Third and fourth degree perineal tears – predictor factors in a referral hospital. Acta Obstet Gynaecol Scand 2001; 80: 229–234
43 de Leeuw JW, Sruijk PC, Vierhout ME, Wallenburg HCS. Risk factors for third degree perineal ruptures during delivery. Br J Obstet Gynaecol 2001; 108: 383–387
44 Fitzpatrick M, McQuillan K, O'Herlley C. Influence of persistent occipito-posterior position on delivery outcome. Obstet Gynecol 2001; 98: 1027–1031
45 Bodner-Adler B, Bodner K, Kaider A *et al.* Risk factors for third degree perineal tears in a vaginal delivery with an analysis of episiotomy types. J Reprod Med 2001; 46: 752–756
46 Richter HE, Brumfield CG, Cliver SP *et al.* Risk factors associated with anal sphincter tear: a comparison of primiparous vaginal births after cesarean deliveries, and patients with previous vaginal delivery. Am J Obstet Gynecol 2002; 187: 1194–1198
47 Christiansen LM, Bovbjerg VE, McDavitt EC, Hullfish KL. Risk factors for perineal injury during delivery. Am J Obstet Gynecol 2003; 189: 255–260
48 Adams EJ, Bricker L, Richmond DH, Neilson JP. Systematic review of third degree tears: risk factors. Int Urogynecol J Pelvic Floor Dysfunct 2001; 71 (Suppl 3): 12
49 Zetterstrom JP, Lopez A, Anzen B, Dolk A, Norman M, Mellgren A. Anal incontinence after vaginal delivery: a prospective study in primiparous women. Br J Obstet Gynaecol 1999; 106: 324–330
50 Macarthur C, Glazener CM, Wilson PD, Herbison GP, Gee H, Lang G. Obstetric practice and faecal incontinence three months after delivery. Br J Obstet Gynaecol 2001; 108: 678—683
51 Faltin DL, Sangalli MR, Roche B, Floris L, Boulvain M, Weil A. Does a second delivery increase the risk of anal incontinence? Int J Gynaecol Obstet 2001; 108: 684–688
52 Moller BK, Laurberg S. Intervention during labour: risk factors associated with complete tear of the anal sphincter. Acta Obstet Gynaecol Scand 1992; 71: 520–524
53 Buchhave P, Flatow L, Rydhstroem H, Thorbert G. Risk factors for rupture of the anal sphincter. Eur J Obstet Gynecol Reprod Biol 1999; 87: 129–132
54 Coats P, Chan K, Wilkins M. A comparison between midline and mediolateral episiotomies. Br J Obstet Gynaecol 1980; 87: 408–413
55 Signorello LB, Harlow BL, Chekos AK, Repke JT. Midline episiotomy and anal incontinence: retrospective cohort study. BMJ 2000; 320: 86–90
56 Tincello DG, Williams A, Fowler GE, Adams EJ, Richmond DH, Alfirevic Z. Differences in episiotomy technique between midwives and doctors. Br J Obstet Gynaecol 2003; 110: 1041–1044
57 Andrew V, Thakar R, Sultan AH, Jones PW. Are mediolateral episiotomies actually mediolateral? Br J Obstet Gynaecol 2005; 112: 1156
58 Donnelly V, Fynes M, Campbell D, Johnson H, O'Herlihy C. Obstetric events leading to anal sphincter damage. Obstet Gynecol 1998; 92: 955–961
59 Varma A, Gunn J, Gardiner A, Lindow SW, Duthie GS. Obstetric anal sphincter injury. Prospective evaluation of incidence. Dis Colon Rectum 1999; 42: 1537–1543
60 Sultan AH, Johanson RB, Carter JE. Occult anal sphincter trauma following randomised forceps and vacuum delivery. Int J Gynaecol Obstet 1998; 61: 113–119
61 Johanson RB, Menon V. Vacuum extraction versus forceps for assisted vaginal delivery. The Cochrane Library, Issue 2, 2004
62 Royal College of Obstetricians and Gynaecologists. Operative vaginal delivery. Guideline No. 26. London: RCOG, 2005
63 Snooks SJ, Swash M, Setchell M, Henry MM. Injury to innervation of pelvic floor sphincter musculature in childbirth. Lancet 1984; ii: 546–550
64 Bannister JJ, Gibbons CP, Read NW. Preservation of faecal continence during rises in intra-abdominal pressure: is there a role for the flap valve? Gut 1987; 28: 1242–1245
65 Snooks SJ, Swash M, Henry MM. Abnormalities in central and peripheral nerve conduction in patients with anorectal incontinence. J R Soc Med 1985; 78: 294–300
66 Snooks SJ, Swash M, Henry MM. Fecal incontinence due to external sphincter division in childbirth is associated with damage to the innervation of the pelvic floor musculature: a double pathology. Br J Obstet Gynaecol 1985; 92: 824–828
67 Kamm MA. Obstetric damage and faecal incontinence. Lancet 1994; 344: 730–733
68 Williams A, Tincello DG, White S, Adams EJ, Alfirevic Z, Richmond DH. Risk scoring

system for prediction of obstetric anal sphincter injury. Br J Obstet Gynaecol 2005; 112: 1066–1069

69 Al-Mufti R, McCarthy A, Fisk NM. Obstetricians' personal choice and mode of delivery. Lancet 1996; 347: 544

70 National Institute for Health and Clinical Excellence. Caesarean section: understanding NICE guidance – information for pregnant women, their partners and the public. London: NICE, 2004

71 MacArthur C, Bick DE, Keighley MRB. Faecal incontinence after childbirth. Br J Obstet Gynaecol 1997; 104: 46–50

72 Fynes M, Donnelly V, O'Connell R, O'Herlihy C. Cesarean delivery and anal sphincter injury. Obstet Gynecol 1998; 92: 496–500

73 Glazener CM, Abdall M, Stroud P, Naji S, Templeton A, Russell IT. Postnatal maternal morbidity: extent, causes, prevention and treatment. Br J Obstet Gynaecol 1995; 102: 282–287

74 MacArthur C, Bick DE, Keighley MR. Faecal incontinence after childbirth. Br J Obstet Gynaecol 1997; 104: 46–50

75 Chaliha C, Kalia V, Stanton SL, Monga A, Sultan AH. Antenatal prediction of postpartum urinary and faecal incontinence. Obstet Gynecol 1999; 94: 689–694

76 Fernando RJ, Sultan AH, Radley S, Jones PW, Johanson RB. Management of obstetric anal sphincter injury: a systematic review and national practice survey. BMC Health Serv Res 2002; 2: 9

77 Glazener CMA. Sexual function after childbirth: women's experiences, persistent morbidity and lack of professional recognition. Br J Obstet Gynaecol 1997; 104: 330–335

78 Glazener CMA, Lang G, Wilson PD, Herbison GP, Macarthur C, Gee H. Postnatal incontinence: a multicentre randomised controlled trial of conservative management. Br J Obstet Gynaecol 1998; 105: 47–50

79 MacArthur C, Lewis M, Knox EG. Health after childbirth: an investigation of long term health problems beginning after childbirth in 11701 women. London, The Stationary Office, 1991; 83–103

80 Haadem K, Ohrlander S, Lingham G. Long-term ailments due to anal sphincter rupture caused by delivery- a hidden problem. Eur J Obstet Gynecol Reprod Biol 1988; 27: 27–32

81 Leigh RJ, Turnberg LA. Faecal incontinence: the unvoiced symptom. Lancet 1982; 1: 1349–1351

82 Giebel GD, Mennigen R, Chalabi KH. Secondary anal reconstruction after obstetric injury. Coloproctology 1993; 1: 55–58

83 Venkatesh KS, Ramanujam PS, Larson DM, Haywood MA. Anorectal complications of vaginal delivery. Dis Colon Rectum 1989; 32: 1039–1041

84 Williams A, Adams EJ, Tincello DG, Alfirevic Z, Walkinshaw SA, Richmond DH. How to repair an anal sphincter injury after vaginal delivery: results of a randomised controlled trial. Br J Obstet Gynaecol 2006; 113: 201–207

85 Fernando RJ, Sultan AH, Kettle C, Radley S, Jones PW, O'Brien PMS. Repair techniques for obstetric anal sphincter injuries. A randomised controlled trial. Obstet Gynecol 2006; 107: 1261–1268

86 Fitzpatrick M, Behan M, O'Connell R, O'Herlihy C. A randomised clinical trial comparing primary overlap with approximation repair of third degree tears. Am J Obstet Gynecol 2000; 183: 1220–1224

87 Royal College of Obstetricians and Gynaecologists. Management of third and fourth degree perineal tears following vaginal delivery. RCOG Guideline No. 29. London: RCOG, 2001

88 Faltin DL, Boulvain M, Irion O, Bretones S, Stan C, Weil A. Diagnosis of anal sphincter tears by postpartum endosonography to predict fecal incontinence. Obstet Gynecol 2000; 95: 643–647

89 Faltin DL, Boulvain M, Floris AL, Irion O. Diagnosis of anal sphincter tears to prevent fecal incontinence. Obstet Gynecol 2005; 106: 6–13

90 Groom KM, Patterson-Brown S. Can we improve on the diagnosis of third degree tears? Eur J Obstet Gynecol Reprod Biol 2002; 101: 19–21

91 Norton C, Christiansen J, Butler U *et al*. Anal incontinence. In: Abrams P, Cardozo L,

Khoury, Wein A. (eds) Incontinence. Plymouth: Health Publication, 2002; 985–1044
92 Royal College of Obstetricians and Gynaecologists. Management of third and fourth degree perineal tears. RCOG Guideline No. 29. London: RCOG, 2007
93 Fernando RJ, Sultan AH, Kettle C, Thakar R, Radley S. Methods of repair for obstetric anal sphincter injury. Cochrane Database of Systematic Reviews 2006; Art No. CD002866
94 Sultan AH, Monga A, Kumar D, Stanton SL. Primary repair of obstetric anal sphincter rupture using the overlap technique. Br J Obstet Gynaecol 1999; 106: 318–323
95 Mahony R, Behan M, O'Herlihy C, O'Connell R. Randomised clinical trial of bowel confinement vs. laxative use after primary repair of a third degree obstetric anal sphincter tear. Dis Colon Rectum 2004; 47: 12–17
96 Garcia V, Rodgers RG, Kim SS, Hall RJ, Kammerer-Doak DN. Primary repair of obstetric anal sphincter laceration: a randomised trial of two surgical techniques. Am J Obstet Gynecol 2005; 192: 1697–1701
97 Katz S, Izhar M, Mirelman D. Bacterial adherence to surgical sutures. A possible factor in suture induce infection. Ann Surg 1981; 194: 35–41
98 Williams A, Adams EJ, Bolderson J, Tincello DG, Richmond DH. Effect of a new guideline on outcome following third-degree perineal tears: results of a 3-year audit. Int Urogynecol J Pelvic Floor Dysfunct 2003; 14: 385–389
99 Sangwan YP, Solla JA. Internal anal sphincter – advances and insights. Dis Colon Rectum 1998; 41: 1297–1311
100 Fernando RJ, Sultan AH, Radley S, Jones PW, Johanson RB. Management of obstetric anal sphincter injury – a systematic and national practice survey. BMC Health Service Res 2002; 2: 1–9
101 Thakar R, Sultan AH, Fernando RJ, Monga A, Stanton S. Can workshops on obstetric anal sphincter rupture change practice? Int Urogynecol J Pelvic Floor Dysfunct 2001; 12: 45–51
102 Nielsen MB, Hauge C, Rasmussen OO, Pedersen JF, Christiansen J. Anal endosonographic findings in the follow-up of primarily sutured sphincteric ruptures. Br J Surg 1992; 79: 104–106
103 Sultan AH, Monga A, Kumar D, Stanton SL. Primary repair of obstetric anal sphincter rupture using the overlap technique. Br J Obstet Gynaecol 1999; 106: 318–323
104 Sander P, Bjarnesen J, Mouitsen L, Fuglsang-Frederiksen A. Anal incontinence in women after third/fourth-degree laceration. One year follow-up after pelvic floor exercises. Int Urogynecol J Pelvic Floor Dysfunct 1997; 10: 177–181
105 Bek KM, Laurberg S. Risks of anal incontinence from subsequent vaginal delivery after a complete obstetric anal sphincter tear. Br J Obstet Gynaecol 1992; 99: 724–726
106 Sultan AH, Thakar R. Lower genital tract and anal sphincter trauma. Best Pract Res Clin Obstet Gynaecol 2002; 16: 99–115
107 Williams A, Lavender T, Richmond DH, Tincello DG. Women's experiences after a third degree obstetric anal sphincter tear: a qualitative study. Birth 2005; 32: 129–136

Marilyn Huang Brian M. Slomovitz
*Thomas A. Caputo Hugh Barber**

Cancer in pregnancy

Cancer-complicating pregnancy is uncommon, estimated at 1 in 1000–1500 live births.[1–3] Currently, cancer is the second leading cause of death in women of reproductive age but, fortunately, a rare cause of maternal mortality.[4] Given the present trend of women delaying childbearing to a later age, the frequency of cancer occurring in pregnancy is likely to increase. When cancer and pregnancy co-exist, the physician must answer difficult questions – questions that they themselves will ask, questions that the patient will ask, and questions the patient's family will ask. Boronow[2] has set up questions as follows:

1. *Does the pregnancy alter prognosis?*
2. *Will termination of the pregnancy be therapeutic?*
3. *May subsequent pregnancies be permitted?*
4. *Will castration be therapeutic?*
5. *Will the malignancy affect the fetus?*
6. *Will the therapy affect the fetus?*
7. *When should therapy be started?*
8. *If started, should therapy be suspended?*

Marilyn Huang MD
Department of Obstetrics and Gynecology, Division of Gynecologic Oncology, New York Presbyterian Hospital-Weill Medical College of Cornell University, 525 East 68th Street, New York, NY 10021, USA

Brian M. Slomovitz MD MS (for correspondence)
Assistant Professor, Department of Obstetrics and Gynecology, Division of Gynecologic Oncology, New York Presbyterian Hospital-Weill Medical College of Cornell University, 525 East 68th Street J-130 New York, NY 10021, USA. E-mail: brs9002@med.cornell.edu

Thomas A. Caputo MD
Professor of Obstetrics and Gynecology, Department of Obstetrics and Gynecology, Division of Gynecologic Oncology, New York Presbyterian Hospital-Weill Medical College of Cornell University, 525 East 68th Street, New York, NY 10021, USA

Hugh Barber MD *
[*Deceased] Emeritus Professor, Department of Obstetrics and Gynecology, Division of Gynecologic Oncology, New York Presbyterian Hospital-Weill Medical College of Cornell University, New York, USA

Major cancers in women include breast, gastrointestinal, and genital. However, when comparing cancer mortality by age group, the predominant causes among US women of reproductive age include leukemia, lymphomas, and brain and central nervous system tumors. Cancer breakdown by age group is as follows:

- under 15 years – leukemia, cancer of the brain and central nervous system, kidney, bone and connective tissue
- 15–34 years – leukemia, Hodgkin's disease and cancer of the breast, brain, central nervous system and uterus
- 35–54 years – cancer of the breast, bone, colon, rectum, uterus and ovary.

The majority of malignant diseases that are associated with pregnancy are breast cancers, lymphomas, malignant melanomas, and cervical cancers.[2,5] Cancer-complicating pregnancy is best divided into pelvic and extra-pelvic malignancy as follows:

1. **Gynecological** – vulva, vagina, cervix, uterus, fallopian tubes, ovaries and choriocarcinoma
2. **Extra-genital** – breast, melanoma, Hodgkin's lymphoma, non-Hodgkin's lymphomas, leukemia, thyroid, gastrointestinal tract, genito-urinary tract, and central nervous system.

Pelvic cancer occurring during pregnancy is most often treated by surgery.

BASIC PRINCIPLES

In the past decades, there has been an overall improvement in therapy for cancer. The impact of greater emphasis on cancer detection remains to be evaluated, although early reports indicate that the discovery of cancer in pregnancy has increased due to diligent screening programs. Shaping appropriate treatment of an individual is a combination of: indication for treatment, ethical issues, cultural and religious attitudes and, most importantly, the patient's wish to continue the pregnancy.

EPIDEMIOLOGY OF CANCER IN GENERAL

Approximately 1 in 4 women will develop cancer and 1 out of 7 will die of cancer. Pregnant women account for less than 0.8% of all cancers in women. Site-related incidences vary dramatically and reports suggest that coincident cancer in pregnancy occurs in fewer than 1 in 1000 pregnancies.[1,6] The incident rates for women are highest in breast, gastrointestinal, genital tract, and thyroid cancers. The leading mortality sites for women are lung, breast, gastrointestinal tract, and the ovaries. Dysplasia and carcinoma *in situ* occur at relatively comparable frequencies among like-populations, pregnant or not. In view of this and of the relatively high frequency of invasive cancers of the cervix in the reproductive years, it is somewhat curious that invasive cancer is found only once in approximately 3000 pregnancies. This inconsistency has not yet been clearly explained.

The criteria for eligibility in this series is that the patient must be pregnant and a diagnosis of malignancy must be made within 1 year of the pregnancy. An appreciable number of cases of cervical cancer associated with pregnancy were discovered during or within the last 4 months of the pregnancy. Similar observations have been made for other gynecological malignancies complicating pregnancy.[1,7,8] This emphasizes the importance of investigating excessive discharge and vaginal bleeding during pregnancy. There is an increasing body of evidence appearing in the current literature that favors primary surgery as the preferred method of treatment for gynecological cancer occurring during pregnancy. Radiation therapy has its optimum effect in highly oxygenated tissue that is undergoing rapid growth. As soon as the pregnancy is treated by radiation, involution results and creates an anoxic type of tissue, which is a poor setting to achieve good radiation effects.

GYNECOLOGICAL MALIGNANCY

Vulvar cancer

There are few cases of vulva-complicated pregnancies recorded in the literature exclusive of melanomas. It occurs at a surprisingly young age (average age is 29 years) and pregnancy does not have an adverse effect upon the malignancy. The prognosis depends on the stage and spread of the disease rather than on whether or not a pregnancy exists.[1] If detected during the first trimester, management is as if the pregnancy did not exist, and radical vulvectomy with or without bilateral lymph node dissection should be undertaken. In the second trimester, the planned procedure should take into account the size of the uterus. In the third trimester, if the lesion is small, it will not interfere with a vaginal delivery. Postpartum follow-up should include necessary procedures. In subsequent pregnancies following vulvectomy, cesarean section should be reserved for patients with excessive vulvovaginal scarring or obstetrical indications.

Following radical vulvectomy, vaginal delivery should be allowed if there is suitable care of the introitus and a timely episiotomy in order to avoid scar tissue from tearing. If there is a significant vaginal stenosis or fibrosis, cesarean section is advisable. If labor occurs before the wound is healed or there has been a degree of dehiscence, then elective cesarean section is advised. Pregnancy has no adverse effect on the prognosis and termination is not indicated in such patients.

Vaginal cancer[9–11]

Vaginal cancer is extremely rare, comprising less than 1% of all genital cancers. The ratio of cervical cancer to vaginal cancer is roughly 50:1. Often, it is difficult to tell if the tumor arises primarily in the vaginal epithelium or extends to it from a primary locus in the cervix. When both are involved, the cervix is considered the primary focus.

Lack of collected experience in managing vaginal cancer-complicating pregnancy makes it difficult to establish a plan for therapy. However, management in general should be similar to that for a patient that is not pregnant. If the fetus is viable, delivery by high vertical cesarean should be performed and therapy should be started as if the pregnant patient were not pregnant. If the fetus is not viable or near viable age, and the lesion looks small, treatment can be delayed until viability of the fetus is established. If it is deemed necessary to treat the lesion, external radiation therapy followed by intracavitary bachytherapy is the treatment of choice. The plan of treatment takes into consideration the location of the lesion. In cases where the patient does not spontaneously abort following external radiation, the uterus should be emptied prior to vaginal treatment. If the lesion is early (stage I) and located in the upper part of the vagina, it can be managed by radical hysterectomy, vaginectomy, and pelvic lymph node dissection.

Herbst *et al.*[9] reported on seven girls, 15–22 years of age, with adenocarcinoma of the vagina of the clear cell Mullerian type. Should adenocarcinoma be diagnosed during pregnancy in a DES exposed patient, management should be the same as in the non-pregnant state (*i.e.* radical hysterectomy, vaginectomy, and bilateral pelvic lymph node dissection with construction of a vagina). If the diagnosis is made at viability, a cesarean section should be carried out and then followed immediately by the treatment outlined above.

Cervical cancer[7,8,12]

In 2007, cervical cancer will be diagnosed in about 11,000 women with 3600 deaths.[13] The average incidence from large centers is 1 in 2500 pregnancies, whereas the incidence of carcinoma *in situ* during pregnancy is approximately 1 in 750. With increased screening programs and the wide-spread availability of PAP smears at antepartum clinics, an increase is anticipated in the incidence of carcinoma *in situ* and in the detection of invasive cancers at a very early stage.

Often, in pregnancy, the diagnosis is delayed. The youth of the patient and the accompanying pregnancy undoubtedly play a role in the reluctance on the part of the responsible physician to examine the patient at the first sign of abnormal bleeding. This emphasizes the importance of investigating excessive discharge and vaginal bleeding during pregnancy. Speculum examination is indicated in all pregnant women, particularly in those with symptoms, and even more so in those with any bleeding. The prognosis depends on the extent of the disease rather than on whether or not a pregnancy exists. Punch biopsy should be performed. If positive, no further biopsies are necessary. Cone biopsy is hazardous in the pregnant patient. Cone biopsy during pregnancy is dangerous because of the possible miscarriage, infection, or hemorrhage. Micro-invasion can be followed carefully during pregnancy; if there is no change on cytological examination, the management can be delayed until after delivery.

Women who are diagnosed with cervical cancer during the first 3 months of pregnancy often are advised to seek immediate treatment although it would require that the pregnancy be terminated. Although surgery is the preferred method of treatment for invasive cervical cancer in pregnancy, radiation therapy is an alternative for many physicians. The surgical treatment for invasive cancer of the cervix in pregnancy is as follows:[1]

1. First trimester and early second trimester – radical hysterectomy and pelvic lymph node dissection with the fetus in utero.

2. Later part of second trimester – wait for viability of the fetus and then perform a classical cesarean section followed immediately by radical hysterectomy and pelvic lymph node dissection.
3. Third trimester – classic cesarean section followed immediately by radical hysterectomy and pelvic lymph node dissection.
4. Postpartum – radical hysterectomy and pelvic lymph node dissection should be performed.

Radiation therapy of invasive cancer of the cervix and pregnancy is best managed as follows:

1. Non-viable fetus, first and second trimesters – treatment is given as if the pregnancy did not exist. External therapy is given to the pelvis. Spontaneous evacuation is preferred to intervention.
2. Viable fetus, late second and third trimester – cesarean section immediately followed by external therapy and brachytherapy.
3. Postpartum – radiation in the non-pregnant give external radiation therapy first followed by intravaginal and intra-uterine radiation.

Micro-invasive disease requires a careful assessment and perhaps a cone biopsy in order to exclude invasion. For patients who have a lesion < 1 cm in diameter and in whom invasion is < 3 mm, the cone biopsy may suffice temporarily as therapy, but will require re-evaluation after delivery. However, if there are multiple foci of invasion, or if there is involvement of vascular lymphatic spaces and penetration is > 3 mm, the patient must be treated as though she has invasive cancer of the cervix and the previously mentioned protocol for either surgery or radiation should be performed.

In the presence of untreated invasive cervical cancer, vaginal delivery is extremely dangerous. Hemorrhage, sepsis, and cervical laceration may result. Whether malignant cells are spread by vaginal delivery remains controversial. However, the complications that may arise give a strong impetus to carrying out a cesarean section in the presence of anything but a small invasive lesion.

If there is dysplasia or a small lesion by biopsy, there is no contra-indication for the patient to delivery vaginally and cesarean section is then only required for an obstetrical indication.

Ovarian cancer[1,2,5,14,15]

Cancer of the ovary accounts for approximately 5–6% of all cancers among women, and occurs in 1 in 18,000 pregnancies. It is estimated that 1 in 70 women will develop ovarian cancer during their life-time. In 2007, approximately 22,400 women will be diagnosed with ovarian cancer and another 15,200 will die from the disease.[13] The malignancy rate of ovarian tumors complicating pregnancy is 2–5% in contrast to an 18–20% malignancy rate in the non-gravid state. Although ovarian cancer ranks second in incidence among gynecological cancers, it causes more deaths than any other cancer of the female reproductive system. Signs and symptoms are essentially the same as in the non-pregnant state. Usually, an adnexal mass is found at the time of the first antepartum visit. If it regresses on follow-up, the diagnosis is that of a functional cyst (corpus luteum). Fortunately, most malignancies that occur during pregnancy are diagnosed at an early stage (stage I) mainly because most patients seek medical advice (antepartum visit) prior to the occurrence of symptoms related to the tumor. The survival rate, which is much the same as for the non-pregnant patient, is determined by the stage and type of tumor. If the tumor is diagnosed during the third trimester, surgery may be delayed until the fetus is viable. The patient must be counseled in detail as to her options before surgery is undertaken.

Common epithelial ovarian cancer is usually seen in women over the age of 40 years, but there is an increasing number seen in younger women as well. Germ cell tumors of the ovary are most commonly seen from birth to age 20 years. Gonadal stromal tumors are usually seen during the child-bearing years. Germ cell and gonadal stromal tumors are more often unilateral than are the common epithelial ovarian cancer. Thus, if the tumor is confined to the ovary, and the other ovary is negative, unilateral salpingo-oophrectomy may be an acceptable treatment during pregnancy.

Unilateral encapsulated freely-movable mass of uniform consistency that is < 20 cm can be kept under observation until the second trimester. Surgical intervention is indicated if a complication occurs. A hard, knobby mass of variegated consistency, bilaterality or signs of fluid are indications for surgical intervention despite the trimester of pregnancy. The presenting symptom may be a complication of the ovarian tumor such as torsion, hemorrhage, or infection. There may be sudden acute abdominal pain with vomiting and possibly shock.

While some advocate immediate attention to surgery despite trimester, clinical judgment determines the plan of management. The diagnostic work-up should include a PAP smear, a pelvic and rectovaginal examination, magnetic resonance imaging of the abdomen and pelvis, and a careful search for distant metastases. If there is widely metastatic disease, a decision on the management at this point is made by clinical judgment along with the wishes of the patient. The toll from cancer will only be lowered if an early diagnosis is made.

Management

- treat as in the non-pregnant state
- perform exploratory laparotomy
- aspirate fluid from the pelvis and the abdomen for cytological assessment
- if tumor is low grade, unilateral and encapsulated, a unilateral salpingo-oophrectomy is performed and the opposite ovary is biopsied. If negative, the treatment at this time is considered to be adequate and pregnancy is allowed to go to term
- if the tumor has extended beyond the ovary, aspiration for cytology, total hysterectomy, bilateral salpingo-oophorectomy, appendectomy, omentectomy, lymph node sampling should be performed. Later, if indicated, chemotherapy should be given
- if the pregnancy is allowed to continue, cesarean section is done only for obstetrical reasons.

Rectal cancer[15–18]

Rectal cancer, though not a gynecological cancer, is a pelvic cancer. The incidence of rectal cancer associated with pregnancy is extremely low, approximately 1 in 50,000 cases. In 2007, rectal cancer will occur in about 17,600 women.[13] Colon cancers are not generally influenced by pregnancy. Early diagnosis and the stage of disease are more important than prognosis and whether a pregnant or non-pregnant state prevails. The symptoms related to cancer may be overshadowed by those that pregnancy produces: nausea, vomiting, colicky abdominal pain, obstipation, constipation, diarrhea, rectal bleeding, and bloody mucus with tenesmis. These patients should be investigated thoroughly rather than assuming that it is simply due to the pregnancy. Lesions have been discovered during all trimesters with equal frequency, as well as during labor, and a few patients have had obviously predisposing factors such as ulcerative colitis, familial polyposis, Gardner's syndrome, or villous tumors. The prognosis for colon cancer during pregnancy has generally been very poor because of the delay in diagnosis.

Management

- first and early second trimester
  - ignore the pregnancy
  - the procedure of choice is either abdominal-perineal or anterior resection depending upon the position of the lesion.
- late second and third trimester
  - conservative management is followed until viability is established cesarean
  - section followed by an *en bloc* hysterectomy and low anterior resection with pelvic lymph node evaluation is considered an ideal treatment.
- during pregnancy, a clinical judgment must be exercised in evaluating the patient's desire for a child, the extent of the cancer, and treatment-related complications. Certain investigators feel that bilateral oophorectomy is indicated in the presence of colon cancer as prophylaxis in eliminating a major site for metastases.

EXTRA-PELVIC MALIGNANCY

Breast cancer[1,19,20]

Breast cancer is the most common cancer in women. One out of every eight women will develop breast cancer in her life-time. About 15% of breast cancers occur in women younger than 40 years; about 3% occur during pregnancy, complicating approximately 1 in over 3000 pregnancies. The incidence of breast cancer has been increasing by more than 1% per year for at least the last 10 years. A particularly steep rise has occurred in women under the age of 40 years. There is a familial incidence of breast cancer so the risk of developing the disease increases by 5–10 times if a first-degree relative has the disease. Breast cancer is the leading site of mortality from cancer in women aged 39–44 years. An estimated 178,480 women will be diagnosed with breast cancer and 40,400 will succumb in the US during 2007.[13] Additionally, breast cancer is the most common cancer to occur during pregnancy.

With more and more women delaying their first pregnancy until after the age of 35 years or more, the number of women that develop breast cancer during pregnancy increases. The dilemma for treatment is acute. Therapeutic abortion does not appear to improve the chances of a cure even though this potentially lethal disease is often considered hormone sensitive. The diagnosis is difficult as physiological changes continue throughout the pregnancy with alterations in vascularity, lymphatic permeation, and hormonal milieu.

The breast is difficult to examine clinically, particularly during pregnancy. Mammograms, which can be performed with little risk to the fetus, can appear negative despite the presence of cancer during pregnancy.[21] Ultrasonography can also be considered to assess a palpable mass or one detected on mammogram; however, it is not appropriate for documenting the extent of disease.[22] There is a higher incidence of positive nodes in pregnancy. The main diagnosis, rather than the pregnancy factor, plays the most important role. The survival is dependent on the stage of disease rather than if a pregnancy is present or not. Subsequent pregnancies are permissible after a 2-year interval following treatment. Breast feeding is a debatable topic. Most surgeons suggest that it should be discouraged. Lactation increases the prolactin secretions, which has a direct affect on the breast tissue.

Management

- treat as in the non-pregnant state – treatment is a radical mastectomy and axillary node dissection (or modified radical mastectomy)
- the role of lumpectomy in pregnancy has not been clarified and there is hesitation to do a lumpectomy because the follow-up treatment, radiation, is probably contra-indicated during pregnancy
- pregnancy is no longer considered a criterion for inoperability
- pregnancy should be discouraged for 3 years after completion of therapy; during this period, those patients with aggressive tumor or decreased host resistance will be eliminated
- no firm answer can be advanced in support of prophylactic oophorectomy; an argument may be made for oophorectomy in the presence of lymph node metastases
- inoperable cases – therapeutic abortion should be considered when it is a part of a planned program of estrogen ablation when uterus with its pregnancy, fallopian tubes, and ovaries are removed. Anti-estrogen therapy and/or chemotherapy should be at the discretion of the physician

* chemotherapy given during the first trimester may result in a marked increase in teratogenicity, but less likely in the second and third trimesters. Some studies indicate that chemotherapy during the second and third trimesters can be given with minimal complications to the pregnancy.[4]

Melanoma[3,24]

In the year 2000, there was an anticipated 20,400 cases of melanoma diagnosed in women, with approximately 2900 deaths. It is estimated that, in 2007, melanoma will be diagnosed in 26,000 women and be the cause of death for 2900 women.[13] Epidemiological studies suggest that there continues to be an increasing incidence of melanoma with an associated decrease in age at presentation for patients in the US. These trends suggest that approximately 35% of women will be diagnosed with melanoma during their child-bearing years.

Classification

1. The same precursor as in the non-pregnant patient.
2. Flat macular lesion.
3. Functional nevus.
4. Pregnancy accompanied by an increased pigmentation of breast, face, vulva, nipples, and so forth.

Melanomas or malignant melanomas are malignancies that generally originate from pre-existing pigmented moles. The malignancy is derived from the melanocyte, the cell involved with melanin pigment formation. The malignant cells usually maintain their function of pigment production. The melanocyte is embryologically derived from the neural crest cells and migrates to sites in the skin, eyes, central nervous system, and occasionally elsewhere during fetal development. The majority of melanomas arise *de novo* from melanocytes and perhaps one-third arise from nevi, many of which are congenital.

With peak incidence in the third and fourth decades of life, melanoma is concentrated among women in their reproductive years. There is controversy on the affect of pregnancy on melanoma. Although some authors advise termination of pregnancy, there seems to be a consensus of opinions in the literature that termination of pregnancy is not considered therapeutic.

Melanoma, it has been suggested, is either induced or exacerbated by pregnancy. The assumption is based on the following observation: melanocyte-stimulating hormone levels increase after the second month of pregnancy, which results in increased pigmentation. Metastatic spread would appear to be more rapid in pregnancy. However, stage for stage, there may be no significant difference in the prognosis for the patient. At puberty, obvious pigmentation occurs in moles, genitalia, and elsewhere. There is also increased pigmentation in pregnancy as evidenced in the nipple, areola, vulva, and linea nigra with occasional changes in pre-existing nevi and in cases of chloasma. MSH of the pituitary has been quantitative and only increases after the second month of pregnancy. Obviously, melanoma remains one of the most erratic malignancies with no conclusive evidence of either a beneficial or deleterious affect of pregnancy on its clinical course. There have been reports of women who had a pregnancy before the melanoma developed who survived longer than women without a previous pregnancy. The explanation suggests that exposure to fetal antigens might protect against the dissemination of melanoma cells that bear similar fetal antigen. However, these findings have not been confirmed by other authors.

Management

- treat as in non-pregnant state
- wide local excision with or without regional node dissection is necessary

- *en bloc* excision with regional lymph node dissection is the treatment of choice
- in order to ensure an adequate excision, the area of excision must be wide enough so that it can be handled by skin graft
- nevi on the feet, hands, and genitalia should be excised, particularly in the pregnant state
- termination of pregnancy is not considered therapeutic.

Thyroid cancer[15,25]

The incidence of thyroid cancer is low. Even though it most often occurs in young women, thyroid cancer is not a common cancer and firm conclusions regarding its relationship to pregnancy are difficult to make. The disease is characterized by a wide variety of pathological patterns that, on sub-division, display further variety. The disease has a markedly different mortality in the young. The young do well and have an overall 10-year survival rate without evidence of disease of about 79%. Reports indicate that thyroid cancer in pregnancy should not be permitted to co-exist. Some clinicians suggest the following:

- thyroid cancer is up to 4 times as frequent in women as it is in men
- TSH is elevated in pregnancy
- a certain percentage of thyroid malignancies are functional and, hence, theoretically, would be responsive to TSH
- the most common type, papillary, has the most favorable prognosis. The second most common, follicular, also has a favorable prognosis.

The prognosis for differentiated thyroid cancer is good; most have a long survival history. Papillary and follicular types account for two-thirds or more of thyroid malignancies. One large series of papillary tumors in young adults revealed 74% living without disease after 10 years. While women do have more thyroid cancer than men, the ratio of the more malignant variety is about even for both sexes. The undifferentiated tumors are highly malignant and usually rapidly fatal.

Management

- treat as in the non-pregnant state
- total thyroidectomy and unilateral or bilateral neck dissection is the treatment of choice
- give 180–240 mg of thyroid daily in an attempt to control TSH output.

Prognosis

- the prognosis is generally good; most patients have a long, natural history
- papillary cancer is the most common type with the most favorable prognosis

- follicular cancer is the second most common type and prognosis is also favorable
- papillary and follicular cancers comprise more than two-thirds of thyroid cancers
- abortion is not therapeutic.

Hodgkin's disease[15,26,27]

In 2007, Hodgkin's lymphoma is expected to account for 3720 new cases and 300 deaths.[13] Hodgkin's disease is the most common of the lymphoma group and constitutes about 40% of malignant lymphomas. It commonly affects young people and is now being cured and controlled with irradiation and chemotherapy. The disease is caused by neoplastic proliferation of lymphoreticular portions of the reticulo-endothelial system that involves lymph nodes, bone marrow, spleen, or liver. The majority of patients present with tumor in the lymph nodes. There have been many recent advances in the management of Hodgkin's disease.

The staging and comprehensive treatment are difficult to achieve during pregnancy without risk to the fetus. Evaluating the abdomen is the obvious handicap. The liver–spleen scan and staging laparotomy should be avoided during pregnancy. Lymphangiography presents a similar problem, but may be carried out followed by a single abdominal film 24 h after the injection of dye.

Hematological malignancies rarely complicate pregnancy. Pregnancy is not thought to affect the course of Hodgkin's lymphoma, non-Hodgkin's lymphoma, or leukemia. The prognosis worsens only if there is a delay in diagnosis or treatment. Both chemotherapy and radiation have been administered during pregnancy with favorable results. The fetus must be completely shielded from the radiation.

Most young women treated for Hodgkin's lymphoma wish to maintain a normal life-style, marry, and have children. Immunogenicity of radiation and chemotherapy with the possibility of long-term damage to gonadal tissue is well-recognized. However, little is known regarding the magnitude of risk of fetal mortality and fetal morbidity that may result from damaged maternal gonadal tissue.

In patients treated for Hodgkin's disease, if the disease remains active for 2 years after the start of treatment, the prognosis is poor. However, if the patient has remained free of disease for three or more years, the prognosis is good. Therefore, the patient should be told to wait for 3 years after treatment for Hodgkin's lymphoma before attempting pregnancy. This delay serves to identify those that do not respond or who have recurrence or poor immunity. When exacerbation occurs in association with pregnancy, the patient is most vulnerable during the postpartum period. There have been at least two documented cases of Hodgkin's disease in infants of mothers with Hodgkin's disease.

The surgical approach to Hodgkin's disease has changed radically in the last few years. The patient usually has an exploratory laparotomy, splenectomy, lymph node sampling, and often the ovaries are moved laterally out of the radiation field above the pelvic brim.

Management

- radiation therapy to involve nodal areas but shielding the pregnancy
- antibiotics as indicated
- supportive therapy – high caloric diet, rest, nursing care, and transfusions
- corticosteroids – prednisone, meticortem (20–100 mg/day) to be used in critically ill patients before instituting chemotherapy
- anti-inflammatory and potent analgesics as needed
- chemotherapy – best delayed until after the first trimester; higher incidence of fetal complications with combinations of drugs than with the application of a single drug.

Non-Hodgkin's lymphoma[2,26,28]

In 2007, non-Hodgkin's lymphoma will account for 28,990 new cases and 9060 deaths in the US.[13] This is a lymphoma comprised by a mixed family of diseases characterized by clonal neoplasms arising from one of the cellular constituents of the lymph node. Approximately 85% of non-Hodgkin's lymphoma are B-cell tumors, 15% are T-cell tumors, and a small percentage are from other cells, primarily macrophages. The diagnosis is usually made after biopsy of enlarged palpable nodes. Non-Hodgkin's lymphomas are cured in less than 25% of patients, although women of reproductive age have reports of 50% cure rates. The treatment is similar to that for Hodgkin's disease. Abortion is not considered therapeutic for either Hodgkin's or non-Hodgkin's lymphoma.

Leukemia[13,27,28]

There are about two cases of acute leukemia in every 75,000 deliveries. In 2007, there will be an estimated 19,440 new cases and 9740 deaths due to leukemia.[13] Of all leukemias, 41% are acute with an average patient age of 28 years. It has been estimated that, during pregnancy, most leukemias are acute – two-thirds are myeloid (AML) and one-third are lymphatic (ALL). Chronic myeloid leukemia (CML) occurs in less than 10% of leukemias in pregnancy. The survival time without treatment is approximately 2.5 months. Today, the remission rates are up to 90% in some medical centers. Chemotherapy is dramatically lengthening survival time, in some cases 10 years or more.

Postpartum hemorrhage occurs in less than 15% of cases. Hypofibrinogenemia occasionally occurs. Fetal maternal transmission of leukemia has been reported.

Management

- the same as in the non-pregnant patient
- corticosteroids – prednisone (20–100 mg/day) to be used in critically ill patients before instituting chemotherapy
- antibiotics as needed

- supportive – high caloric diet, rest, nursing care, and transfusions
- chemotherapy – should be avoided in the first trimester
- weekly CBC with differential
- cesarean section reserved only for obstetrical indications
- abortion is not therapeutic.

Acute leukemia can be treated in the second and third trimesters with little affect on the pregnancy or fetus. If the fetus is viable, an amniocentesis reveals fetal lung maturity, delivery should be expedited before definitive therapy is undertaken. In patients cured of acute leukemia, potential for subsequent pregnancy exists with little likelihood of increased fetal malformation. However, the long-term affects of chemotherapy on infants exposed *in utero* are not completely known.

Chronic leukemia[27,28]

Chronic leukemia is characterized in pregnancy by the following:

- low maternal and fetal mortality
- rare maternal hemorrhage
- pregnancy not being adversely affected and vice versa
- abortion is not therapeutic.

Management

- chemotherapy is the treatment of choice
- X-ray may be administered to involved nodes; the fetus must be shielded
- treatment is best withheld during the first trimester; it may result in abortion or malformation.

Myeloproliferative disease[27]

Myeloproliferative disease occurrence in pregnancy is unusual. Pregnancy has no adverse affect on the course of the mother's hematological disease. However, the myeloproliferative disease, especially if uncontrolled, results in increased fetal prematurity and mortality. The treatment of the pregnant patient should be conservative, and chemotherapy should be avoided until at least after the first trimester of pregnancy.

Gastrointestinal tract tumors[18,29]

There are a significant number of cases of stomach cancers associated with pregnancy in the literature. Fortunately, the incidence of stomach cancer has dropped dramatically in the US in the past 15 years. However, a high index of suspicion for making an early diagnosis in women with symptoms is the key to successful management of these patients.

Liver tumors have been reported as a result of contraceptive pill use. There are some cases that have complicated pregnancy. Management is surgery. Pregnancy is contra-indicated in the presence of an unresected liver adenoma or in one that has been partially resected.

Central nervous system tumors[1,14,15]

Tumors of the central nervous system that are most commonly adversely affected by pregnancy are pituitary adenomas, craniopharyngiomas, and meningiomas. Pituitary tumors may or may not be associated with endocrinopathy.

Pregnant women with malignant brain tumors are usually misdiagnosed or there is a delay in diagnosis because many of the early symptoms are identical to complaints encountered in normal pregnancy. Pregnancy is normally associated with an enlarged pituitary gland, many as a result of hyperplasia of the acetophilic cells concerned with prolactin secretion and existent pituitary tumors. The resulting symptoms include headache and visual disturbances, primarily increased visual disturbances and decreased visual acuity with diminished visual fields.

Early diagnosis offers the patient maximal chance of salvage from an otherwise fatal or disabling outcome. A high index of suspicion in patients with headache, visual disturbance, or other cerebral symptoms that do not improve should suggest a work-up. A diagnosis may be established by complete physical and neurological examination, CT scans, electroencephalography, by testing visual acuity and visual fields, and angiography, if indicated.

Meningiomas predominate in women and have been reported to enlarge rapidly with pregnancy. They have been found to have estrogen receptors and, thus, may be associated with hormone sensitivity. Meningiomas that are asymptomatic or do not enlarge can most likely be observed until viability of the fetus.

Treatment of malignant brain tumor during pregnancy is the same as in the non-pregnant patient. Surgical excision with or without radiation therapy is usually chosen. There is little information, if any, in the literature on the treatment of brain tumors with a gamma probe in pregnancy. Vaginal delivery is preferred, while cesarean section is reserved for obstetrical indications or when instantaneous delivery is necessary. The increase in intra-abdominal pressure associated with bearing down efforts in the second stage of labor markedly elevates cerebrospinal fluid pressure. This should be minimized by the use of outlet forceps. If the fetus has reached viability, delivery should be offered prior to surgical intervention or radiation therapy for the brain tumor.

Pituitary adenomas have received considerable attention in the literature. These are often microadenomas. During pregnancy, there is a physiological enlargement of the pituitary and an asymptomatic patient with a small pituitary tumor, even though not pregnant, may develop acute neurological symptoms during pregnancy. Therefore, the question arises of whether to treat the patients with known prior-to-pregnancy adenoma or not. Some patients became pregnant and it is only at that time that the tumor becomes apparent. Since it is not possible to predict which tumors may enlarge and cause symptoms during pregnancy, it is probably safer to treat all patients with a complicating pituitary tumor before pregnancy is attempted.

Pheochromocytomas[4,30]

These are extremely rare tumors but very dangerous during pregnancy with a 50% maternal and fetal mortality. Pheochromocytoma is a catecholamine-secreting tumor that consists of neuro-ectoderm or neural crest derived cells that affect 1 in 200,000 of the general population and is responsible for 0.1% of all cases of diastolic hypertension. The presentation of pheochromocytoma in pregnancy is rare, but well-described in more than 150 cases reported in the literature. The majority of these tumors occur sporadically. Approximately 5% are familial and they are usually bilateral. Alpha-blocker control with phenoxybenzamine is required and surgical removal is attempted only after localizing the tumor. It is preferable to do this in the postpartum period.

If a pheochromocytoma is diagnosed during early pregnancy, phenoxybenzamine should be started and therapeutic termination should be carried out. Additionally, attempts should be made to localize the tumor using the radiological techniques that have been associated with this diagnosis and then the tumor should be surgically removed. Should the diagnosis not be made until the second or third trimester, pregnancy should be allowed to continue under phenoxybenzamine control and with careful monitoring until induction or cesarean section is indicated. If progress is satisfactory, localizing investigations can be postponed until after the delivery.

Sarcoma[1]

Sarcoma-complicating pregnancy is very rare. The management of the pregnant patient with a sarcoma depends upon the type of lesion, anatomical location, stage of disease, and age of gestation. The question frequently asked is whether or not pregnancy will have an adverse affect on the growth of the sarcoma. A report on 57 patients who were pregnant simultaneously with or subsequent to the treatment to a variety of soft tissue tumors and found that there was no difference in the survival rate from the non-pregnant patients.

Several soft tissue tumors may be influenced by hormonal factors. These include angiosarcoma, cystosarcoma, sarcoma phylloides and, more specifically, giant intra-canicular myxoma that arise from fibroadenomas most frequently in women of multiparity and suppressed lactation. Desmoids frequently arise or occur during pregnancy. They should be treated with surgery as in the non-pregnant state.

FETAL AND PLACENTAL TRANSMISSION OF MALIGNANCY[1,31]

The fear of transmission of malignant disease to the fetus is always of concern to the patient and her family. Such a phenomenon is extremely rare and it is uncommon even to find metastases localized only to the placenta. In a study of at least 100 placentas of patients delivered of malignant disease, none had malignancy invading the placenta proper. In those cases in which the tumor cells were found, they were found outside of the villi. No clearly defined time period has been found to designate the occurrence of metastatic disease in the fetus and newborn. One year of age is selected as the limiting period.

Concern that the maternal cancer may metastasize to the fetus is not justified because an accumulated series is extremely rare. The infrequency of fetal involvement has led to the speculation about the biological protective mechanism that may exist for the placenta and the fetus and the role that may be played by circulatory separation in the placenta or immunological responses of the fetus. Despite the fact that the incidence is rare, routine gross and microscopic examination of the placenta of women who have had or have cancer is desirable as is careful examination of the infant, particularly if the maternal tumor was melanoma, leukemia, or lymphoma.

ANTI-NEOPLASTIC THERAPY AND RADIOTHERAPY[12,32]

Surgery and radiation are effective forms of treatment for localized cancer. Chemotherapy, the treatment of cancer by means of drugs and hormones, can be used for disseminated as well as localized tumors. The treatment of cancer with drugs is a relatively new development that dates from 1945 when nitrogen mustard was found to be effective in treating lymphomas. Since that time, many drugs have been added to the therapeutic armamentarium.

The major goal of current chemotherapy is to achieve cures by the prompt and vigorous treatment of these malignancies. Combinations of anti-neoplastic drugs have been used with success, particular when each drug acts on the cancer cell at a different part of the cycle. Progress has been made by using different drugs simultaneously as well as in sequence.

If employed only in the second and third trimester of pregnancy, single drug chemotherapy gives rise to few problems. Various problems may arise from use of anti-cancer drugs in the first trimester; however, the risk is small, but ever present, if a single drug is used. The physician must be cautious concerning the side effects of new agents, especially in combination, and particularly prior to completion of organogenesis.

The delayed consequences of chemotherapy remain controversial and it may be some time before enough data are accumulated to make a positive statement. In women who have had chemotherapy, the fetus and future pregnancies may be at risk. In approximately 100 pregnancies on follow-up in women who had chemotherapy, about 16% terminated in abortion and 3% in still-birth. Three of the pregnancies resulted in birth defects with significant general malformations.

Exposure of the developing embryo to ionizing radiation may cause abortion, malformation or possibly leukemia. Animal and atomic bomb studies clearly demonstrate the teratogenic and carcinogenic effect of radiation. Radiation injury sustained late in fetal life is less harmful than that sustained early when organogenesis and differentiation are more active. Some abortions are not a direct effect of radiation, but may be indirectly produced by hormonal imbalances initiated by therapeutic radiation of the mother. Fetal structures, particularly the central nervous system, the eye and the mesenchymal tissues appear to be more radiosensitive than the same structures in adults. This is probably on account of more rapid growth and greater metabolic activity of the fetus. It is strongly suggested that the pregnant woman not be exposed to any radiation during the first 16 weeks of pregnancy.

KEY POINTS FOR CLINICAL PRACTICE

- With assisted reproduction technology (*e.g.*, IVF) allowing women to reproduce at a later age, the incidence of cancer in pregnancy, particularly ovarian and breast cancer, is likely to rise.
- Cervical cancer is the most common gynecologic malignancy diagnosed during pregnancy. Women with microinvasive disease can be managed with uterine preserving treatment (*e.g.*, cervical conization).
- The patient, her family, the obstetrician and the oncologist must work together to best treat women who are diagnosed with cancer during pregnancy.

References

1 Barber HRK. Malignant disease in the pregnant woman. In: Coppleson M. (ed) Gynecology Oncology, 2nd edn, vol 2. New York, Churchill Livingstone, 1992; 68
2 Boronow RC. Extrapelvic malignancy and pregnancy. Obstet Gynecol Surv 1964; 19: 1
3 Squartrito RC, Harlow SP. Melanoma complicating pregnancy. Obstet Gynecol Clin North Am 1998; 25: 407
4 Gifford RW, Kvala WF, Maher FT, Roth GM, Priestley JT. Clinical features, diagnosis and treatment of pheochromocytoma: a review of 76 cases. Mayo Clin Proc 1964; 39: 281
5 Barber HRK, Brunschwig A. Gynecologic cancer complicating pregnancy. Am J Obstet Gynecol 1962; 85: 156
6 Sorosky JL. Preface, cancer complicating pregnancy. Obstet Gynecol Clin North Am 1998; 25: xi
7 Hannigan EV. Cervical cancer in pregnancy. Clin Obstet Gynecol 1990; 33: 837
8 Method MW, Brost BC. Management of cervical cancer in pregnancy. Semin Surg Oncol 1999; 16: 251
9 Herbst A, Ulfedler H, Poscanger DC. Adenocarcinoma of the vagina. Association of maternal stilbestrol therapy with tumor appearance in young women. N Engl J Med 1971; 284: 878
10 Sadan O, Kruger S, Van Iddehinge B. Vaginal tumors in pregnancy. Acta Obstet Gynecol Scand 1987; 66: 559
11 Senekjian EK, Hubby M, Bell DA, Anderson D, Herbst AL. Clear cell adenocarcinoma (CCA) of the vagina and cervix in association with pregnancy. Gynecol Oncol 1986; 24: 207
12 Mayr NA, Chen Wen B, Saw CB. Radiation therapy during pregnancy. Obstet Gynecol Clin North Am 1998; 25: 301
13 American Cancer Society. <http://www.cancer.org>
14 Bertson JR, Golden ML. Cancer and pregnancy. Am J Obstet Gynecol 1961; 81: 719
15 Falkenberry SS. Cancer in pregnancy. Surg Oncol Clin North Am 1998; 7: 375
16 Barber HRK, Brunschwig A. Carcinoma of the bowel, radiation, surgical management and pregnancy. Am J Obstet Gynecol 1968; 100: 926
17 Shillin JS. Colorectal cancer complicating pregnancy. Obstet Gynecol Clin North Am 1998; 25: 417
18 Walsh C, Fazio VW. Cancer of the colon, rectum, and anus during pregnancy. The surgeon's perspective. Gastroenterol Clin North Am 1998; 27: 257
19 Holleb A, Farrow JH. The relation of carcinoma of the breast and pregnancy in 283 patients. Surg Gynecol Obstet 1962; 115: 65
20 Marchant DJ. Breast cancer in pregnancy. Clin Obstet Gynecol 1994; 37: 993
21 National Institutes of Health. <http://www.nci.nih.gov>
22 Nicklas AH, Baker ME. Imaging strategies in the pregnant cancer patient. Semin Oncol 2000; 27: 623

23 Berry DL, Theriault RL, Holmes FA *et al*. Management of breast cancer during pregnancy using a standardized protocol. J Clin Oncology 1999; 17: 855
24 Thorney SD, McCullough LB, Chervenak FA. Ethical and spiritual considerations for treatment. Decisions associated with cancer in pregnancy. Cancer Bull 1994; 46: 3
25 Morris PC. Thyroid cancer complicating pregnancy. Obstet Gynecol Clin North Am 1998; 25: 401
26 Fisher PM, Hancock BW. Hodgkin's disease in the pregnant patient. Br J Hosp Med 1996; 56: 529
27 Smith SE. Hematologic malignancies during pregnancy. Clin Obstet Gynecol 1995; 38: 535
28 Peleg D, Ben-Ami M. Lymphoma and leukemia complicating pregnancy. Obstet Gynecol Clin North Am 1998; 25: 365
29 Cappel MS. Colon cancer during pregnancy. The gastroenterologist's perspective. Gastroenterol Clin North Am 1998; 27: 25
30 Harper MA, Murnaghan GA, Kennedy L, Hadden DR, Atkinson AB. Pheochromocytoma in pregnancy. Five cases and a review of literature. Br J Obstet Gynaecol 1989; 99: 594
31 Dildy GA, Moise KJ, Carpenter RJ, Kilma T. Maternal malignancy metastatic to the products of conception: a review. Obstet Gynecol Surv 1989; 44: 535
32 Bueckers TE, Lallas TA. Chemotherapy in pregnancy. Obstet Gynecol Clin North Am 1998; 25: 323

William J. Ledger

Human papilloma virus (HPV) infections

Human papilloma virus (HPV) infections can cause a variety of health problems for women. They can cause new growths, genital warts (condyloma acuminata), on the cornified squamous skin of the perineum or on the mucous membranes of the introitus, the vagina, or the cervix. The appearance of these visible lesions is not a trivial event for the patient involved. To many women, these genital warts are a continued marker of a sexual indiscretion in which they have acquired a sexually transmitted disease (STD). Understandably, they would like their doctor to remove these signs of infection as soon as possible. For those women who have acquired mucous membrane warts, the first early sign is often dyspareunia. To add more tension to the situation, current treatment options are limited. Haste can make waste. The methods most often employed by physicians today can be uncomfortable; occasionally, post-treatment scarring can result in loss of personal esteem and long-term sexual problems, because of pain. These are all difficult quality-of-life issues.

More serious from a medical viewpoint, there are high-risk oncogenic HPV types that are the cause of all, or nearly all, invasive cervical cancers, both the squamous cell and adenocarcinoma. One study quoted a figure of 99.7%.[1] High-risk HPV types also contribute to vulvar and vaginal cancer. This creates a new basis for medical thought. Cervical cancer, vulvar cancer, vaginal cancer are infectious diseases. Physician awareness of this needs to be paralleled by an understanding of the mechanisms of disease progression. This knowledge will guide the new and improved methods of care for these women today and in the future.

NATURAL HISTORY OF HPV INFECTION AND ITS CONSEQUENCES

Because of their biological background, physicians reflexively turn to classification to bring order out of the chaos of nature. The relationship of HPV

William J. Ledger MD
Professor and Chairman Emeritus, Department of Obstetrics and Gynecology, Weill Medical College of Cornell University, 525 East 68th Street, J-130, New York, NY 10021, USA
E-mail: wjledger@med.cornell.edu

to subsequently identified disease is complex. To date, over 100 HPV types have been identified, and they can cause visible benign lesions (condyloma acuminata) or more serious pre-invasive or invasive cancers of the lower genital tract. Different HPV types have different risk factors for women, and the viruses have been characterized as low-risk, related to wart formation, and high-risk, related to cellular abnormalities. The majority of research focus to date has been upon the high-risk viruses.

HPV is a small, DNA virus that targets the epithelial cells of the lower genital tract. The genome of approximately 8000 base pairs is divided into early (E) and late (L) genes. The late genes control the formation of the capsid coat, which in exposed humans results in an antibody response. The high-risk oncogenic viruses are potentially dangerous to the human host, for they contain two early genes that can result in vulvar, vaginal, or cervical neoplasms. E6 and E7 encode transforming proteins that induce cell proliferation and prevent apoptosis of these infected epithelial cells by binding to the tumor suppressor gene products p53 and pRB.[2] The result, over time, for some infected women is disease. Over the short term, weeks or months, visible lesions appear, the condyloma. Over months and years, pre-invasive and invasive cancers of the genital tract can be discovered on the vulva, vagina, or cervix.

There is a disconnect here between this unrelenting progression of disease and reality. On the one hand, HPV infections are very common. One estimate for the US is that there are approximately 6.2 million new HPV infections each year and that about 20 million individuals are currently infected.[3] Compare these millions with infection with the many thousands of people who get warts each year and the estimate for 2002 that approximately 13,000 women would get invasive cervical cancer and about 4100 would die of the disease in the US.[4] Another estimate is that on a point-in-time analysis, 10% of the US population has an HPV infection, 4% have cervical cytological abnormalities, and 1% have visible genital warts.[5] How do we account for these variances?

EPIDEMIOLOGY

Most patients, both men and women, will acquire one or more of these viruses during their life-time and eliminate them without symptomatology. This is primarily a disease of young adults, and obstetricians and gynecologists need to be aware of this. Surveys indicate that the peak age of HPV infection for women is 20–29 years.[6] This is true in all Western societies. One study from Manchester, UK, collected data from 242 women who were attending a family planning clinic and reported having their first sexual intercourse within the past 6 months. These women ranged in age from 15–19 years and reported only one sexual partner. During the 3 years after first intercourse, the risk of an HPV infection was 46% despite the fact that 74% of these women reported using barrier contraception.[7] Similar results were found in a study of 444 women in the US with a mean age at enrollment of 19.2 years who were HPV-negative at enrollment. Of special interest, there was no difference in the acquisition of HPV for those who were virgins and non-virgins at the time of enrollment. The initiation of sexual activity was associated with a high risk of HPV infection. The cumulative 24-month incidence of HPV among women

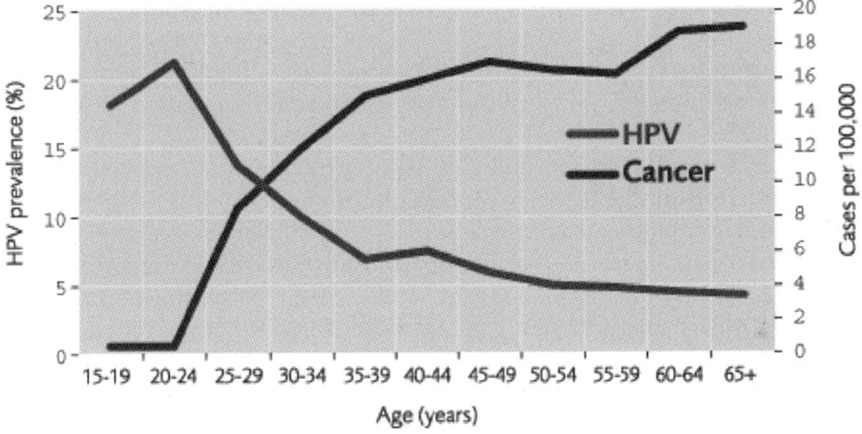

Fig. 1 HPV and cervical cancer prevalence. National Cancer Institute SEER Data, 1990–1994 (with permission).

who were sexually active at enrollment was 38.8% compared with 38.9% among virgins who subsequently began heterosexual activity.[8]

These frequent HPV infection rates among the young are balanced by the biological fact that young women with intact immune systems are highly efficient in eliminating these viruses without symptoms or disease. One study of sexually active co-eds found that 70% had cleared the HPV after 1 year and 91% after 2 years.[9] This is fortunate, because acquiring more than one HPV infection is so common in these young, sexually active women. Of those who eliminated one high-risk HPV type, 70% had become infected with another high-risk type within 24 months.[10] This clinical observation suggests that, in addition to being common, HPV infections produce an immunity that is usually very type-specific. Comparing the incidence of HPV infection and cervical cancer in women indicates two diverging pictures when an arbitrary cut-off point of 30 years is used (Fig. 1).[11] In women under 30 years of age, there is a high incidence of HPV infection and a low incidence of invasive cervical cancer. After age 30 years, these two line tangents change course. The incidence of HPV infection lessens, and the incidence of cervical cancer increases.

There are a wide variety of influences on the acquisition of these viruses. There is an increased risk of HPV infection associated with sexual contact with a new partner.[8] Although it is logical to believe that male condom use would reduce the risk of HPV infection for women, this has not been a consistent finding.[8] One recent study of young women initiating sexual activity, however, showed a benefit for both HPV-acquisition and the development of cervical squamous intra-epithelial lesions.[12] The incidence of genital HPV infection was 37.8 per 100 patient-years at risk among women whose partners used condoms for all instances of intercourse during the 8 months before testing as compared to 89.3 per 100 patient-years at risk in women whose partners used condoms less than 5% of the time.[12] This is a significant reduction but, obviously, there is still a risk of infection for these are field infections, *i.e.* in a woman, the virus can often be isolated from multiple sites, the cervix, vagina, and perineum. In men as well, perineal shedding of the virus can result in infection, even when a condom is used. The protection that the condom affords extends beyond the acquisition of an HPV infection. No cervical squamous intra-epithelial lesions were detected in 32 patient-years at risk in women reporting 100% condom use by their partners, as compared to 14 incident lesions, in 97 patient-years at risk among women whose partners did not use condoms or used them less consistently.[12]

There are a number of factors that influence the rate of patient elimination of HPV. Women younger than 24 years are more efficient in ridding themselves of the virus than women over the age of 30 years.[13] Persistence of high-risk HPV types is usually more prolonged than with low-risk HPV types.[14] The current standard of care that creates local tissue damage, for example, colposcopy with biopsy, or hot-wire excision of a larger area of the cervix, conization, enhances the rate of spontaneous regression of low-grade squamous intra-epithelial lesions (LSILs).[15] This concept of enhancing the local immune response is further buttressed by the observations of patient response after conization for pre-invasive cervical disease. HPV is a wide-spread infection with infected cells present beyond the tissue removed by conization. This treatment of pre-invasive disease of the cervix breaks the one basic tenet of the operative care of cancer, *i.e.* that all abnormal tissue must be excised. In this instance, incomplete removal of the abnormal pre-invasive tissue is uncommonly a treatment failure. One study showed complete regression of disease in 70% of women in whom the margins of the removed tissue were not free of disease.[16] These operative interventions, biopsy or conization, enhance the woman's local immune response. Although condom use does not always eliminate the possibility of HPV acquisition,[12] one study showed that continued use of a condom by the male sexual partner aided the woman's clearance of HPV and the regression of cervical intra-epithelial neoplasia.[17] Finally, cigarette smoking has been associated with an increased risk of cervical intra-epithelial neoplasia (CIN) and invasive cervical cancer through its adverse impact upon the host's immune response.[18] Taken together, this is a complex clinical picture of a common infection, with many influences on an individual patient's prognosis. Knowledge of all of these factors by responsible physicians should play an important role when making judgments about patient care.

DIAGNOSIS

There have been remarkable improvements in both the sensitivity and specificity of HPV testing in the last three decades. In the past, changes in the individual cells, either on a cytological screen, such as a Papanicolau smear, or pathological microscopic sections were often labeled as viral effect, probably due to HPV. Too often, there was little correlation between laboratories, when more than one microscopist attempted to determine if biopsy specimens showed condyloma with HPV changes. There was more specificity added using DNA probes of the tissue specimens to determine the presence of HPV, but these were insensitive tests that too often tested negative when HPV was there. They have been replaced by more effective testing methods. More sensitive and more specific HPV testing is currently in vogue. Polymerase chain reaction testing has been employed in many clinical observational studies.[9,10] It has the advantages of being very sensitive and specific in the identification of individual HPV types. It has the disadvantages of being expensive and not approved by the Food and Drug Administration (FDA), so currently unavailable as a clinical tool in the US. Despite this, it is a useful test in determining disease progression or regression and has been widely used in many research studies. Currently, the only FDA-approved testing system in the US is the second-generation hybrid capture system. The test employed today in the US screens for five low-risk HPV types and 13 high-risk HPV types. It tests fresh cells obtained with a cytology brush and is primed to register a positive result when there are 5000 or more HPV copies present. The test often results in difficult-to-resolve questions of interpretation for the physician and the patient. On the one hand, the specimen collection is easy and the results are seemingly simple and straightforward. The test is either positive or negative for low-risk and high-risk HPV types. On the other hand, it is not quantitative. This can make the evaluation of results difficult. A patient who is developing increasing immunity over time and is now shedding 10^4 viral copies as compared to an earlier stage in the infection when she was shedding 10^6 or more copies, has the same positive test result. The other problem of interpretation occurs when a patient has cleared herself of one low-risk or high-risk HPV type and then becomes infected with a different strain. This has been reported to occur frequently in young, sexually active women.[10] In this case, a patient who was initially HPV-positive, then negative, becomes positive again. The patient asks: 'Is this a recurrence?' It is probably a new infection, but the current tests cannot determine this. Finally, as is true with any sensitive testing technology, there is the possibility of a false positive test. Cross-well contamination of test samples can occur during processing and influence interpretation of some borderline positives. One study reported the proportion of these cases at risk to be low (< 3%).[19]

The role of HPV testing in clinical practice has not been defined to my satisfaction. The problems are many. HPV infections are common, many more women are infected than are those who will develop manifestations of clinical disease such as 'warts' or abnormal cervical cytological changes, and the treatment options for the HPV-positive patient are limited and unsatisfactory. Because of this, the current focus has been to use HPV testing to improve the specificity of cytological screening. There is good justification for this, for cytology screens are neither sensitive nor specific. Despite this, the standard for years has been to use abnormal cytology testing as the screen that leads to colposcopy and directed biopsies to be sure more advanced lesions are not present than had been noted in the cytology report. Keeping a focus upon cytology, the current logic is that, since a cytology report of low-grade or high-grade intra-epithelial lesion dictates colposcopy, HPV testing need not be used to determine whether colposcopy should be done. This has resonance, for in one study LSIL or HSIL abnormal tissue was frequently obtained by biopsy in women who were Digene HPV negative.[20] The biggest problem for physician decision-making is the large number of women, 3–4% in most surveys, with the report of atypical squamous cells of undetermined significance (ASCUS). What is the best course of care for these patients? This ASCUS report predicts subsequent abnormal biopsy findings with little specificity; the results are usually benign but, rarely, more advanced lesions are found. In this instance, HPV testing has become a valuable adjuvant to the ASCUS report with the positive HPV test dictating colposcopic evaluation. This results in far fewer colposcopic examinations than if all ASCUS patients were subjected to this procedure. In addition, the HPV test is currently recommended to be used as a screen in one population. Since HPV infection is so common in sexually active women under the age of 30 years and nearly all of these young women clear the virus and any low-grade cervical cytological changes if present without treatment, HPV testing is not recommended for this group.[14] In women over 30 years, the incidence of HPV infection is much lower, spontaneous clearance of the virus is slower, and the risk of high-grade cervical changes is higher. Because of this, in 2003 the US FDA approved hybrid capture II HPV testing combined with Pap smear testing in women over the age of 30 years.[21] It was further recommended that those women who have normal cytology and a negative HPV test need not have a repeat Papanicolau screening done for 3 years. Those with a positive HPV test and normal cytology should have both tests repeated in 6–12 months with colposcopy done for those with persistently positive, high-risk HPV types.

I am troubled by these recommendations for a number of reasons. They are based upon the current reality that the only approved treatment option for the woman with an abnormal Pap smear is colposcopy and biopsy. That is true today, but all physicians must acknowledge that this is an expensive and uncomfortable procedure for women. In addition, colposcopy is a flawed diagnostic technique with a high failure rate in identifying the most advanced disease of the cervix.[22,23] In the earlier study comparing paired punch biopsy with the loop excision specimen in which the loop specimen showed CIN 3 or greater severity, 41% of the punch biopsy specimens showed a lesion of lesser severity.[22] Similarly, in the Atypical Squamous Cell of Undetermined Significance/Low-Grade Squamous Intraepithelial Triage Study (ALTS), approximately one-third of the patients had more advanced disease than noted by the colposcopy biopsy.[23] Obviously, alternatives to this intervention are needed. If high-risk, HPV-positive women could be given local immune enhancers to speed the elimination of these viruses, that would be a stimulus for major modifications of the current HPV testing protocol. Also, the current guidelines to some extent ignore the pathophysiology of HPV infection and subsequent pathology when they opt for 3-year intervals for screening. An HPV-negative patient can acquire an HPV infection from a new sexual contact or from her assumed monogamous partner days or weeks after a negative HPV test. The rationale for this 3-year interval is the knowledge that it is unlikely that such a patient acquiring a high-risk HPV infection in this test-free time-frame will have developed an invasive cervical cancer by the time she is tested again. That is re-assuring, but the reality is that she will have the strong likelihood of needing colposcopy and biopsy, possibly conization, repeated cytology screens, and much emotional turmoil and concern. We need to do better than this when planning care for women. Detection and elimination of high-risk HPV seems to me a better choice and should be a future goal. If effective, it would either eliminate or markedly reduce the subsequent development of abnormal cervical cytology and the necessity for colposcopy. This would be a major public health benefit, both improving the comfort of patients and lowering medical costs.

Finally, screening for HPV infections today opens a Pandora's box for physicians. Patients are obviously anxious when told they have an infection that can cause cancer and are told to come back in 6–12 months to be checked again. This does not sit well with them. I have had patient after patient ask: 'You're not going to do anything about those atypical cells'? The medical terminology is disquieting to the lay public. In addition, many of the women whom I have cared for with a history of normal Pap smears for years who turn up with a newly discovered HPV infection are not aware of their partners' dalliances. There are social as well as medical questions, and this results in difficult counseling situations.

PREVENTION

A frustration of living in the US in these early years of the 21st century is to see how often political and religious beliefs at the personal level outweigh scientific fact, and this raised my concerns about the introduction of an HPV vaccine. The Terri Schiavo case and the US Government's emphasis upon abstinence, not condoms, in trying to prevent the spread of HIV in Africa and Asia are two prime examples of politics trumping science. As the *Financial Times* noted in a 3 June 2006 editorial, 'the US Government backs prevention programs that promote the virtues of abstinence before marriage and fidelity in marriage, even though the evidence in Africa and Asia is that most women catch the HIV virus from their husbands'.[24] In contrast to the failed abstinence HIV prevention programs sponsored and supported by the US, there is the example of an aggressive Government program in Brazil, encouraging the use of condoms that has slowed the spread of this virus and has helped contain that country's HIV epidemic.[25] Fortunately, in the case of prevention of HPV infection, the public emphasis in the US to date has been almost entirely upon the use of a vaccine that will prevent cancer, not a sexually transmitted disease. Thus far, none of the large, organized, social or religious groups in the US have taken a stand against an HPV vaccine.

Recognizing a need for a vaccine as the primary and most effective tool for prevention of HPV infections, there were many problems that delayed the development of an effective immunization tool. There were difficulties in both propagating HPV in tissue culture and in infecting non-human species. Natural infection with HPV in the human produces an immune response to the L_1 protein. To develop a safe vaccine, the problem was to obtain an L_1 protein that was immunogenic and not infective. Eventually, this material was obtained by the use of microbial expression systems. Expression of the L_1 gene in yeast produced the formation of virus-like particles (VLPs) that are so close to native virions that immunization with VLPs elicits virus-neutralizing antibodies that prevent infection with the same virus type. An early study showed a high percentage of women immunized with HPV-11 VLPs produced serum antibodies capable of neutralizing large numbers of HPV-11 virions.[26]

This was followed by studies to see if VLP immunization would protect against genital HPV infection in women. The evidence to date from a number of studies is that this is indeed an effective protective technique. One early double-blind trial in the US evaluated 2392 women aged 16–23 years who received either three doses of placebo or a three-dose HPV-16 virus-like particle vaccine.[27] After a median follow-up interval of 17.4 months, the incidence of persistent HPV-16 infection was 3.3 per 100 woman-years at risk in the placebo group and 0 per 100 woman-years at risk in the vaccine group. All nine cases of HPV-16-related cervical intra-epithelial neoplasia (CIN) were observed in the placebo population. In this study, the specificity of the immunological response seemed apparent. There were an additional 44 cases of CIN not associated with HPV-16 infection, and these were equally divided – 22 among placebo and 22 among vaccine recipients.[27] This vaccine reduced the numbers, but did not eliminate CIN. This highly successful and promising study was followed by a preliminary evaluation of a quadrivalent human papillomavirus (types 6, 11, 16, and 18) L1 virus-like particle vaccine. A total of 277 women received three doses of the quadrivalent HPV-vaccine or three doses of placebo. The combined incidence of persistent infection or disease due to HPV-6, -11, -16, or -18 fell by 90% ($P < 0.0001$) in those who received the active vaccine as compared to those who received placebo.[28] This was a vaccine designed to protect against genital warts by including HPV types 6 and 11 as well as HPV types 16 and 18, which contribute to cervical cellular abnormalities. Another immunogenic strategy being studied is a bivalent HPV-16 or HPV–18 virus-like particle vaccine. The women in this study ranged in age between 15–25 years and had no evidence of a current or post-HPV-16 or HPV–18 infection. A total of 1013 women were randomized to the three-dosage trial, 560 to receive the vaccine, and 553 to receive the placebo. There was 100% vaccine efficacy in preventing persistent HPV-16 and HPV-16/18 infection, detected in both cervical and combined cervical and cervicovaginal samples.[29] Another study looked at the long-term efficacy for up to 4.5 years of a bivalent L_1-virus-like particle vaccine.[30] It was highly effective. More than 98% seropositivity for HPV-16/18 antibodies was maintained during this extended follow-up period, and there was 100% efficacy against cervical intra-epithelial neoplasia lesions associated with HPV-16 or HPV-18. This was another positive result, confirming the hope of long-term protection. What was not anticipated, but just as exciting, was the evidence of protection against HPV-45 and HPV-31 as well. There was only one incident of infection with HPV-45 among 528 women receiving the vaccine compared to 17 incident infections with HPV-45 among 518 women receiving the placebo. There were also statistically significant differences when HPV-31 infections were noted. There were 14 incident HPV-31 infections seen in 528 women who received the vaccine compared to 30 incident HPV-31 infections among 516 women who received the placebo.[30] These latter findings were unexpected, although studies of natural HPV infection have shown type-specific response with cross-reactivity between phylogenetically related types.[31] In addition, there is the possibility of cell-mediated T-helper cell response.[32] More studies of all the vaccines in trial are needed to see if this cross-protection is real and, if so, what mechanisms are involved. The 'bottom-line' is that these vaccines are effective and will be available for clinical use.

Even though these vaccines seem effective, safe, and well-tolerated, a number of questions remain to be resolved over the coming years. Although high antibody levels have been noted among the recipients of the quadrivalent (HPV-6, -11, -16, -18) vaccine and the bivalent (HPV-16, HPV-18) vaccine, it is not known how long this immunity will last. Will it be life-time or will a booster dose be required in 10–20 years? This is a particularly important point, because all of the evidence from observational studies suggest that heterosexual activity begins at an early age for females, and this activity is associated with a high rate of high-risk HPV acquisition.[6–8] The primary target group for this vaccine will be young girls ages 9–13 years who will be less likely to have had any heterosexual contact as yet. Who will give the vaccine? I see no problem with this pre-teen population. Primary care physicians and pediatricians are the providers of care for these young girls, and they are experienced in immunization techniques that require more than one dose. The problem will be with the teenagers and young adult females who will usually present to obstetricians and gynecologists to receive this vaccine. This is a real clinical problem, for on 8 June 2006, the US FDA approved the quadrivalent HPV vaccine (HPV-6, -11, -16, -18) for 9–26-year-old girls and women. In late June 2006, a Federal vaccine advisory panel in the US voted unanimously to recommend that all girls and women aged 11–26 years receive this vaccine. Teenagers and young adults are often cared for by obstetricians and gynecologists, a physician group that generally has little experience or interest in immunizing patients. Their focus to date has been upon immunizing the few Rubella-susceptible women post-partum and offering the influenza vaccine to pregnant women during the winter months. My own experience with obstetricians and gynecologists reinforces this concern. A number of years ago at Cornell, we evaluated post-partum immunization of susceptible women with the hepatitis B vaccine. This required a similar dosing schedule as the current HPV vaccines and was shown to be successful.[33] The study showed measurable antibodies to hepatitis B in 96% of the women who received all three doses of the vaccine. These are comparable figures to other studies of hepatitis B immunization in adults. The striking thing to me was the lack of obstetrician response to this study. There was not a single reprint request from an American obstetrician and, currently, not a single obstetrician at the New York Presbyterian Hospital/Weill Cornell Medical Center screens for hepatitis B susceptibility during pregnancy so that post-partum immunization can be performed.

Finally, the question remains, what to do with males? Their future risk of oncogenic activity with HPV infection is very low, probably restricted to those who have receptive anal sex with other males. Immunizing all males would certainly decrease the spread of HPV infection in women but, to date, this has not been employed as an indication for this use of the HPV vaccine in the US. Although the quadrivalent vaccine would diminish the number of genital warts in males, the 8 June 2006 approval was limited to females.

TREATMENT

This is the currently deficient aspect of care of women with HPV infections. Today, the most commonly used treatments are usually destructive, painful, expensive, and often result in tissue changes that have an adverse impact on the future health of the patient involved. For patients with condyloma acuminata, the focus has been almost entirely upon destructive techniques to remove warts, by burning, freezing, local acid application, or podophyllin application. These are effective in removing the warts, but the scarring, particularly on mucous membrane lesions, can be a continued source of social disruption due to the disfiguring scars and dyspareunia. In addition, most of these interventions are expensive, because they require a visit to the doctor. An alternative to these destructive techniques, the local injection of interferon α-2β into the base of mucous membrane warts has been very effective. The major advantage is that it causes regression of the warts over time without scar formation. The disadvantages are that it requires repeated visits to the doctor, is expensive, the injections are painful, and women have a flu-like reaction to the first injection with fever, chills, and muscle- and joint-aches.[34]

Patient self-treatments are also available. One is the product podofilox, which is a self-applied pododylline derivation that destroys the cells of the wart.[35] A new direction is the use of imiquimod, which also is applied locally but, instead of destroying the lesion of the warty tissue, enhances the patient's own local immune system by stimulating the host's production of interferon and tumor necrosis factor.[36] Unfortunately, it also causes an intense local inflammatory tissue response, so it is a poor choice for lesions on mucous membranes.

The major medical concern is the prevention of lower genital tract malignancies. Currently, the mode of treatment for women persistently infected with high-risk HPV types is colposcopy and biopsy with conization reserved for patients with CIN II or III proven by biopsy. This is a highly effective method of treatment that has contributed to the remarkable diminution in the numbers of women with invasive cervical cancer and death from cervical cancer in the US in the past three decades. The problem is that this is expensive, uncomfortable for women, and those who need a conization are at increased risk for preterm labor and delivery in future pregnancies.[37] The current focus of the HPV testing guidelines is to reduce the number of women needing colposcopy by restricting this intervention in patients with an ASCUS report to those who are also high-risk HPV-positive. All of this could change if safe, effective alternative methods of treatment become available. Women who are high-risk HPV-positive with normal Pap smears could be given other therapies to speed up their clearance of the virus and avoid progression to an abnormal Pap smear. There are a number of therapeutic possibilities. Imiquimod has proven effective in clearing high-grade vaginal epithelial lesions from the vagina.[38] Intramuscular interferon has been successful in eliminating abnormal cervical tissue cells.[39] It could be used locally as well. There are other potential agents on the horizon that are currently being evaluated in animal models. An effective agent with few side-effects is the goal of these trials. It would be a great step forward if one could limit the use of colposcopy to the occasional patient who has neglected personal care.

KEY POINTS FOR CLINICAL PRACTICE

- Human papillomavirus causes condyloma acuminata and invasive squamous cell and adenocarcinoma of the cervix.
- HPV is usually cleared by the human host.
- The quadrivalent HPV vaccine is preventive, not therapeutic.

References

1 Walboomers JM, Jacobs MV, Manos MM *et al*. Human papilloma virus is a necessary cause of invasive cervical cancer world-wide. J Pathol 1999; 189: 12–19
2 Kirwan MJK, Herrington CS. Human papilloma virus and cervical cancer: Where are we now? Br J Obstet Gynaecol 2001; 108: 1202–1213
3 Centers for Disease Control and Prevention. Genital HPV infection – CDC fact sheet. 2004
4 American Cancer Society. Cancer facts and figures 2002. Atlanta, GA: American Cancer Society, 2002
5 Koutsky LA. Epidemiology of genital human papillomavirus infection. Am J Med 1997; 102 (Suppl): 3–8
6 Syrjänen KJ. Human papillomavirus lesions in association with cervical dysplasias and neoplasias. Obstet Gynecol 1983; 62: 617–624
7 Collins S, Mazloomzadeh S, Winter H *et al*. High incidence of cervical human papillomavirus infection in women during their first sexual relationship. Br J Obstet Gynaecol 2002; 109: 96–98
8 Winer RL, Lee S-K, Hughes JP *et al*. Genital human papillomavirus: infection incidence and risk factors in a cohort of female university students. Am J Epidemiol 2003; 157: 218–226
9 Ho GYF, Bierman R, Beardsby L *et al*. Natural history of cervicovaginal human papillomavirus (HPV) infection in young women. N Engl J Med 1998; 338: 423–428
10 Ho GYF, Studentsou Y, Hall CB *et al*. Risk factors for subsequent cervicovaginal human papillomavirus (HPV) infection and the protective role of antibodies to HPV-16 virus-like particles. J Infect Dis 2002; 186: 737–742
11 National Cancer Institute SEER Data, 1990–1994
12 Winer RL, Hughes JP, Feng Q *et al*. Condom use and the risk of genital human papillomavirus infection in young women. N Engl J Med 2006; 354: 2645–2654
13 Hildesheim A, Schiffman MH, Gravitt PE *et al*. Persistence of type-specific human papillomavirus among cytologically normal women. J Infect Dis 1994; 169: 235–240
14 Van Ranst M, Kaplan JB, Burk RD. Phylogenetic classification of human papillomaviruses: correlation with clinical manifestation. J Gen Virol 1992; 73: 2653–2660
15 Nasiell K, Nasiell M, Vaclavinkova V *et al*. Behavior of moderate cervical dysplasia during long-term follow-up. Obstet Gynecol 1983; 61: 609–614
16 Ahlgren M, Ingemersson I, Lindberg LG *et al*. Conization as a treatment of carcinoma *in situ* of the uterine cervix. Obstet Gynecol 1975; 46: 135–140
17 Hogewoning CJA, Bleeker MCG, Vanden Brule AJC *et al*. Condom use promotes regression of cervical intraepithelial neoplasia and clearance of human papillomavirus: a randomized clinical trial. Int J Cancer 2003; 107: 811–816
18 Wigle PT, Mao Y, Grace M. Smoking and cancer of the uterine cervix: hypothesis. Am J Epidemiol 1980; 111: 125–127
19 Federschneider JM, Yuan L, Brodsky J *et al*. The borderline or weakly positive Hybrid Capture II HPV test: a statistical and comparative (PCR) analysis. Am J Obstet Gynecol 2004; 191: 757–761
20 Ledger WJ, Gee R, Genc M *et al*. Human papillomavirus testing in women with an abnormal Pap smear. Int J Gynaecol Obstet 2004; 16: 103–109
21 Spitzer M, Burk RD. ACOG Practice Bulletin. Human papillomavirus. Obstet Gynecol 2005; 105: 905–918
22 Buxton EJ, Luesley DM, Shafi MI *et al*. Colposcopically directed punch biopsy: a potentially misleading investigation. Br J Obstet Gynaecol 1991; 98: 1273–1276
23 Cox JT, Schiffman M, Solomon D *et al*. Prospective follow-up suggests similar risk of subsequent cervical intraepithelial neoplasia grade 2 or 3 among women with cervical intraepithelial neoplasia grades 1 or negative colposcopy and directed biopsy. Am J Obstet Gynecol 2003; 188: 1406–1412
24 Editorial: More aid against Aids. Financial Times, 2006 (3 June), 6
25 Okie S. Fighting HIV: lessons from Brazil. N Engl J Med 2006; 354: 1977–1981
26 Brown DR, Bryan JT, Schroeder JM *et al*. Neutralization of human papillomavirus type II (HPV-II) by serum from women vaccinated with yeast-derived HPV-II L_1 virus-like particles: correlation with competitive radioimmunoassay titer. J Infect Dis 2001; 184: 1183–1186

27 Koutsky LA, Ault KA, Wheeler CM *et al.* A controlled trial of a human papillomavirus type 16 vaccine. N Engl J Med 2002; 347: 1645–1651
28 Villa LI, Costa RIA, Petta CA *et al.* Prophylactic quadrivalent human papillomavirus (types 6, 11, 16, and 18) L_1 virus-like particle vaccine in young women: a randomized double-blind placebo-controlled multicentre phase II efficacy trial. Lancet Oncol 2005; 6: 271–278
29 Harper DM, Franco EI, Wheeler C *et al.* Efficacy of a bivalent L1 virus-like particle vaccine in prevention of infection with human papillomavirus types 16 and 18 in young women: a randomized controlled trial. Lancet 2004; 364: 1757–1765
30 Harper DM, Franco EI, Wheeler CM *et al.* Sustained efficacy up to 4.5 years of a bivalent L_1 virus-like particle vaccine against human papillomavirus types 16 and 18: follow-up from a randomized control trial. Lancet 2006; 367: 1247–1255
31 Wideroff L, Schiffman M, Horderer P *et al.* Seroreactivity to human papillomavirus types 16, 18, 31, and 45 virus-like particles in a case-control study of cervical squamous intraepithelial lesions. J Infect Dis 1999; 180: 1424–1428
32 Stanley M. Immune response to human papillomavirus. Vaccine 2005 (doi: 10,1016/j.vaccine.2005.09.002)
33 Jurema MW, Polaneczky M, Ledger WJ. Hepatitis B immunization in postpartum women. Am J Obstet Gynecol 2001; 185: 355–358
34 Eron LT, Judson F, Tucker S *et al.* Interferon therapy for condyloma acuminata. N Engl J Med 1986; 315: 1059–1064
35 Greenberg MD, Rutledge LH, Reid R *et al.* A double-blind randomized trial of 0.5% podofilox and placebo for the treatment of genital warts in women. Obstet Gynecol 1991; 77: 735–748
36 Tyring SK, Arany I, Stanley MA *et al.* A randomized, controlled, molecular study of condyloma acuminata clearance during treatment with imiquimod. J Infect Dis 1998; 178: 551–555
37 Crane JMG, Delaney T, Hutchens D. Transvaginal ultrasonography in the prediction of preterm birth after treatment for cervical intraepithelial neoplasia. Obstet Gynecol 2006; 106: 37–44
38 Diakomandis E, Haidopoulos P, Stefandis K. Treatment of high-grade vaginal intraepithelial neoplasia with imiquimod cream. N Engl J Med 2002; 347: 374
39 Gonzalez-Sanchez JL, Martinez-Chequer JC, Hernandez-Celaya ME *et al.* Randomized placebo-controlled evaluation of intramuscular interferon beta treatment of recurrent human papillomavirus. Obstet Gynecol 2001: 97: 621–624

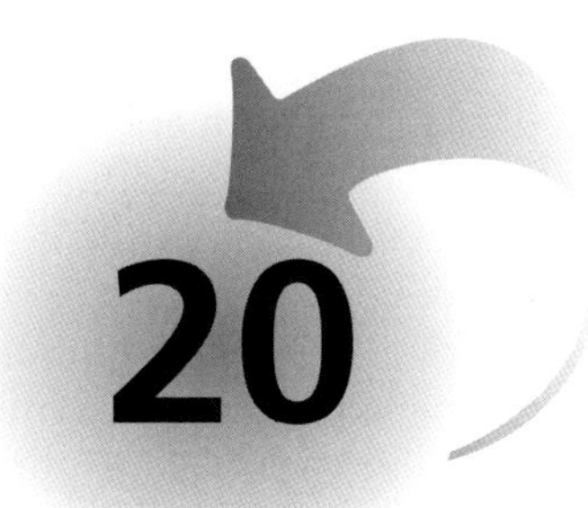

Maha Ragunath Sujit Mukhopadya Susan J. Ward

A review of pediatric gynecology

Gynecologic diseases in childhood are common. The paramount issue in the management of these patients is to appreciate the anatomical and physiological differences in the pelvis of young girls and adult women.

The onus of treating pediatric gynecologic problems often falls on gynecologists. With increasing patient load and the heavier demand on consultants' time, there are increasing opportunities for such patients to be seen at the initial consultation by a specialist registrar (SpR). This review is intended for the SpR, to enable careful and sound management of pediatric patients as the initial assessment is paramount to proper management.

Childhood gynecologic problems may be short-lived, affecting only one part of development, or long-standing resulting from tumors or congenital abnormalities. This can have varied repercussions in terms of continuing problems into adult life with subsequent gynecologic or even psychiatric consequences.

The following chapter elucidates the common conditions encountered in clinical practice with respect to problems in early childhood, puberty and adolescence.

PROBLEMS IN EARLY CHILDHOOD

Vulvovaginitis

Etiopathogenesis and clinical features

Prior to puberty, the milieu is hypo-estrogenic with a flattened vulva, attenuated

Maha Ragunath MRCOG MSc (for correspondence)
Senior Registrar in Obstetrics & Gynaecology, Queen's Medical Centre, Derby Road, Nottingham, UK
E-mail: maharagunath@doctors.org.uk

Sujit Mukhopadya MRCOG
Specialist Registrar in Obstetrics & Gynaecology, King's Mill Hospital, Mansfield Road, Sutton-in-Ashfield, Mansfield NG17 4JL, UK

Susan J. Ward FRCOG MD
Consultant in Obstetrics & Gynaecology, King's Mill Hospital, Mansfield Road, Sutton-in-Ashfield, Mansfield NG17 4JL, UK

labia minora and a small uterus. The vaginal epithelium is thin and red with little vaginal secretion which is relatively alkaline. Both of these factors result in an increased susceptibility to vulvovaginitis, with symptoms ranging from mild discomfort to severe pruritis sometimes associated with a serous/purulent discharge. On examination, the vulva and introitus are red and inflamed with or without accompanying discharge.

A variety of organisms have been reported with *Haemophilus influenzae*, *Staphylococcus aureus*, Group A streptococci and *Escherichia coli* being the most common.[1] *Candida* spp. are rare and may be found in girls with predisposing factors, such as prolonged antibiotic treatment in 90% of cases, diabetes mellitus in 0.3%, steroid therapy in 0.2%, deficient hygiene in 5% and a diet rich in carbohydrates in 9%.[2] The isolation of organisms that are sexually transmitted, such as *Trichomonas* spp. and *Chlamydia* spp., should prompt a careful evaluation for sexual abuse.[3]

Other causes

Infestation with thread worms (*Entrobius vermicularis*) can cause vulvar/vaginal irritation especially at night. Diagnosis is by the Graham technique (peri-anal adhesive sellotape test) to perform a parasitological diagnosis.[4] This involves using adhesive sellotape on the underwear to retrieve eggs that have been deposited in the peri-anal region at night.

Rarely, allergy producing an atopic or irritant dermatitis, constipation and skin diseases such as lichen sclerosus can present in a similar fashion and needs proper evaluation and treatment.[5]

Management

Clinical examination with gentle separation and inspection of the vulva is paramount to confirm presence of discharge and exclude dermatological conditions. Bacteriological swabs are usually unhelpful as fecal contamination is likely. Recurrent vaginal discharge, unresponsive to symptomatic or antibiotic treatment, needs further evaluation to exclude a retained foreign body. Examination under anesthetic with vaginoscopy using a pediatric cystoscope is imperative, and allows for the identification of not only a retained foreign body but may facilitate diagnosis of unusual conditions such as dermatitis, lymphatic duct chylous drainage and non-specific vulvovaginitis.[6]

Treatment is symptomatic in non-specific vulvovaginits, with advice on vulval hygiene, avoidance of tight-fitting clothes and irritant soaps, front-to-back wiping after defecation and antibiotic treatment with recurrent vulvovaginitis if organisms are isolated. The use of salt baths and bland emollients such as Sudacrem or E45 may be beneficial. Sometimes, a short course of treatment with topical estrogen cream will ease irritation and discharge especially when mixed organisms are grown on culture, but should be used with caution.[7]

Labial adhesions

Etiopathogenesis and clinical features

Labial fusion is a common pediatric problem often associated with a low estrogenic status, but can exist even when estrogen levels are normal.[8] The peak incidence was found to be 3.3% at 13–23 months of age in a retrospective Canadian study.[9]

In younger children, findings are usually reported by the mother, but the condition sometimes presents with asymptomatic bacteriuria and urinary infections.[10] Rarely, it can cause voiding difficulty and urinary incontinence.

Management

Most of the retrospective studies done to review treatment of labial adhesions agree that, after the initial gynecologic evaluation, treatment should include topical estrogen, followed by manual separation on a regular basis done by the mother. Surgical separation is reserved for resistant cases refractory to medical treatment. This involves sharp incision through the adhesion under general anesthetic with regular use of estrogen cream to prevent re-adhesion at cut surfaces.[11]

Other dermatological conditions

Lichen scelerosus

Lichen sclerosus is a chronic skin condition affecting men, women and children and usually occurs in the anogenital area. The underlying cause is unknown but there is a strong association with autoimmune disorders and immunogenetic studies have demonstrated a link with HLA DQ7. An Oxford study, published in 2001, found a prevalence of 1 in 900 and confirmed an increasing incidence of the condition. There was a positive family history in a minimum of 17% of cases with associated autoimmune disease occurring in 14%.[12] Unlike the adult form of the disease, the condition is self-limiting, with no risk of malignancy and resolves at or just after menarche.

Symptoms are usually of vulval itching and soreness. Sometimes skin changes such as discrete white papules, white plaques and hemorrhagic areas similar to bruising may be seen. This may be confused with the changes seen in sexual abuse and needs careful exclusion.[13] Childhood anogenital lichen sclerosus often presents with recalcitrant constipation and other gastro-intestinal complaints.[14]

Careful hygiene together with the use of potent topical corticosteroids, such as clobetasol propionate, are effective management and give relief from itching pain and inflammation.

Lichenoid eruptions

These are quite common in children and can result from different origins. The precise pathophysiology is unknown but is believed to be immunologic in nature. Lichen striatus, lichen nitidus and lichen spinulosus are examples of lichenoid lesions that are commoner in children than in adults. Distinguishing this diagnosis is necessary for optimal management. In most cases, clinical characteristics enable a diagnosis, but may sometimes require a biopsy. Most lesions are self-limited and only require symptomatic treatment.[15]

Vulvar warts

Anogenital warts can occur in children and may be due to an HPV-2-induced condylomata which can co-exist with cutaneous common warts. Whilst it is

Table 1 Tanner staging of breast and pubic hair development

	Breast	Pubic hair
Stage I	Infantile breasts	No pubic hair
Stage II	Development of breast bud – median age 9.8 years	Sparse, long, pigmented hair along L Majora – median age 10.5 years
Stage III	Enlargement of the breasts and areola, with rounded breast contour – median age 11.2 years	Dark, coarse, curled hair sparsely spread over mons – median age 12 years
Stage IV	Nipple and areola enlarge to produce secondary projection above the breast contour – median age 12.1 years	Adult-type hair, abundant but limited to mons – median age 12 years
Stage V	Normal adult breast with rounded contour and assimilation of nipple and areola into the whole breast – median age 14.6 years	Adult-type spread in quantity and distribution – median age 13.7 years

Adapted from Speroff *et al.*[17]

important to exclude sexual abuse, non-sexual transmission can also occur by persons with lesions taking care of children. Perinatal transmission appears to be an important route of infection.[16] Treatment with 10–20% podophyllin, depending on the age of the child ,is useful with a maximum of three applications taking care not to damage the normal surrounding skin.

PROBLEMS AT PUBERTY

Puberty is defined as a period of maturation during which a child develops both physically and mentally into adulthood. The physical changes follow an orderly sequence with an initial acceleration of growth followed by breast budding (thelarche) occurring at a median age of 9 years. This is followed by the growth of pubic hair at 10.5 years and axillary hair at 12.5 years (adrenarche). Menarche is a late event occurring at 12.8 years. The process of puberty thus starts at 9 years of age and is completed by the age of 16 years (Table 1).

Precocious puberty

Etiopathogenesis and clinical features

Pubertal changes with menarche before the age of 10 years and development of secondary sex characteristics occurring before the age of 8 years is regarded as precocious. There are two main causes of precocious puberty – GnRH-dependent and GnRH-independent. The former is responsible for 80% of cases and is due to premature activation of the hypothalamo-pituitary axis which is either idiopathic in 10%, or due to an inherent pathology in the central nervous system. This can be due to tumors such as harmartomas, craniopharyngiomas or meningitis, hydrocephalus or skull injury. Features of CNS involvement may include seizures, mental retardation, raised intracranial pressures or focal neurological deficits.[18] Constitutional precocity runs in families and occurs closer to the borderline age of 8 years, whereas idiopathic sexual precocity presents with changes much earlier in childhood.

The GnRH-independent causes can be due to ovarian tumors (10%) such as granulosa cell and theca cell tumors, adrenal tumors, ectopic gonadotrophin production and drugs such as contraceptives and anabolic steroids.

Management

A detailed physical examination is important and should include a Tanner staging. Bone age must be determined, with hormonal assays to include gonadotropin levels, thyroid function tests and assays of adrenal steroids. An MRI/CT scan of the head is usually necessary,[19] as is an ultrasound examination of the abdomen and pelvis to exclude adrenal/ovarian tumors.

The treatment is usually of the cause and can involve thyroxine or testosterone replacement, neurosurgery/radiotherapy for central nervous system tumors or surgical excision for ovarian/adrenal masses. Idiopathic precocious puberty is treated with GnRH agonists which causes a substantial regression of pubertal characteristics and reduction of growth velocity. Treatment is continued until epiphyseal fusion occurs or until the appropriate pubertal/chronological ages are matched. The intellectual and psychological implications of precocious puberty on the child should be recognised and support offered.

Delayed puberty

Though a wide variation exists, most adolescent girls begin to mature by the age of 13 years. Delayed puberty is a rare condition and occurs in about 2–5% of the population. Constitutional delay, genetic defects or hypothalamic-pituitary disorders are common causes.[20]

Amenorrhea

Amenorrhea and oligomenorrhoea are conditions frequently seen in an out-patient clinic and the investigations leading up to a diagnosis are best dealt with from an anatomical standpoint with systematic evaluation at each level of the hypothalamo-pituitary-ovarian(HPO)-uterine axis. At the same time, treatment should be tailored to the age and needs of the young adolescent.

Amenorrhea is considered to be primary in a girl who has never menstruated and secondary when there is absence of a period for more than 6 months. Primary amemorrhea is, therefore, best described as the absence of menstruation by 16 years of age irrespective of the presence or absence of secondary sexual characteristics (Table 2).

Examination of the amenorrhoeic patient is performed to establish presence of secondary sexual characteristics, and exclude anatomical causes as well as stigmata of chromosomal conditions. A knowledge of the body mass index as well as signs of virilisation and hirsutism should be looked for. As most of these patients are young and may not be sexually active, an ultrasound scan can be a useful alternative to a pelvic examination.

Table 2 Causes of primary amemorrhea

Level 1 – Extrinsic to the HPO axis	
	Thyroid and adrenal disorders
	Systemic disease
	Physiological
	Pregnancy and lactation
Level 2 – Hypothalamic	
	Congenital – Kallman's syndrome
	Acquired – pituitary stalk disconnection syndromes (craniopharyngioma), excessive weight loss, excessive exercise, cranial radiotherapy
Level 3 – Pituitary	
	Tumors – prolactinomas, non-functional tumors
	Infection – tuberculosis
	Radiotherapy, surgery
Level 4 – Ovarian	
	Polycystic ovary syndrome
	Ovarian failure (premature menopause)
	Resistant ovary syndrome
	Ovarian agenesis, dysgenesis (Turner's syndrome)
	Chemo/radiotherapy and surgery
Level 5 – Uterovaginal	
	Uterine agenesis
	Testicular feminisation
	Imperforate hymen
	Radiotherapy

Adapted from Speroff *et al.*[17]

The initial investigations should include a baseline FSH and LH, TFT and prolactin levels. Further investigations should then be based on abnormal results and should be directed at the suspected diagnosis.

A progesterone challenge test is a useful means of evaluating the level of endogenous estrogen as well as the integrity of the outflow tract. This involves giving a 5-day course of medroxyprogesterone acetate. A positive bleed confirms a functional outflow tract, while no bleed suggests either outflow tract obstruction or absent estrogenic endometrial proliferation. Estrogen can be supplemented as estrogen valerate 2 mg for 21 days followed by progesterone for 10 mg for 5 days. If this is followed by bleed, a hypo-estrogenic state can be established and an assay done for FSH and LH levels. Normal/low levels of gonadotropic hormones necessitate a CT imaging of the sella turcica to exclude a pituitary tumor in the absence of which hypothalamic amemorrhea can be diagnosed. High levels of gonadotropins indicate primary ovarian failure.

Management

Management is based on the etiology, and the presence or absence of secondary sexual characteristics. With conditions like gonadal dysgenesis and hypothalamic amemorrhea, treatment is based on hormone replacement given in a way that mimics natural hormone production to induce breast development and induce withdrawal bleeds and also long term to prevent osteoporosis and cardiovascular disease.

With abnormalities of the outflow tract and normal secondary sexual differentiation, like imperforate hymen, a careful history may reveal cyclical lower abdominal pain and, rarely, urinary retention caused by vaginal distension. General examination may reveal a lower abdominal mass, with a distended blue-colored membrane on separating the labia. The diagnosis of hematocolpos can be made on an ultrasound scan. Treatment is with a cruciate incision of the membrane under general anesthetic to release chocolate-colored, tarry material.

Absence of the uterus is usually associated with an absence of the vagina owing to failure of development of the Mullerian duct system as in Rokitansky-Kuster-Hauser syndrome or the complete androgen-insensitivity syndrome. The latter is an X-linked disorder where the affected are phenotypically female with well-developed breasts and external genitalia, but are genetically male with an XY karyotype. The testes will be found in the abdomen, inguinal canal or vulva and should be removed because of the risk of malignancy. The girl and the parents need the appropriate support with counselling and hormone replacement therapy will be required.

PROBLEMS AT ADOLESCENCE

Dysfunctional uterine bleeding

Etiopathogenesis and clinical features

In about 95% cases of dysfunctional uterine bleeding in adolescents, late maturation of the HPO axis with a lack of E2 positive feedback on LH, leading to anovulatory cycles is the causative factor.[21] This results in the over-stimulation and proliferation of the endometrium from unopposed estrogen which eventually breakdown to cause heavy irregular bleeding.

Management

The diagnosis of anovulatory bleeding, though one of exclusion, should have excluded pregnancy in the first instance. A satisfactory history and physical examination is paramount. Other disorders to be excluded are thyroid disease, Cushing's syndrome, hypoprolactinemia, acromegaly and coagulation defects. If periods do not improve with therapy, organic causes such as pelvic inflammatory disease, endometriosis, genital tract tumors and, rarely, hematological disorders such as von Willebrand's disease need exclusion.

It is worth asking the young girl to keep a diary of the frequency and heaviness of her periods prior to treatment. If the periods do fall within normal limits, re-assurance may be all that is needed. The initial laboratory tests need not be extensive but must include a hemoglobin estimation, coagulation screen and thyroid function tests.[22]

With regular periods, prostaglandin synthetase inhibitors such as mefenamic acid or tranexamic acid taken during the days of heavy flow are useful. If bleeding is irregular, hormone treatment with norethisterone or dydrogestrone 5 mg tds from day 15 to day 25 of the cycles usually helps to regulate the cycle and decrease bleeding. Rapid saturation of the endometrium with conjugated equine estrogens used intravenously is effective, through its stimulation of fibrinogen production, Factors V and IX and platelet aggregation. Progestogens are a highly effective mode of treatment for excessive bleeding caused by dysfunctional uterine bleeding in adolescents. In one study, oral medroxyprogesterone acetate tablets administered at a dose of 60–120 mg at admission followed by 20 mg/day for 10 days reduced blood loss to acceptable levels in all patients.[23] The oral contraceptive pill is often the panacea with its ease of use and ability to regulate the cycle. Oral iron should be concomitantly prescribed to prevent anemia. The use of GnRH analogues is controversial, but may be useful in patients with hematologic disorders and when coagulopathy is predictable, as in patients undergoing chemotherapy and bone-marrow transplantation.[24] The most important issue with treatment of adolescent dysfunctional uterine bleeding is that these patients require education about the problem and re-assurance in conjunction with treatment.

Dysmenorrhoea

Etiopathogenesis and clinical features

This is a common problem in adolescence. At the start of menarche, the cycles may be painless as they are anovulatory. With the onset of ovulation, dysmenorrhoea is an increasingly common problem, with spasmodic and colicky pain beginning premenstrually and lasting until day 2–3 of the cycle. Pain affects the lower abdomen and back and occasionally radiates to the thighs. In severe cases, vomiting and diarrhoea may be experienced.

Management

Treatment is usually with simple analgesics such as aspirin or codeine in the first instance. If ineffective, prostaglandin synthetase inhibitors such as mefenamic acid 250–500 mg three times a day can be tried. Treatment should start at the beginning of menstruation and taken regularly during the days affected. In severe cases, the oral contraceptive pill can be used. Endometriosis is unusual in this age group, but must be considered as a possibility if there is no response to therapy and must be excluded by a diagnostic laparoscopy. Uterosacral nerve ablation can be tried for intractable dysmenorrhoea.

Secondary amemorrhea

This is defined as the absence of menstruation for longer than 6 months. The commonest reason in an adolescent that first needs exclusion is pregnancy (Table 3).

Etiopathogenesis and clinical features

Hypothalamic amemorrhea caused by excessive weight loss is common in the west, and is one of the cardinal signs of anorexia nervosa in women with a steady increase in prevalence over the last 20 years. A low body mass index (BMI) frequently produces secondary amemorrhea in the absence of psychological disease. Intense sustained exercise leads to cessation of GnRH pulses and amemorrhea, but less intense exercise in combination with dieting

Table 3 Causes of secondary amemorrhea

Physiological	Pregnancy
Pathological	Hypothalamic/pituitary Stress Weight loss Hypogonadotropic hypogonadism Prolactinoma Panhypopituitarism
Ovarian	Polycystic ovarian disease Hormone secreting tumor Chemotherapy, radiotherapy and surgery
Uterine	Absence
Systemic causes	Thyroid Adrenal

seems to produce similar effects. Patients present with low/normal levels of FSH, LH and estrogen. Rare, space-occupying lesions in the hypothalamus can present with secondary amemorrhea as can tumors causing pituitary stalk compression. Hyperprolactinemia caused by a prolactin secreting micro- or macro-adenoma can cause both primary and secondary amemorrhea depending on the timing of presentation, being responsible for nearly 15% of secondary amemorrhea. As 10% of patients will have macro-adenomas, it is important to diagnose these lesions by means of an MRI, since they can cause optic nerve damage at the levels of the optic chiasma. Medication causing secondary amemorrhea is rare in children.

The pituitary can also be damaged by surgery and radiotherapy with resultant pan-hypopituitarism. Polycystic ovarian syndrome (PCOS) is the most common endocrinopathy in young women frequently causing oligomenorrhoea and secondary amemorrhea in 25%. Associated features include obesity, hirsutism, acne, with reduced fertility presenting variably in adulthood. There is strong evidence of insulin resistance with the risk of developing type II diabetes in later life. Diagnosis is confirmed by a raised LH: FSH ratio (> 3), total and free testosterone, reduced SHBG and hyperprolactinemia. A pelvic ultrasound may show larger than normal ovaries, with a dense stroma showing a number of small circumferentially arranged cysts.

Premature ovarian failure is rare in this age group though occasional cases have been reported. Rarer causes include galactosemia and Turner's mosaicism leading to early-onset secondary amemorrhea and autoimmune oophoritis.

Management

Initial basic investigations should include FSH, LH, thyroid function tests, prolactin and a pelvic ultrasound. Further investigations will be determined by the suspected diagnosis and should be dealt with in a systematic manner. If hypothalamic following stress or weight loss, re-assurance that periods will resume once a critical body weight is attained and support may be all that is required. In cases of prolonged amemorrhea, hormone replacement is needed to protect from osteoporosis. Space-occupying lesions of the hypothalamus and pituitary require neurological/neurosurgical assessment.

Treatment of PCOS depends on the clinical presentation. Menstrual regulation with cyclical estrogen/progesterone or the oral contraceptive pill may be needed. This can be combined with cyproterone acetate if control of hirsutism is needed as well.

PEDIATRIC GYNECOLOGICAL TUMORS

Gynecological tumors in childhood and adolescents are fortunately rare, and represent 1.5–2% of all malignancies in this age group. However, it is important to consider this an entity needing exclusion, as procrastination will inevitably delay diagnosis.

Non-epithelial tumors predominate, while carcinomas are rare and their incidence rises with increasing age. Malignancies of the external genitalia are rare with vaginal malignancies which are usually embryogenic, rhabdomyosarcoma, yolk sac tumors and vaginal adenocarcinomas all of which are highly malignant. Uterine tumors are rare and ovarian tumors represent 1.5% of all childhood tumors, germinal and gonadal stromal tumors being typical of this age.[25] Only the commonest of the tumors will be considered in this review

Cervical vaginal tumors

Botryoid sarcoma (rhabdomyosarcoma)

This the one of the most commonly occurring and the most serious childhood vaginal tumor, frequently affecting girls of below 2 years of age, with 90% occurring in girls below 5 years of age, though it may occur in the cervix in older girls and adolescents. The presenting features are usually of blood-stained vaginal discharge and, sometimes, with frank bleeding. Examination usually reveals a fleshy hemorrhagic lesion, classically described as grape-like, though it may be seen as a simple polyp.

The tumor originates in the sub-epithelial layer of the cervical/vaginal epithelium and spreads widely within this layer producing a classical polypoid appearance before invading the vaginal wall. Later spread is via the lymphatic and blood-stream.

A good EUA is essential for all blood-stained discharge from the vagina with biopsy for histological diagnosis. Treatment is by combination chemotherapy over a period of 6 months, followed by extended hysterectomy and vaginectomy. If response to chemotherapy is very good, it can be continued for a further 6–12 months.

Clear-cell adenocarcinoma

This affects the vagina and the cervix and is usually secondary to diethylstilbestrol (DES) exposure whilst *in utero*. Approximately two-thirds of girls exposed to DES have congenital abnormalities of the cervix, like pseudopolyp formation and hypertrophy of the endocervical tissue and vaginal abnormalities including incomplete septa, fibrous bands and vaginal adenosis. The predominant symptom is vaginal bleeding and the risk of cancer is 0.14–1.4 per 1000 and, therefore, merits colposcopy follow-up from early teens.

Treatment if clear-cell adenocarcinoma develops is by extended hysterectomy and vaginectomy, though tumor excision gave an excellent outcome in one series.[26] Radiotherapy can be used as an adjunct following surgery.

Ovarian tumors

Functional ovarian cysts/benign tumors

These are among the most common ovarian masses in adolescents. The commonest presenting complaint is abdominal pain and ultrasonography can be used to define the size and well as to characterise its gross morphological condition as solid, cystic or complex cystic. Treatment often involves only a simple cyst resection of the mass and, rarely, salpingo-oopherectomy, if there is torsion with loss of tissue viability.[27]

Teratomas

These are usually benign and may be unilateral or bilateral (10%). They are derived from totipotent primordial germ cells and contain ectodermal, mesodermal and endodermal tissue in varying amounts, with a preponderance of skin, sebum and hair (dermoid cysts). Mature differentiated teratomas are usually benign, but decreasing differentiation means worse biological effects.

Presentation is usually as an asymptomatic abdominal mass although abdominal pain might be present. An ultrasound examination confirms the presence of a multicystic tumor with mixed solid and cystic areas, and an X-ray examination may show areas of calcification or teeth-like structures. Treatment is by surgical removal taking care to preserve as much of the affected ovary as possible, especially where the tumor is bilateral.

Dysgerminomas

These tumors develop from primordial germ cells and are termed malignant, though generally not of high malignant potential. They are relatively more common in childhood than in adults, with 60% developing in the first two decades of life. They occur more frequently in Y-chromosome karyotypes and have malignant progression with early propagation to lymph nodes.

The clinical presentation is usually of a rapidly growing tumor presenting as an asymptomatic abdominal mass, with ascites being a feature of advanced disease. Treatment is based on the degree of malignancy. Where there is obvious malignancy with involvement of the opposite ovary, peritoneal involvement and ascites, total abdominal hysterectomy with bilateral salpingo-oopherectomy is required, followed by postoperative radiation if necessary as the tumor is radiosensitive. In less aggressive tumors, unilateral oopherectomy and lympadenectomy of the affected side followed by chemotherapy may be sufficient, together with careful long-term follow-up.

Yolk sac tumors

These are common among germ cell tumors presenting in the pediatric age group and presents a spectrum of cytomorphological features. These tumors typically secrete α-fetoprotein and HcG and present as pelvi-abdominal masses. They are highly malignant with short survival.[28]

Granulosa cell tumors

Granulosa cell tumors are rare, accounting for < 5% of ovarian tumors occurring in childhood and adolescence. The tumor secretes estrogen and sometimes prolactin, thereby resulting in symptoms of precocious pseudo-puberty, pelvic mass and, rarely, galactorrhoea. Most present at the first stage and have a good prognosis. Treatment usually involves unilateral oopherectomy, with careful, long-term follow-up for signs of contralateral disease.

FERTILITY PRESERVATION IN CHILDREN AND ADOLESCENTS

Advances in cancer therapy have improved long-term survival of young patients, who face the bleak prospect of loss of gonadal function and sterility as a consequence of treatment. With the rapid progress in IVF techniques, this can be addressed by various means including the substitution of alkylating agents, cyclical rather than continuous regimens, surgically tacking the ovaries out of the field of radiation like laparoscopic suspension of ovarian tissue and ovarian transplantation in an ectopic site, and the cryopreservation of oocytes and ovarian tissue prior to treatment.

KEY POINTS FOR CLINICAL PRACTICE

- Initiate a careful assessment of the patient taking into account the anatomical and physiological differences in the pelvis of young girls and adult women.
- Think of common problems first with a systematic approach to excluding more serious conditions.
- Adopt a multidisciplinary outlook with early involvement of other specialists if needed.

References

1 Jacquiery A, Stylionopoulus A, Hogg G, Grover S. Vulvovaginitis: clinical features, aetiology and microbiology of genital tract. Arch Dis Child 1999; 81: 64–67
2 Felea D, Matasaru S, Nistor S *et al*. Aspects of children's candidiasis in outpatient practice. Rev Med Chir Soc Med Nat Iasi 2004; 108: 151–154
3 Deligeoroglou E, Salakos N, Makrakis E *et al*. Infections of the lower female genital tract during childhood and adolescence. Clin Exp Obstet Gynaecol 2004; 31: 175–178
4 Acosta M, Cazorla D, Gaevett M. Enterobiasis among school children in a rural population from Estado Falcon, Venezuela and its relation with socioeconomic level. Invest Clin 2002; 43: 173–181
5 Fischer G, Rogers M. Vulvar disease in children: a clinical audit of 130 cases. Pediatr Dermatol 2000; 17: 1–6
6 Smith YR, Berman DR, Quint EH. Premenarchal vaginal discharge: findings of procedures to rule out foreign bodies. J Pediatr Adolesc Gynaecol 2002; 15: 227–230

7 Jones R. Childhood vulvovaginitis and vaginal discharge in general practice. Fam Pract 1999; 13: 369–372
8 Dapagianni M, Stanhope R. Labial adhesions in a girl with isolated premature thelarche: the importance of estrogenization. J Pediatr Adolesc Gynecol 2003; 16: 31–32
9 Leung AK, Robson WH, Tay-Uyboco J. The incidence of labial fusion in children. J Paediatr Child Health 1993; 29: 235–236
10 Leung AK, Robson WL. Labial fusion and asymptomatic bacteriuria. Eur J Pediatr 1993; 152: 250–251
11 Nurzia MJ, Eickhorst KM, Ankem MK, Barone J. The surgical treatment of labial adhesions in pre-pubertal girls. J Pediatr Adolesc Gynecol 2003; 16: 21–23
12 Powell J, Wojnarowska F. Childhood vulvar lichen sclerosus: an increasingly common problem. J Am Acad Dermatol 2001; 44: 803–806
13 Attaran M, Rome E, Gidwani GP. Unusual presentation of LS in an adolescent. J Paediatr Adolesc Gynecol 2000; 13: 99
14 Maronn ML, Esterly NB. Constipation as a feature of anogenital lichen sclerosus in children. Paediatrics 2005; 115: e230–e232
15 Tittly JJ, Drolet BA, Esterly NB. Lichenoid eruptions in children. J Am Acad Dermatol 2004; 51: 606–624
16 Obalek S, Misiewicz J, Jablonska S, Favre M, Orth G. Childhood condyloma acuminatum: associated with genital and cutaneous human papilloma viruses. Pediatr Dermatol 1993; 10: 101–106.
17 Speroff L, Glass RH, Kase NG. Clinical Gynecologic Endocrinology and Infertility. Baltimore, MD: Williams & Wilkins, 1989; 165–213
18 Bajpai A, Sharma J, Kabra M, Kumar Gupta A, Menon PS. Precocious puberty: clinical and endocrine profile and factors indicating neurogenic precocity in Indian children. J Pediatr Endocrinol Metab 2002; 15: 1173–1181
19 Ng SM, Kumar Y, Cody D, Smith CS, Aidi M. Cranial MRI scans are indicated in all girls with central precocious puberty. Arch Dis Child 2003; 88: 414–418
20 Hoffman B, Bradshaw KD. Delayed puberty and amenorrhea. Reprod Med 2003; 21: 353–362
21 Deligeoroglou E. Dysfunctional uterine bleeding. Ann NY Acad Sci 1997; 816: 158–164
22 Spence JE. Menstrual abnormalities in the adolescent abuse of the birth control pill. Pediatr Adolesc Gynecol 1983; 1: 125–148.
23 Aksu F, Madazli R, Budak E, Cepni I, Bernian A. High dose medroxyprogesterone acetate for the treatment of DUB in 24 adolescents. Aust NZ J Obstet Gynecol 1997; 37: 228–231
24 Laufer MR, Rein MS. Treatment of abnormal uterine bleeding with gonadotrophin-releasing hormone analogues. Clin Obstet Gynecol 1993; 36: 668–678
25 Horejsi J, Rob L. Malignant tumours of the female genitalia in childhood – yesterday, today and tomorrow. Cas Lek & Cesk, 2003; 142: 84–87
26 McNall RY, Nowicki PD, Miller B, Billups CA, Liu T, Daw NC. Adenocarcinoma of the cervix and vagina in paediatric patients. Pediatr Blood Cancer 20004; 43: 289–294
27 Skiadas JT, Koutoulidis V, Eleytheriades M *et al.* Ovarian masses in young adolescents: imaging findings with surgical confirmation. Eur J Gynaecol Oncol 2004; 25: 201–206
28. Afroz N, Khan N, Chana RS. Cytodiagnosis of yolk sac tumour. Indian J Pediatr 2004; 71: 939–942

Ivica Zalud Raydeen Busse

Gynecologic ultrasound: a primer for clinicians

Ultrasound use in gynecologic practice has become standard and valuable for the clinician in many aspects of daily practice. This is due to the ease of use of the equipment and relative low cost compared with other available imaging modalities. With proper training, ultrasound can be an important adjunct to clinical practice for everyday decision-making for gynecologic patients.

The American Institute of Ultrasound in Medicine (AIUM) lists indications for gynecologic ultrasound that include, but are not limited to, pelvic pain, dysmenorrhea, menorrhagia, metrorrhagia, menometrorrhagia, follow-up of previously detected abnormality (*e.g.* hemorrhagic cyst), evaluation and/or monitoring of infertile patients, delayed menses or precocious puberty, postmenopausal bleeding, abnormal pelvic examination, further characterization of a pelvic abnormality noted on another imaging study (*e.g.* computed tomography or magnetic resonance imaging), evaluation of congenital anomalies, excessive bleeding, pain, or fever after pelvic surgery or delivery, localization of an intra-uterine contraceptive device, and screening for malignancy in patients with an increased risk.[1] In addition, gynecologic ultrasound encompasses the realm of early pregnancy failures or pregnancies of uncertain outcome and, of course, ectopic pregnancies.

There have been numerous studies reported in the literature that assess the accuracy of ultrasound in gynecology. The purpose of this review is to determine which cases warrant ultrasound evaluation in general gynecologic

Ivica Zalud MD PhD FACOG FAIUM (for correspondence)
Associate Professor and Chief, Obstetrics and Gynecology Imaging Division, Department of Obstetrics and Gynecology and Women's Health, John A. Burns School of Medicine, University of Hawaii, Kapiolani Medical Center for Women and Children, Suite 540, 1319 Punahou Street, Honolulu, Hawaii 96826, USA
E-mail: Ivica@hawaii.edu

Raydeen Busse MD FACOG
Assistant Professor, Department of Obstetrics and Gynecology and Women's Health, John A. Burns School of Medicine, University of Hawaii, Kapiolani Medical Center for Women and Children, Honolulu, Hawaii, USA

practice. The sensitivity and specificity of ultrasound for certain gynecologic conditions, diseases, and symptoms will be presented in a selective way.

NORMAL FINDINGS

Uterus

Ultrasound is an excellent method to evaluate the uterus and its contents. It is important to note the timing of a woman's cycle for the proper interpretation of normal and its variants. It is also notable if the woman is premenopausal or postmenopausal. Evaluation of the uterus can be performed transabdominally, preferably with at least a partially distended bladder that displaces the small bowel and gaseous intestines from the area being viewed or, more precisely, via transvaginal scanning with the bladder emptied. Not infrequently, both modalities are useful in cases of overly large uterus or large pelvic mass. The transabdominal scan can serve as a 'roadmap' to guide the sonographer in the location of adnexal structures.

Uterine size is depicted by uterine length (measured in the long axis from the fundus to the cervix, depth via antero-posterior measurement perpendicular to the length and width via the coronal view (Fig. 1). Uterine shape and orientation is also noted. Documentation of the endometrium, myometrium and cervix should also take place. The normal postpubertal nulliparous uterus is 5–8 cm long, 1.5–3.0 cm deep and 2.5–5.0 cm wide.[2] In terms of volume, as determined by the prolate ellipse formula of length x width x depth x 0.53, the normal uterus is < 100 cm^3. The myometrium is hypoechogenic and homogeneous and the endometrium is well demarcated from the myometrium (Fig. 2). The endometrium deserves additional description as

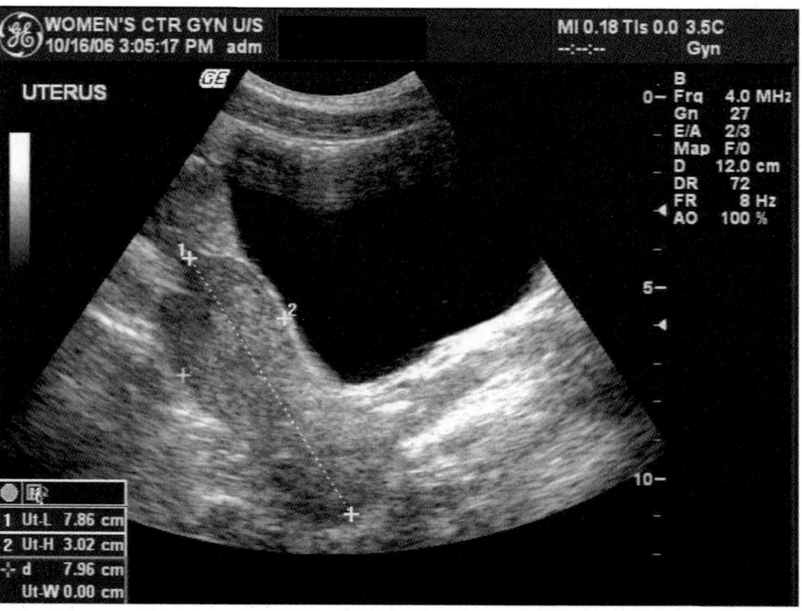

Fig. 1 Normal anteverted uterus seen by transabdominal ultrasound.

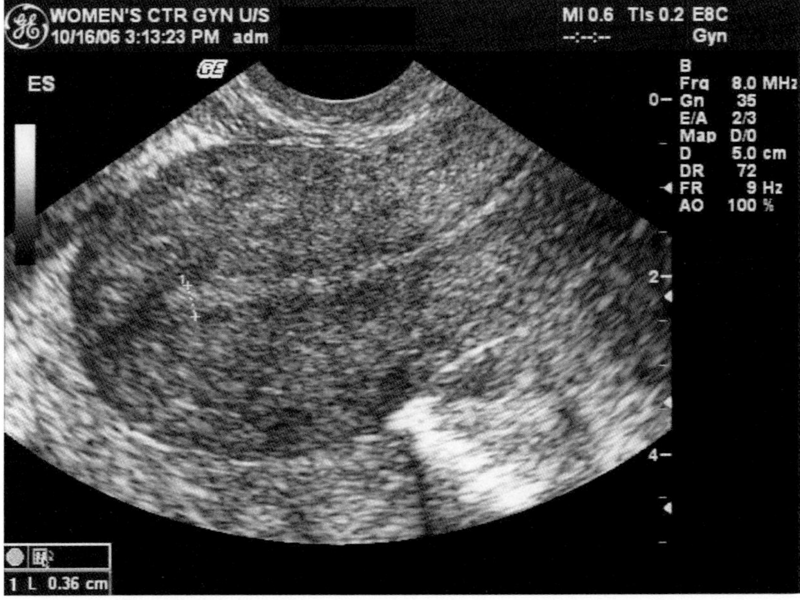

Fig. 2 Normal myometrium and endometrium in a postmenopausal woman visualized by transvaginal ultrasound.

it depends heavily the timing of the menstrual cycle. The endometrium is thinnest during menses and is usually 1–4 mm thick visualized as a single hyperechogenic line. During the follicular phase, the thickness increases to 8–15 mm and develops a 'trilaminar' appearance of two outer proliferating bands and a central canal echo. During the secretory phase, the endometrial thickness does not increase but the canal echo and out proliferating bands blend to form a single hyperechogenic band. The postmenopausal uterus is generally smaller than the premenopausal uterus and the endometrium has a maximum thickness of < 5 mm.[3]

Ovary

The normal resting ovary is moderately echogenic, well-demarcated and located just above the iliac vessels and lateral to the edge of the broad ligament (Fig. 3). Due to its mobility, it can also be found in the posterior cul de sac and also in the lower abdomen. The ovary goes through many changes during the menstrual cycle and even into the first few years of menopause. The cyclic ovarian changes that occur in the premenopausal ovary are dependent on numerous and complex hormonal factors and interplays. During the follicular phase, a group of antral follicles begin to develop; anywhere from 4–8 antral follicles measuring 3–5 mm in size by mid-proliferative phase (day 6–7). Usually only one developing follicle is selected to become the dominant follicle and ovulate so that by day 7, the dominant follicle begins to grow at a more rapid rate and reaches a maximum of 18–24 mm just prior to ovulation (day 14). The rest of the follicles can reach a maximum size of 10 mm before becoming atretic as the dominant follicle matures. At the time of ovulation,

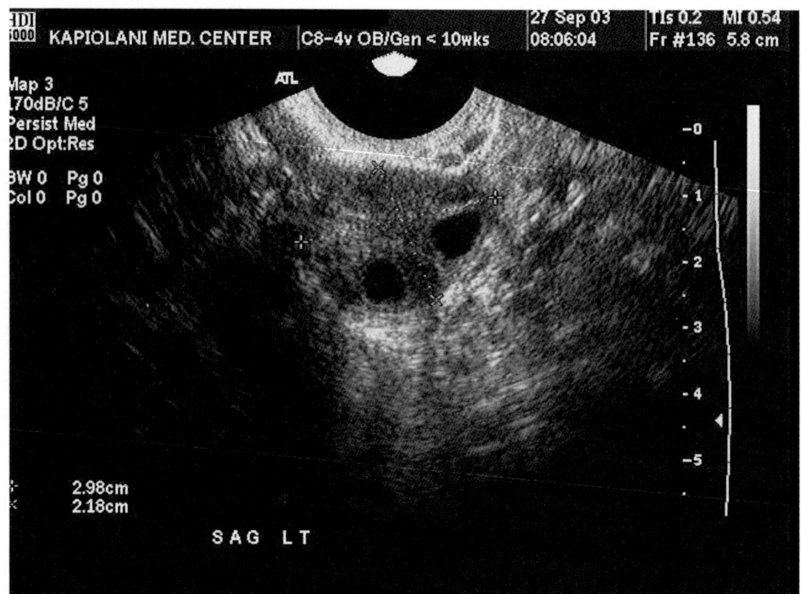

Fig. 3 Normal ovary in a menstruating woman.

there is a loss of the follicular fluid as the oocyte is expelled and the follicular cyst can disappear or diminish in size. There is further change in this follicle in which it becomes a corpus luteum and sometimes a hemorrhagic corpus luteum. The corpus luteum can take the shape of a cyst or a more solid, echogenic appearing structure within the ovary. The corpus luteum usually disappears within a day or two of menstruation.

UTERINE ABNORMALITIES

Fibroids

Ultrasound is an excellent method for diagnosing uterine myomas. Uterine leiomyomata are the most common uterine pathology. Uterine contour irregularity and enlargement are the most common features seen transabdominally and upon closer visualization transvaginally, the most common appearance is of a hypo-echoic or heterogeneous uterine mass (Fig. 4). When distinct uterine masses are not visualized, the myometrium can take on a heterogeneous, thickened appearance. Degenerative changes in a fibroid can take on differing echogenic patterns such as irregular, central anechoic areas as seen in cystic degeneration or as bright and highly echogenic areas with distal shadowing seen in calcified degeneration.

Location is also important to note due to the varied locations in which fibroids are found. Pedunculated myomas can mimic adnexal masses but visualizing a vascular 'bridge' connecting the mass in question to the uterus can help to confirm the diagnosis of a pedunculated myoma. Submucosal fibroids near the uterine fundus can distort the endometrium mimicking a bicornuate uterus but saline infusion sonography with excellent ultrasound

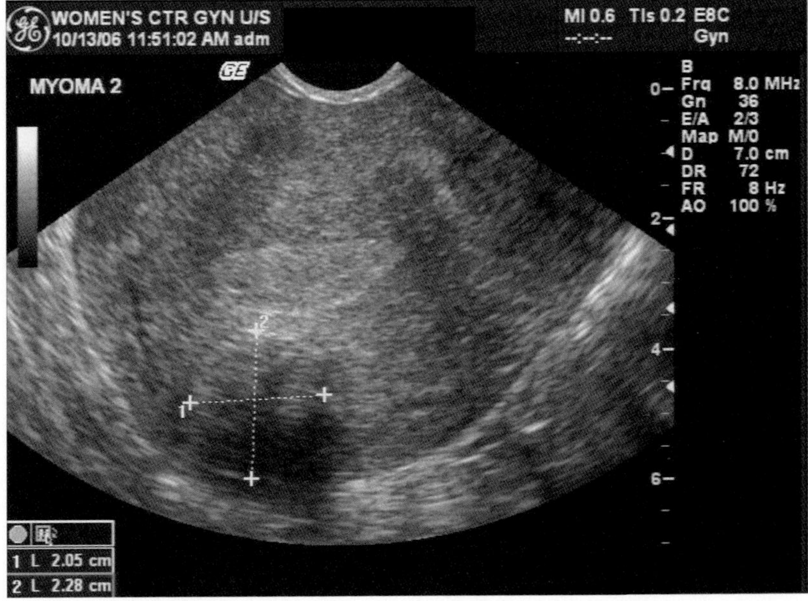

Fig. 4 Small intramural uterine fibroid.

technique can distinguish between a truly anomalous uterus and a submucosal fibroid.

Adenomyosis

Adenomyosis is a condition whereby endometrial glands and stroma deep in the myometrium are associated with surrounding myometrial hypertrophy. The clinical presentation classically associated with adenomyosis is excessive uterine bleeding accompanied by worsening dysmenorrhea. Ultrasound features of adenomyosis include: 'rainy' pattern of acoustic shadowing, normal vessels, enlarged uterus (AP diameter) and asymmetry. Adenomyosis is often seen along with leiomyomata uteri and fibroids can make it more difficult to diagnose adenomyosis. Reinhold *et al.*[4] showed that transvaginal ultrasound was able to correctly diagnose 25 of 29 pathologically proven cases of adenomyosis. Additionally, adenomyosis was correctly ruled out in 61 of 71 patients. In their hands, transvaginal ultrasound had a sensitivity of 86%, a specificity of 86%, and a positive and negative predictive value of 71% and 94%, respectively. Myometrial cysts characterized by cystic spaces ranging from 2–7 mm in diameter located within the myometrium were found in up to 52% of uteri with adenomyosis. Using the presence of myometrial cysts for diagnosing adenomyosis resulted in a sensitivity of 45%, a specificity of 100%, a positive predictive value of 100%, and a negative predictive value of 82%. The importance of this paper is not so much about the sensitivity but more so about the high negative predictive value for adenomyosis with the goal that it may prevent unnecessary surgery.

A few papers have described the more common diagnostic features of adenomyosis which include: diffuse heterogeneous echo texture of

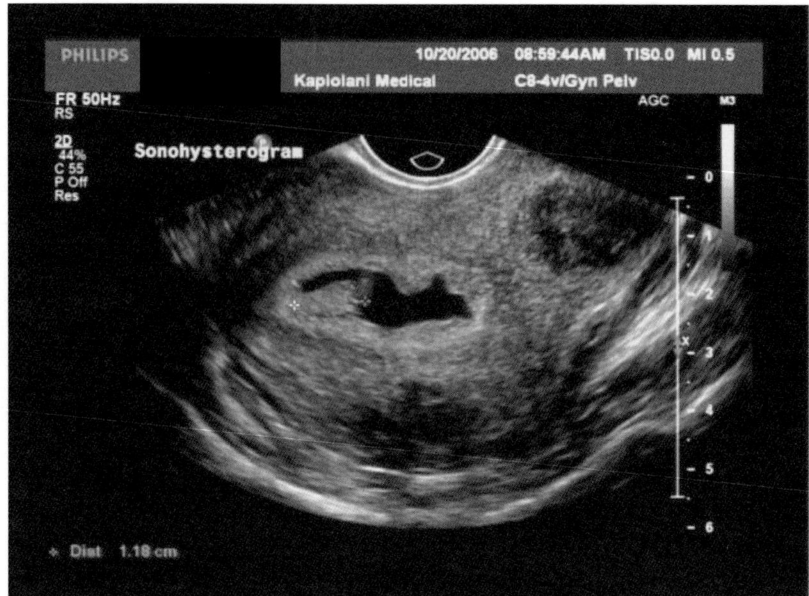

Fig. 5 Saline infusion sonography (SIS) in a patient with menorrhagia: endometrial polyps were visualized. Myometrium was shown with several intramural fibroids.

myometrium, asymmetric thickening of either the anterior or posterior wall of the uterus, subendometrial myometrial cysts which cause the endometrial–myometrial junction to be poorly defined, subendometrial echogenic nodules, subendometrial echogenic linear striations, and a globular, enlarged uterus without a definitive mass.[5,6]

Endometrial pathology

Endometrial pathology is suspected when a patient presents with abnormal uterine bleeding which includes irregular menstruation, menorrhagia, metrorrhagia, and menometrorrhagia. Anatomic abnormalities such as a submucous leiomyomata and endometrial polyps may be seen by ultrasound to explain the cause of the patient's symptoms (Fig. 5). There have been numerous studies that have compared the use of transvaginal ultrasound (TVS) and saline infusion sonography (SIS) with the 'gold standard' hysteroscopy. The advantage of SIS when compared to hysteroscopy is that it is well-tolerated, easily performed, with low cost and low risk, and minimally invasive. In the studies where SIS findings were compared with surgical findings and histological assessment (hysteroscopy + biopsy or hysterectomy), it was found that SIS has a high sensitivity (87–96%) and even higher specificity (91–100%) for evaluation of abnormal uterine bleeding.[7,8] Kamel *et al.*[9] reported that SIS is significantly more accurate than transvaginal sonography in the detection of endometrial polyps in cases with abnormal uterine bleeding. Combining both techniques did not significantly improve the diagnostic accuracy. For the detection of submucous fibroids, Farquhar *et al.*[10] reviewed 19 relevant studies and concluded that all 3 diagnostic tests were moderately accurate in detecting intra-uterine pathology. However, SIS and hysteroscopy performed better than transvaginal ultrasound in detecting submucous fibroids.

Postmenopausal bleeding

The challenge for the gynecologist is in determining which diagnostic approach to consider for a patient with postmenopausal bleeding. The traditional 'gold standard' is to perform a dilation and curettage but due to its invasiveness, discomfort and need for anesthesia, it has largely been replaced by an office endometrial biopsy as an equivalent diagnostic test. Reports show sensitivity rates for the use of a pipelle for endometrial biopsy in patients with postmenopausal bleeding to be greater than 95% for endometrial cancer and 88% for atypical hyperplasia, with specificity being greater than 98%.[11] Office endometrial biopsy remains an invasive procedure. However, it is poorly tolerated by some patients.

A meta-analysis of 35 studies which included 5892 women found that a thin (< 5 mm) endometrial stripe (double thickness measurement) on TVS can exclude endometrial disease in the majority of postmenopausal women with vaginal bleeding, regardless of hormone replacement use.[12] TVS has similar sensitivity as endometrial biopsy and can be used when endometrial biopsy is not available, non-diagnostic, or unsuccessful. Women on hormone replacement therapy (HRT) can also follow the > 5 mm cut-off for considering the endometrium abnormal and requiring further studies although it would increase the false positive rate. Some data support that it may be safe to refrain from endometrial biopsy in women with postmenopausal bleeding and endometrial thickness < 5 mm, but recurrence of bleeding should be an indication for endometrial biopsy regardless of endometrial stripe measurement.[3,12] As far as SIS is concerned, Epstein *et al.*[13] found it to be as good as hysteroscopy at detecting intra-uterine lesions in women with postmenopausal bleeding. They also concluded that neither hysteroscopy nor SIS could reliably discriminate between benign and malignant focal lesions. Gull *et al.*[3] found that no endometrial cancer cases were missed in about 400 women when the endometrial stripe was ≤ 4 mm on transvaginal sonography, even if the subjects were followed for 10 years. Women with recurrent bleeding were a high-risk group but women without recurrent bleeding were not at higher risk to develop endometrial cancer or atypia up to 10 years later. Lastly and importantly, they emphasized that a thick endometrium, with histopathology of atrophy or tissue insufficient for diagnosis, requires a guided biopsy or SIS.

Localization of intrauterine device (IUD)

Localizing an IUD by 2-D sonography has limitations and there is a paucity of data in this regard. The brightness of all arms of the IUD is very distinctive when visualized. Palo[14] reported that transabdominal and preferably transvaginal sonography could detect both proximal and distal ends of the vertical arm of the IUD. Shadowing of surrounding tissues also facilitated IUD detection. 3-D transvaginal sonography using multiplanar views has proven to be superior with full visualization of the complete IUD in about 95% of patients.[15]

OVARIAN/ADNEXAL ABNORMALITIES

Pelvic masses

Whether feeling a pelvic mass on routine examination or on examination as a result of a gynecologic complaint, frequently, if not always, raises the anxiety level of both the patient and clinician. More specifically, the concern is that it may be a malignancy. Ultrasound can offer a safe, quick, inexpensive and, in skilled hands, a relatively reliable method to help distinguish between most benign and malignant conditions of the adnexa (Figs 6 and 7). The goal is to avoid unwarranted and unnecessary invasive procedures (*i.e.* laparoscopy or laparotomy) and to prevent undue anxiety but at the same time not to miss or, at the least, delay the diagnosis of pelvic malignancy when it is, in fact, present.

Numerous studies have been published to help look at the sensitivity and specificity of ultrasound in differentiating benign versus malignant disease. Timmerman *et al.*[16] found that experienced ultrasonographers using some clinical information and subjective assessment of sonographic images can differentiate malignant from benign masses in most cases. Valentin[17] likewise found subjective evaluation of the gray-scale ultrasound image and color Doppler ultrasound examination ('pattern recognition'), to be superior to logistic regression models. Of course, not all pelvic masses are so easily classified, such as borderline malignancies. Clearly, certain morphological characteristics increase the risk for malignancy, especially if found contemporaneously. These could include, but are not limited to, solid components (*i.e.* excrescences or papillary projections) and any other irregularities, decreased resistance index, neovascularization and ascites. Of course, following changes over a short interval of time is also an important

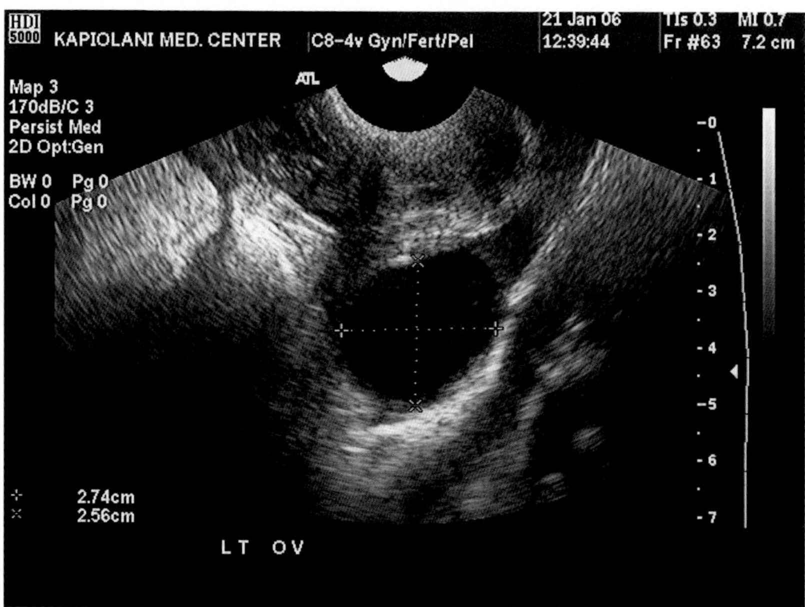

Fig. 6 Simple ovarian cyst in an asymptomatic postmenopausal woman. The size is less than 5 cm, thin walls, no internal echoes or papillary projections.

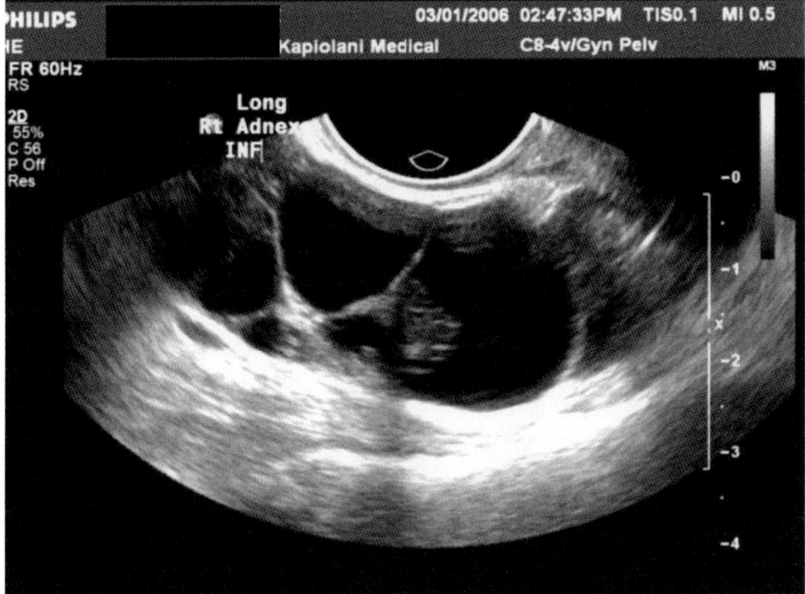

Fig. 7 Enlarged ovary in a postmenopausal woman, complex predominantly cystic ovarian mass with solid components and internal echoes. Ovarian malignancy was suspected on ultrasound and confirmed after surgery (cystadenocarcinoma).

component to any abnormal, suspicious finding that is not clear upon first examination. Doppler ultrasound can give information about vascularization of the adnexal mass.

Ectopic pregnancy

First trimester bleeding is common accounting for up to 30% of all diagnosed pregnancies.[18] Important causes of first trimester bleeding include spontaneous abortion/missed or threatened abortion, ectopic pregnancy, and gestational trophoblastic disease. Ultrasound evaluation of patients with first trimester bleeding is the mainstay of the examination. One of the greatest dilemmas in early pregnancy ultrasound is to determine the cause of pain or bleeding accurately. The clinician's goal is to first determine if a pregnancy exists in a woman of reproductive age who presents with abdominal/pelvic pain, vaginal bleeding, syncope, or hypotension. If the patient is pregnant, the next crucial step is to determine where the pregnancy is located. The differential diagnosis lies between an intra-uterine pregnancy that may be too early to detect, a complete miscarriage or an ectopic pregnancy. The β-human chorionic gonadotropin (β-hCG) radioimmunoassay is a crucial adjunct to assist the clinician in the interpretation of transvaginal ultrasound. However, delay in more definitive treatment (*i.e.* surgery) should not occur if a ruptured ectopic pregnancy is suspected. If β-hCG levels are followed, it should be noted that 85% of normal intra-uterine pregnancies exhibit the expected 66% rise in titer in 48 hours. β-hCG levels have a sensitivity of 85% with a false positive rate of 15%.[18] A less than expected rise may be indicative of an ectopic

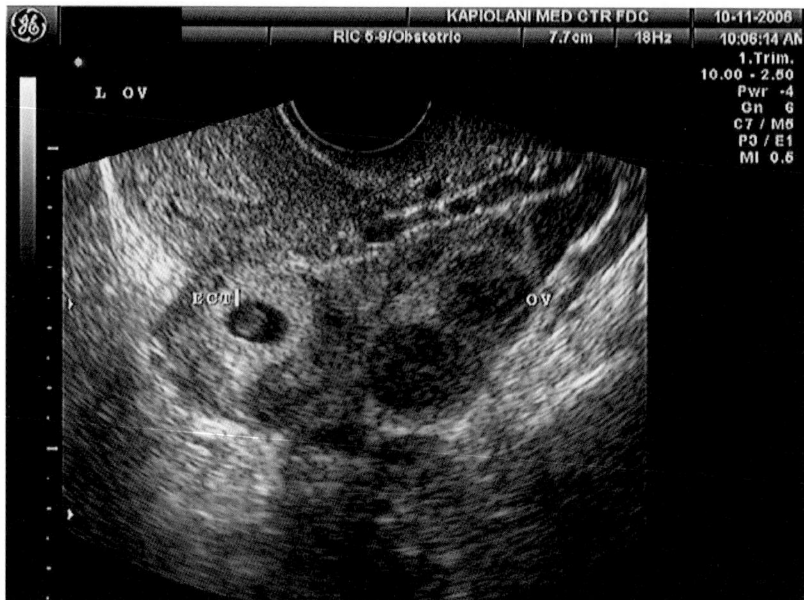

Fig. 8 Ectopic pregnancy with an embryo (ECT). Empty uterus was seen above the left adnexal mass and ovary (OV) visualized to the left.

pregnancy or an abnormal/failed intra-uterine pregnancy. With that in mind, equivocal ultrasound results should be combined with quantitative β-hCG levels; if the level is ≥ 1500 mIU/ml or greater, ectopic pregnancy should be suspected.[19] Intra-uterine gestational sac visualization by transvaginal with β-hCG levels between 1000–2000 mIU/ml should be present. Yolk sac visualization within the gestational sac is definitive evidence of intra-uterine pregnancy. Embryonic cardiac activity can usually be seen with CRL of > 5 mm. Conversely, a gestational sac (GS) with a mean sac diameter (MSD) of 8 mm or more without a yolk sac and a GS with an MSD of 16 mm or more without an embryo, are predictive of pregnancy failure.[19]

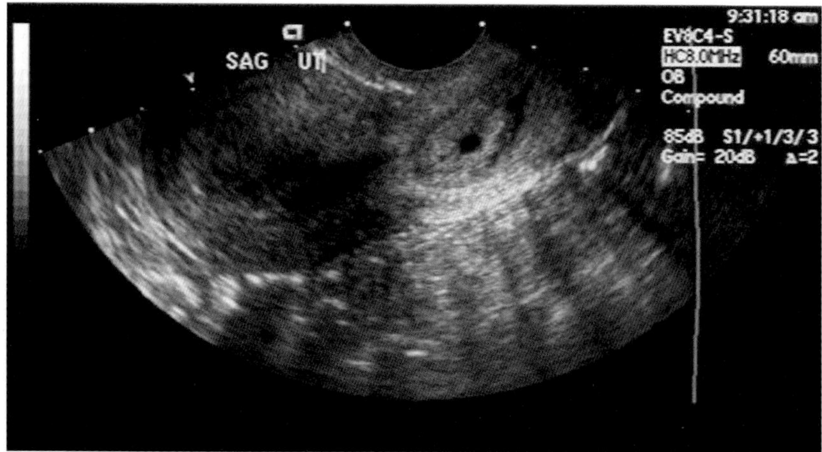

Fig. 9 Cervical ectopic pregnancy. Embryo not visualized.

The most telling ultrasound finding in an ectopic pregnancy is a live embryo in the adnexae (seen in 20–25% of ectopic pregnancies by transvaginal scan), followed by a tubal ring (doughnut or bagel sign) with or without hemorrhage, intra-uterine pseudosac along with complex adnexal mass, free fluid (especially of low level echogenicity) in the adnexa or cul de sac, and thickened endometrium with no viable intra-uterine pregnancy at discriminatory levels of serum β-hCG (Figs 8 and 9). It must be borne in mind that two conditions exist whereby visualization of confirmatory signs of an intra-uterine pregnancy would be delayed beyond achieving the discriminatory level of β-hCG. These conditions are early multiple gestation and heterotopic pregnancy. Care must be taken to consider these possibilities especially if the patient is hemodynamically stable and offer repeat ultrasound in 7–10 days and/or repeat quantitative β-hCG levels to assure normally rising titers. The rise in titer may actually exceed this minimum in the above two scenarios.

PELVIC PAIN

Acute or chronic pelvic pain accounts for up to 10% of all gynecologic referrals/visits and is a very common reason for an emergency room (ER) visit.[20] The most common concern for acute pelvic pain is ovarian torsion and pelvic inflammatory disease (PID) or tubo-ovarian abscess (TOA). The most sensitive and reproducible diagnostic criterion for PID is pelvic pain. The following gives an assessment of the utility of transvaginal ultrasound and color Doppler for sorting through the differential diagnoses of acute and chronic pelvic pain.

Ovarian torsion

Ovarian torsion is a surgical emergency especially if ovarian conservation is being contemplated; but the dilemma has been in accurately making this diagnosis pre-operatively on the basis of imaging studies. Ultrasound features include: enlarged ovary that appears edematous, heterogeneous echo texture, small cystic areas towards the periphery and some free fluid. Comparison with the morphologic appearance and blood flow patterns (by Doppler ultrasound) of the contralateral ovary is very important for diagnosis (Fig. 10). Here are some helpful hints: (i) palpatory information provides added value at no extra cost; (ii) have the patient use pain scale in order to determine the site most likely to be the source of pain; and (iii) distinguish between the unpleasant pressure of examination and focal pain.

A number of studies have demonstrated the utility of ultrasound in the pre-operative determination of ovarian torsion with varying reliability. Tepper *et al.*[21] found that the combination of Doppler flow imaging along with the morphologic assessment improves the diagnostic accuracy of ovarian torsion. In this study, the authors displayed no blood flow within 8 of 22 ovaries suspected of ovarian torsion, which was confirmed by laparoscopy. Ben-Ami and co-authors[22] prospectively investigated the ability of color flow Doppler to predict ovarian torsion and had 15 surgically proven ovarian torsion patients exhibit abnormal color and spectral Doppler studies. In 5 cases, there was no venous blood flow but peripheral arterial flow was detected. Conversely,

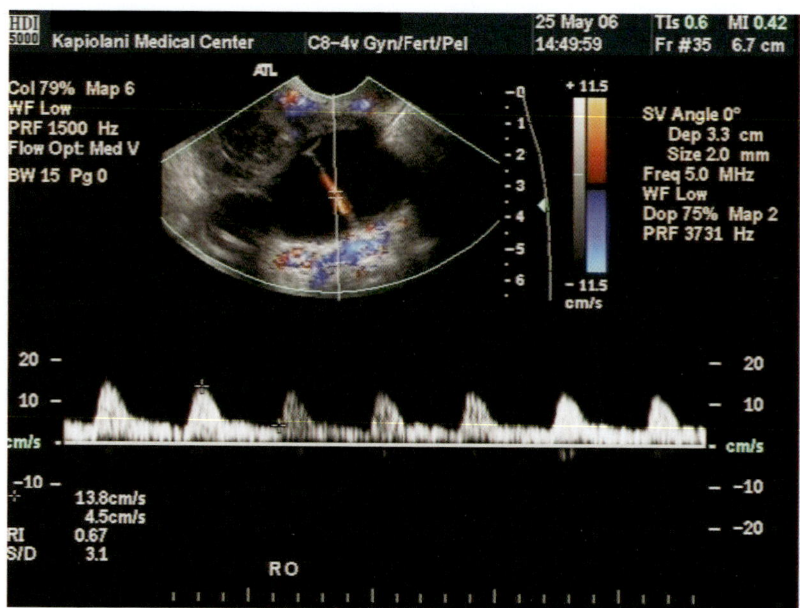

Fig. 10 Abundant arterial (shown) and venous blood flow visualized by Doppler ultrasound in a patient with severe acute pelvic pain and multicystic ovarian mass. Ovarian torsion was excluded.

torsion was very unlikely if Doppler studies showed venous flow. They found that the sensitivity, specificity, positive and negative predictive values of the color and spectral Doppler examinations in detecting ovarian torsion were 100, 98, 94 and 100, respectively. This study demonstrated that the visualization of arterial flow by color Doppler does not rule out ovarian torsion. Pena[23] had similar findings and additionally found that normal flow detected by Doppler sonography missed 60% of the cases of ovarian torsion and led to delay in this subsequent diagnosis. Lee *et al.*[24] showed an 87% rate of detecting twisted ovarian vessels pre-operatively by color Doppler studies.

Endometriosis

Endometriosis is by far the most common etiology of chronic pelvic pain. The diagnosis of endometriosis is made either by laparoscopy or laparotomy but the clinician's challenge is to have high degree of suspicion for this diagnosis pre-operatively as proper assessments and patient pre-operative preparations (*i.e.* bowel preparation, informed consent issues) can improve outcomes. Endometriotic cysts seen on ultrasound are usually multilocular and characterized by homogeneous low to medium level echoes and they have thick walls (Fig. 11). Hemorrhagic cyst should be on differential diagnosis list.

There have been a number of studies that have clearly shown the efficacy and accuracy of sonography for the differentiation of ovarian endometriomas and other ovarian neoplasms especially when transvaginal ultrasound was employed.[25] The 'typical' sonographic appearance of endometriotic ovarian cysts has been described as containing low-level internal echoes, multiloculations and hyperechoic, thickened cyst walls. To

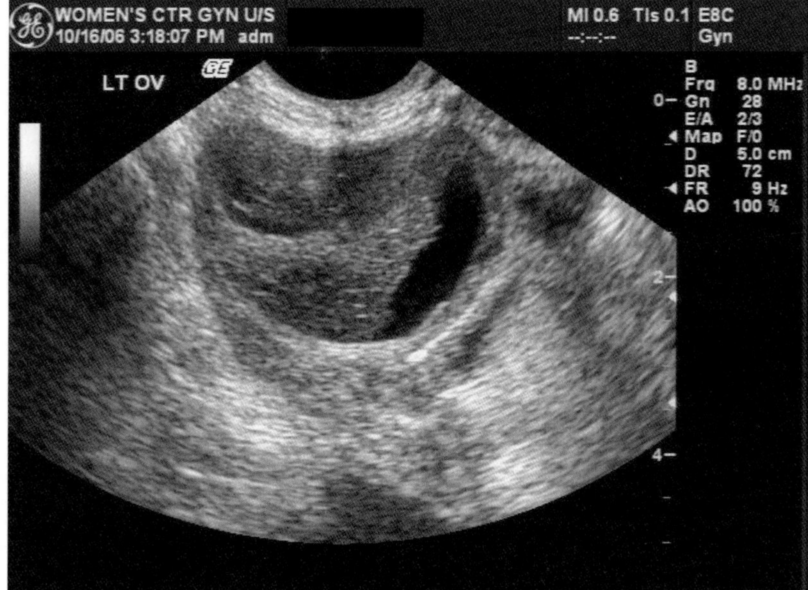

Fig. 11 Endometriosis of the ovary. Multilocular cysts with homogeneous low to medium level echoes and thick walls are visualized.

confuse the issue, there are numerous cases of a variety of sonomorphologic appearances for endometriomas. Nevertheless, Mais *et al.*[26] noted a sensitivity of 75% and a specificity of 99% in the screening for ovarian endometriosis, and a sensitivity of 84% and specificity of 90% in screening for other ovarian masses. The utility of Doppler ultrasound in distinguishing ovarian endometriosis from other ovarian masses was also investigated.[27] In a validation study of non-surgical diagnosis of endometriosis, Eskenazi *et al.*[28] found that ovarian endometriosis could be reliably predicted with transvaginal sonography. Ultrasound and physical examination best predicted ovarian endometriosis, with a 100% correct diagnoses and no false positives in this study sample of 21 ovarian endometriosis cases. Non-ovarian endometriosis did not have good correlation with examination or ultrasound with only 38% of the non-ovarian endometriosis being accurately predicted by a combination of indicators. Examination findings that Eskenazi considered 'positive' for the study above were uterosacral pain, fixed adnexal mass, painful adnexal mass, pain in the posterior cul de sac, nodularity in the posterior cul de sac or uterosacral ligaments, scarring in the uterosacral ligaments, pain on movement of uterus and vaginal or endometriotic lesions.

As stated above, transvaginal sonography is poor at detecting the presence of adhesions and mild endometriotic implants on peritoneal surfaces. In deep infiltrating disease, where endometriosis involves the posterior cul de sac, hypo-echoic linear thickening, or nodules/masses can be seen. The posterior cul de sac can also be obliterated with or without free fluid. With this in mind, Bazot *et al.*[29] found a 79%, 95%, 95% and 78% sensitivity, specificity, positive and negative predictive values, respectively for TVS predicting deep infiltrating pelvic endometriosis in women who had clinical signs of endometriosis. A prospective study by Exacoustos *et al.*[30] of 121 women concluded that ultrasonographic findings can predict extent and stage of endometriosis. Prior to laparoscopy, all women had ultrasonographic 'staging' done for their presumed endometriosis (using ovarian endometriomas and other sonographic markers such as peritoneal nodules). There was 83.5% concordance between sonographic and laparoscopic staging for endometriosis. With a high degree of suspicion and with experienced sonographers, severe endometriosis and ovarian endometriosis can be predicted to a fair degree of accuracy and reliability.

Pelvic inflammatory disease

Pelvic inflammatory disease (PID) can cause acute or chronic pelvic pain (mainly in the form of adhesive disease). Hydrosalpinx is seen by ultrasound as tubular adnexal structure with septations or nodules in its wall (Fig. 12). There is a paucity of studies that attempt to diagnose acute or chronic PID by sonographic criteria. Boardman *et al.*[31] conducted a study of 55 women who either met the Centers for Disease Control and Prevention's minimal criteria for acute pelvic inflammatory disease or were being evaluated for non-classic signs of upper genital tract infection. PID was confirmed by laparoscopic visualization or by histological or microbiological evidence of salpingitis or endometritis. In this study, ultrasound showed a sensitivity of 36% and specificity of 48%, and a likelihood ratio of 1.33 for diagnosing PID. Based on these results, the authors of this study could not recommend the routine use of ultrasound in the evaluation of patients with suspected PID.

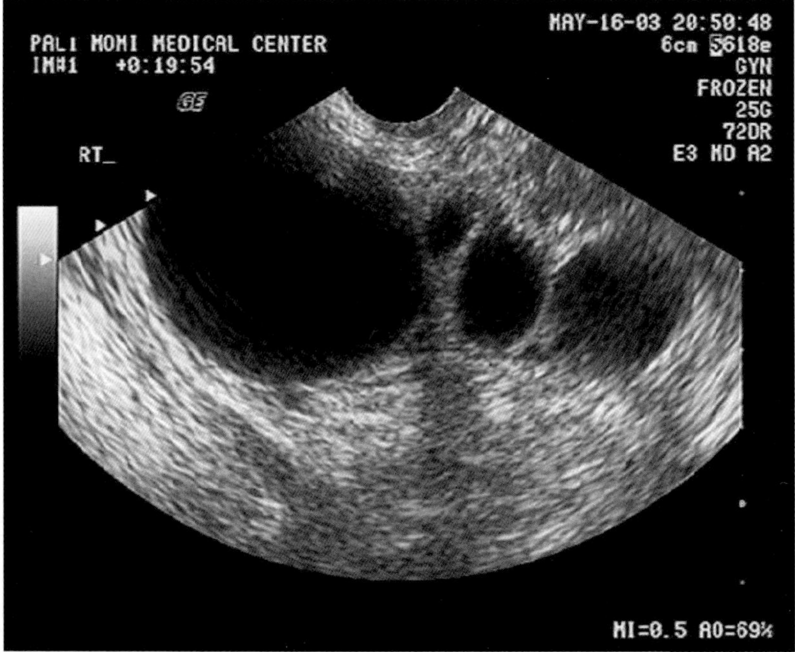

Fig. 12 Tubular adnexal structure with septations was seen in a patient with chronic pelvic pain. Hydrosalpinx was suspected and confirmed on surgery.

CONCLUSIONS

Gynecologic ultrasound brings 'light' into female pelvis, making the uterus and ovaries visible to a practicing clinician. This modality can help in diagnosis and management of many uterine and ovarian/adnexal disorders. Ultrasound evaluation of the female pelvis can give information about morphology, hormonal status, sensation (pain mapping), pelvic organ mobility and vascular anatomy. The ultrasound examination must be technically adequate and all of the uterus, ovary and pelvic mass if present should be clearly visualized. Most pelvic masses can be characterized by B-mode and Doppler ultrasound and this can significantly influence management plans. Gynecologic ultrasound is among the most important advances in modern obstetrics and gynecology. Its simplicity and ease of operation is changing the gynecologic office and ER practice. It is now the new era of image-based gynecology.

KEY POINTS FOR CLINICAL PRACTICE

- Ultrsound brings 'light' into the female pelvis visualizing the uterus and adnexa.
- This imaging modality can help in diagnosis and management of many uterine and ovarian or adnexal disorders.
- Clinical information is obtained about morphology, hormonal status, sensation (pain mapping), pelvic organ mobility and vascular anatomy.
- The ultrasound exam must be technically adequate.
- Most of pelvic masses can be characterized by B-mode and Doppler ultrasound.

References

1 AIUM Practice guidelines for the performance of the ultrasound examination of the female pelvis. 2006, <http://www.aium.org/publications/clinical/pelvis.pdf>

2 Sample WF, Lippe BM, Gyepes MT. Gray-scale ultrasonography of the normal female pelvis. Radiology 1977; 125: 477–483

3 Gull B, Karlsson B, Milsom I, Granberg D. Can ultrasound replace dilation and curettage? A longitudinal evaluation of postmenopausal bleeding and transvaginal sonographic measurement of the endometrium as predictors of endometrial cancer. Am J Obstet Gynecol 2003; 188: 401–408

4 Reinhold C, Atri M, Mehio A, Zakarian R, Aldis AE, Bret PM. Diffuse uterine adenomyosis: morphologic criteria and diagnostic accuracy of endovaginal sonography. Radiology 1995; 197: 609–614

5 Atri M, Reinhold C, Mehio AR, Chapman WB, Bret PM. Adenomyosis: US features with histologic correlation in an *in-vitro* study. Radiology 2000; 215: 783–790

6 Chopra S, Lev-Toaff A,Ors F, Bergin D. Adenomyosis: common and uncommon manifestations on sonography and magnetic resonance imaging. J Ultrasound Med 2006; 25: 617–627

7 Widrich T, Bradley LD, Mitchinson AR, Collins RL. Comparison of saline infusion sonography with office hysteroscopy for the evaluation of the endometrium. Am J Obstet Gynecol 1996; 174: 1327–1334

8 Schwarzler P, Concin H, Bosch H *et al*. An evaluation of sonohysterography and

diagnostic hysteroscopy for the assessment of intrauterine pathology. Ultrasound Obstet Gynecol 1998; 11: 337–342
9 Kamel HS, Darwish AM, Mohamed SA. Comparison of transvaginal ultrasonography and vaginal sonohysterography in the detection of endometrial polyps. Acta Obstet Gynecol Scand 2000; 79: 60–64
10 Farquhar C, Ekeroma A, Furness S, Arroll B. A systematic review of transvaginal ultrasonography, sonohysterography and hysteroscopy for the investigation of abnormal uterine bleeding in premenopausal women. Acta Obstet Gynecol Scand 2003; 82: 493–504
11 Gupta JK, Wilson S, Desai P, Hau C. How should we investigate women with postmenopausal bleeding? Acta Obstet Gynecol Scand 1996; 75: 475–479
12 Smith-Bindman R, Kerlikowske K, Feldstein VA *et al.* Endovaginal ultrasound to exclude endometrial cancer and other endometrial abnormalities. JAMA 1998; 280: 1510–1517
13 Epstein E, Ramirez A, Skoog L, Valentin L. Transvaginal sonography, saline contrast sonohysterography and hysteroscopy for the investigation of women with postmenopausal bleeding and endometrium > 5 mm. Ultrasound Obstet Gynecol 2001; 18: 157–162
14 Palo P. Transabdominal and transvaginal ultrasound detection of levonorgestrel IUD in the uterus. Acta Obstet Gynecol Scand 1997; 76: 244–247
15 Lee A, Eppel W, Sam C, Kratochwil A, Deutinger J, Bernaschek G. Intrauterine device localization by three-dimensional transvaginal sonography. Ultrasound Obstet Gynecol 1997; 10: 289–292
16 Timmerman D, Schwarzler P, Collins WP *et al.* Subjective assessment of adnexal masses with the use of ultrasonography: an analysis of interobserver variability and experience. Ultrasound Obstet Gynecol 1999; 13: 11–16
17 Valentin L, Hagen B, Tingulstad S, Eik-Nes S. Comparison of 'pattern recognition' and logistic regression models for discrimination between benign and malignant pelvic masses: a prospective cross validation. Ultrasound Obstet Gynecol 2001; 18: 357–365
18 Dogra V, Paspulati RM, Bhatt S. First trimester bleeding evaluation. Ultrasound Q 2005; 21: 69–85
19 Lozeau A, Potter B. Diagnosis and management of ectopic pregnancy. Am Fam Physician 2005; 72: 1707–1714
20 Reiter RC. A profile of women with chronic pelvic pain. Clin Obstet Gynecol 1990; 33: 130–136
21 Tepper R, Zalel Y, Goldberger S, Cohen I, Markov S, Beyth Y. Diagnostic value of transvaginal color Doppler flow in ovarian torsion. Eur J Obstet Gynecol Reprod Biol 1996; 68: 115–118
22 Ben-Ami M, Perlitz Y, Haddad S. The effectiveness of spectral and color Doppler in predicting ovarian torsion: a prospective study. Eur J Obstet Gynecol Reprod Biol 2002; 104: 64–66
23 Pena JE, Ufberg D, Cooney N, Denis AL. Usefulness of Doppler sonography in the diagnosis of ovarian torsion. Fertil Steril 2000; 73: 1047–1050
24 Lee EJ, Kwon HC, Joo HJ, Suh JH, Fleischer AC. Diagnosis of ovarian torsion with color Doppler sonography: depiction of twisted vascular pedicle. J Ultrasound Med 1998; 17: 83–89
25 Fleischer AC, Entman SS. Differential diagnosis of pelvic masses. In: Chervenak FA, Isaacson GC, Campbell S. (eds) Ultrasound in Obstetrics and Gynecology. Boston, MA: Little, Brown, 1993; 1643–1653
26 Mais V, Guerriero S, Ajossa S, Angiolucci M, Paoletti AM, Melis GB. The efficiency of transvaginal ultrasonography in the diagnosis of endometrioma. Fertil Steril 1993; 60: 776–780
27 Kurjak A, Kupesic S. Scoring system for prediction of ovarian endometriosis based on transvaginal color and pulsed Doppler sonography. Fertil Steril 1994; 62: 81–88
28 Eskenazi B, Warner M, Bonsignore L, Olive D, Samuels S, Vercellini P. Validation study of nonsurgical diagnosis of endometriosis. Fertil Steril 2001; 76: 929–935
29 Bazot M, Thomassin I, Hourani R, Cortez A, Darai E. Diagnostic accuracy of transvaginal sonography for deep pelvic endometriosis. Ultrasound Obstet Gynecol 2004; 24: 180–185
30 Exacoustos C, Zupi E, Carusotti C *et al.* Staging of pelvic endometriosis: role of sonographic appearance in determining extension of disease and modulating surgical approach. J Am Assoc Gynecol Laparosc 2003; 10: 378–382
31 Boardman LA, Peipert JF, Brody JM, Cooper AS, Sung J. Endovaginal sonography for the diagnosis of upper genital tract infection. Obstet Gynecol 1997; 90: 54–7

Kevin M. Holcomb Thomas A. Caputo
Robert C. Knapp

Diagnosis of ovarian cancer

Epithelial ovarian cancer (EOC) has long been thought to be a silent killer, offering little or no characteristic symptoms until advanced disease has developed. While recent studies have questioned the validity of this long-held belief, early diagnosis of EOC has remained an elusive goal. The disease is presently detected in three situations: (i) the screening of asymptomatic women; (ii) screening of high-risk women; and (iii) the diagnostic evaluation of women with characteristic symptoms. The diagnostic modalities utilized differ between these three conditions as well as the definition of an abnormal test result. The following chapter is a review of the performance of the various EOC screening tests in the general and high-risk populations as well as the search for symptoms that characterize early-stage disease. Both areas of research seek to attain the same goal: an improvement in survival for one of the deadliest gynecological malignancies.

OVARIAN CANCER SCREENING

The purpose of cancer screening is to decrease the morbidity and mortality associated with a specific disease through early detection. This aim is achieved through the performance of cost-effective tests applied to an asymptomatic population that is at significant risk for the disease. The screen is not diagnostic of the disease itself, but identifies a population that requires more specific

Kevin M. Holcomb MD
Associate Professor, Department of Obstetrics and Gynecology, Weill Medical College of Cornell University 525 East 68th Street, Suite J-130, New York, NY 10021, USA

Thomas A. Caputo MD
Professor Obstetrics and Gynecology, Department of Obstetrics and Gynecology, Division of Gynecologic Oncology, Weill Medical College of Cornell University, 525 East 68th Street, Suite J-130, New York, NY 10021, USA

Robert C. Knapp MD (for correspondence)
Professor Emeritus, Harvard Medical School, Boston, Massachusetts, USA. E-mail: rknapp@nyc.rr.com

testing to determine if treatment is required. The ideal screening test is inexpensive and is not associated with significant discomfort or inconvenience to the patient. The yield per test is expected to be low. Diagnostic tests differ from screening tests in that they are applied to symptomatic populations, tend to be more expensive, and have a higher yield per test. Certain characteristics make particular cancers good candidates for screening programs. These cancers are associated with significant morbidity and mortality in the population being screened. In addition, the cancers must have a prevalent and identifiable preclinical state during which diagnosis leads to an improvement in survival. Finally, there must be an available screening test with sufficient sensitivity and specificity to achieve the goal of decreased morbidity and mortality. Although there are more than 100 different types of cancer, only cancers of the cervix, breast, colon-rectal, and skin have widely accepted screening tests.

The validity of a screening test is determined by its ability to predict accurately the presence or absence of preclinical disease or at the earliest stage of the malignancy. A true positive screening test is an abnormal test for cancer in an individual who is subsequently found to have cancer within a defined period after the test. The sensitivity of a screening test is its ability to detect those individuals with cancer in the population while the specificity is the ability of the test to identify those individuals free from cancer in the population. The predictive values are a function of the sensitivity and specificity of the test as well as the prevalence of the disease in the population. Table 1 outlines the cross tabulation between disease status and test results and gives formulas for the calculation of sensitivity, specificity, positive, and negative predictive values. The sensitivity and specificity of a screening test may be altered by the definition of an 'abnormal' test result. The determination of a cut-off for normal is a compromise between increasing sensitivity and decreasing specificity. For example, lowering the threshold for an abnormal test will result in fewer false negatives and a more sensitive test. The same manipulation, however, also increases the probability of false positive results and, therefore, decreases specificity. Effective screening tests require a very high specificity while the sensitivity is less critical. In ovarian cancer, a specificity of 99.6% is necessary to achieve a positive predictive value of 10% (9 false-positive results for each true-positive detected).[1]

Table 1 Evaluation of the validity of screening tests

	True disease status	
Screening test results	Present	Absent
Positive	TP	FP
Negative	FN	TN

TP, true positive; FP, false positive; FN, false negative; TN, true negative.
Sensitivity = TP/(TP + FN) x 100.
Specificity = TN/(TN + FP) x 100.
Positive predictive value = TP/(TP + FP) x 100.
Negative predictive value = TN/(TN + FN) x 100.

There are several sources of potential bias that may explain an apparent improved survival in cases of a cancer detected by screening. The most important are lead-time, length, and selection bias. Lead-time bias occurs when the screening test advances the date of diagnosis but has no effect on the natural history of the disease. In this scenario, the interval between cancer detection by screening and the time it would have presented with symptoms is included in the calculation of survival. This leads to the false impression of increased survival in screen-detected cancers and must be considered when evaluating any screening test. Another potential source of bias is length-time bias. This occurs when screening is more likely to detect less aggressive tumors that have a longer preclinical period. These tumors would likely have a relatively good prognosis even in the absence of screening as compared to the highly aggressive interval cancers. In an extreme example of length bias, lesions that meet the clinical criteria of malignancy but are of no clinical significance are detected. Finally, patients who elect to undergo cancer screening may differ from patients who do not in ways that effect survival leading to a selection bias. When evaluating cancer screening programs, a comparison of mortality in the screened and unscreened populations is the most valid study end-point because it avoids both lead-time and length-time biases. Prospective, randomized, controlled trials and case-control studies using mortality and other end-points such as survival and quality of life have been used to evaluate the efficacy of screening tests.

Ovarian cancer is the 6th leading cause of death due to cancer and the 7th most frequent site of cancer in women in the developed world. There are an estimated 192,000 cases per year world-wide[2] and there is great variation in the geographic distribution of the disease. The highest incidence is found in North America and Europe, especially the Nordic countries and the UK.[3] It is generally a disease of postmenopausal women that develops between 60 and 64 years of age. The overall 5-year survival is 48.4% but ranges from 89.9% for patients with stage IA disease to only 16.8% for patients with stage IV disease.[4] Unfortunately, about 75% of patients are diagnosed with advanced stage disease (III or IV). These findings suggest that an effective screening program that could shift toward an earlier stage at diagnosis would have a significant impact on survival in this disease. While this is theoretically true, ovarian cancer presents some unique challenges for the development of such a screening program.

Unlike cervical or colon carcinoma, where known pre-clinical and pre-malignant lesions have been identified, no such entity has been identified in the ovary. There has even been some debate regarding the origin of ovarian carcinoma. The fact that apparent early stage ovarian cancer can involve both ovaries at presentation has led some to suggest that ovarian cancer 'metastases' may represent a polyclonal process with multifocal carcinogenesis. If this were the case, screening would be unlikely to result in survival benefit due to the lack of a localized preclinical period. For example, a study of allelic loss and mutational patterns of the P53 gene in patients with primary peritoneal serous carcinoma showed variation at multiple tumor sites, suggesting a polyclonal origin of this disease.[5] Tsao *et al.*,[6] however, found identical patterns of allelic deletion and X-chromosome inactivation at various tumor sites in 16 patients with stage III ovarian cancer, offering strong evidence of the clonal nature of the disease.

Another challenge of ovarian cancer screening is its low prevalence, even in the highest risk areas. The ovarian cancer incidence in Denmark between 1978 and 1998, one of the highest in Europe, was only 23/100,000.[7] This low prevalence has its main impact on the positive- and negative-predictive values of the screening test being evaluated and requires a exceedingly specific test to reach an acceptable level of false-positive results. Epidemiological studies have identified specific genetic, reproductive, and environmental factors that increase the risk of ovarian cancer. The efficacy of screening is more likely to be proven in high-risk populations due to the increased prevalence of the disease. Epithelial ovarian cancer is primarily a disease of postmenopausal women and 90% of cases occur in women older than 50 years. Screening trials performed in the general population, therefore, usually target these women.

Family history has consistently been proven to be a significant factor in determining a woman's risk of developing ovarian cancer. For example, the baseline risk of developing ovarian cancer in a woman with no family history of the disease is 1.6%. A woman with one first-degree relative with ovarian cancer has about a 4–5% risk of developing the disease.[8] The risk is further increased to approximately 7% when two first-degree relatives are affected.[9] It should be noted that the majority of ovarian cancers are sporadic and only 7% of ovarian cancer patients report a family history of the disease.

It has been estimated that about 10% of ovarian cancer cases are part of a hereditary cancer syndrome. Three distinct syndromes have been described – breast–ovarian cancer syndrome, site-specific ovarian cancer syndrome, and hereditary non-polyposis colon cancer syndrome (HNPCC). The first two are associated with germ line mutations in the BRCA-1 and BRCA-2 tumor suppressor genes and account for about 90% of hereditary ovarian cancers. HNPCC is associated with mutations in germ line DNA mismatch repair genes, primarily hMLH1 and hMSH2, and accounts for about 10% of hereditary ovarian cancer. The cumulative life-time risk of ovarian cancer is 40–50% for BRCA-1 mutation carriers and 20–30% for BRCA-2 mutation carriers. HNPCC is associated with a greater than 12% risk of ovarian cancer.[10] Data from the US, Israel, and Australia indicate that 1–2% of Ashkenazi Jews carry a pathogenic ancestral mutation of the BRCA-1 gene. These prevalence estimates were determined by DNA testing of individuals without selection by family or personal history of cancer. In the following sections, we will review the efficacy data for the available screening tools in both the general and high-risk populations.

Pelvic ultrasound

Pelvic sonography has long been the primary technique used to evaluate adnexal masses palpable on pelvic examination and it was one of the earliest modalities evaluated as a potential ovarian cancer screen. Sonography, particularly by the transvaginal route, is very sensitive for the detection of ovarian pathology and it was hypothesized that it could detect the earliest morphological changes associated with ovarian carcinogenesis. DePriest *et al.*[11] performed pelvic ultrasounds on 121 women undergoing exploratory laparotomy for ovarian masses and found no cancers with a volume less than 10 cm^3. Ovarian wall structure, however, was the most reliable morphological characteristic in distinguishing ovarian cancers from benign lesions. In this study,[11] a morphological index including ovarian volume, wall and septal structure provided a positive predictive value of 45% for the detection of ovarian cancer.

One of the largest studies examining the efficacy of transvaginal sonographic screening in asymptomatic women at risk for ovarian cancer was performed through the University of Kentucky Ovarian Cancer Screening Project.[12] Between 1987 and 1999, 14,469 women were screened with annual transvaginal sonograms. Entry criteria included age ≥ 50 years or age ≥ 25 years with a history of ovarian cancer in a first or second degree relative. Annual transvaginal sonogram was performed and ovarian volume calculated using the prolate ellipsoid formula (length x width x height x 0.523). Ovarian volumes greater than 10 cm^3 and 20 cm^3 were considered abnormal postmenopausal and premenopausal women, respectively. In addition, any cystic ovarian mass with a solid or papillary projection into the lumen was considered abnormal. Patients with an abnormal sonogram underwent a repeat TVS in 4–6 weeks and those with persistent abnormalities were recommended surgical exploration. The enrolled women underwent over 57,000 sonograms and 180 women underwent surgical exploration (1.2%) due to persistent abnormalities. Seventeen ovarian cancers were detected (11 epithelial, 3 granulosa cell tumors, 3 borderline tumors), 14 of which were stage I or II at the time of diagnosis. The sensitivity of TVS for the detection of ovarian cancer in this trial was 81%, the specificity 98.9%, and the positive predictive value 9.4%. When borderline tumors, stromal tumors and advanced epithelial ovarian cancers were excluded, however, the sensitivity of TVS for the detection of stage I epithelial cancers was only 31%. The survival of ovarian cancer patients in the screened group was 88% at 5 years, far higher than the 50% survival typical of unscreened populations. This finding, however, is subject to length bias in that TVS screening may have preferentially detected biologically less aggressive tumors. This study confirmed the observations of many of the prior ovarian cancer screening trials that TVS is not ideally sensitive and may result in many unnecessary surgical interventions for each ovarian cancer detected.

Other radiological modalities

Computed tomography, magnetic resonance imaging, and positron emission tomography have all been proven to have efficacy in the detection of ovarian cancer. The high costs and limited availability of these tests, however, preclude their use as primary screening modalities and no prospective screening trials utilizing these modalities have been performed to date. They may be used in a multimodal screening program as second-line tests to follow-up abnormal tumor markers or ultrasound.

Serum tumor markers

In 1983, Bast *et al.*[13] developed the first clinically useful serum tumor marker for the monitoring of patients with ovarian cancer. A murine monoclonal antibody (OC 125) directed against a high molecular weight glycoprotein common to most non-mucinous epithelial ovarian cancers (CA-125) was developed through the somatic hybridization of spleen cells from mice immunized with an ovarian cancer cell line. Using a cut-off of 35 U/ml, the CA-125 radioimmunoassay was found to be elevated in only 1% of apparently healthy women, but in 82% of women with histologically proven ovarian cancer.[13] It is important to consider that the original purpose of the assay was the monitoring of known ovarian cancer patients and not the screening of an asymptomatic population. Of ovarian cancer patients in this study, 85% were stage III or IV when the assay was performed. The first study to evaluate the sensitivity of CA-125 for the detection of occult ovarian cancer was performed by Zurawski *et al.*[14] Serum from 105 women who subsequently developed ovarian neoplasia was compared to that of 323 matched controls in the Norwegian serum bank. Overall, 50% of patients had serum CA-125 levels > 30 U/ml in the 18 months preceding diagnosis; however, only 33% of patients with stage I had CA-125 levels > 35 U/ml during the same interval. At 30 and 35 U/ml, the respective specificities were 92.6% and 95.4%. These levels are insufficient for a clinically useful screen and would be associated with an unacceptable false-positive rate. For this reason, no prospective ovarian cancer screening trials employing serum CA-125 as a single modality have been conducted.

Another method to increase the relatively low sensitivity of CA-125 for early-stage ovarian cancer is the simultaneous use of multiple markers. More than 30 serum proteins have been evaluated alone or in combination with CA-125 as potential markers for early stage disease. These include human epididymis protein 4 (HE4),[15] macrophage colony stimulating factor (M-CSF),[16] OVX1 (16), and soluble mesothelin related (SMR) marker.[17] The combination of CA-125, CA-15-3, CA-72-4, and M-CSF was found to increase the sensitivity of early stage ovarian cancer detection from 45% with CA-125 alone to 70% when analyzing the four markers simultaneously.[18] No prospective screening trial using a panel of tumor markers has been conducted to confirm the efficacy of this strategy.

Multimodal screening

Recognizing the unacceptable positive predictive value of CA-125 and transvaginal ultrasound (TVS) as single modalities for ovarian cancer screening, several large trials incorporated the two tests into multimodal and sequential protocols. The Stockholm Screening Study on Ovarian Cancer was the earliest study to examine the specificity of CA-125 and TVS in a prospective manner.[19] A total of 5550 apparently healthy women aged 37–85 years were randomly chosen from the Stockholm population registry. Each woman underwent an initial CA-125 test to determine the need for intensive surveillance. A cut-off value of 35 U/ml was initially used; however, this was subsequently decreased to 30 U/ml. Of these, 175 patients had abnormal CA-125 levels and underwent an additional CA-125 level test every 3 months with transabdominal ultrasound and pelvic examinations every 6 months. The clinicians caring for these women were blinded to the CA-125 results and management was based on clinical and sonographic findings alone. Ovarian cancer was detected in 6 women with abnormal CA-125 levels with 4 cancers being early stage. The specificities for distinguishing women with ovarian cancer were 95.7% and 97.6% when using cut-off values of 35 and 30 U/ml, respectively. In a long-term follow-up of the Stockholm screening study, the median survival of the patients identified through screening was 100 months. Twenty additional patients were diagnosed with ovarian cancer subsequent to the screening period and had a median survival of only 20 months ($P = 0.059$).[20] This apparent survival advantage did not reach statistical significance and was subject to length-time bias.

The Royal London Hospital Study, a randomized controlled trial, was then performed to assess multimodal ovarian cancer screening with sequential CA-125 and pelvic ultrasound.[21] Nearly 22,000 postmenopausal women were randomized to control and screening groups. The screening regimen consisted of three annual CA-125 levels. Pelvic sonography was performed if the CA-125 was greater than 30 U/ml and referral to a gynecologist made if the ovarian volume was greater than 8.2 ml on sonogram. Of 468 women in the screened group with elevated CA-125, 29 were referred for gynecological opinion. Twenty-three women had no pathology, benign pathology, or adenocarcinoma of unknown primary (false positive results). Six women were diagnosed with ovarian cancer. Interestingly, half of the screen-detected cancers were stage III at the time of diagnosis. The positive predictive value of this screening regimen was 27% with 99.9% specificity. During the 8 years of follow-up, 10 more ovarian cancers were detected in the screened group and 20 index cancers were detected in the control group. There was a tendency toward earlier stage at diagnosis and grade in the screen-detected cancers. The median survival of women with index cancers in the screened and control groups were 72.2 months and 41.2 months, respectively ($P = 0.112$). There was no significant difference, however, in mortality from ovarian cancer between the two groups.

Both the Royal London and Stockholm studies utilized a specific cut-off value of CA-125 level to determine the need for pelvic sonography. Observations from these studies demonstrated that women with ovarian cancer tended to have rising CA-125 levels prior to diagnosis while women without cancer had static or falling levels, even when greater than 30 U/ml. Skates *et al.*[22] re-analyzed the serial CA-125 levels of several women in the Stockholm screening study and performed a linear regression of the log [CA-125] on time since the first sample for both cases and controls. The slope and the intercept of this regression summarized the data. Baye's Theorem was used to calculate the risk of ovarian cancer (ROCA) using the slope, intercept and assay variability. The ROCA algorithm was then applied to a training set of participants on the trial and proved to have excellent specificity (99.7%) and a positive predictive value of 16%. Menon *et al.*[23] utilized the ROCA algorithm in conjunction with pelvic sonography to screen 6682 postmenopausal women aged 50 years and older. After the initial CA-125 screen, 91 women were calculated to have a high risk of ovarian cancer (> 1/500) and an additional 1228 women were considered to be at intermediate risk (1/2000 to 1/500). After further testing of the intermediate risk group, an additional 53 women were determined to have a high risk of ovarian cancer. All 144 high-risk women underwent TVS (2.2% referral rate) and 16 women underwent surgery as a result of the screening results. Primary ovarian cancer was detected in 3 patients; 1 patient was diagnosed with a borderline serous tumor and 1 patient with an ovarian recurrence of breast cancer. This screening strategy achieved a positive predictive value of 19% for the detection of primary ovarian cancer and specificity of 99.7%. The purpose of this study was to aid in the study design of a definitive ovarian cancer screening trial using ovarian cancer mortality as the primary endpoint. This trial, named United Kingdom Collaborative Trial of Ovarian Cancer Screening (UKCTOCS), aims to recruit 200,000 postmenopausal women over a 3-year period. One hundred thousand women will be randomly assigned to either annual transvaginal sonogram screening or multimodal screening using the ROCA algorithm. The other 100,000 women will be randomized to the control group. A psychosocial component will be included to examine the emotional, social, and sexual effects of ovarian cancer screening. Results are expected in 2014.

Another on-going multimodal screening trial is the Prostate, Lung, Colorectal and Ovarian (PLCO) cancer screening trial. The objectives of this randomized prospective trial are to determine in healthy subjects aged 55–74 years at entry whether: (i) screening with flexible sigmoidoscopy can reduce mortality from colorectal cancer in males and females; (ii) screening with chest X-ray can reduce mortality from lung cancer in males and females; (iii) screening with digital rectal examination plus serum prostate specific antigen (PSA) can reduce mortality from prostate cancer; and (iv) screening with CA-125 and transvaginal ultrasound can reduce mortality from ovarian cancer. The results of the baseline ovarian cancer screening examinations of were recently published.[24] Between 1993 and 2001, 78,237 females were enrolled into the trial and 39,115 were randomized to the intervention arm. Ovarian cancer screening consists of annual serum CA-125 examinations for 6 years and annual TVS for 4 years. CA-125 values ≥ 35 U/ml are considered abnormal. An abnormal sonogram is defined as any ovarian volume > 10 cm^3, any ovarian cyst volume > 10 cm^3, or any papillary projection or mural nodule extending into the cyst. A total of 28,816 women received at least one screening test and 28,506 received both. Five hundred and seventy surgical procedures were performed due to abnormal screening tests, including 325 laparotomies. Twenty-nine malignancies were identified, 26 of which arose in the ovary. These included 16 invasive epithelial ovarian cancers, 9 low malignant potential tumors , and 1 granulosa cell tumor. In addition, 2 fallopian tube carcinomas and 1 primary peritoneal carcinoma were diagnosed. Of the 16 invasive epithelial ovarian cancers detected, 13 were stage III or greater at diagnosis. The positive predictive values for TVS, CA-125, and multimodal screening were 1%, 3.7%, and 23.5%, respectively. Interestingly, 31% of malignancies detected in this trial were low-malignant potential tumors, which usually comprise no more than 15% of ovarian malignancies. This finding suggests that ovarian cancer screening, as performed in the PLCO study, may preferentially detect low-grade tumors which may have otherwise gone undetected. Since ovarian cancer mortality is the primary end-point of the PLCO trial, the potential for length bias will be eliminated. Hopefully, the UKCTOCS and PLCO trial results will finally determine whether multimodal screening using CA-125 and TVU can significantly reduce the mortality from ovarian cancer in the general population.

Although multimodal screening may lack sufficient specificity to reduce mortality from ovarian cancer in the general population due to the low prevalence of the disease, this screening strategy may prove effective in a high-risk population. As stated earlier, several factors, including age, family history, germ-line tumor suppressor gene mutations, and Ashkenazi Jewish ethnicity, may increase a woman's life-time risk of ovarian cancer. A recent meta-analysis examined the efficacy of multimodal screening in the high-risk patient population.[25] Eleven studies including about 6000 screened women were included. The entry criteria were variable but generally included known BRCA-1 or BRCA-2 mutations as well as personal and family history of breast or ovarian cancer. Thirty-eight primary ovarian cancers were detected, excluding borderline and germ-cell tumors. Of these, 9 were stage I, 5 were stage IIA or IIB, and 24 were stage IIC or higher. The authors estimated at least 15 interval cancers occurred; however, 13 of these occurred after the last screen. Screening the high-risk population, therefore, apparently gives 94% sensitivity for the detection of ovarian cancer at 1 year of follow-up; however, only 45% of these tumors are early stage at diagnosis. The role of screening versus prophylactic bilateral salpingo-oophorectomy in the high-risk population remains unclear; however, many women will be unwilling or not ready to undergo prophylactic surgery. The United Kingdom Familial Ovarian Cancer Screening Study (UKFOCSS) is a study designed to establish the optimal screening regimen in women with a > 10% life-time risk of ovarian cancer. All patients will receive annual CA-125 and TVS as well as 4-monthly blood tests for CA-125. The ROC algorithm will be used retrospectively to calculate a familial ROC index. The study is presently funded until 2011. Serum samples are also being stored for retrospective analysis for novel tumor markers.

Serum proteomic screening

Serum biomarkers have proven to be important tools in the detection and monitoring of cancer. They are the hallmarks of the physiological state of a cell and can signal early changes caused by genetic mutations, alterations in gene expression, and abnormal metabolism that often accompanies carcinogenesis. The enzyme-linked immunosorbent assay (ELISA) method is one of the most reliable and widely available protein-based tests for the detection of cancer but it is limited by a number of factors. It requires the identification of a single, highly validated, protein biomarker of disease and a high-affinity antibody used to detect the protein. The protein must be detectable in an accessible body fluid such as blood, urine, or saliva. In the past, the search for new biomarkers for ovarian cancer screening has been performed in a one-at-a-time fashion. Although this process has yielded more than 30 tumor-associated proteins, it is laborious and no single marker or panel of markers has proven to be an effective screen for the detection of early-stage EOC. Serum proteomic applications are novel approaches to cancer screening and the detection of new biomarkers of the disease.

The serum proteome is the total distribution of the various proteins and protein fragments that circulate throughout the body. As blood enters the microcirculation of a tumor, various altered proteins are deposited thereby making slight changes to the serum proteomic pattern. These alterations offer a diagnostic signature that is potentially disease-specific. The proteomic spectrum can be produced using surface-enhanced laser desorption ionization time of flight (SELDI-TOF) mass spectrometry. In this process, a small amount of raw, unfractionated serum is applied to a protein-binding chip which binds a subset of the proteins. The chip is then rinsed of unbound proteins and dried with a matrix compound. The chip is placed within a vacuum chamber and irradiated with a laser. The bound proteins are desorbed from the chip as charged ions and are propelled down a cylinder before being detected by an electrode. The time-of-flight (TOF) of each protein is a function of the mass to charge ratio (*m/z*) of the ion and the entire proteome will produce a spectral pattern containing a data point for each protein or protein fragment. SELDI-TOF mass spectrometry produces tens of thousands of data points per sample. This massive amount of data must be analyzed with sophisticated bioinformatics to detect the subset of proteins that discriminate patients with and without the disease in question.

Petricoin *et al.*[26] performed the first study describing the use of proteomic pattern analysis for the detection of ovarian cancer. Proteomic spectral patterns were produced using mass spectrometry utilizing serum from 50 women with ovarian cancer and 50 healthy controls. High-order data mining software was used to determine a discriminatory proteomic pattern and this pattern was applied to a set of 116 masked serum samples. The discriminatory pattern correctly identified all 50 ovarian cancer cases in the masked set, including 18 patients with stage I disease. While identification of the specific discriminatory proteins was not necessary to distinguish between cases and controls, serum proteomic analysis has been used to identify novel biomarkers. Zhang *et al.*[27] analyzed the proteomic spectral patterns of 153 patients with invasive epithelial ovarian cancer, 42 with other ovarian cancers, 166 with benign pelvic masses, and 142 healthy women. Three biomarkers were identified including apolipoprotein A1 (down-regulated), a truncated form of transthyretin (down-regulated), and a cleavage fragment of inter-α-trypsin inhibitor heavy chain H4 (up-regulated). A panel of these 3 markers and CA-125 was found to be more sensitive for the detection of ovarian cancer when compared to CA-125 alone (74% versus 65%, respectively). The potential benefit of serum proteomic analysis over traditional biomarker screening has prompted the National Cancer Institute Clinical Proteomics Program to launch a diagnostic study that is currently following women in remission from ovarian cancer. The study seeks to compare the sensitivity and specificity of serum proteomics and CA-125 for the detection of recurrent EOC.

Detection of ovarian cancer in the symptomatic patient

The lack of proven efficacy in screening asymptomatic women for ovarian cancer and the relatively good prognosis associated with early stage disease has focused attention on the symptoms of early ovarian cancer. The disease has traditionally been taught to be a 'silent killer' with a lack of associated symptoms until late into the course of the disease. Several recent studies have shown that this is not the case and the new battle-cry of many ovarian cancer support groups is 'it whispers, so listen!'. Smith *et al.*[28] reviewed the histories of 83 women diagnosed with ovarian cancer with regard to symptomatology and delay in diagnosis. Of early-stage patients, 75% reported symptoms prior to diagnosis and were more likely than late-stage patients to complain of fatigue and urinary complaints. However, 90% attributed the symptoms to non-serious medical conditions like menopause or aging. Only menstrual irregularity was more likely to convince these patients to seek a diagnosis. Interestingly, no association was found between the degree of the symptoms, the perceived cause, delay in seeking medical attention, and the stage at diagnosis. In an attempt to elucidate further the early symptoms of ovarian cancer and the causes for delayed diagnosis, Goff *et al.*[29] distributed a 2-page survey to 1500 subscribers of *CONVERSATIONS!*, a newsletter about ovarian cancer. Over 1700 responses were received from the US and Canada. As expected, 70% of respondents were stage III or IV at the time of diagnosis. Only 11% of early-stage patients and 3% of late-stage patients reported no symptoms prior to diagnosis. The reported symptoms were categorized as abdominal (77%), gastrointestinal (70%), pain (58%), constitutional (50%), urinary (34%), and pelvic (26%). Women who ignored their symptoms were significantly more likely to be diagnosed with advanced stage disease compared to those that did not. After presentation to a physician, 37% of patients experienced a delay in diagnosis of 6 months or more. The design of this study, however, was subject to recall and selection biases. In addition, many healthy women present to primary care physicians with the same non-specific complaints that were associated with ovarian cancer. In order to address these weaknesses, a prospective case-control study was performed to determine the frequency of ovarian cancer symptoms in women presenting to primary care clinics.[30] A total of 1709 women presenting to two primary care clinics completed an anonymous survey of symptoms experienced over the past year. An identical survey was also completed by 128 women prior to surgery for a pelvic mass (84 benign, 44 malignant). Women with ovarian cancer were 7.4 times more likely to experience increased abdominal girth, 3.6 times more likely to have abdominal bloating, 2.5 times more likely to experience urinary urgency, and 2.2 times more likely to experience pelvic pain compared to clinical controls. The symptoms tended to be more frequent and of greater severity than those experienced by women with benign masses and in clinical controls. The combination of increased abdominal girth, abdominal bloating, and urinary urgency was found in 43% of women with ovarian cancer but in only 8% of women presenting to the primary care clinic. While the majority of women who noted symptoms of ovarian cancer did not have the disease, the study helped to define the roles of symptom severity, frequency, and duration in the detection of ovarian cancer. It remains to be proven that earlier detection of ovarian cancer through a heightened awareness of symptoms can decrease the mortality of the disease.

CONCLUSIONS

Ovarian cancer remains the deadliest gynecological malignancy in developed nations and the poor prognosis is largely attributable to the late stage at diagnosis for the majority of patients. Attempts to screen asymptomatic women at average and high-risk for the disease have yet to determine the optimal screening strategy or to demonstrate a significant reduction in mortality due to these efforts. Large trials of multimodal screening are underway but are not likely to yield results before 2012. Advances in the analysis of the currently known serum tumor markers as well advances in techniques to discover novel markers will surely impact future screening strategies. In the meantime, a heightened awareness of the symptoms of early ovarian cancer on the part of patients and practitioners may help to reduce the delay in diagnosis typically experienced by women with ovarian cancer and hopefully result in an improvement in outcome for some.

References

1 Droegemueller W. Screening for ovarian carcinoma: hopeful and wishful thinking. Am J Obstet Gynecol 1994; 170: 1095–1098

2 Parkin DM, Bray F, Ferlay J, Pisani P. Estimating the world cancer burden: Globocan 2000. Int J Cancer 2001; 94: 153–156

3 La Vecchia C. Epidemiology of ovarian cancer: a summary review. Eur J Cancer Prev 2001; 10: 125–129

4 Heintz APM, Odicino F, Maisonneuve P. Carcinoma of the ovary. J Epidemiol Biostat 2001; 6: 108–138

5 Muto MG, Welch WR, Mok SC *et al*. Evidence for a multifocal origin of papillary serous carcinoma of the peritoneum. Cancer Res 1995; 55: 490–492

6 Tsao SW, Mok CH, Knapp RC *et al*. Molecular genetic evidence of a unifocal origin for human serous ovarian carcinomas. Gynecol Oncol 1993; 48: 5–10

7 Bray F, Loos AH, Tognazzo S, La Vecchia C. Ovarian cancer in Europe: cross-sectional trends in incidence and mortality in 28 countries, 1953–2000. Int J Cancer 2005; 113: 977–990

8 Carlson KJ, Skates SJ, Singer DE. Screening for ovarian cancer. Ann Intern Med 1994; 121: 124–132

9 Whittemore AS. Characteristics relating to ovarian cancer risk: implications for prevention and detection. Gynecol Oncol 1994; 55: S15–S19

10 Prat J, Ribe A, Gallardo A. Hereditary ovarian cancer. Hum Pathol 2005; 36: 861–870

11 DePriest PD, Shenson D, Fried A *et al*. A morphology index based on sonographic findings in ovarian cancer. Gynecol Oncol 1993; 51: 7–11

12 van Nagell Jr JR, DePriest PD, Reedy MB *et al*. The efficacy of transvaginal sonographic screening in asymptomatic women at risk for ovarian cancer. Gynecol Oncol 2000; 77: 350–356

13 Bast Jr RC, Klug TL, St John E *et al*. A radioimmunoassay using a monoclonal antibody to monitor the course of epithelial ovarian cancer. N Engl J Med 1983; 309: 883–887

14 Zurawski Jr VR, Orjaseter H, Andersen A, Jellum E. Elevated serum CA 125 levels prior to diagnosis of ovarian neoplasia: relevance for early detection of ovarian cancer. Int J Cancer 1988; 42: 677–680

15 Hellstrom I, Raycraft J, Hayden-Ledbetter M *et al*. The HE4 (WFDC2) protein is a biomarker for ovarian carcinoma. Cancer Res 2003; 63: 3695–3700

16 Woolas RP, Xu FJ, Jacobs IJ *et al*. Elevation of multiple serum markers in patients with stage I ovarian cancer. J Natl Cancer Inst 1993; 85: 1748–1751

17 McIntosh MW, Drescher C, Karlan B *et al*. Combining CA 125 and SMR serum markers for diagnosis and early detection of ovarian carcinoma. Gynecol Oncol 2004; 95: 9–15

18 Skates SJ, Horick N, Yu Y *et al*. Preoperative sensitivity and specificity for early-stage ovarian cancer when combining cancer antigen CA-125II, CA 15-3, CA 72-4, and macrophage colony-stimulating factor using mixtures of multivariate normal distributions. J Clin Oncol 2004; 22: 4059–4066

19 Einhorn N, Sjovall K, Knapp RC *et al*. Prospective evaluation of serum CA 125 levels for early detection of ovarian cancer. Obstet Gynecol 1992; 80: 14–18

20 Einhorn N, Bast R, Knapp R, Nilsson B, Zurawski Jr V, Sjovall K. Long-term follow-up of the Stockholm screening study on ovarian cancer. Gynecol Oncol 2000; 79: 466–470

21 Jacobs IJ, Skates SJ, MacDonald N *et al*. Screening for ovarian cancer: a pilot randomised controlled trial. Lancet 1999; 353: 1207–1210

22 Skates SJ, Xu FJ, Yu YH *et al*. Toward an optimal algorithm for ovarian cancer screening with longitudinal tumor markers. Cancer 1995; 76: 2004–2010

23 Menon U, Skates SJ, Lewis S *et al*. Prospective study using the risk of ovarian cancer algorithm to screen for ovarian cancer. J Clin Oncol 2005; 23: 7919–7926
24 Buys SS, Partridge E, Greene MH *et al*. Ovarian cancer screening in the Prostate, Lung, Colorectal and Ovarian (PLCO) cancer screening trial: findings from the initial screen of a randomized trial. Am J Obstet Gynecol 2005; 193: 1630–1639
25 Hogg R, Friedlander M. Biology of epithelial ovarian cancer: implications for screening women at high genetic risk. J Clin Oncol 2004; 22: 1315–1327
26 Petricoin EF, Ardekani AM, Hitt BA *et al*. Use of proteomic patterns in serum to identify ovarian cancer. Lancet 2002; 359: 572–577
27 Zhang Z, Bast Jr RC, Yu Y *et al*. Three biomarkers identified from serum proteomic analysis for the detection of early stage ovarian cancer. Cancer Res 2004; 64: 5882–5890
28 Smith EM, Anderson B. The effects of symptoms and delay in seeking diagnosis on stage of disease at diagnosis among women with cancers of the ovary. Cancer 1985; 56: 2727–2732
29 Goff BA, Mandel L, Muntz HG, Melancon CH. Ovarian carcinoma diagnosis. Cancer 2000; 89: 2068–2075
30 Goff BA, Mandel LS, Melancon CH, Muntz HG. Frequency of symptoms of ovarian cancer in women presenting to primary care clinics. JAMA 2004; 291: 2705–2712

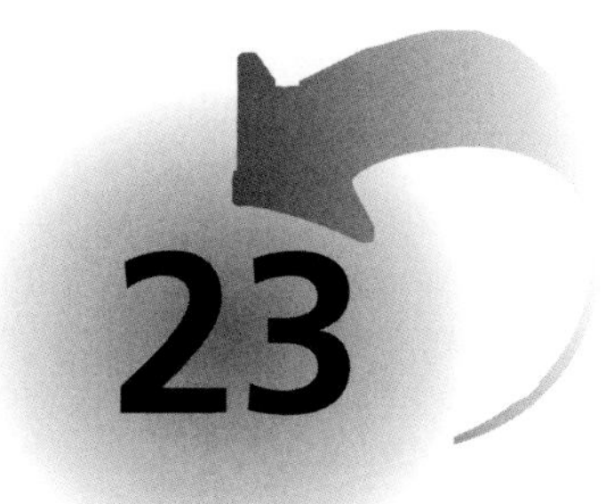

Padma Vanga Anga S. Arunkalaivanan

Painful bladder syndrome/interstitial cystitis and its management

Painful bladder syndrome is the complaint of suprapubic pain related to bladder filling, accompanied by other symptoms, such as increased day-time and night-time frequency, in the absence of proven urinary infection or other obvious pathology. Interstitial cystitis is painful bladder syndrome with typical cystoscopic and/or histological features in the absence of infection or other pathology.[1] Painful bladder syndrome/interstitial cystitis was a neglected disease for many years but, recently, has received increasing attention. The pathophysiology of interstitial cystitis pain is poorly understood, but is thought to be a complex entity including nociceptive, visceral and neuropathic components. Its etiology is multifactorial, involving microbiological, immunological, mucosal, neurogenic and other yet unidentified agents. History, physical examination, urine analysis and culture as well as cystoscopy and hydrodistension are useful diagnostic tools but the final diagnosis tends to be one of exclusion. The quality of life of patients with painful bladder syndrome/interstitial cystitis is significantly debilitating. Treating interstitial cystitis is one of the greatest challenges facing physicians and other healthcare providers who manage patients with this condition. Though there are currently no universally effective therapies, multiple forms of therapy are available including self-care and dietary changes, medical and intravesical treatments, neuromodulation and surgical intervention. Oral treatments, however, are frequently used, including non-steroidal anti-inflammatory drugs, antihistamines, tricyclic antidepressants and pentosan polysulphate, all of which have shown varying degrees of efficacy. Intravesical

Padma Vanga MBBS
Specialist Registrar, City Hospital, Dudley Road, Birmingham B18 7QH, UK

Anga S. Arunkalaivanan MD MRCOG (for correspondence)
Consultant Urogynaecologist and Obstetrician, City Hospital, Dudley Road, Birmingham B18 7QH, UK
E-mail: anga.arunkalaivanan@swbh.nhs.uk

therapies include dimethyl sulphoxide, heparin, hyaluronic acid and bacille Calmette-Guérin. Bladder augmentation cystoplasty has been used for refractory interstitial cystitis/painful bladder syndrome for many years. Among the potentially effective new treatment modalities currently under investigation are suplatast tosilate, resiniferatoxin, and botulinum toxin and gene therapy to modulate the pain response. Non-pharmacological approaches, such as bladder training, biofeedback and dietary changes, can provide supplemental relief. As knowledge of the pathogenesis of interstitial cystitis increases through intensified research, the ability to provide effective treatment to patients with this disease will improve.

Skene and Hunner were pioneers in the discovery of interstitial cystitis. It was first described in medical textbooks back in the late 19th century. The name interstitial cystitis was given to the disease by A.J.C. Skene. Guy Hunner, a Boston surgeon, described this inflammatory bladder disorder in a number of patients in 1914. He described the lesions as ulcers in the bladder wall of some patients and later they were known as 'Hunner's ulcers'. In recent years, painful bladder syndrome/interstitial cystitis has been classified into two types – classical or ulcerative and non-ulcerative. It has been estimated that approximately 5–10% of painful bladder syndrome/interstitial cystitis patients have the classical type. Therefore, painful bladder syndrome/interstitial cystitis has been under-diagnosed for many decades. The most successful attempt to define a clinically useful definition of interstitial cystitis was the National Institute of Diabetes and Digestive and Kidney Diseases (NIDDK) criteria established at a workshop in 1987 and later revised in 1988 (Table 1).

The NIDDK criteria were only fulfilled by one-third of patients thought to have the disease. The European Society for the Study of IC/PBS (ESSIC) has approached the problem of defining and classifying the disease from a different angle (Table 2).

Interstitial cystitis is a clinical diagnosis primarily based on symptoms of urgency, frequency and pain in the bladder and or pelvis. The International Continence Society (ICS) prefers the term painful bladder syndrome defined as: 'the complaint of suprapubic pain related to bladder filling, accompanied by other symptoms such as increased day-time and night-time frequency, in the absence of proven urinary infection or other obvious pathology'. ICS reserves the diagnosis interstitial cystitis to typical cystoscopic and histological features, without further specifying these. Logically, interstitial cystitis should include some form of demonstrable inflammation in the bladder wall, while painful bladder syndrome should include pain in the region of the bladder.[2]

The ESSIC obtained consensus on a new classification and proposes to replace the term interstitial cystitis with bladder pain syndrome followed by a type indication (Table 2). During this transition period, the name painful bladder syndrome/interstitial cystitis (BPS/IC) could be used in parallel with BPS.

EPIDEMIOLOGY

Available data on the epidemiology are heterogeneous. The wide ranges of prevalence estimates can be attributed to problems including lack of a uniform definition of painful bladder syndrome/interstitial cystitis, lack of readily available diagnostic marker(s), unknown etiology, uncertain pathophysiology, lack of

Table 1 National Institute of Diabetes and Digestive and Kidney Diseases (NIDDK) diagnostic criteria for interstitial cystitis

To be diagnosed with interstitial cystitis, patients must have either glomerulations on cystoscopic examination or a classic Hunner's ulcer, and they must have either pain associated with the bladder or urinary urgency. The presence of any one of the following excludes a diagnosis of interstitial cystitis:

- Bladder capacity greater than 350 ml on awake cystometry, using either gas or liquid as a filling medium
- Absence of an intense urge to void with the bladder filled to 100 ml of gas or 150 ml of water during cystometry, using a fill rate of 30–100 ml/min
- Demonstration of phasic involuntary bladder contractions on cystometry, using the fill rate of 30–100 ml/min
- Duration of symptoms less than 9 months
- Absence of nocturia
- Symptoms relieved by antimicrobials, urinary antiseptics, anticholinergics, or antispasmodics (musculotropic relaxants)
- Frequency of urination, while awake, less than 8 times per day
- Diagnosis of bacterial cystitis or prostatitis within a 3-month period
- Bladder or lower ureteral calculi
- Active genital herpes
- Uterine, cervical, vaginal, or urethral cancer
- Urethral diverticula
- Cyclophosphamide or any type of chemical cystitis
- Tuberculous cystitis
- Radiation cystitis
- Benign or malignant bladder tumors
- Vaginitis
- Age younger than 18 years

Adapted from Wein AJ, Hanno PM *et al.* Interstitial cystitis: an introduction to the problem. In: Hanno PM, Staskin DR, Krane RJ, Wein AJ. (eds) Interstitial Cystitis. London: Springer, 1990; 13–15.

Table 2 ESSIC classification of bladder pain syndrome types

Biopsy	Cystoscopy with hydrodistension			
	Not done	Normal	Glomerulations[a]	Hunner's lesions[b]
Not done	XX	1X	2X	3X
Normal	XA	1A	2A	3A
Inconclusive	XB	1B	2B	3B
Positive[c]	XC	1C	2C	3C

[a]Cystoscopy: glomerulations grade 2–3.
[b]With or without glomerulations.
[c]Histology showing inflammatory infiltrates and/or detrusor mastocytosis and/or granulation tissue and/or intrafascicular fibrosis.
Types XX, XA, XB, 1X, 1A, and 1B were formerly known as painful bladder syndrome.
Types XC, 1C and all types 2 and 3 were formerly known as interstitial cystitis.

standardised methodology, differences in the populations studied, and overlapping conditions and definitions. The true prevalence of painful bladder syndrome/interstitial cystitis is hard to determine because most patients remain undiagnosed, although it is now thought to occur in up to 7.5% of the general female population and in 38–85% of women who present with chronic pelvic pain.[3] In the literature, the reported incidence varies from 1.6–158 per 100,000 women. Self-report, as part of the National Household Interview Survey, found a rate of 450 per 100,000; three studies that used O'Leary-Sant scores found prevalences of approximately 300 per 100,000. A recent survey from Finland indicated the prevalence of clinically confirmed probable interstitial cystitis in women was 230 per 100,000 and that of possible/probable interstitial cystitis 530 per 100,000.[4] In Japan, comparable estimates were 1.2 per 100,000 patients and 4.5 per 100,000 female patients with a male:female ratio of 1:5.8.[5]

The prevalence of interstitial cystitis in The Netherlands was calculated to be 8–16 per 100,000 female patients which is in line with that of other reports from Europe but low compared to findings in the US.[6] Generally, it is more frequently diagnosed in developed countries than in developing ones. The overall prevalence of interstitial cystitis was highest in middle-aged women (40–59 years) at 464 per 100,000.[7] A pilot study conducted on members of the Interstitial Cystitis Association (ICA) in the US concluded that the adult, female, first-degree relatives of patients with interstitial cystitis may have a prevalence of interstitial cystitis 17 times that found in the general population.[8] Interstitial cystitis has been rarely reported in children, though it is recognisable and should not be confused with dysfunctional voiding in which complaints are secondary to involuntary bladder contractions.[9]

QUALITY OF LIFE

Once thought to be a rare condition, painful bladder syndrome/interstitial cystitis is being increasingly recognised as an important cause of chronic pelvic pain. Women with interstitial cystitis have significantly lower quality of life scores in 4 of the 7 quality of life dimensions, including role/physical, bodily pain, vitality and social function compared to women without interstitial cystitis. Women with interstitial cystitis experienced greater differences in vitality and mental health than women with rheumatoid arthritis or hypertension.[10] Interstitial cystitis can masquerade as, and co-exist with, other causes of pelvic pain, particularly endometriosis. Early diagnosis and treatment of interstitial cystitis can improve the patient's prognosis and quality of life. In a voluntary health survey project in Vienna using the O'Leary-Sant interstitial cystitis questionnaire, about two-thirds of the women with moderate-to-high risk for interstitial cystitis reported an impairment of quality of life and 35% reported an effect on their sexual life.[11]

ETIOPATHOGENESIS

The cause of interstitial cystitis remains unknown. Potential causes including infection, vascular alterations, psychological aberrations, bladder surface alterations, toxic agents, neurological disorders, and autoimmune responses, all of which have been investigated. A unified understanding of the pathogenesis of interstitial cystitis is emerging. Multiple theories as to the cause of interstitial cystitis have been proposed with varying degrees of evidence. The current body of evidence supports the idea that interstitial cystitis is associated with an intrinsic pathology of the bladder urothelial cells. Although the epidemiology of this disorder is similar to that of bacterial cystitis, prospective studies using sensitive culture techniques and polymerase chain reaction assay for a variety of micro-organisms have failed to identify a specific infectious etiology for interstitial cystitis. Keay and Warren[13] have identified a low-molecular-weight peptide termed anti-proliferative factor (APF) in the urine of interstitial cystitis patients that inhibits the proliferation of normal bladder epithelial cells *in vitro*. The chronically damaged epithelium is prone to colonisation with various micro-organisms, and the resulting exposure to these micro-organisms, other urinary antigens, and/or damaged epithelial cells prompts the low-level inflammatory response commonly seen in this disorder. Furthermore, APF regulates expression of other cytokines, including up-regulating heparin-binding epidermal growth factor-like growth factor and down-regulating epidermal growth factor by bladder urothelial cells. These cytokine abnormalities were also related to increases in purinergic (adenosine triphosphate) signaling, which could mediate increased bladder sensation.[14] An increased number of mast cells have been associated with interstitial cystitis, but the published reports are inconclusive and often conflicting. It was found that mast cells from interstitial cystitis patients averaged as high as 34 cells/mm^2 as compared to less than 16/mm^2 in controls. Electron microscopy revealed that over 90% of mast cells from interstitial cystitis patients were activated to various degrees and it was concluded that mast cell activation is a pathological characteristic for interstitial cystitis.[15] It has been shown in animal models that bladder mast cells are located close to neuronal processes, and are activated *in situ* by acetylcholine and substance P. Such activation is augmented by estradiol, which acquires significance in view of the fact that human bladder mast cells express estrogen receptors, but few progesterone receptors; this may explain the worsening of interstitial cystitis symptoms during ovulation.[16]

DIAGNOSIS AND INVESTIGATIONS

Diagnosis is made on the basis of pain related to the urinary bladder, accompanied by at least one other urinary symptom such as: (i) day-time and night-time frequency; (ii) exclusion of confusable diseases (*see* Table 3) as the cause of the symptoms; (iii) cystoscopy with hydrodistension; and (iv) biopsy, if indicated.

Symptoms

The most typical symptom of interstitial cystitis is pelvic pain. The pain is relieved by voiding small amounts of urine from the bladder, but soon recurs as the bladder fills. Other common symptoms are an uncomfortable, constant urge to void that does not go away even after the patient has voided and deep dyspareunia. Sometimes, the symptoms of interstitial cystitis are exacerbated after patients consume certain foods, especially coffee, alcohol, carbonated drinks, citrus fruits, tomatoes and chocolate.[17] Patients should be asked to keep a 24-h log of voiding activity for frequency of urination and voiding patterns for at least 3 days. O'Leary-Sant Symptom Score supplemented with the Quality of Life Score from the

Table 3 List of relevant confusable diseases and how they can be excluded or diagnosed

Confusable disease	Excluded or diagnosed by
Carcinoma	Cystoscopy and biopsy
Carcinoma *in situ*	Cystoscopy and biopsy
Infection with	
common intestinal bacteria	Routine bacterial culture
Chlamydia trachomatis	Special culture
Ureaplasma urealyticum	Special culture
Mycoplasma hominis	Special culture
Mycoplasma genitalium	Special culture
Corynebacterium urealyticum	Special culture
Mycobacterium tuberculosis	Dipstick; if 'sterile' pyuria culture for *M. tuberculosis*
Candida spp.	Special culture
Herpes simplex	Physical examination
Human papilloma virus	Physical examination
Radiation	Medical history
Chemotherapy, including immunotherapy with cyclophosphamide	Medical history
Anti-inflammatory therapy with tiaprofenic acid	Medical history
Bladder neck obstruction	Flowmetry and ultrasonography
Neurogenic outlet obstruction	Medical history, flowmetry and ultrasonography
Bladder stone	Imaging or cystoscopy
Lower uretic stone	Medical history and/or hematuria (→ upper urinary tract imaging, such as CT or IVP)
Urethral diverticulum	Medical history and physical examination
Endometriosis	Medical history and physical examination
Vaginal candidiasis	Medical history and physical examination
Cervical, uterine and ovarian cancer	Physical examination
Incomplete bladder emptying (retention)	Post-void residual urine volume measured by ultrasonography
Overactive bladder	Medical history and urodynamics
Prostate cancer	Physical examination and PSA
Benign prostatic obstruction	Flowmetry and pressure-flow studies
Chronic bacterial prostatitis	Medical history, physical examination, culture
Chronic non-bacterial prostatitis	Medical history, physical examination, culture
Pudendal nerve entrapment	Medical history, physical examination, nerve block may prove diagnosis
Pelvic floor muscle related pain	Medical history and physical examination

The diagnosis of a confusable disease does not necessarily exclude a diagnosis of bladder pain syndrome.

Nordling J, Anjum F, Bade J *et al*. Primary evaluation of patients suspected of having interstitial cystitis (IC). Eur Urol 2004; 45: 662–669.
van de Merwe JP, Nordling J. Interstitial cystitis: definitions and confusable diseases. ESSIC Meeting 2005 Baden. Eur Urol Today March 2006; p6, 7, 16.

International Prostate Symptom Score and a Visual Analogue Scale are helpful to evaluate pain.

Physical examination

A careful pelvic examination is needed to rule out vaginitis, vulvar lesions and urethral diverticulae. Pelvic examination in women often reveals tenderness of the bladder base.

Urinalysis

Findings on urinalysis may be entirely normal or may show microscopic hematuria or pyuria. Urine culture results are usually sterile. However, patients with interstitial cystitis may also have a concurrent bladder infection. Urine cytology may be helpful in ruling out transitional cell carcinoma of the bladder. If indicated, tuberculosis may be ruled out with urine testing for acid-fast bacillus, or bladder biopsy.[18]

Urodynamics

The current consensus is that urodynamic evaluation is not required for diagnosis of interstitial cystitis but may provide useful information regarding the differential diagnosis of painful voiding disorders and the symptoms of the overactive bladder. There is a significant overlap between the symptoms of the overactive bladder syndrome and interstitial cystitis (*i.e.* frequency, urgency, and urge incontinence). On urodynamic evaluation, many interstitial cystitis patients have sensory urgency and overactivity, reduced bladder capacity and pain with bladder filling at low volumes. Subjective measurements of symptoms associated with interstitial cystitis can be confirmed objectively with urodynamic studies.[19]

Cystoscopy and biopsy

Cystoscopy under anesthesia, either spinal or general, is mandatory in cases with suspected interstitial cystitis.

The Hunner's lesions are circumscribed, reddened mucosal areas with small vessels radiating towards a central scar, with a fibrin deposit or coagulum attached to this area. This site ruptures with increasing bladder distension, with petechial oozing of blood from the lesion and the mucosal margins in a waterfall manner. A rather typical, slightly bullous oedema develops post-distension with varying peripheral extension (Fig. 1).

Glomerulations are pin-point hemorrhages (petechiae) seen in the bladder mucosa following hydrodistension of the bladder. This term should be replaced by the following classification grading:[20]

Grade 0	Normal mucosa.
Grade I	Petechiae in at least two quadrants.
Grade II	Large submucosal bleeding (ecchymosis).
Grade III	Diffuse global mucosal bleeding.
Grade IV	Mucosal disruption, with or without bleeding/oedema.

The severity of cystoscopic findings observed during hydrodistension with

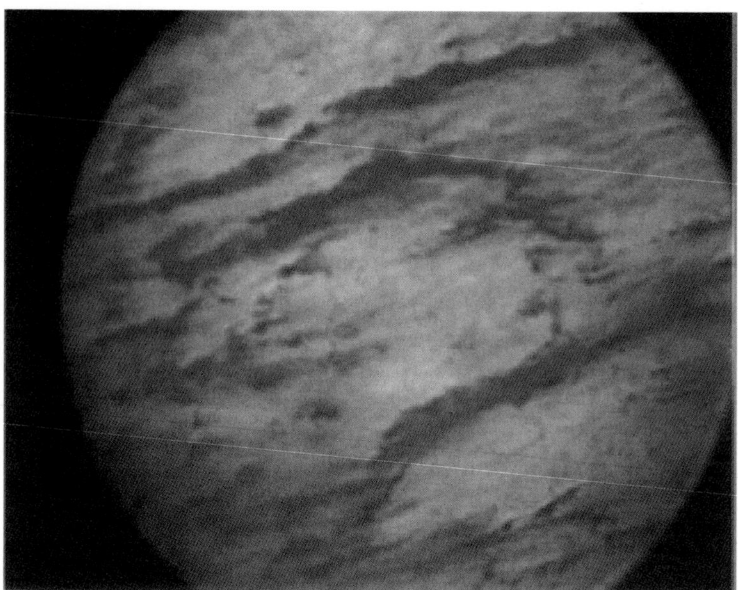

Fig. 1 Petechial hemorrhage following hydrodistension typical of interstitial cystitis.

anesthesia does not appear to correlate with the degree of inflammation identified histologically in patients with suspected interstitial cystitis.[21]

Intravesical potassium sensitivity test

The potassium test, which was studied for some time as a possible diagnostic tool for interstitial cystitis, is no longer considered to be sufficiently reliable and is, therefore, not internationally recommended as part of a diagnostic algorithm.

Urinary markers

The search for non-invasive techniques for diagnosis of interstitial cystitis has led to the study of urinary markers. The markers that have been the focus of the most research in the recent literature are APF, epidermal growth factor, heparin-binding epidermal growth factor-like growth factor, glycosaminoglycans, and bladder nitric oxide. Urine of interstitial cystitis patients specifically contains APF that inhibits primary bladder epithelial cell proliferation and has significantly decreased levels of heparin-binding epidermal growth factor-like growth factor (HB-EGF) and increased levels of epidermal growth factor (EGF) compared with urine from asymptomatic controls and patients with bacterial cystitis. APF activity was present significantly more often in interstitial cystitis than control urine specimens ($P < 0.005$ for interstitial cystitis versus any control group; sensitivity, 94%; specificity, 95%). HB-EGF levels were also significantly lower and EGF levels significantly higher in interstitial cystitis urine than in specimens from controls. Therefore, APF, HB-EGF, and EGF are promising markers for interstitial cystitis.[22]

MANAGEMENT

The management of patients with interstitial cystitis remains a challenge because no single agent has proven universally effective.

Non-pharmacological treatments

Complementary and alternative therapies are a classic addition to the pharmacological management of interstitial cystitis. A diet low in acidic foods, and avoiding beverages (such as coffee, tea, carbonated and/or alcoholic drinks) may be helpful in reducing interstitial cystitis symptoms. Balanced fluid intake, behavioral therapy, stress reduction and pelvic floor relaxation are found to improve clinical response.

Pharmacological treatments

The multifactorial etiology of interstitial cystitis has led to the development of a multimodality therapy for the disease. This includes agents that will treat glycosaminoglycan (GAG) layer dysfunction, mast cell abnormalities, neurogenic inflammation and pain control.

Oral medication

Antihistamines

The central role of the mast cell in interstitial cystitis is clear. Antihistamines have been beneficial in the symptomatic treatment of interstitial cystitis especially in women with documented allergies and/or bladder mast cell activation.[23] Hydroxyzine is a heterocyclic piperazine histamine-1 receptor antagonist; it acts by inhibiting the release of histamine from mast cells but has not been proven to be efficacious. Cimetidine is a histamine-2 antagonist. The clinical effect of Cimetidine (400 mg twice daily) was confirmed in a prospective, randomised, double-blind, placebo-controlled trial in 34 patients with non-ulcerative interstitial cystitis. Those receiving cimetidine had a significant improvement in symptoms, with median symptom scores decreasing from 19 to 11 ($P < 0.001$). Suprapubic pain and nocturia were the most improved symptoms.[24]

Amitriptyline

Amitriptyline is the commonly used tricyclic antidepressant agent used in the treatment of interstitial cystitis. It exerts central and peripheral anticholinergic activity, has antihistamine sedation effect, and inhibits serotonin and norepinephrine re-uptake. The recommended dose for interstitial cystitis is 25–100 mg daily, subject to self-titration. A statistically significant change in the symptom score and improvement of pain and urgency intensity in interstitial cystitis patients were observed when compared with placebo. Anticholinergic side-effects constitute the major drawback of amitriptyline treatment.[25]

Sodium pentosanpolysulphate (Elmiron)

Pentosan polysulphate (PPS) remains the corner-stone of drug therapy for most patients with interstitial cystitis. It is the only US FDA-approved oral treatment for the relief of bladder pain and is the only oral therapy for the treatment of interstitial cystitis symptoms that has been studied in placebo-controlled trials. PPS is a heparin-like synthetic, sulphated polysaccharide available in an oral form that is excreted into the urine. It acts by coating the bladder lining, re-establishing normal GAG layer function and decreasing potassium leak into the interstitial space. On a long-term basis, 6.2–18.7% of patients with interstitial cystitis benefit from PPS and the commonest side effect reported is diarrhoea.[26] A recent meta-analysis of all major studies comparing PPS to placebo, concluded that PPS was more efficacious than placebo in the treatment of pain, urgency and frequency associated with interstitial cystitis but not significantly different from placebo in treating nocturia associated with interstitial cystitis.[27] A small, placebo-controlled study has also proved intravesical PPS as an effective option for the treatment of interstitial cystitis.[28]

L-Arginine

Nitric oxide (NO) is involved in host defence reactions; NO production is elevated in various inflammatory disorders and also with very high levels detected intraluminally in the urinary bladder of patients with interstitial cystitis. Oral treatment with low doses of L-arginine, the substrate for NO production, has been reported to alleviate symptoms in patients with interstitial cystitis. A recently conducted, randomised, controlled, double-blinded trial suggested that the effects of L-arginine are clinically insignificant in the treatment of interstitial cystitis.[29]

Intravesical treatment

Hyaluronic acid (Cystistat)

Cystistat is for temporary replacement of the GAG layer in the bladder. Hyaluronic acid is an important compound present in many tissues, including the mucous lining of the bladder and might also work as a scavenger of free radicals and as an immune modulator. It is recommended that the product be instilled into the bladder as 6–8-weekly instillations, then monthly treatments. Many patients begin to experience relief after the fifth or sixth instillation; patients who respond positively may be able to increase the interval between treatments once the symptoms have stabilised. The reported side-effects with Cystistat are mainly initial exacerbation of urinary urgency and frequency due to catheterisation. Hyaluronic acid produced a 71% positive response rate at the end of 12 weeks in a trial on refractory interstitial cystitis, although this response rate decreased after 6 months.[30]

Chondroitin sulphate (Uracyst-S)

Immunohistochemistry studies by Hurst *et al.*[31] has shown a deficiency of chondroitin sulphate from the luminal surface of bladder from interstitial cystitis patients. Chondroitin sulphate is a naturally occurring mucopolysaccharide which acts by replenishing the glycosaminoglycans at the luminal surface of the bladder. The results from an open-label study on the effect of chondroitin sulphate on 18 interstitial cystitis patients (based on NIH criteria and a positive potassium test) have shown good response in 46% of cases and 45% patients had moderate response at 13 months' follow-up.[32]

Dimethyl sulphoxide (DMSO)

DMSO has both anti-inflammatory and analgesic properties. It is believed to inhibit free-radical production, thus reducing pain and inflammation. A 50%

solution of DMSO is instilled intravesically (*i.e.* via catheter) directly into the bladder. It is then held in the bladder for 10–20 min. One treatment is given every 1–2 weeks for 4–8 treatments, depending on the patient's response to the medication. After this initial series, many patients do find some relief, both in pain and frequency. Additional treatments may be necessary, should symptoms recur. Improvement may not be seen until the third or fourth treatment. Common side-effects are garlic halitosis for 24 h after DMSO instillation and temporary worsening of bladder symptoms (chemical cystitis) lasting 24–72 h after treatment. Intravesical therapy with DMSO has been proved to be a feasible option to treat both subtypes of interstitial cystitis with the treatment effect lasting 16–72 months with a reasonably low degree of discomfort.[33]

Heparin

The anticoagulant, heparin, is a heterogeneous group of straight-chain, anionic mucopolysaccharides called glycosaminoglycans. Heparin is known to mimic the GAG layer structure. It has anticoagulant properties and inhibits angiogenesis and proliferation of fibroblast and smooth muscle. In a study consisting of 48 patients with interstitial cystitis treated with self-administered intravesical heparin, 56% had good clinical remission with continued improvement even after 1 year.[34] Intravesical maintenance therapy with heparin in patients treated with DMSO significantly reduced the relapse rates in symptomatic patients with detrusor mastocytosis.[35]

Bacillus of Calmette-Guérin (BCG)

The use of intravesical BCG for interstitial cystitis was first reported by Zeidman and colleagues. The exact mode of action is still unclear; however immunological and/or anti-inflammatory actions have been postulated. A large, multicenter, randomized, controlled trial by NIDDK comparing BCG to placebo found a 12% response rate for placebo compared to a 21% response for BCG. The positive response rate in this large study of 265 patients followed for 34 months failed to reach statistical significance indicating that BCG has no place in the treatment of moderate-to-severe bladder syndrome/interstitial cystitis.[36] Though the BCG safety profile was considered acceptable in the NIDDK trial, adverse events were not uncommon, and rare hypersensitivity reactions to intravesical BCG have been reported.[37]

Hydrodistension

Cystoscopy with hydrodistension is used for the diagnosis and treatment of interstitial cystitis. Indeed, hydrodistension of the bladder is one of the oldest treatments used for interstitial cystitis. The reported improvement of symptoms is seen in just over 50% of patients but the effect is short-lived (mean duration 2 months).[38] It is hypothesised that stretching may injure nerve endings in the bladder and, thereby, reduce pain. Stretching detrusor smooth muscle cells is known to stimulate heparin-binding epidermal growth factor-like growth factor (HB-EGF) production.[39] Prolonged distension probably has little or no benefit over a short-term distension measured in minutes. Bladder vascular necrosis and rupture are two rare, but serious, complications described in the literature with therapeutic hydrodistension.

Hyperbaric oxygen

Hyperbaric oxygen therapy (HBO) has been used extensively and successfully in the treatment of chronic radiation cystitis, which shows similarities with interstitial cystitis regarding symptoms, various histological alterations and therapeutic approaches. Symptoms commonly associated with both bladder diseases include urinary frequency, urgency, incontinence and pelvic pain. A randomised, sham-controlled, double-blind study on 21 patients using 100% oxygen in pressurised chambers at 2.4 atmospheres for 90 min for 30 sessions concluded that 3 out of 14 patients improved on hyperbaric oxygen therapy, and 0 out of 7 on 'placebo'. The treatment with hyperbaric oxygenation appeared to be a safe, efficacious, well-tolerated and resulted in a sustained decrease of pelvic pain and urgency, improvement of voiding patterns and increase of functional bladder capacity for at least 12 months.[41]

Surgical treatment

Neuromodulation

Neuromodulation is defined as the therapeutic alteration of activity in the central, peripheral or autonomic nervous systems, electrically or pharmacologically, by means of implanted devices. Neuromodulation has been used for decades in the form of behavioral modification, biofeedback, drug therapy and physical therapy. These modalities have all been used for the treatment of urinary frequency, urgency and urge incontinence. Those patients in whom all medical and behavioral therapies have been tried and failed may then be candidates for neuromodulation. Electrical neuromodulation with surface electrodes or with implantable systems has become a valuable addition to the therapeutic options in the last two decades. Interstitial cystitis is an emerging indication. The main drawback is the high surgical revision rate and cost of the treatment.

Women with intractable interstitial cystitis respond favorably to percutaneous sacral stimulation with significant improvement in pelvic pain, day-time frequency, nocturia, urgency and average voided volume. Permanent sacral implantation may be an effective treatment modality in refractory interstitial cystitis but further long-term evaluation is required. Mean voided volume during treatment increased from 90 ml to 143 ml ($P < 0.001$). Mean day-time frequency and nocturia decreased from 20 to 11 and 6 to 2 times ($P = 0.012$ and 0.007, respectively). Mean bladder pain decreased from 8.9 to 2.4 points on a scale of 0 to 10. Of the women, 73% requested to proceed to complete sacral nerve root implantation.[42]

Botulinum toxin-A (BTX-A)

The role of botulinum toxin-A (BTX-A) in painful bladder syndrome/ interstitial cystitis is still under investigation. The therapeutic value of BTX-A is due to its ability to inhibit acetylcholine release temporarily and cause flaccid paralysis in a dose-related manner. By modulating afferent C-fibre activity within the bladder walls, BTX-A significantly improves urodynamic parameters and reduces bladder pain and urinary frequency. The results of a small pilot study suggest that BTX-A intravesical injections are effective in the short-term management of painful bladder syndrome.[43]

Other procedures

Complex surgical procedures for painful bladder syndrome/interstitial cystitis should be reserved for the motivated and well-informed patient who falls into the category of extremely severe, unresponsive disease, a group which comprises fewer than 10% of patients. Transurethral resection of visible ulcers in patients with classic interstitial cystitis showed 90% had amelioration of symptoms; in 40%, symptom relief lasted for more than 3 years.[44] Neurosurgical denervation and perivesical denervation like cystoplasty and cystolysis are considered in those whose bladder capacity (general anesthetic) is greater than 400 ml. If the bladder capacity (general anesthetic) is less than 400 ml, supratrigonal cystectomy and substitution cystoplasty is the treatment of choice.[45] Supratrigonal and subtrigonal cystectomy resulted in similar relief of symptoms but the former appears to provide better functional bladder rehabilitation.[46] Diversion and/or total cystourethrectomy is recommended if the trigone is affected by interstitial cystitis.

CONCLUSIONS

Diagnosis of painful bladder syndrome/interstitial cystitis requires the exclusion of all other causes of bladder discomfort or pain and urinary frequency. The work-up includes a urinary diary, urine microscopy and culture, and usually a cystoscopy. If indicated, urine cytology, urodynamics, imaging, bladder biopsy or laparoscopy may also be required. A symptom questionnaire can be helpful to monitor progress. The etiology is most likely multifactorial, with epithelial dysfunction and neurogenic inflammation being the most studied and proposed mechanisms. Management options include information regarding the condition, direction toward self-help strategies, and oral, intravesical and possibly surgical treatment. Evidence based on randomised trials to date supports the use of amitryptyline, Elmiron®, and intravesical DMSO. However, many treatments are available, (including analgesics, anti-inflammatories, physical therapies including electrical stimulation, other oral and intravesical instillations, and even surgery) which are used widely and require evaluation. However, patients should be encouraged to attend support groups, such as those for interstitial cystitis (<www.ic-network.com>, <www.cobfoundation.org>) and the International Painful Bladder Syndrome Foundation (<www.painful-bladder.org>).

KEY POINTS FOR CLINICAL PRACTICE

- The cause of painful bladder syndrome/interstitial cystitis remains unknown. Potential causes including infection, vascular alterations, psychological aberrations, bladder surface alterations, toxic agents, neurological disorders, and autoimmune responses.
- The diagnosis of painful bladder syndrome/interstitial cystitis is based on clinical symptoms, exclusion of confusable diseases, and cystoscopy with hydrodistension and/or biopsy if indicated.

KEY POINTS FOR CLINICAL PRACTICE *(continued)*

- Currently, no single agent has been proven universally effective; multiple forms of therapy are recommended including self-care and dietary changes, medical and intravesical treatments, neuromodulation, multimodality treatment and surgical intervention.
- New treatment modalities currently under investigation are suplatast tosilate, resiniferatoxin, and botulinum toxin; gene therapy has been used to modulate the pain response.

References

1 ICS definition 2002, modified ESSIC 2005
2 Nordling J. Professor of Urology, Department of Urology, Copenhagen University Hospital in Herlev, Denmark, Personal communication
3 Forrest JB. Epidemiology and quality of life. J Reprod Med 2006; 51 (Suppl): 227–233
4 Leppilahti M, Sairanen J, Tammela TL *et al*. Finnish Interstitial Cystitis-Pelvic Pain Syndrome Study Group. Prevalence of clinically confirmed interstitial cystitis in women: a population based study in Finland. J Urol 2005; 174: 581–583
5 Ito T, Miki M, Yamada T. Interstitial cystitis in Japan. BJU Int 2000; 86: 634–637
6 Bade JJ, Rijcken B, Mensink HJ. Interstitial cystitis in The Netherlands: prevalence, diagnostic criteria and therapeutic preferences. J Urol 1995; 154: 2035–2037
7 Temml C, Wehrberger C, Riedl C, Ponholzer A, Marszalek M, Madersbacher S. Prevalence and correlates for interstitial cystitis symptoms in women participating in a health screening project. Eur Urol 2007; 51: 803–809
8 Warren JW, Jackson TL, Langenberg P, Meyers DJ, Xu J. Prevalence of interstitial cystitis in first-degree relatives of patients with interstitial cystitis. Urology 2004; 63: 17–21
9 Close CE, Carr MC, Burns MW *et al*. Interstitial cystitis in children. J Urol 1996; 156: 860–862
10 Michael YL, Awachi I, Stampfer MJ, Colditz GA, Curham GC. Quality of life among women with interstitial cystitis. J Urol 2000; 164: 423–427
11 Temml C, Wehrberger C, Riedl C, Ponholzer A, Marszalek M, Madersbacher S. Prevalence and correlates for interstitial cystitis symptoms in women participating in a health screening project. Eur Urol 2007; 51: 803–809
12 Lavelle JP, Meyers SA, Ruiz WG, Buffington CA, Zeidel ML, Apodaca G. Urothelial pathophysiological changes in feline interstitial cystitis: a human model. Am J Physiol 2000; 278: F540–F553
13 Keay S, Warren JW. A hypothesis for the etiology of interstitial cystitis based upon inhibition of bladder epithelial repair. Med Hypotheses 1998; 51: 79–83
14 Graham E, Chai TC. Dysfunction of bladder urothelium and bladder urothelial cells in interstitial cystitis. Curr Urol Report 2006; 7: 440–446
15 Letourneau R, Sant GR, el-Mansoury M, Theoharides TC. Activation of bladder mast cells in interstitial cystitis. Int J Tissue React 1992; 14: 307–312
16 Theoharides TC, Pang X, Letourneau R, Sant GR. Interstitial cystitis: a neuroimmunoendocrine disorder. Ann NY Acad Sci 1998; 840: 619–634
17 Erickson DR, Davies MF. Interstitial cystitis. Int Urogynecol J Pelvic Floor Dysfunct 1998; 9: 174–183
18 Mobley DF, Baum N. Interstitial cystitis. When urgency and frequency mean more than routine inflammation. Postgrad Med J 1996; 99: 201–204, 207–208, 214
19 Kirkemo A, Peabody M, Diokno AC *et al*. Associations among urodynamic findings and symptoms in women enrolled in the Interstitial Cystitis Data Base (ICDB) Study. Urology 1997; 49 (Suppl): 76–80
20 Nordling J, Anjum F, Bade J *et al*. Primary evaluation of patients suspected of having interstitial cystitis (IC). Eur Urol 2004; 45: 662–669
21 Denson MA, Griebling TL, Cohen MB, Kreder KJ. Comparison of cystoscopic and histological

findings in patients with suspected interstitial cystitis. J Urol 2000; 164: 1908–1911
22 Keay SK, Zhang CO, Shoenfelt J *et al*. Sensitivity and specificity of antiproliferative factor, heparin-binding epidermal growth factor-like growth factor, and epidermal growth factor as urine markers for interstitial cystitis. Urology 2001; 57(Suppl 1): 9–14
23 Theoharides TC, Sant GR. Hydroxyzine therapy for interstitial cystitis. Urology 1997; 49(Suppl): 108–110
24 Thilagarajah R, Witherow RO, Walker MM. Oral cimetidine gives effective symptom relief in painful bladder disease: a prospective, randomized, double-blind placebo-controlled trial. BJU Int 2001; 87: 207–212
25 van Ophoven A, Pokupic S, Heinecke A, Hertle L. A prospective, randomized, placebo controlled, double-blind study of amitriptyline for the treatment of interstitial cystitis. J Urol 2004; 172: 533–536
26 Jepsen JV, Sall M, Rhodes PR, Schmidt D, Messing E, Bruskewitz RC. Long-term experience with pentosanpolysulfate in interstitial cystitis. Urology 1998; 51: 381–387
27 Hwang P, Auclair B, Beechinor D *et al*. Efficacy of pentosan polysulfate in the treatment of interstitial cystitis: a meta-analysis. Urology 1997; 50: 39–43
28 Bade JJ, Laseur N, Nieuwenburg A, van der Weele LT, Mensink HJ. A placebo-controlled study of intravesical pentosanpolysulphate for the treatment of interstitial cystitis. Br J Urol 1997; 79: 168–171
29 Cartledge JJ, Davies AM, Eardley I. A randomized double-blind placebo-controlled crossover trial of the efficacy of L-arginine in the treatment of interstitial cystitis. BJU Int 2000; 85: 421–426
30 Morales A, Emerson L, Nickel JC. Intravesical hyaluronic acid in the treatment of refractory interstitial cystitis. Urology 1997; 49 (Suppl): 111–113
31 Hurst RE, Roy JB, Min KW *et al*. A deficit of chondroitin sulfate proteoglycans on the bladder uroepithelium in interstitial cystitis. Urology 1996; 48: 817–821
32 Steinhoff G, Ittah B, Rowan S. The efficacy of chondroitin sulfate 0.2% in treating interstitial cystitis. Can J Urol 2002; 9: 1454–1458
33 Rossberger J, Fall M, Peeker R. Critical appraisal of dimethyl sulfoxide treatment for interstitial cystitis: discomfort, side-effects and treatment outcome. Scand J Urol Nephrol 2005; 39: 73–77
34 Parsons CL, Housley T, Schmidt JD, Lebow D. Treatment of interstitial cystitis with intravesical heparin. Br J Urol 1994; 73: 504–507
35 Perez-Marrero R, Emerson LE, Maharajh DO, Juma S. Prolongation of response to DMSO by heparin maintenance. Urology 1993; 41 (Suppl): 64–66
36 Mayer R, Propert KJ, Peters KM *et al*. A randomized controlled trial of intravesical bacillus Calmette-Guérin for treatment refractory interstitial cystitis. J Urol 2005; 173: 1186–1191
37 Parker C, Steele S, Raghavan R *et al*. Hypersensitivity reaction associated with intravesical bacillus Calmette-Guérin for interstitial cystitis. J Urol 2004; 172: 537
38 Ottem DP, Teichman JM. What is the value of cystoscopy with hydrodistension for interstitial cystitis? Urology 2005; 66: 494–499
39 Chai TC, Zhang CO, Shoenfelt JL, Johnson Jr HW, Warren JW, Keay S. Bladder stretch alters urinary heparin-binding epidermal growth factor and antiproliferative factor in patients with interstitial cystitis. J Urol 2000; 163: 1440–1444
40 McCahy PJ, Styles RA. Prolonged bladder distension: experience in the treatment of detrusor overactivity and interstitial cystitis. Eur Urol 1995; 28: 325–327
41 van Ophoven A, Rossbach G, Pajonk F, Hertle L. Safety and efficacy of hyperbaric oxygen therapy for the treatment of interstitial cystitis: a randomized, sham controlled, double-blind trial. J Urol 2006; 176: 1442–1446
42 Maher CF, Carey MP, Dwyer PL, Schluter PL. Percutaneous sacral nerve root neuromodulation for intractable interstitial cystitis. J Urol 2001; 165: 884–886
43 Giannantoni A, Costantini E, Di Stasi SM, Tascini MC, Bini V, Porena M. Botulinum A toxin intravesical injections in the treatment of painful bladder syndrome: a pilot study. Eur Urol 2006; 49: 704–709
44 Peeker R, Aldenborg F, Fall M. Complete transurethral resection of ulcers in classic interstitial cystitis. Int Urogynecol J Pelvic Floor Dysfunct 2000; 11: 290–295
45 Webster GD, Galloway N. Surgical treatment of interstitial cystitis. Indications, techniques, and results. Urology 1987; 29 (Suppl): 34–39
46 Linn JF, Hohenfellner M, Roth S *et al*. Treatment of interstitial cystitis: comparison of subtrigonal and supratrigonal cystectomy combined with orthotopic bladder substitution. J Urol 1998; 159: 774–778

Togas Tulandi Sharifa Al Mahrizi

24

Bowel obstruction after hysterectomy: inform your patients

Donna's case

Donna was a 48-year-old woman who had had a total abdominal hysterectomy for symptomatic uterine fibroids. The operation and postoperative recovery were uneventful. Two years after the hysterectomy, her gynecological surgeon was surprised to receive a letter from a litigation attorney for 'uninformed consent and inappropriate surgical technique'. The gynecologist learned that a general surgeon recently operated on Donna for bowel obstruction.

Adhesion after an abdominal operation is very common. It is a consequence of tissue trauma and healing. In fact, 94% of patients develop intra-abdominal adhesions following a laparotomy.[1,2] Adhesions may cause abdominal pain, infertility, or lead to bowel obstruction.

The importance of adhesions is illustrated in a large retrospective cohort study.[2] The authors reported that 5.7% of all re-admissions following pelvic or abdominal surgeries were directly related to adhesions. Of 29,790 patients who underwent open abdominal or pelvic surgery, 34.6% were re-admitted with an average of 2.1 times over the 10-year period following initial surgery; 22.1% of these admissions were within first year.

Adhesions are also associated with increased medicolegal claims.[3] Using the information from the Medical Defence Union (MDU), Ellis[3] reported that, between 1994 and 1999, it received 77 claims pertaining to abdominal adhesions. They were due to failure to detect or delay in diagnosis, visceral injury at surgery, pain, dyspareunia, infertility, failure to use adhesion-reducing substance, failure

Togas Tulandi MD MHCM FRCSC FACOG (for correspondence)
Professor of Obstetrics and Gynecology and Milton Leong Chair in Reproductive Medicine, McGill University, Montréal, Québec, Canada
E-mail: togas.tulandi@mcgill.ca

Sharifa Al Mahrizi MD
Fellow of Reproductive Endocrinology and Infertility, McGill University, Montréal, Québec, Canada

to warn of risk, and miscellaneous (including death during adhesiolysis). Over an 11-year period, the MDU settled 14 cases out of court.

The presence of intra-abdominal adhesions increases operating times and the risk of bowel injury at subsequent surgery. Surprisingly, not many surgeons advise their patients about the potential risk of adhesion formation prior to surgery.

ADHESIONS AFTER HYSTERECTOMY

The long-term risks of post-surgical adhesions have been under-appreciated. In a study on small bowel obstruction (SBO), the authors[4] reported that the most common causes of bowel obstruction were intra-abdominal adhesions and abdominal malignancy with equal frequency (40%). After excluding oncological cases, they found that of 135 cases of adhesion-related SBO, gynecological operations played the largest role in the occurrence of bowel obstruction (50%).

Among all gynecological operations for benign conditions, total abdominal hysterectomy (TAH) was the most common cause of SBO (13.6 per 1000 TAHs). However, SBO occurs long after the initial surgery (median of 4 years after a hysterectomy).

TYPE OF HYSTERECTOMY

Overall, the incidence of adhesion-related SBO was 2.8% after hysterectomy for benign conditions, 5% after radical hysterectomy, and 20% following a radical hysterectomy and radiation therapy.

Al-Sunaidi and Tulandi,[4] studying SBO after hysterectomy for benign conditions, reported that TAH-related adhesions accounted for 98% of SBO. More than two-thirds of cases were complete obstruction requiring further surgery suggesting the severity of the bowel obstruction. Partial SBO was encountered in a patient after a vaginal hysterectomy.

No SBO was found after laparoscopic supracervical hysterectomy. It is unlikely that this is related to the supracervical nature of the procedure. The most likely explanation is that laparoscopy is associated with less serosal injury and less adhesion formation than laparotomy. This is due to minimal tissue handling by laparoscopy. Also, at laparoscopy we perform surgery in a closed environment maintaining tissue moistness, and contamination with glove powders or lint is non-existent. In addition, the tamponade effect of CO_2 pneumoperitoneum facilitates hemostasis. Compared to laparotomy, it is also associated with a lower incidence of infection.

It appears that hysterectomy by laparoscopy is associated with the least amount of adhesion-related SBO, followed by vaginal hysterectomy and TAH.

SURGICAL TECHNIQUE

SBO-causing adhesions were adhered to previous laparotomy incision in over three-quarters of cases and to the vaginal vault in the remainder. Whether it is related to peritoneal closure is unclear. Several randomized trials have shown that closing either parietal or visceral peritoneum is unnecessary. Closing the peritoneum is associated with a longer operating time, more postoperative pain, and there is a suggestion that it might cause more adhesion formation than non-closure.

The adhesion formation after laparotomy with peritoneal closure was 22.2% and without peritoneal closure 16%. In a recent study, we found that closure of the parietal peritoneum does not seem to contribute to the occurrence of adhesion-related SBO.[4] A larger series is needed for confirmation.

In any event, basic principles of surgery minimizing adhesion formation have to be followed. These include gentle handling of the tissue, meticulous hemostasis, the use of fine instruments and non-reactive sutures, removal of necrotic tissue, minimization of thermal injury or strangulation of tissue, and the use of liberal irrigation. We recommend prophylactic antibiotics.

ADHESION-REDUCING SUBSTANCES

There are two site-specific devices approved by the US Food and Drug Administration (FDA) for adhesion reduction after a laparotomy – oxidized regenerated cellulose (Interceed®; Gynecare, Sommerville, NJ, USA) and sodium hyaluronate-carboxymethylcellulose (CMC) absorbable adhesion barrier (Seprafilm®; Genzyme, Cambridge, MA, USA.[1,5] For reduction of adhesion reformation, one can use 4% icodextrin solution (Adept®; Baxter BioSurgery, Deerfield, IL, USA).[6] In a study on adhesion-related SBO, the use of CMC was associated with a significant reduction in adhesive small bowel obstruction requiring re-operation (1.6% absolute reduction). However, its use at the site of anastomosis might be problematic due to increased incidence of anastomotic leaks.

Despite a large effort in improving anti-adhesive agents, postoperative adhesion formation remains a problem. As a result, the cost of adhesion-related problems to health care is high.

DIAGNOSIS OF BOWEL OBSTRUCTION

Intestinal obstruction leads to dilatation of stomach and small bowel proximal to the site of obstruction, and collapse of the distal bowel (Fig. 1). Dilatation of small bowel can compromise its blood flow and lead to strangulation. The latter increases the mortality from 5% to 37%.

Diagnosis of SBO is based on clinical and radiological findings. The symptoms of SBO include abdominal distension, abdominal pain, nausea and vomiting, inability to pass flatus and constipation. Nausea and vomiting are more pronounced in proximal SBO, and abdominal distension in distal SBO. A history of abdominal or pelvic surgery is highly suggestive of adhesive SBO. The progression of pain from colicky to constant, fever and tachycardia are suggestive of strangulation. Auscultation of bowel sounds is not useful, it may reveal high-pitched or hypo-active sounds.

Laboratory studies are useful to evaluate the severity of dehydration, but not for establishing the diagnosis. Plain abdominal X-ray is diagnostic in about three-quarters of cases. However, the most useful diagnostic tool is computerized tomography (CT). It provides information about the presence, level, severity, and possible cause of SBO. CT scan has a sensitivity and specificity of 93% and 100%, respectively.

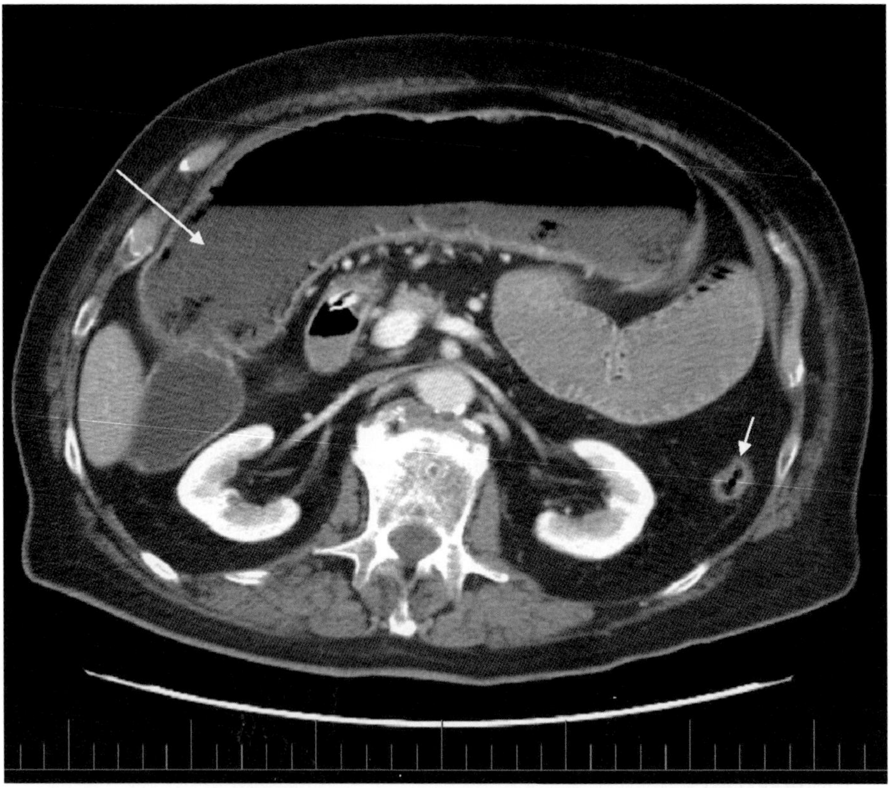

Fig. 1 Computerized tomography scan showing dilated proximal loops of small bowel (long arrow) and collapsed distal loops of large bowel (short arrow).

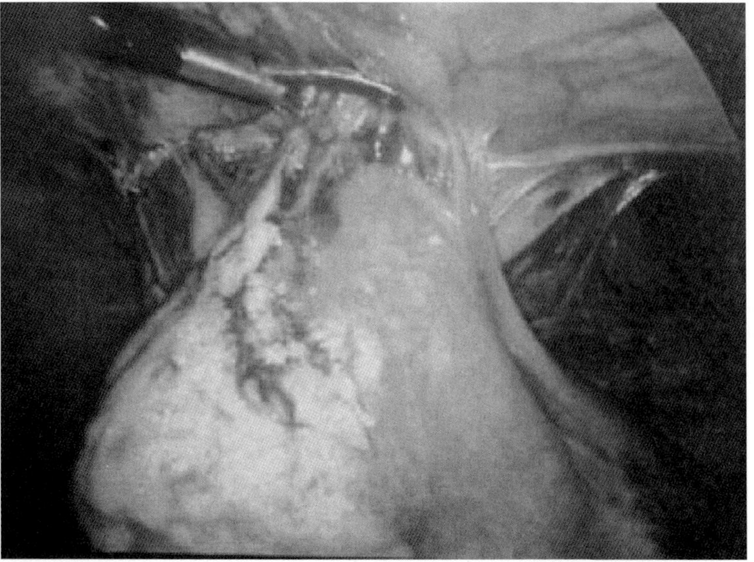

Fig. 2 A loop of small bowel adhered to the site of a previous abdominal incision.

Women who are suspected or diagnosed to have SBO should be consulted to a general surgeon. Further treatment is better conducted by the consulting general surgeon. The treatment could be conservative treatment for incomplete SBO, or surgery for complete SBO. Depending on the familiarity of the consulting surgeon, laparoscopic adhesiolysis could be done in selected cases (Fig. 2).

INFORMED CONSENT

Informed consent is an ethical concept that has become integral to medical ethics and medical practice. It is a process rather than a signature on a form. It includes on-going, shared information and developing choices as long as one is seeking medical assistance (American College of Obstetricians and Gynecologists [ACOG], 2004). If informed consent was not obtained, the surgeon is at risk when a complication occurs despite rendering standard and appropriate care.

In surgical specialties, the surgeon should discuss the goals of surgery, the expected outcome, and the risks and potential complications of the procedure. For hysterectomy, alternatives to hysterectomy, and their advantages and disadvantages, should be discussed. Similarly, discussion about different types of hysterectomy should take place. Besides discussion on possible immediate complications such intra-operative and postoperative bleeding, infection, injury to intra-abdominal organs and thrombosis, patients should also be informed about long-term complications such as adhesion-related SBO.

KEY POINTS FOR CLINICAL PRACTICE

- The most common cause of small bowel obstruction is intra-abdominal adhesions – half of them occur following an abdominal hysterectomy.
- The most common hysterectomy associated with small bowel obstruction is abdominal hysterectomy, followed by vaginal hysterectomy and laparoscopic hysterectomy.
- The median time of onset of small bowel obstruction is 4 years after a hysterectomy. At this time, a general surgeon usually manages the patient, and the treating gynecologist might not be aware of this complication.
- Gynecologists should be aware that hysterectomy, especially by abdominal approach, could lead to small bowel obstruction. They should adhere to basic principles of surgery, minimizing adhesion formation.
- Adhesion-related small bowel obstruction plays a role in the increase of both malpractice lawsuits and healthcare cost.
- Gynecological surgeons should advise their patients about the potential risk of adhesion formation prior to surgery.

References

1 Tulandi T, Al-Shahrani A. Adhesion prevention in gynecologic surgery. Curr Opin Obstet Gynecol 2005; 17: 395–398
2 Ellis H, Moran BJ, Thompson JN *et al*. Adhesion-related hospital readmissions after abdominal and pelvic surgery: a retrospective cohort study. Lancet 1999; 353: 1476–1480
3 Ellis H. Medicolegal consequences of postoperative intra-abdominal adhesions. J R Soc Med 2001; 94: 331–332
4 Al-Sunaidi M, Tulandi T. Adhesion-related bowel obstruction after hysterectomy for benign conditions. Obstet Gynecol 2006; 108: 1162–1166
5 Fazio VW, Cohen Z, Fleshman JW *et al*. Reduction in adhesive small-bowel obstruction by Seprafilm® adhesions barrier after intestinal resection. Dis Colon Rectum 2006; 49: 1–11
6 Menzies D, Pascual MH, Walz MK *et al* ARIEL Registry. Use of icodextrin 4% solution in the prevention of adhesion formation following general surgery: experience from the multicentre ARIEL Registry. Ann R Coll Surg Engl 2006; 88: 375–382

Maya Basu Jonathan R.A. Duckett

Management of the overactive bladder syndrome

Urinary incontinence[1] is one of the most common chronic problems affecting women. Although urinary incontinence is not a life-threatening condition it can severely affect quality of life (QoL). The treatment and containment of urinary incontinence causes a considerable socio-economic burden for society as a whole, as well as for individuals. Interest in urinary incontinence is now increasing but, unfortunately, it is not a political priority. In this review, we examine the current evidence surrounding the treatment of the overactive bladder syndrome (OAB). This is defined[1] as urinary urgency with or without urge incontinence usually with frequency and nocturia, if there is no infection or proven pathology, *i.e.* it is a diagnosis based on symptoms alone, rather than urodynamic findings. OAB can be further classified as 'OAB wet' (with incontinence) or 'OAB dry' (without incontinence).

Whilst studies have attempted to find the prevalence of OAB, the true number of women living with these symptoms is difficult to define. This is because of the so-called 'iceberg phenomenon' whereby only a small number of patients with a condition seek help whilst the greater proportion cope with their symptoms. This is either because of embarrassment or poor access to healthcare services. A recent study of six European countries (France, Germany, Italy, Spain, Sweden and the UK) estimated that 16.6% of the population aged over 40 years had OAB symptoms, this equated to approximately 20–22 million people, of whom only 60% had consulted a

Maya Basu MBBS BSc(Hons)
Specialty Registrar, Department of Obstetrics and Gynaecology, Medway Maritime Hospital, Windmill Road, Gillingham, Kent ME7 5NY, UK
E-mail: mayabasu@aol.com

Jonathan R.A. Duckett FRCOG (for correspondence)
Consultant Urogynaecologist, Medway Maritime Hospital, Windmill Road, Gillingham, Kent ME7 5NY, UK
E-mail: jraduckett@hotmail.com

medical practitioner and only 27% were receiving treatment for their problem.[2,3]

Urinary incontinence is known to have a profound impact on QoL,[4,5] affecting all domains including physical, social, psychological, occupational, activities of daily living and sexual functioning. A study examining a cohort of patients with OAB in the US reported that OAB had a significant impact on QoL, sleep quality and mental health.[4] A 2005 cross-sectional survey of 11,521 individuals with OAB across six European countries (France, Germany, Italy, Spain, Sweden and the UK) found that 76% stated that their symptoms interfered with daily activities.[6] Individuals with 'OAB wet' were more likely to report that symptoms impacted on social situations and home- and work-related activities. Of those with OAB, 32% stated that these symptoms made them feel depressed, with 28% reporting them as a source of stress.

Due to its high prevalence, urinary incontinence causes a significant economic burden.[7] Costs can be divided into direct costs (*e.g.* treatment and diagnosis, pad costs, and drugs) and indirect costs (*e.g.* lost wages). In the year 2000, the estimated cost of OAB in the US was US$12.6 billion, which is similar to the costs of both asthma and osteoporosis. A European study across five countries found the average annual direct cost to be between 269–706 € per patient per year.[3] The largest cost was for the use of incontinence pads, which accounted for 63% of the total cost. The total cost to healthcare systems across all five countries was estimated at 4.2 billion euros in 2000, projected to increase by 1 billion euros by the year 2020. The overall burden also includes indirect costs, which contain lost days at work as well as more subtle, intangible costs related to the QoL impact. These are difficult to quantify. One thing that is certain is that, as the population ages, this burden is likely to increase, making focused and effective management even more important.

Urinary incontinence may be due to a number of factors including systemic diseases, conditions within the bladder or extravesical causes (Table 1). Once local structural and metabolic factors have been excluded, the underlying cause is most often detrusor overactivity. It is important to remember that detrusor overactivity is a urodynamic diagnosis, whereas OAB is a clinical diagnosis. Detrusor overactivity is defined as a urodynamic observation characterised by involuntary detrusor contractions during the bladder filling phase which may be spontaneous or provoked. Phasic detrusor overactivity has a characteristic waveform, which may or may not lead to urinary incontinence. Terminal detrusor overactivity is a single involuntary detrusor contraction, which occurs at cystometric capacity, cannot be suppressed and is often associated with incontinence. Neuropathic detrusor overactivity describes detrusor overactivity, which occurs as a component of a neurological condition. Obstructive detrusor overactivity occurs secondary to any downstream obstruction (*e.g.* prolapse, mid-urethral slings). Idiopathic detrusor overactivity describes detrusor overactivity, which has no obvious cause, and is a diagnosis of exclusion. It usually has a phasic waveform. Bladder function involves a filling and storage phase followed by an emptying phase. Normal detrusor function permits bladder filling with negligible changes in detrusor pressure,[8] via inhibition of detrusor contraction upon stretch of muscle fibers. During filling, pelvic afferent pathways send information about bladder fullness to the pontine micturition center.[9] As

Table 1 Causes of overactive bladder syndrome

Systemic causes	Diabetes mellitus Diabetes insipidus Chronic renal failure Neurological disease Heart failure Sleep apnea Excess fluid intake
Intravesical and urethral causes	Ideopathic detrusor overactivity Urinary tract infection Stones Bladder cancer Tuberculosis Diverticulae Chronic cystitis (interstitial) Radiation cystitis Urodynamic stress incontinence Obstructed voiding – idiopathic, post surgical Post surgical – cause undefined Urethral diverticulae
Extravesicle causes	Fibroids Pelvic mass Pregnancy

bladder volume increases, urethral resistance increases, external urethral sphincter contractions increase and urethral pressure rises. When 75% of bladder capacity is reached, the desire to urinate is triggered. Normal voiding reflexes involve spinal pathways under voluntary control. Spinal parasympathetic outflow is increased, which leads to bladder contraction via acetylcholine activation of muscarinic (predominantly M3) receptors. Sympathetic output to urethral smooth muscle and somatic outflow to urethral and pelvic floor striated muscles are inhibited. There is an increase in bladder pressure allowing urine to flow through a relaxed urethra.

The pathophysiology of idiopathic detrusor overactivity remains obscure, but several observations have been made which may provide some insight. The overactive bladder has increased coupling of smooth muscle.[10] These are known to lead to increased excitability in the face of low-level efferent stimuli, which trigger the sense of urgency and lead to an involuntary contraction. This effect may be age-related or due to nerve damage from injury, disease or obstruction.[11] A possible molecular trigger for changes in bladder afferents or synaptic transmission centrally may be nerve growth factor.[12] This is a naturally occurring substance, which stimulates growth and differentiation of sympathetic and sensory nerves. Patients with OAB and interstitial cystitis have been shown to have elevated levels of nerve growth factor in their bladders; it is unclear the exact role this may play in the pathophysiology of detrusor overactivity.

Whatever the underlying etiology may be, the overactive detrusor exhibits a classical set of signs including a sudden increase in intravesical pressure at low volumes during filling, increased spontaneous muscle activity, altered responsiveness to stimuli and changes in smooth muscle structure.[10]

MANAGEMENT PRINCIPLES

The principles of management of the woman presenting with urgency and/or urge incontinence are based on the basic escalating measures of conservative, medical and interventional. A greater understanding of the role of detrusor contractions in the disease process, as well as increasing availability of urodynamic studies, has lead to a treatment model based on life-style modifications and behavioral measures. These treatments may be combined with pharmacotherapy to modulate the detrusor muscle's activity.

Conservative measures and behavioral therapy

Women with OAB and detrusor overactivity may benefit from simple advice regarding fluid intake (when high) and weight loss (if applicable). Weight loss in the morbidly obese improves incontinence and there is likely to be some improvement in the moderately obese. Caffeine reduction may help, although the evidence is scant. Unlike drug therapy, behavioral therapy has very little in the way of side-effects and complications.

Bladder retraining involves gradually increasing intervals between voiding in the hope of rediscovering central control of continence using an operant learning model.[13] This allows higher centers in the brain to suppress the dominant stimuli which precipitate detrusor contraction via a voluntary pathway. There are four different schedules for bladder retraining – prompted voiding, timed voiding, habit retraining and bladder drill. There is limited evidence concerning the role of bladder retraining. A recent meta-analysis of current available evidence suggests that bladder retraining is a useful tool in the management of adults with urinary incontinence. However, the trials used for the analysis were subject to high levels of bias and with wide confidence intervals.[14] There is some evidence to suggest that initial bladder drill in the hospital is superior to out-patient regimens.

Pelvic floor muscle training (PFMT) has long been regarded as an effective adjunct in the treatment of stress incontinence. PFMT can also be used for the treatment of urge incontinence. There is level 1 evidence that PMFT is better than placebo treatments for urge incontinence. Electrical therapy can be used to treat OAB but the different stimulation types and protocols used in the previous trials make it very difficult to combine the findings in a meaningful way. The biological rationale behind the use of electrical stimulation is difficult to explain and hence many different regimens have been produced. Currently, there is insufficient evidence to judge whether electrical stimulation is better than no treatment for women with detrusor overactivity.

Pharmacotherapy

Drug treatments of detrusor overactivity involve blocking of cholinergic stimulation to the detrusor muscle. The detrusor muscle is supplied by the parasympathetic nerves via spinal segments S2, S3 and S4. The predominant neurotransmitter at the nerve endings on the detrusor muscle is acetylcholine acting via muscarinic M3 receptors. Blocking of these receptors leading to a reduction in detrusor overactivity is the concept that underpins the pharmacotherapy for detrusor overactivity. The major drawback with these drugs is the fact that acetylcholine is a neurotransmitter in many other organs (via five different receptor subtypes named M1–M5); therefore, administration of anticholinergic medications will have adverse effects related to other systems throughout the body. The M3 receptors are mainly responsible for the detrusor contraction.[15] M3 receptors are also present in the salivary glands, smooth muscle, eyes and brain,[16] which explains the difficulties behind the development of bladder-selective medications. The presence of the M3 receptor in these organs gives rise to the adverse effects of constipation, dry mouth, blurred vision, drowsiness and cognitive impairment.

Anticholinergics are the recommended first-line drug treatment for overactive bladder symptoms.[17] The aims of treatment are to decrease incontinence episode frequency and number of voids per day, ultimately leading to improvements in clinical parameters and QoL. The choice of drug will be a balance between clinical efficacy and adverse effects.

Oxybutynin

Oxybutynin is a tertiary amine, which has anticholinergic effects on smooth muscle, including the bladder. It was the first anticholinergic drug used for overactive bladder symptoms, although a number of newer drugs have been developed over recent years. Oxybutynin has muscle relaxant and local anesthetic effects in addition to an antimuscarinic action. It is selective for M1 and M3 receptors over M2 receptors. Oxybutynin is available in immediate release, once daily extended release and transdermal formulations. The immediate release form has an onset of action within 30–60 min of administration with peak effects at 3–6 h. The immediate release preparations are particularly useful for women wish to use medication 'as required' to control symptoms in a certain situation. Randomised control trials have shown oxybutynin to be superior to placebo in terms of reduction of voiding episodes and incontinence episodes.[18,19] However, in normal clinical practice, the marked adverse effects, (particularly dry mouth) are frequently dose-limiting and only a minority of patients are able to persist with treatment beyond 6 months.[20] More worryingly, cognitive impairment has been associated with oxybutynin and it has been suggested that it should not be taken by elderly patients. The side effects are principally caused by metabolites of oxybutynin. These difficulties highlighted a need for modified formulations and drug delivery systems. The extended release formulation was approved by the US Food and Drug Administration in 1999. Published evidence suggests that there are no significant differences in efficacy between immediate release and extended release oxybutynin; however, the extended release formulation is better tolerated with a lower incidence of dry mouth.[21] A newer transdermal preparation has recently been introduced to the market. The great advantage of this over any oral preparation is that it completely bypasses hepatic first-pass metabolism, leading to greater bioavailability. Transdermal systems avoid peaks and troughs in drug concentration, with a steady concentration maintained in the therapeutic range. Because a lower total dose is required to achieve the same plasma concentration, there is a lower incidence of side effects. There have been several, large, controlled trials evaluating the use of transdermal oxybutynin. Studies have shown beneficial effects over placebo in terms of incontinence episodes and QoL measures.[22,23] A head-to-head trial compared immediate release oxybutynin to transdermal oxybutynin.[24] Each was found to be similar in terms of efficacy, with over 20% of patients in each group becoming totally dry. In terms of side effects, 94% of patients in the immediate release group reported dry mouth, as compared to 32% in the transdermal group. Skin reactions limit the use of transdermal oxybutynin. These range from mild erythema to severe cutaneous reactions which may lead to treatment discontinuation. Allowing the alcohol to evaporate for a few minutes before applying the patch may reduce this side effect

Tolterodine

Tolterodine was launched in 1998 in an attempt to introduce a drug with higher bladder selectivity and fewer antimuscarinic side effects. *In vivo* studies have shown tolterodine to be bladder selective leading to a longer and more pronounced effect on the bladder than on salivary glands.[25] As with oxybutynin, both twice daily immediate release and a once daily extended release formulations are available.

Studies comparing immediate release tolterodine to oxybutynin show similar efficacy but less side effects in the tolterodine arm. However, extended release tolterodine has largely replaced the immediate release preparations because the extended release preparation has been shown to be more effective.[26] It was found that both the immediate release and extended release formulations significantly reduced the number of urge incontinence episodes per week ($P = 0.0005$ and $P = 0.0001$, respectively), but extended release tolterodine was 18% more effective than immediate release tolterodine ($P < 0.05$). The rate of dry mouth for patients taking tolterodine extended release was 23% lower than those taking tolterodine immediate release ($P < 0.02$). All other adverse effects were seen with similar frequency in all the groups, including the placebo arm. Interestingly, despite the higher rates of dry mouth in the immediate release arm, the withdrawal rates for each arm of the study were essentially the same (extended release 5%, immediate release 5%, placebo 6%). A longer term study has shown that extended release tolterodine maintains similar efficacy and favorable incidence of side effects over longer treatment periods of up to a year.[27]

Trospium chloride

Trospium is a quaternary amine with predominantly peripheral antimuscarinic activity, leading to smooth muscle relaxation in the bladder. It is thought to lack CNS side effects since it is unable to cross the blood–brain barrier.[28] A Phase 3 study of a total of 658 patients randomised to trospium or placebo showed it to significantly decrease urgency symptoms – an effect that was seen at the end of week one, and was sustained throughout the 12-week study period.[29] Dry mouth was the most common side effect (19.8% in trospium group, placebo 5.2%). The overall discontinuation rate due to adverse effects was 7.3% in the treatment arm (versus 4.6% in the placebo group); the most common reason for discontinuation was dry mouth. Trospium was found to improve health-related QoL significantly, as measured by the incontinence impact questionnaire at 12 weeks.[30]

Solifenacin

Solifenacin is an anticholinergic which was released in 2004, and was reported to be more bladder selective than any of the alternative medications available at the time. A Phase 3 trial found solifenacin to be significantly superior to placebo in terms of incontinence episode reduction and urgency symptoms. Of patients who were incontinent at the start of the trial, 50% were fully dry at the end of the 12-week study period. As with all of the other medications, the most frequently reported side effect was dry mouth, although this was reported to be mild in severity. The incidence at a 5 mg o.d. starting dose was 7.7% and at a 10 mg dose was 23%.[31] This study did not, however, assess impact on QoL. A longer term open label study which was an extension of two Phase 3 studies showed that 81% of participants were willing to continue with solifenacin over a treatment period of 40 weeks. The pooled data showed significant improvements in 9 of the 10 domains of the King's Health Questionnaire, although patient satisfaction had dropped to only 48% after 40 weeks' treatment.[32]

Darifenacin

This is the newest drug in a growing market. Darifenacin is a tertiary amine derivative and is the most selective M3 receptor antagonist available.[33] A double-blind, randomised, cross-over study showed darifenacin to be as effective as oxybutynin in terms of urodynamic outcome, but superior in terms of salivary side effects.[34] A pooled analysis of Phase 3 studies involving 1059 participants found significant, dose-dependent, positive effects on urgency symptoms, incontinence and bladder capacity.[35] The most common side effects were dry mouth and constipation, although these lead to few discontinuations (darifenacin 7.5 mg in 0.6% of patients; darifenacin 15 mg in 2.1% of patients; placebo in 0.3% of patients). A 2-year open label study showed that this favorable efficacy and safety profile was maintained over a longer treatment period.[36]

Other drug therapies

Propiverine has been shown in clinical trials to be effective in the treatment of frequency. Imipramine may be used to treat nocturia or when bladder pain is a significant factor in the history. Desmopressin (DDAVP) is an antidiuretic hormone derivative that can be used for women with nocturia. Unfortunately, it should not be used in the elderly – the exact group most likely to suffer from nocturia and to be able to benefit. Duloxetine may have some application in women with mixed incontinence. The side-effect profile is different to anticholinergics and this may give therapeutic options when anticholinergics are contra-indicated. Some drugs can be instilled directly into the bladder. Intravesicle oxybutynin can be used in resistant cases but is expensive. Capsaicin and resiniferatoxin are neurotoxins which can also be instilled directly into the bladder. Bladder instillations are time consuming, require catheterisation and are not likely to become widely used when in competition with oral medication.

Choice of drug

As can be seen, there are a number of drugs available for the treatment of OAB. A recent meta-analysis of 56 trials of anticholinergic medications found the drugs to all be safe and efficacious. Apart from oxybutynin immediate release,

Table 2 Comparison of different drugs used for treatment of overactive bladder syndrome

Drug	Benefits	Weaknesses
Generic oxybutynin	Cheap Recommended by NICE Well established	Poorly tolerated
Slow release oxybutynin	Improved side-effect profile Escalating dose regimen possible	More expensive than immediate release
Oxybutynin patches	Reduced side-effect profile	Patches may cause skin irritation limiting use
Tolterodine	First of newer anticholinergics Robust trial evidence	Trial suggests not as effective as solifenacin
Trospium	Does not cross blood–brain barrier May have benefits in the elderly or patients with polypharmacy	Broad spectrum anticholinergic side effects
Propiverine	Calcium antagonist action	Recommended for frequency but not urge incontinence
Solifenacin	STAR study suggests some benefits over tolterodine at normal dose	Commonest side effect – dry mouth
Darifenacin	M3 selective	Limited direct clinical experience outside of trials

Data adapted from NICE, UK National Institute for Health and Clinical Excellence.[17]

all were well tolerated, and no drug was associated with increases in any serious adverse events. There were significant differences in terms of withdrawal rates and efficacy outcomes.[37] However, comparison of different drugs using this type of meta-analysis carries certain problems, mainly relating to the heterogeneity of the trials and different methodology and patient populations. Some of the benefits and limitations of each drug are listed in Table 2. With this in mind, a number of head-to-head studies have been carried out, although these should also be interpreted with caution. The OPERA (Overactive bladder: Performance of Extended Release Agents) trial compared oxybutynin extended release with tolterodine extended release in 790 women.[38] Oxybutynin extended release was found to be significantly superior to tolterodine extended release in terms of reduction in frequency (P = 0.003) and urge incontinence episodes (P = 0.03). Both groups had a low incidence of adverse effects and comparable discontinuation rates, although dry mouth was more common in the oxybutynin group (P = 0.02). The ACET (Antimuscarinic Clinical Effectiveness Trial) study again compared oxybutynin extended release and tolterodine extended release.[39] In contrast to the OPERA trial, this trial showed tolterodine 4 mg once daily to be superior to oxybutynin extended release 5 mg or 10 mg and tolterodine 2 mg in terms of patient perception of improvement in bladder symptoms ($P < 0.01$). Incidence of dry mouth was significantly lower in the tolterodine group.

The Solifenacin (flexible dosing with 5 mg and 10 mg o.d. doses) and Tolterodine 4 mg o.d. as an Active comparator in a Randomised (STAR) trial aimed to compare the effectiveness and side-effect profile of the two newer anticholinergics solifenacin and tolterodine extended release.[40] The investigators found solifenacin, with a flexible dosing regimen, to be superior to tolterodine extended release in terms of urgency ($P = 0.035$), urge incontinence ($P = 0.001$) and overall incontinence ($P = 0.006$). Of incontinent patients in the solifenacin group, 59% became continent at the study's end, compared with 49% in the tolterodine extended release group ($P = 0.006$). Discontinuation rates due to side effects were 3.5% in the solifenacin group and 3.0% in the tolterodine extended release group. Discontinuation rates due to lack of efficacy were 2.0% in the tolterodine group versus 1.2% in the solifenacin group.

One essential question is whether any of these trials are actually of any help in deciding which antimuscarinic to use in a particular patient. For example, the two trials comparing oxybutynin extended release to tolterodine extended release outlined above reported opposite results in terms of efficacy. It is debatable whether trial data can actually help clinicians in practice when it is often so conflicting. It is also important to remember that what clinicians deem to be important in determining a drug's efficacy may differ significantly from the opinion of individual patients. It is arguably more important, therefore, to place more emphasis on patient perceived outcomes and QoL than absolute numbers in terms of voiding episodes, incontinence episodes, *etc*. A major factor in choice of drug is the side-effect profile. Indeed, this seems to be the driving force behind new drug development for OAB symptoms. As the population ages and OAB symptoms become more prevalent, the quest for more bladder-selective drugs becomes even more critical. It is clear that with each new generation of antimuscarinic, the incidence of side effects is dropping. Drug trials in urinary incontinence are arguably a 'false' situation; thus, the true efficacy and acceptability of a drug is only really seen once it is in use in real-life situations. This is highlighted by the relatively large placebo response that is a characteristic of trials of drugs for lower urinary tract symptoms. Participation in a randomised, controlled trial (RCT) protocol may be highly intensive with frequent interaction with study investigators and clinical staff. Completion of patient diaries and QoL questionnaires may give patients better insight into their condition. Participating in the trial protocol may thus confer behavioral interventions that benefit the patient and will, in themselves, lead to improvements in QoL.

Ultimately, the choice of drug for a particular patient is a balance between efficacy and side-effect profile. Some patients may be willing to trade off a rapid onset of action against a higher incidence of side effects; for example, taking oxybutynin immediate release to ensure that they are dry for a social engagement or work event. Drug treatment should be tailored to each patient's life-style and symptom profile.

Non-drug interventional treatments

Conservative and pharmacotherapy remain the mainstay of treatment for urgency symptoms. However, there is a subset of patients with intractable symptoms, who fail to respond to multiple therapies. For these patients, other, more invasive, treatments have been developed.

Neuromodulation

Neuromodulation using sacral nerve stimulation (SNS) became available in 1994 as a treatment for refractory urge incontinence. It involves surgical implantation of a generator to provide electrical stimulation to the sacral nerves, thus modulating output to the detrusor muscle. It has been found to produce prolonged subjective benefit in a group of patients with therapy-resistant urgency and urge incontinence. A retrospective analysis of 107 patients with urgency who underwent implantation for SNS found that 63.6% had a 'good result' (based on patient satisfaction) at the time of their last follow-up. Approximately 48.3% had a re-operation for an adverse event, most frequently changes in stimulation sensation, loss of efficacy and pain at the implantation site.[41] The investigators reported a significant 'learning curve' effect with results improving as the study period progressed. This treatment is expensive and provided in very few specialist centres.

Botulinum toxin (Botox)

This is a neurotoxin produced by the bacterium *Clostridium botulinum* and is one of the most poisonous substances known to man. It binds to peripheral cholinergic terminals and inhibits acetylcholine release at the neuromuscular junction. Seven distinct botulinum toxins (A–G) have been isolated, but it is botulinum toxin A that is of most interest to the medical community. It has been shown to inhibit afferent nerve mediated bladder strip contractions,[42] and thus is thought to be of use in conditions associated with overactivity. Injections of botulinum toxin A into the detrusor muscle in patients with OAB symptoms and detrusor overactivity have been shown to result in significant increases in cystometric capacity and detrusor compliance, with a significant fall in mean maximum detrusor pressures. This has lead to subjective and objective improvements lasting 9–12 months.[43] To qualify for Botox treatment, these women have needed to show resistance or poor tolerance to most conventionally used anticholinergics. Hence, they are a group of women who are particularly difficult to treat and may have been offered a clam ileocytoplasty in the past. These results are promising but there are currently no RCTs evaluating the use of Botox in OAB and detrusor overactivity. The beneficial effect of Botox is also responsible for its side effects. Thus, Botox may be so successful in suppressing detrusor activity, that patients cannot empty their bladders or contract the detrusor muscle at all. This side effect is seen in approximately 20% of women; therefore, patients must be able and willing to self-catheterise before being offered this treatment. Fortunately, this side effect is usually short-lived in the majority of women and usually lasts for less than 6 weeks. When counselling women prior to treatment, it is also important to stress that there are no long-term studies of this treatment.

Surgery

Surgical options for urgency symptoms refractory to other treatments are highly specialised and include augmentation (clam) cystoplasty and diversion procedures. A cure rate of up to 90% has been claimed[44] for augmentation cystoplasty but the operation is not without significant morbidity and even mortality. During the procedure, a loop of bowel is resected and sewn into the top of the bladder to increase the bladder capacity. Leakage of feculant material from the bowel anastomosis may be unusual but very dangerous. Patients need to be taught self-catheterisation as there is a significant risk of postoperative voiding dysfunction. Mucus produced by the mucosa of the bowel may be difficult to pass urethrally and may cause distress to the patient. There are risks of stone formation, electrolyte disturbance and chronic urinary infection. Malignant change has also been reported in the ileal segment. This procedure has largely been superseded by Botox therapy. However, as difficulties with long-term Botox therapy emerge, there may be recurrent interest in this operation in future years.

CONCLUSIONS

OAB is a common, distressing and bothersome condition that carries substantial co-morbidity and impacts significantly on individuals and society as a whole. After many years of little interest in the development of new treatments, there are now many new drugs which improve symptoms. The use of these agents in many patients will be limited, or at least guided, by their side-effect profiles. It is also important to remember the essential role that life-style measures and bladder retraining will play in producing a lasting improvement in symptoms. As the population ages, these conditions will become ever more prevalent, necessitating greater awareness of OAB and its treatment amongst the medical community. The future looks promising for OAB sufferers with newer, more bladder-selective agents appearing on the market, as well as research into other therapies such as SNS and Botox. It should always be remembered that treatment should be tailored to the individual, with the emphasis on quality of life being paramount.

KEY POINTS FOR CLINICAL PRACTICE

- Urinary incontinence has a profound impact on quality of life and carries substantial socio-economic costs.
- Overactive bladder syndrome (OAB) is defined as urinary urgency with or without urinary incontinence, usually with frequency and nocturia. It is a clinical diagnosis and the most common underlying cause is detrusor overactivity.
- Initial management is conservative, consisting of weight loss, modification of fluid and caffeine intake, bladder retraining and physiotherapy.
- The next step is anticholinergic treatments, which block muscarinic stimulation of the detrusor muscle.
- The choice of drug is a balance between clinical efficacy and adverse effects.

KEY POINTS FOR CLINICAL PRACTICE *(continued0*

- Anticholinergic medications are associated with the side effects of dry mouth (most commonly), constipation, blurred vision, drowsiness and cognitive impairment.
- Side effects may be reduced by using extended release or transdermal preparations.
- Options for women with intractable symptoms include neuromodulation, botulinum toxin A, and surgical interventions such as clam cystoplasty.

References

1 Abrams P, Cardozo L, Fall M *et al.* The standardisation of terminology of lower urinary tract function: report from the standardisation sub-committee of the International Continence Society. Neurourol Urodyn 2002; 21: 167–178

2 Milson I, Abrams P, Cardozo L *et al.* How widespread are the symptoms of an overactive bladder and how are they managed? A population based prevalence study. BJU Int 2001; 87: 760–766

3 Reeves P, Irwin D, Kelleher C. The current and future burden and cost of overactive bladder in five European countries. Eur Urol 2006; 50: 1050–1057

4 Stewart W, Van Rooyen J, Cundiff G *et al.* Prevalence and burden of overactive bladder in the United States. World J Urol 2003; 20: 327–336

5 Jackson S. The patient with an overactive bladder – symptoms and quality of life issues. Urology 1997; 50 (Suppl 6A): 18–22

6 Irwin D, Milson I, Kopp Z. Impact of overactive bladder symptoms on employment, social interactions and emotional well being in six European countries. BJU Int 2005; 97: 96–100

7 Kobelt G. Economic considerations and outcome measurement in urge incontinence. Urology 1997; 50 (Suppl 6A): 100–107

8 Abrams P. Describing bladder storage function: overactive bladder syndrome and detrusor overactivity. Urology 2003; 62 (Suppl 2): 28–37

9 Fowler C. Bladder efferents and their role in the overactive bladder. Urology 2002; 59 (Suppl 1): 37–42

10 Chu F, Dmochowski R. Pathophysiology of overactive bladder. Am J Med 2006; 119: 35–55

11 Yoshida M, Miyamae K, Iwashita H *et al.* Management of detrusor dysfunction in the elderly: changes in acetylcholine and adenosine triphosphate release during aging. Urology 2004; 63: 17–23

12 Steers W. Pathophysiology of overactive bladder and urge incontinence. Rev Urol 2002; 4: S7–S18

13 Toozs-Hobson P, Parsons M. The overactive bladder syndrome. Cardozo L, Staskin D. (eds) *Textbook of female urology and urogynaecology*, 2nd edn. London: Informa, 2006.

14 Wallace S, Roe B, Williams K, Palmer M. Bladder training for continence in adults. Cochrane Database Syst Rev 2004; 1: CD001308

15 Chapple C, Yamonishi T, Chess-Williams R. Muscarinic receptor subtypes and management of the overactive bladder. Urology 2002; 60 (5 Suppl 1): 82–88

16 Scarpero H, Dmochowski R. Muscarinic receptors: what we know. Curr Urol Report 2003; 4: 421–8

17 National Collaborating Centre for Women's and Children's Health. *NICE Clinical Guideline number 40: The management of urinary incontinence in women*. London: National Institute for Health and Clinical Excellence, 2006

18 Tapp A, Cardozo L, Versi E, Cooper D. The treatment of detrusor instability in post-menopausal women with oxybutynin chloride: a double blind placebo controlled study. Br J Obstet Gynaecol 1990; 97: 521–526
19 Thusoff J, Bunke B, Ebner A *et al.* Randomised double-blind multicenter trial on treatment of frequency, urgency and incontinence related to detrusor hyperactivity: oxybutynin versus propantheline versus placebo. J Urol 1991; 145: 813–816
20 Kelleher C, Cardozo L, Khullar V, Salvatore S. A medium term analysis of the subjective efficacy of treatment for women with detrusor instability and low bladder compliance. Br J Obstet Gynaecol 1997; 104: 988–993
21 Anderson R, Mobley D, Blank B *et al.* Once daily controlled versus immediate release oxybutynin chloride for urge urinary incontinence: OROS oxybutynin study group. J Urol 1999; 161: 1809–1812
22 Dmochowski R, Davila G, Zinner N *et al.* Efficacy and safety of transdermal oxybutynin in patients with urge and mixed urinary incontinence. J Urol 2002; 168: 580–586
23 Sand P, Zinner N, Newman D *et al.* Oxybutynin transdermal system improves the quality of life in adults with overactive bladder: a multicentre, community-based, randomised study. BJU Int 2006; 99: 836–844
24 Davila G, Daugherty C, Sanders S, Transdermal oxybutynin study group. A short term multicenter, randomised, double-blind dose titration study of the efficacy and anticholinergic side effects of transdermal compared to immediate release oral oxybutynin treatment of patients with urge urinary incontinence. J Urol 2001; 166: 140–145
25 Stahl M, Eckstrom B, Sparf A *et al.* Urodynamic and other effects of tolterodine: a novel antimuscarinic drug for the treatment of detrusor overactivity. Neurourol Urogyn 1995; 14: 647–655
26 van Kerrbroek P, Kreder K, Jonas U *et al.* Tolterodine once-daily: superior efficacy and tolerability in the treatment of the overactive bladder. Urology 2001; 57: 414–420
27 Kreder K, Mayne C, Jonas U. Long term safety, tolerability and efficacy of extended release tolterodine in the treatment of overactive bladder. Eur Urol 2002; 41: 588–595
28 Todorova A, Vonderheid-Guth B, Dimpfel W. Effects of tolterodine, trospium chloride and oxybutynin on the central nervous system. J Clin Pharmacol 2001; 41: 636–644
29 Rudy D, Cline K, Harris R *et al.* Multicenter phase 3 trial studying trospium chloride in patients with overactive bladder. Urology 2006; 67: 275–280
30 Zinner N, Giffelman M, Harris R *et al.*; for the Trospium Study Group. Trospium chloride improves overactive bladder symptoms: a multicenter phase 3 trial. J Urol 2004; 171: 2311–2315
31 Cardozo L, Lisec M, Millard R *et al.* Randomised, double blind placebo controlled trial of the once daily antimuscarinic agent solifenacin succinate in patients with overactive bladder. J Urol 2004; 172: 1919–1924
32 Haab F, Cardozo L, Chapple C, Ridder A; for the Solifenacin Study Group. Long term open label solifenacin treatment associated with persistence with therapy in patients with overactive bladder syndrome. Eur Urol 2005; 47: 376–384
33 Napier C, Gupta P. Darifenacin is selective for the human recombinant M3 receptor subtype. Neurourol Urodyn 2002; 21: A445
34 Chapple C, Abrams P. Comparison of darifenacin and oxybutynin in patients with overactive bladder: assessment of ambulatory urodynamics and impact on salivary flow. Eur Urol 2005; 48: 102–109
35 Chapple C, Steers W, Norton P *et al.* A pooled analysis of three phase 3 studies to investigate the efficacy, tolerability and safety of darifenacin, a muscarinic M3 selective receptor antagonist, in the treatment of overactive bladder. BJU Int 2005; 95: 993–1001
36 Haab F, Corcos J, Siami P *et al.* Long term treatment with darifenacin for overactive bladder: results of a 2 year, open-label extension study. BJU Int 2006; 98: 1025–1032
37 Chapple C, Khullar V, Gabriel Z, Dooley J. The effects of antimuscarinic treatments in overactive bladder: systematic review. BMJ 2003; 326: 841–844
38 Diokno A, Appell R, Sand P *et al.* Prospective, randomised, double-blind study of the efficacy and tolerability of the extended-release formulation of oxybutynin and tolterodine for overactive bladder: results of the OPextended releaseA trial. Mayo Clin Proc 2003; 78: 687–695

39 Sussman D, Gareley A. Treatment of overactive bladder with once daily extended-release tolterodine or oxybutynin: the antimuscarinic clinical effectiveness trial (ACET). Curr Med Res Opin 2002; 18: 177–184
40 Chapple C, Martinez-Garcia R, Selvaggi L *et al.*; for the STAR study group. A comparison of the efficacy and tolerability of solifenacin succinate and extended release tolterodine at treating overactive bladder syndrome: results of the STAR trial. Eur Urol 2005; 48: 464–470
41 van Voskuilen A, Oerlmans D, Weil E *et al.* Long term results of neuromodulation by sacral nerve stimulation for LUT symptoms: a retrospective single center study. Eur Urol 2006; 49: 366–372
42 Smith C, Fraser M, Bartho L *et al.* Botulinum toxin A inhibits afferent nerve evoked bladder strip contractions [Abstract]. J Urol 2002; 167: 41
43 Sahai A, Khan M, Fowler C, Dasgupta P. Botulinum toxin for the treatment of lower urinary tract symptoms: a review. Neurourol Urodyn 2005; 24: 2–12
44 Westney OL, McGuire EJ. Surgical procedures for the treatment of urge incontinence. Tech Urol 2001; 7: 126–132

Shai E. Elizur Ri-Cheng Chian Hananel E.G. Holzer Yariv Gidoni Ezgi Demirtas Seang Lin Tan

In vitro maturation of oocytes for treatment of infertility and preservation of fertility

ENDOCRINOLOGY OF OOCYTE MATURATION

Oocyte maturation *in vivo*

Follicles, in the human female ovary, begin to form at 18–20 weeks of fetal life. The first follicle formed, the primordial follicle, contains an oocyte, enveloped by a single layer of spindle-shaped pregranulosa cells enclosed by a basement membrane. The primordial follicle can develop into the primary follicle (the pregranulosa layer changes to cuboidal layer of granulosa cells), pre-antral follicle (more complete granulosa cells proliferation) and antral follicle (characterized by a fluid-filled space). At any point in this development, individual follicles may become arrested and eventually regress in an apoptotic process. This follicular development is believed to be independent of gonadotropin stimulation. Consequently, large numbers of follicles die at the early antral stage. All together, out of the 6-7 million oogonia present by 16–20 weeks of fetal life, only about 400–500 mature oocytes will be ovulated from the ovary to the fallopian tube for potential fertilization throughout a woman's reproductive life. After the onset of puberty, only a portion from the growing cohort of antral follicles, will respond to the rising levels of follicle-stimulating hormone (FSH) and luteinizing hormone (LH). During each menstrual cycle,

Shai E. Elizur MD, **Yariv Gidoni** MD, **Ezgi Demirtas** MD
Clinical/Research Fellows in Reproductive Endocrinology and Infertility, Department of Obstetrics and Gynecology, McGill University Royal Victoria Hospital, 687 Pine Avenue West, Montréal, QC 113 1A1, Canada

Ri-Cheng Chian MSc PhD, **Hananel E.G. Holzer** MD,
Assistant Professors, Department of Obstetrics and Gynecology, McGill University Royal Victoria Hospital, 687 Pine Avenue West, Montréal, QC 113 1A1, Canada

Seang Lin Tan MBBS FRCOG FRCSC FACOG MMed(O&G) MBA (for correspondence)
James Edmund Dodds Professor and Chairman, Department of Obstetrics and Gynecology, McGill University Royal Victoria Hospital, 687 Pine Avenue West (Room F4.29), Montréal, QC 113 1A1, Canada
E-mail: seanglin.tan@muhc.mcgill.ca

approximately 20 antral follicles respond to the rising levels of gonadotropins, and usually one of them continues through all of the pre-ovulatory stages of development and ovulates.[1] It is estimated that it takes approximately 85 days for the primordial stage follicle to achieve pre-ovulatory status. As mentioned, gonadotropins are necessary for part of the follicular development *in vivo* and both these hormones use the cyclic adenosine monophosphate (cAMP) pathway as an intracellular second messenger. In addition, there are many other growth factors and cytokines that modulate the action of gonadotropins.

The process of follicular development, from the primordial to the pre-ovulatory follicle, entails both granulosa cell and oocyte development:

1. **Granulosa cell development**: the pregranulosa spindle shaped layer of the primordial follicle proliferates and differentiates into two populations – the mural granulosa cells that are adjacent to the basement membrane and the cumulus cells that surround the oocyte.

2. **Oocyte development**: the oocyte itself grows in size from the primordial to the pre-ovulatory follicle stage (reaching a maximum of ~100 μm) and, thereafter, undergoes a process of maturation, which begins at the pre-ovulatory mid-cycle LH surge.

The mid-cycle LH surge triggers a series of changes in the ovarian follicle critical for ovulation and oocyte maturation. LH receptors are located mainly on the mural granulosa cells. Therefore, the mechanism(s) by which LH stimulates oocyte maturation is mainly indirect. Although much is known about LH signaling in the mural granulosa cells, how the LH signal is passed on to the oocyte is incompletely understood.[2] Ultimately, the action of LH on the mural granulosa cells translates to a change in signaling molecules within the oocyte to initiate meiotic resumption. Recent work[3] has shown that mural granulosa cells express RNA encoding epidermal growth factor (EGF)-like proteins within 1–3 h of LH receptor stimulation, and these proteins, in particular amphiregulin and epiregulin, cause follicle-enclosed as well as cumulus-enclosed oocytes to mature as effectively as LH, though with a faster time-course. They do not cause maturation of isolated oocytes. However, the signaling pathway between cumulus cells and oocytes remains unknown.

Oocyte maturation requires changes in both the nucleus and cytoplasm of the oocyte. The nucleus of the oocyte is arrested at the prophase stage of the first meiotic division from the primordial follicle to the pre-ovulatory stage follicle. It is well established that relatively high levels of cAMP within the oocyte are essential to keep the meiotic cycle on hold, whereas a drop in intra-oocyte concentrations of this nucleotide enables resumption of meiosis. Prior to the mid-cycle surge of LH, the growing oocyte acquires the ability to undergo oocyte maturation. The acquisition of meiotic competence occurs around the time of antrum formation. Nevertheless, the source of the inhibitory cAMP is still a matter of controversy. One theory suggests that the oocyte generates the inhibitory cAMP on its own,[4] whereas another claims that meiotic arrest is dependent on the cumulus/granulosa cells for the supply of this inhibitor.[5] According to the first theory, self-production of cAMP by the oocyte takes place in response to a ligand continuously generated by the granulosa cells that, in turn, activates an oocyte membrane-bound G_s protein which stimulates oocyte adenylyl cyclase. In this case, the spontaneous maturation that occurs upon the release of the oocyte from the ovarian follicle may represent the termination of their exposure to the granulosa-derived, G_s-activating ligand.[4,6] The second theory proposes that cAMP produced in the surrounding granulosa cells is transferred into the oocyte via gap junctions, thereby maintaining meiotic arrest. This hypothesis further suggests that LH-induced oocyte maturation occurs subsequently to interruption of gap junction communication. According to this hypothesis, the release of the oocyte from the ovarian follicle, which results in its spontaneous maturation, actually mimics the effect of LH, in that it terminates the supply of the inhibitory cAMP from the granulosa cells to the oocyte.[5]

Oocytes at the pre-ovulatory follicle are at the germinal vesicle (GV) stage. Following the LH surge, the resumption of meiosis begins at the oocyte nucleus; the nuclear membrane dissolves and the chromosomes progress from the metaphase I to the telophase I stage. This is known as the germinal vesicle breakdown (GVBD). After the first meiotic division, which is characterized by the extrusion of the first polar body, the second meiotic division begins and a secondary metaphase plate (metaphase II) is formed. Therefore, oocyte maturation is defined morphologically as the re-initiation and completion of the first meiotic division from the GV stage to the metaphase II stage (M II).

Oocyte nuclear maturation is accompanied by a process of cytoplasmic maturation. These ultrastructural and functional modifications, which are mainly invisible, are crucial for oocyte fertilization and early embryonic development. Among others, these include changes in the distribution of the organelles, with movement of the endoplasmic reticulum, mitochondria, and cortical granules just below the oolemma.[7] In addition, formation and localization of cell microfilaments and specific cytoplasmic protein synthesis may be involved in cytoplasmic maturation.

Oocyte maturation *in vitro*

As mentioned previously, cumulus-oocyte complexes can be spontaneously induced to resume meiosis when they are released from follicles into culture *in vitro*. Therefore, the action of endocrine factors that affect the oocyte maturation *in vitro* may be quite different from *in vivo* conditions. Immature oocytes with or without surrounding cumulus cells can be matured to the M II stage. However, the capacity for early development of denuded oocytes is questionable. The beneficial effects of cumulus cells on early embryonic development have been reported in many species including human.[8] The actions of endocrine, paracrine and autocrine factors that control oocyte maturation *in vitro*, either directly or indirectly, are mediated by the cumulus cells. Although FSH and LH play an important role in the development and maturation of pre-antral, antral and pre-ovulatory follicles *in vivo*, these gonadotropins may not play the same role in promoting oocyte maturation *in vitro*. Currently, most *In vitro* maturation (IVM) protocols supplement FSH or LH into a culture medium for oocyte maturation.[9] However, the effects of these hormones on oocyte maturation and subsequent fertilization as well as early embryonic development are still controversial. The idea of supplementing these hormones into a culture medium is based on their physiological role in oocyte maturation *in vivo*. The contradictory reports that FSH or LH are major hormones involved in IVM may be related to cross contamination of FSH with LH, or LH with FSH, since each preparation derives from urinary extracts.[10] While it has been reported that using the combination of recombinant FSH with recombinant LH in IVM of immature oocytes resulted in significantly higher developmental competence, evident by increased development to the blastocyst stage compared with recombinant FSH alone or no gonadotropins,[11] conclusive results require further study. In addition, recently it has been shown that recombinant human chorionic gonadotropin (hCG) or recombinant LH are equally effective in promoting oocyte maturation *in vitro*, although there was no proper control group in the study to confirm this conclusion.[12] In *in vitro* conditions, it was initially considered that FSH and LH probably act to induce oocyte maturation by an indirect action mediated by cumulus cells, because it has been hitherto believed that there are no FSH or LH receptors on the oocytes. However, recent reports[13,14] indicate that messenger RNA for FSH and LH hormone receptors is present in mouse and human oocytes, zygotes and pre-implantation embryos indicating a potential role for gonadotropins in the modulation of meiotic resumption and the completion of oocyte maturation. In addition, it has been known that culture medium supplemented with a physiological concentration of FSH or LH stimulates steroid (estradiol and progesterone) secretions from the cultured granulosa and cumulus cells.[15] Therefore, it is likely that one of the actions of gonadotropins is mediated by either estradiol or progesterone, which may control oocyte maturation *in vitro*. A recent report indicated that LH receptor formation in the cumulus cells that surround porcine oocytes had an important role in oocyte cytoplasmic maturation.[16] However, its importance in oocyte maturation *in vitro* and how this action was linked to other signal transduction pathways are still largely unknown.

Estradiol and progesterone are mediators of normal mammalian ovarian function. Inhibition of steroid synthesis in whole, cultured follicles impairs subsequent fertilization and developmental capacity of the oocytes in sheep.[17] The presence of estradiol in the culture medium of *in vitro* matured human oocytes had no effect on the progression of meiosis but improved the fertilization and cleavage rates.[18] However, it may not be necessary to add estradiol to the oocyte maturation medium when the oocytes are cultured with cumulus cells because the culture medium supplemented with gonadotropins stimulates estradiol secretion from the granulosa and cumulus cells during culture *in vitro*.[15] There is little information about the effect of progesterone contained in the culture medium on oocyte maturation. However, we have found a negative effect of progesterone on bovine oocyte maturation *in vitro*.

It is well known that there are many growth factors contained in follicular fluid. These growth factors must be secreted from the granulosa and cumulus cells that respond to gonadotropins, and subsequently act on the oocyte via paracrine and autocrine pathways. Although a growing number of studies have indicated that there are beneficial effects of growth factors on oocyte maturation, it seems that only denuded oocytes require the supplementation of growth factors in the culture medium for proper oocyte maturation.[19] This suggests that the granulosa and cumulus cells can secrete some growth factors during culture and play some functional roles during oocyte maturation *in vitro*.

IVM of oocytes from women with PCO and PCOS

Research into the maturation of oocytes goes back to 1935 when Pincus and Enzman[20] showed that mammalian oocytes removed from their follicle spontaneously resumed meiosis. Although Edwards *et al.*[21] described IVM of human oocytes, it was not until 1991 when this procedure was incorporated as a treatment for human infertility. Cha *et al.*[22] reported that human oocytes harvested from unstimulated ovaries during a gynecological operation were matured *in vitro* and fertilized. Five embryos were then transferred to a woman with premature ovarian failure, who subsequently delivered healthy triplet girls.

IVM was initially considered as a treatment for patients with polycystic ovarian syndrome (PCOS).[23] This is a very heterogeneous syndrome, which consists of oligo or amenorrhea, clinical and/or biochemical evidence of hyperandrogenism and, typically, the ultrasonic feature of numerous antral follicles in the ovaries. Some women have only the typical ultrasonic feature of the polycystic ovaries (PCO) without menstrual irregularities or hyperandrogenism. Conventional *in vitro* fertilization (IVF) treatment requires that the ovaries be stimulated with FSH and LH in order to increase the number of mature oocytes retrieved and, consequently, to improve pregnancy rate. IVF today results in higher pregnancy rates than spontaneous conception.[24,25] However, ovarian stimulation protocols are associated with high costs, daily injection of gonadotropins and the need for close monitoring. Moreover, they carry a risk of causing ovarian hyperstimulation syndrome (OHSS). Although a mild or moderate degree of OHSS may not be very dangerous, severe OHSS may be associated with significant morbidity. The most severe manifestation of OHSS involves massive ovarian enlargement and multiple cysts, hemoconcentration and third-space accumulation of fluid. The syndrome may be further complicated by renal failure and thrombo-embolic episodes. Women with PCO only or PCOS have the highest risk (up to 6%) of developing OHSS.[26] Several methods have been proposed in order to minimize the risk of OHSS in high-risk patients. Among these are intravenous administration of human albumin at the time of oocyte retrieval,[27] withholding gonadotropins and hCG injections until serum estradiol levels decrease (coasting),[28] administration of glucocorticoids,[29] reduction of hCG dosage given to trigger ovulation,[30] elective cryopreservation of all embryos[31] and others. However, to date, no precise method has been developed to eliminate severe OHSS completely following ovarian stimulation. Thus, the best course of action would be to avoid ovarian stimulation with gonadotropins altogether. Therefore, IVM of oocytes seems to be an appealing alternative for women with PCO or PCOS. It has been shown that the main clinical determinant of success rates of IVM treatment is antral follicle count.[32] As women with PCO or PCOS have a high antral follicle count (usually more than 20), they are prime candidates for IVM treatment. When hCG priming is used before oocyte retrieval, it has been found that immature oocytes retrieved from patients with normal ovaries, PCO or PCOS have similar high maturation, fertilization, and cleavage potential.[33,34] These results suggest that IVM is a promising alternative to conventional IVF treatment for those women requiring assisted conception.

IVM for hyper-responders to gonadotropin ovarian stimulation

As mentioned previously, there is no precise method to prevent severe OHSS completely during ovarian stimulation treatment. However, in women that over-respond to ovarian stimulation treatment, the risk of severe OHSS can be reduced by withholding the ovulation-inducing trigger of hCG and canceling the treatment. It is known that high levels of serum estradiol, on the day of hCG administration, is associated with severe OHSS. Thus, in conventional ovarian stimulation for IVF, where there has been an over-response and there is a high risk for OHSS, early administration of hCG, when estradiol serum levels are still low, may prevent severe OHSS. Lim *et al.*[35] reported 17 patients with a high risk to develop OHSS during conventional IVF. Instead of canceling the cycle, they administered hCG when the leading follicle was 12–14 mm diameter and matured *in vitro* the oocytes. Of 233 oocytes, 27 (11.6%) were at the M II stage on the day of collection and, following 48 h, 75.9% of oocytes matured. Eight out of the 17 patients conceived and none of the patients developed OHSS. Therefore, in cases at high risk for developing OHSS during conventional IVF, early administration of hCG followed by IVM can be an alternative to cycle cancellation.

Fertility preservation

Tremendous progress in treatment over the past three decades has resulted in a steady increase in the survival rates of cancer patients. Therefore, because these patients live longer, they are exposed to the long-term effects of chemo- and radiotherapy. Unfortunately, since many of the anti-tumor agents have a detrimental effect on the gonads, many young cancer patients carry a considerable risk of losing their future fertility potential. In addition, some patients with advanced connective tissue maladies require chemotherapy in order to control their disease. Therefore, fertility preservation is becoming an integral part of patient consultation prior to gonadotoxic treatment.[36] Among the available fertility preservation options, it is possible to offer embryo, ovarian tissue or oocyte cryopreservation. Although IVF followed by embryo cryopreservation is the established method of fertility preservation, it is not feasible for women with no partner, in cases when hormonal ovarian stimulation is contra-indicated or when there is insufficient time for ovarian stimulation. Another alternative is ovarian tissue cryopreservation which offers the special benefit of providing estrogen activity following ovarian auto-transplantation. However, this option requires two surgical procedures – excision of the ovarian tissue and autografting. Moreover, the survival time of the ovarian graft following transplantation is unknown. In addition, orthotopic ovarian tissue transplantation has only produced two live births to date[37,38] and is relatively inefficient.[39] Finally, it carries a very small risk of re-introducing malignant cells, if the original procedure was performed for fertility preservation for cancer.

In order to cryopreserve embryos or oocytes, mature oocytes could be harvested from the ovaries of cancer patients after controlled ovarian stimulation. However, there are two major drawbacks associated with conventional IVF in patients facing gonadotoxic treatment. First, the time interval needed for IVF treatment ranges from 2–6 weeks and in some cases there is insufficient time for ovarian stimulation. Second, ovarian stimulation is associated with relatively high estradiol serum levels, which may not be deemed totally safe for some cases of estrogen-sensitive breast cancer or systemic lupus erythematosus (SLE). Therefore, IVM is a promising fertility preservation option for many patients facing gonadotoxic treatment who are unable to undergo controlled ovarian stimulation. We recently reported the retrieval of immature oocytes from unstimulated ovaries before gonadotoxic therapy for oocyte vitrification.[40] In addition, we have shown that immature oocytes aspirated at the luteal phase are able to mature, fertilize and cleave properly.[41] Therefore, in extreme cases, when gonadotoxic treatment is urgent, oocyte collection can be performed on any day of a woman's menstrual cycle. We have recently performed both follicular and luteal-phase oocyte collection in several women about to undergo urgent gonadotoxic treatment. In young, single women, mature oocytes can be vitrified for future use or, if a partner is available, embryos can be vitrified following fertilization. As mentioned previously, ovarian tissue cryopreservation offers the special benefit of providing estrogen activity following ovarian auto-transplantation. We have recently combined ovarian tissue cryobanking with IVM of immature oocytes collected from the ovarian tissue, followed by vitrification of the matured oocytes.[42] Therefore, it seems that, due to the recent major breakthroughs in oocyte vitrification, IVM is likely to become a major form of treatment for fertility preservation in the near future.

Oocyte donation

Oocyte donation has become a standard treatment for women: (i) with diminished ovarian reserve and/or who are of advanced reproductive age; (ii) affected by, or who are carriers of, a significant genetic defect; and (iii) with poor oocyte and/or embryo quality. Oocyte donation results in a high pregnancy rate for patients with an otherwise grave reproductive prognosis. However, there is a world-wide shortage of egg donors and, in most countries, the waiting list for egg donation programs is daunting. The inconvenience and possible long-term side effects of hormone injections and the risk of OHSS are a major source of concern to potential egg donors. As mentioned previously, IVM treatment eliminates the risk of OHSS and reduces the cost of medication for ovarian stimulation required in an egg donation program. We have recently reported[43] on 12 oocyte donors (mean age, 29.3 ± 4.0 years) with high antral follicle count (29.6 ± 8.7), who underwent immature oocyte collection without ovarian stimulation. Six of the 12 recipients (50%) conceived and four delivered. These preliminary results suggest that collecting immature oocytes from a donor's unstimulated ovaries in an oocyte donation program may be worthwhile in selected cases.

Combination of natural cycle IVF with IVM

The first live birth following IVF treatment resulted from natural cycle IVF. However, this has been gradually replaced by hormonal ovarian stimulation combined with IVF in order to increase the number of mature oocytes retrieved and pregnancy rates. Recently, there is an increasing interest in natural cycle IVF, primarily because it is more comfortable to patients, has fewer side effects, avoids OHSS and possible long-term hormonal effects and reduces treatment costs. As mentioned previously, during the follicular phase of the menstrual cycle usually only a single dominant follicle grows to the pre-ovulatory stage and releases one oocyte for potential fertilization. However, approximately 20 additional small antral follicles respond to the rising levels of gonadotropins and continue developing through different stages of the pre-ovulatory follicle. It seems that, even after the selection of the dominant follicle, atresia does not occur in the non-dominant follicles; therefore, an appealing option for enhancing the success of natural cycle IVF treatment is combining it with immature oocyte retrieval and IVM. In order to prevent ovulation from the dominant follicle, due to the natural LH surge, a 10,000 IU hCG injection is given when the dominant follicle had reached 12–14 mm in diameter and oocyte retrieval is performed 36–38 h later. Lim *et al.*[44] reported a 35% clinical pregnancy rate for 82 women who underwent a natural cycle IVF/IVM treatment. All had regular menstrual cycles and normal ovaries with more than 7 antral follicles. Natural cycle IVF/IVM treatment should be considered for women wishing to avoid hormonal ovarian stimulation for various reasons.

IVM for poor responders

There is no universally accepted definition for poor ovarian response to gonadotropins stimulation. However, the most common criterion for poor responders is a low number of dominant follicles (usually 3 or less) developed on the day of hCG administration after a standard dose ovarian stimulation protocol. Poor response to gonadotropin stimulation may be expected to occur more often in older women or those with high basal serum levels of FSH and estrogen, and low basal serum levels of antimullerian hormone (AMH) or inhibin B, and women with low antral follicle count (AFC). Some poor responders appear to respond to stimulation but have a low estrogen level or few or slow-growing follicles. Normally, these groups of patients require a prolonged stimulation time and higher doses of gonadotropins. Moreover, following gonadotropin stimulation, the number of follicles may be normal, but their size may be smaller than in the usual treatment cycles. These patients experienced a higher cancellation rate because of the smaller number or size of follicles. Many different ovarian stimulation protocols have been tried for treatment of poor responders in IVF; however, no single protocol seems to benefit all poor responders.[45] Check *et al.*[46] reported that two pregnancies were established following IVM when germinal vesicle or metaphase I stage oocytes were retrieved after hCG administration from such poor responders. In another study reported by Child *et al.*,[47] eight women with a previous poor response to IVF underwent oocyte collection without ovarian stimulation. hCG was administered 36 h before collection. Six of these women underwent embryo transfer and one became pregnant and delivered. In addition, Liu *et al.*[48] reported a 37.5% (3 of 8) pregnancy rate following immature oocyte retrieval and IVM. Although oocyte donation would be the ideal treatment for those patients, some will not accept this option. Therefore, based on the results of these preliminary studies, it seems that IVM may be a possible option for patients with poor ovarian response wishing to avoid oocyte donation treatment.

GUIDELINES FOR IVM TREATMENT CYCLE

Follicle monitoring

As in conventional IVF treatments, patient follow-up during IVM cycles is mainly performed using ultrasound scans of the ovaries and endometrium. However, in contrast to conventional IVF, there is no need for serum hormonal levels (estradiol, progesterone) follow-up in IVM cycles. The first ultrasound scan in performed between days 2–5 of the menstrual cycle. In amenorrheic women, withdrawal bleeding is induced with progesterone. At this base-line ultrasound scan, the number and size (average of two perpendicular dimensions) of all antral follicles is recorded along with endometrial thickness. A second scan is performed on days 6–8 of the cycle and, in addition to all the above described measurements, the presence and size of the dominant follicle is recorded. In some centers, IVM cycles are cancelled if a dominant follicle is identified.[49] However, we have recently reported that, when a dominant follicle is present, atresia does not occur in the other non-dominant follicles.[50] In most patients with PCOS, a dominant follicle will not develop; in other patients, including those with PCO, we give hCG priming when the dominant follicle has reached 12 mm in diameter and the endometrial thickness is 8 mm. By doing so, we can aspirate one or two mature oocytes on the day of collection in addition to several immature oocytes and increase pregnancy rates.[51]

Priming with hCG and pretreatment with FSH

Some studies suggest that pretreatment with FSH during the early follicular phase will enhance the number of oocyte retrieved and their rate of maturation. We have shown that hCG priming prior to IVM oocyte collection increases the maturation rate of oocytes *in vitro*;[52] therefore, it is our practice to administer 10,000 IU of hCG 38 h prior to collection. A prospective, randomized control trial demonstrated no improvement in oocyte maturation rates with 20,000 IU of hCG; therefore, there is no benefit from the higher dose.[53]

Endometrial preparation and luteal support

The role of the endometrium in the implantation process is well established. Although it is not clear whether ultrasound measurement of endometrial thickness can predict outcome of IVF cycles, an endometrial thickness of less than 7 mm is probably associated with a reduced pregnancy rate. In our IVM program, in order to achieve optimal endometrial growth, exogenous 17β-estradiol (micronized) is given in a dosage depending on the endometrial thickness starting on the day of oocyte retrieval. If the endometrium is less than 6 mm, a 12 mg/day is started; if the thickness is between 6–8 mm, a 10 mg/day is started; and if the thickness is more than 8 mm, 6 mg is used, all in three divided doses. We are currently investigating an alternative approach, where when a thin endometrium (< 6 mm) is identified at the second ultrasound scan, HMG 150 IU/day is administered for 3 days along with 12 mg of exogenous 17β-estradiol (micronized). In anovulatory women, it is possible to follow-up by ultrasound scan every 3–4 days, without HMG

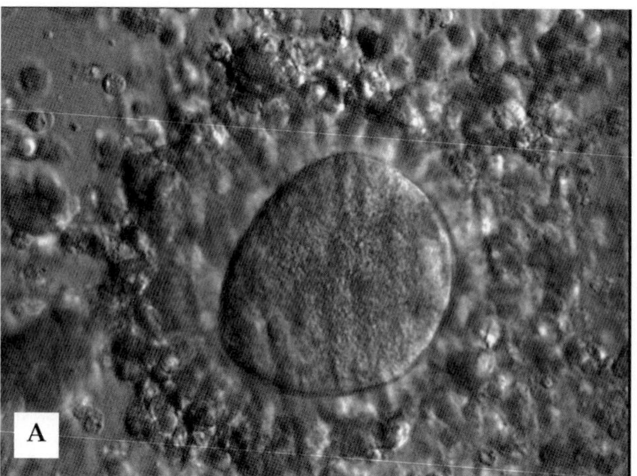

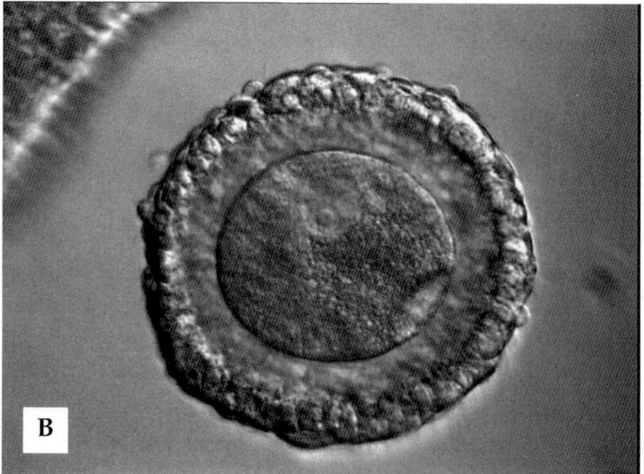

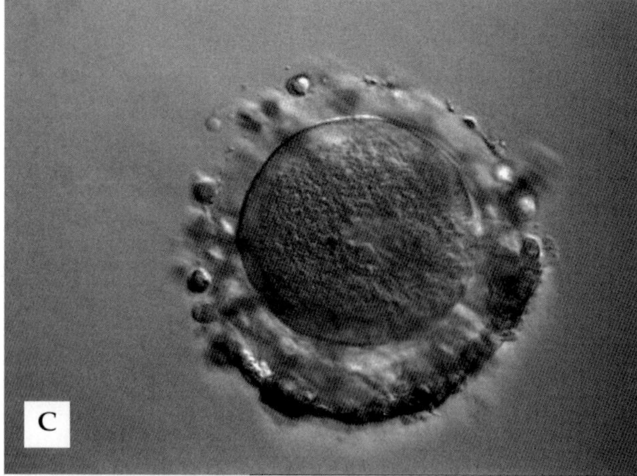

Fig. 1 Human immature oocytes at the time of retrieval. (A) A germinal vesicle (GV)-stage oocyte with dispersed cumulus cell appearance. (B) A GV-stage oocyte with compacted cumulus cell appearance. (C) A GV-stage oocyte with sparse cumulus cell appearance. Original magnification x400. Reprinted from an article in *Reproductive BioMedicine Online* by W-Y Son *et al.*[54] with permission from Reproductive Healthcare Ltd.

supplementation, until the endometrium thickens. In all our IVM cycles, both intracytoplasmic sperm injection (ICSI) and assisted hatching (AHA) are performed. On the day of oocyte retrieval, we begin treatment with doxycycline 100 mg BID for 7 days along with methylprednisolone 16 mg QD for 4 days. Progesterone luteal support, either as intramuscular injection 50 mg daily or vaginal tablets (Prometrium) 200 mg TID, is started on the day that oocyte maturation is achieved. Estradiol and progesterone supplementation is continued until the 12th week of pregnancy.

Immature oocyte retrieval

Oocyte retrieval is performed under general or spinal anesthesia or intravenous sedation using fentanyl and midazolam (1–2 mg). Intravenous fentanyl is administered at intervals of 15–20 min up to a total dose of 150–200 μg. Local infiltration of bupivacaine 0.5% in the vaginal fornix reduces the discomfort of multiple needle puncture. Retrieval is performed under ultrasound guidance with a 19-G, single-lumen aspiration needle. The aspiration pressure is reduced to 87–90 mmHg to avoid damage to the immature oocytes. The follicular fluid is collected in culture tubes containing 0.9% saline with 2 U/ml of heparin. In contrast to conventional IVF, in IVM oocyte collection, several needle punctures are needed to each ovary. Owing to the low aspiration pressure and the small-gauged needle, the bloodstain aspirate may occasionally block the needle. Therefore, following aspiration of several follicles, the needle is withdrawn from the vagina to flush and avoid any blockage. The procedure is repeated until all follicles are aspirated.

IVM FERTILIZATION AND EMBRYO TRANSFER

Immature oocytes are incubated in a culture dish containing maturation medium supplemented with 75 mIU/mL of FSH and LH. The oocytes are cultured at 37°C in an atmosphere of 5% carbon dioxide and 95% air with high humidity. Immediately following collection, the cumulus-oocyte complex (COC) pattern and oocyte maturity is evaluated. It has been shown that COC showing dispersed cumulus cells is associated with faster maturation, a higher fertilization rate and improved embryonic development compared to a COC with compacted or sparse cumulus cell (Fig. 1).[54] Oocytes are checked for maturity 24 h and 48 h after culture. Oocytes, which are matured on the day of oocyte retrieval or in the following 24 h, result in better quality embryos compared to late matured oocytes.[55] Mature oocytes are fertilized. It has been demonstrated that *in vitro* matured human oocytes fertilize without ICSI when sperm parameters are within normal limits. However, in order to avoid unexpected poor fertilization, it is our policy to fertilize the *in vitro* matured oocytes using ICSI. After ICSI, the oocytes are transferred into 1 ml of IVF medium in a tissue culture dish. Fertilization is assessed 18 h following the ICSI procedure. The fertilized oocytes are further cultured up to day 2 or 3 and then embryo transfer is performed. AHA is performed to avoid reduced implantation due to a possible hardened zona pellucida. It has been shown that embryos derived from *in vitro* matured oocytes can develop to the blastocyst stage; therefore, blastocyst or double transfer is an alternative approach.

Table 1 Results of fresh *in vitro* maturation cycles (excluding oocyte donation cycles)

	Age	
	< 35 years	35–40 years
Number of cycles	54	20
Number of oocytes collected (mean)	17.1	16.1
Number of embryos transferred (mean)	3.6	4.0
Pregnancy rate per collection (%)	37.0	35.0
Pregnancy rate per embryo transfer (%)	37.0	35.0
Implantation rate (%)	11.5	6.3
Clinical pregnancy rate per collection (%)	25.9	25.0

Source : McGill Reproductive Center (1 January to 31 December 2006).

IVM TREATMENT OUTCOME

Pregnancy rates with IVM are correlated with the number of immature oocytes retrieved. In women younger than 35 years, we have achieved a pregnancy rate of 37% per cycle (Table 1). The implantation rate is approximately 12%. A recent analysis of the obstetric, neonatal and infant outcome in our IVM conception showed pregnancy rates of 73% singleton, 24% twin and 2.7% triplet. The median gestation age was 39 weeks for singleton and 37 weeks for multiple pregnancies.[50] There was no increase in relative risk of malformation when IVM pregnancies were compared with IVF and spontaneous pregnancies.[56]

CONCLUSIONS AND FUTURE CONSIDERATIONS

IVM is an evolving technique, which was initially indicated for patients with PCO and PCOS in order to avoid ovarian stimulation, thus eliminating the risk of OHSS. However, this technology is now being extended to various fertility treatments. IVM cycles requires less monitoring and fewer clinical visits, lessening the burden on patient, and further reducing costs which are already lower due to the lack of gonadotropin stimulation. In addition to PCO and PCOS patients, IVM may be offered today for poor responders wishing to avoid egg donation and for egg donors. Moreover, IVM is a promising fertility preservation option for many patients facing gonadotoxic treatment and who are unable to undergo controlled ovarian stimulation. IVM can be also used occasionally for women who had primarily poor quality embryos for no obvious reasons in repeated IVF cycles (*e.g.* young women with normal AFC, normal basal serum levels of FSH and E_2). Long-term follow-up of the children conceived following IVM is of crucial importance to establish this treatment modality. Altogether, IVM is a promising technique, which will have increasing application in the coming years.

KEY POINTS FOR CLINICAL PRACTICE

- IVM is an evolving technique, which was initially indicated for patients with PCO and PCOS in order to avoid ovarian stimulatin, thus eliminating the risk of OHSS.

KEY POINTS FOR CLINICAL PRACTICE *(continued)*

- IVM cycles require less monitoring and fewer clinical visits, lessening the burden on the patient, and further reducing costs which are already lower due to lack of gonadotrpon stimulation.
- This technology is now being extended to various fertility treatments and is a promising fertility preservation option for many patients facing gonadotoxic treatment who are unable to undergo controlled ovarian stimulation.

References

1 Hillier SG. Current concepts of the roles of follicle stimulating hormone and luteinizing hormone in folliculogenesis. Hum Reprod 1994;9:188–91
2 Richards JS, Russell DL, Ochsner S, Espey LL. Ovulation: new dimensions and new regulators of the inflammatory-like response. Annu Rev Physiol 2002;64:69–92
3 Park JY, Su YQ, Ariga M, Law E, Jin SL, Conti M. EGF-like growth factors as mediators of LH action in the ovulatory follicle. Science 2004;303:682–4
4 Mehlmann LM, Jones TL, Jaffe LA. Meiotic arrest in the mouse follicle maintained by a G_s protein in the oocyte. Science 2002;297:1343–5
5 Sela-Abramovich S, Edry I, Galiani D, Nevo N, Dekel N. Disruption of gap junctional communication within the ovarian follicle induces oocyte maturation. Endocrinology 2006;147:2280–6
6 Mehlmann LM, Saeki Y, Tanaka S *et al*. The G_s-linked receptor GPR3 maintains meiotic arrest in mammalian oocytes. Science 2004;306:1947–50
7 Ducibella T. The cortical reaction and development of activation competence in mammalian oocytes. Hum Reprod Update 1996;2:29–42
8 Cha KY, Chian RC. Maturation *in vitro* of immature human oocytes for clinical use. Hum Reprod Update 1998;4:103–20
9 Chian RC, Lim JH, Tan SL. State of the art in *in-vitro* oocyte maturation. Curr Opin Obstet Gynecol 2004;16:211–9
10 Bevers MM, Fieleman SJ, Van den Hurk R, Izadyar F. Regulation and modulation of oocyte maturation in the bovine. Theriogenology 1997;47:13–22
11 Anderiesz C, Ferraretti A, Magli C *et al*. Effect of recombinant human gonadotrophins on human, bovine and murine oocyte meiosis, fertilization and embryonic development *in vitro*. Hum Reprod 2000;15:1140–8
12 Hreinsson J, Rosenlund B, Friden B *et al*. Recombinant LH is equally effective as recombinant hCG in promoting oocyte maturation in a clinical *in-vitro* maturation programme: a randomized study. Hum Reprod 2003;18:2131–6
13 Patsoula E, Loutradis D, Drakakis P, Kallianidis K, Bletsa R, Michalas S. Expression of mRNA for the LH and FSH receptors in mouse oocytes and preimplantation embryos. Reproduction 2001;121:455–61
14 Patsoula E, Loutradis D, Drakakis P, Michalas L, Bletsa R, Michalas S. Messenger RNA expression for the follicle-stimulating hormone receptor and luteinizing hormone receptor in human oocytes and preimplantation-stage embryos. Fertil Steril 2003;79:1187–93
15 Chian RC, Ao A, Clarke HJ, Tulandi T, Tan SL. Production of steroids from human cumulus cells treated with different concentrations of gonadotropins during culture *in vitro*. Fertil Steril 1999;71:61–6
16 Shimada M, Nishibori M, Isobe N, Kawano N, Terada T. Luteinizing hormone receptor formation in cumulus cells surrounding porcine oocytes and its role during meiotic maturation of porcine oocytes. Biol Reprod 2003;68:1142–9
17 Moor RM, Polge C, Willadsen SM. Effect of follicular steroids on the maturation and fertilization of mammalian oocytes. J Embryol Exp Morphol 1980;56:319–35

18 Tesarik J, Mendoza C. Nongenomic effects of 17 beta-estradiol on maturing human oocytes: relationship to oocyte developmental potential. J Clin Endocrinol Metab 1995;80:1438–43
19 Chian RC, Tan SL. Maturational and developmental competence of cumulus-free immature human oocytes derived from stimulated and intracytoplasmic sperm injection cycles. Reprod Biomed Online 2002;5:125–32
20 Pincus G, Enzmann EV. The comparative behavior of mamalian eggs *in vivo* and *in vitro*. J Exp Med 1935;62:655–75
21 Edwards RG, Bavister BD, Steptoe PC. Early stages of fertilization *in vitro* of human oocytes matured *in vitro*. Nature 1969;221:632–5
22 Cha KY, Koo JJ, Ko JJ, Choi DH, Han SY, Yoon TK. Pregnancy after *in vitro* fertilization of human follicular oocytes collected from nonstimulated cycles, their culture *in vitro* and their transfer in a donor oocyte program. Fertil Steril 1991;55:56–60
23 Trounson A, Wood C, Kausche A. *In vitro* maturation and the fertilization and developmental competence of oocytes recovered from untreated polycystic ovarian patients. Fertil Steril 1994;62:353–62
24 Tan SL, Royston P, Campbell S *et al*. Cumulative conception and livebirth rates after *in-vitro* fertilisation. Lancet 1992;339:1390–4
25 Engmann L, Maconochie N, Bekir JS, Jacobs HS, Tan SL. Cumulative probability of clinical pregnancy and live birth after a multiple cycle IVF package: a more realistic assessment of overall and age-specific success rates? Br J Obstet Gynaecol 1999;106:165–70
26 MacDougall MJ, Tan SL, Jacobs HS. *In-vitro* fertilization and the ovarian hyperstimulation syndrome. Hum Reprod 1992;7:597–600
27 Aboulghar M, Evers JH, Al-Inany H. Intravenous albumin for preventing severe ovarian hyperstimulation syndrome: a Cochrane review. Hum Reprod 2002;17:3027–32
28 Mansour R, Aboulghar M, Serour G, Amin Y, Abou-Setta AM. Criteria of a successful coasting protocol for the prevention of severe ovarian hyperstimulation syndrome. Hum Reprod 2005;20:3167–72
29 Tan SL, Balen A, el Hussein E, Campbell S, Jacobs HS. The administration of glucocorticoids for the prevention of ovarian hyperstimulation syndrome in *in vitro* fertilization: a prospective randomized study. Fertil Steril 1992;58:378–83
30 Nargund G, Hutchison L, Scaramuzzi R, Campbell S. Low-dose HCG is useful in preventing OHSS in high-risk women without adversely affecting the outcome of IVF cycles. Reprod Biomed Online 2007;14:682–5
31 Awonuga AO, Pittrof RJ, Zaidi J, Dean N, Jacobs HS, Tan SL. Elective cryopreservation of all embryos in women at risk of developing ovarian hyperstimulation syndrome may not prevent the condition but reduces the live birth rate. J Assist Reprod Genet 1996;13:401–6
32 Tan SL, Child TJ, Gulekli B. *In vitro* maturation and fertilization of oocytes from unstimulated ovaries: predicting the number of immature oocytes retrieved by early follicular phase ultrasonography. Am J Obstet Gynecol 2002;186:684–9
33 Child TJ, Abdul-Jalil AK, Gulekli B, Tan SL. *In vitro* maturation and fertilization of oocytes from unstimulated normal ovaries, polycystic ovaries, and women with polycystic ovary syndrome. Fertil Steril 2001;76:936–42
34 Child TJ, Phillips SJ, Abdul-Jalil AK, Gulekli B, Tan SL. A comparison of *in vitro* maturation and *in vitro* fertilization for women with polycystic ovaries. Obstet Gynecol 2002;100:665–70
35 Lim KS, Son WY, Yoon SH, Lim JH. IVM/F-ET in stimulated cycles for the prevention of OHSS. Fertil Steril 2002;78:s10
36 Holzer HEG, Tan SL. Fertility preservation in oncology. Minerva Ginecol 2005;57:99–109
37 Donnez J, Dolmans MM, Demylle D *et al*. Livebirth after orthotopic transplantation of cryopreserved ovarian tissue. Lancet 2004;364:1405–10
38 Meirow D, Levron J, Eldar-Geva T *et al*. Pregnancy after transplantation of cryopreserved ovarian tissue in a patient with ovarian failure after chemotherapy. N Engl J Med 2005;353:318–21
39 Oktay K, Buyuk E, Veeck L *et al*. Embryo development after heterotopic transplantation of cryopreserved ovarian tissue. Lancet 2004;363:837–40
40 Rao GD, Chian RC, Son WY, Gilbert L, Tan SL. Fertility preservation in women undergoing cancer treatment. Lancet 2004;363:1829–30
41 Oktay K, Demirtas E, Son WY, Lostritto K, Chian RC, Tan SL. *In vitro* maturation of germinal vesicle oocytes recovered post premature LH surge. Description of a novel approach to fertility

preservation. Fertil Steril 2007; In press
42 Huang J, Holzer HEG, Tulandi T, Tan SL, Chian RC. Combining ovarian tissue cryobanking with retrieval of immature oocytes by *in vitro* maturation and vitrification: a noble method of fertility preservation. Fertil Steril 2007; In press
43 Holzer HEG, Scharf E, Chian RC, Demirtas E, Buckett WM, Tan SL. *In vitro* maturation of oocytes collected from unstimulated ovaries for oocyte donation. Fertil Steril 2007;88:62–7
44 Lim JH, Yang SH, Chian RC. New alternative to infertility treatment for women without ovarian stimulation. Reprod Biomed Online 2007;14
45 Elizur SE, Aslan D, Shulman A, Weisz B, Bider D, Dor J. Modified natural cycle using GnRH antagonist can be an optional treatment in poor responders undergoing IVF. J Assist Reprod Genet 2005;22:75–9
46 Check ML, Brittingham D, Check JH, Choe JK. Pregnancy following transfer of cryopreserved-thawed embryos that had been a result of fertilization of all in vitro matured metaphase or germinal stage oocytes. Clin Exp Obstet Gynecol 2001;28:69–70
47 Child TJ, Chian RC, Abdul-Jalil K, Tan SL. *In vitro* maturation (IVM) of oocytes from unstimulated normal ovaries of women with previous poor response to IVF. Fertil Steril 2000;74 (Suppl. 1):s45
48 Liu J, Lu G, Qian Y, Mao Y, Ding W. Pregnancies and births achieved from *in vitro* matured oocytes retrieved from poor responders undergoing stimulation in *in vitro* fertilization cycles. Fertil Steril 2003;80:447–9
49 Le Du A, Kadoch IJ, Bourcigaux N *et al*. *In vitro* oocyte maturation for the treatment of infertility associated with polycystic ovarian syndrome: the French experience. Hum Reprod 2005;20:420–4
50 Chian RC, Buckett WM, Abdul Jalil AK *et al*. Natural-cycle *in vitro* fertilization combined with *in vitro* maturation of immature oocytes is a potential approach in infertility treatment. Fertil Steril 2004;82:1675–8
51 Son WY, Chung J, Cui S, Dean N, Tan SL, Chian RC. Comparison of embryology and clinical outcome between IVM cycles with and without mature oocytes collected following HCG priming. Fertil Steril 2006;86 (Suppl. 1):s394–5
52 Chian RC, Gulekli B, Buckett WM, Tan SL. Priming with human chorionic gonadotropin before retrieval of immature oocytes in women with infertility due to polycystic ovary syndrome. N Engl J Med 1999;341:1624–6
53 Gulekli B, Buckett WM, Chian RC, Child TJ, Abdul-Jalil AK, Tan SL. Randomized, controlled trial of priming with 10,000 IU versus 20,000 IU of human chorionic gonadotropin in women with polycystic ovary syndrome who are undergoing *in vitro* maturation. Fertil Steril 2004;82:1458–9
54 Son WY, Yoon SH, Lim JH. Effect of gonadotrophin priming on in-vitro maturation of oocytes collected from women at risk of OHSS. Reprod Biomed Online 2006;13:340–8
55 Son WY, Lee SY, Lim JH. Fertilization, cleavage and blastocyst development according to the maturation timing of oocytes in *in vitro* maturation cycles. Hum Reprod 2005;20:3204–7
56 Buckett WM, Chian RC, Holzer HEG, Dean N, Usher R, Tan SL. Obstetric outcomes and congenital abnormalities after *in-vitro* maturation, *in-vitro* fertilization and intracytoplasmic sperm injection. Obstet Gynecol 2007; In press

Jai B. Sharma

Tuberculosis and obstetric and gynecological practice

About 2 billion people (one-third of the world's population) are infected with *Mycobacterium tuberculosis* and are at risk of developing the disease. Each year, almost 8 million people develop active tuberculosis (TB) out of which about 2 million die.[1] Over 95% of new TB cases and deaths occur in developing countries with 75% patients being in the most economically productive age group (15–54 years) causing great economic burden on the family and the nation. There has been a 2–3-fold increase in TB cases in sub-Saharan Africa due to co-infection with human immunodeficiency virus (HIV) which significantly increases the risk of developing TB.[1] More liberal immigration from high-risk to low-risk areas has been responsible for increased incidence even in North America and Western Europe. Multidrug resistant (MDR) and extreme drug resistant (XDR) TB, which are caused by poor case management, are a cause of serious concern throughout the world.[1]

Alarmed by the high prevalence, high mortality and morbidity due to TB globally (indirectly reflecting the failure of various TB control programs of different countries), the World Health Organization's Global Tuberculosis Programme (WHO, GTB) took an unprecedented step and declared TB a global emergency in 1993 and promoted a new effective TB control based on five essential elements called the Directly Observed Treatment Shortcourse (DOTS) strategy (Table 1).[2] WHO's World Health Assembly (WHA) set two targets for TB control to be reached by 2000: (i) to detect 70% of all new sputum-smear positive cases arising each year (70% case detection rate); and (ii) to treat 85% of these cases successfully.[2] These targets were not met by 2000 and were deferred to 2005.[3] A total of 183 countries and territories were

Jai B. Sharma MD DNB FRCOG MFFP MAMS FICOG FIMSA
Assistant Professor of Obstetrics and Gynaecology, All India Institute of Medical Sciences, New Delhi–110029, India
E-mail: jbsharma2000@gmail.com

Table 1 Five components of the DOTS strategy[3,4]

- Continued political commitment from governments
- Case detection through quality-assured bacteriology (sputum microscopy for pulmonary TB and other standard diagnostic modalities for extrapulmonary TB including genital TB)
- Standardized short-course chemotherapy (6–8 months) for all cases of TB under proper case management conditions and directly observing the treatment
- An effective drug supply and management system ensuring uninterrupted supply of quality-assured drugs
- Monitoring and evaluation system and measurement of impact by recording and reporting assessment of all patients and overall program performance.

implementing the DOTS strategy during 2004 covering almost 83% of the world's population.[3] The United Nations' Millennium Development Goals (MDGs) for TB control are to halve and to begin to reverse the TB incidence by 2015 while Stop TB Partnership's target is to halve the 1990 prevalence and death rates by 2015 and to eliminate TB as a public health problem (less than one case per million population) by 2050.[3] Many countries including India adopted these as national targets. The Revised National Tuberculosis Control Programme (RNTCP) of India incorporating DOTS strategy covered 87% of the population (947 million) in 2004 with a 72% case detection rate and 86% treatment success rate with a 7-fold reduction in death rate (from 29% to 4%).[4]

Among women of reproductive age group, TB is a leading cause of death, surpassing all causes of maternal mortality. TB-infected women run the risk of being abandoned by their families as a result of their disease. Although pulmonary TB (PTB) remains the commonest and the most infectious type of TB, extrapulmonary TB (EPTB) is becoming more prevalent especially in young women throughout the world.[5] Female genital TB (FGTB), being non-infectious, has been neglected by healthcare providers but is an important cause of both significant morbidity and short- and long-term sequelae for the affected women.[5,6]

EPIDEMIOLOGY OF FEMALE GENITAL TUBERCULOSIS

FGTB was first described by Morgagni in 1744 on autopsy of a young lady who died of TB peritonitis, while a detailed study of its course and treatment was reported by Hager in 1886.[5] The exact incidence of FGTB is not accurately known as it is under-reported due to asymptomatic cases and lack of reliable confirmatory investigations.[5,6] The reported incidence varies in different countries from 1% in US to 1–19% in various parts of India.[7,8] Bazaz-Malik *et al.*[9] observed a 2.3% prevalence of TB endometritis in 42,770 specimens of non-pregnant endometrial curettings and biopsies examined in Delhi. Genital TB was responsible for 0.02% and 1% of all gynecological admissions in Sweden and India, respectively.[5,10] In women presenting with infertility, prevalence of genital TB was found to be < 1% of women in the US, but was 5–10% world-wide with about 10% in India.[7,8,11,12] At All India Institute of Medical Sciences

(AIIMS) in New Delhi, we found a 16% prevalence of FGTB in women of infertility and incidence of infertility in FGTB to be 42.5%, which may be due to referral of difficult and intractable cases to this apex hospital from the whole of India, especially from states like Bihar where prevalence of TB is very high (Sharma JB, Gupta N, Mittal S. unpublished data from hospital statistics). Genital TB is observed in up to 8% cases of abnormal uterine bleeding.[13] Genital TB was found on autopsy in 1–12% of women dying with pulmonary TB.[7] We observed a high prevalence of genital TB (30%) in sputum-positive pulmonary TB cases on endometrial sampling (Sharma JB, Singh UB, Kumar S, Roy KK, Gupta P, unpublished data, study ongoing). Even in extrapulmonary TB, we observed 10% prevalence of genital TB (Sharma JB, Singh UB, Kumar S, Roy KK, Malhotra N, Karmakar D, unpublished data, study ongoing). Tripathy and Tripathy[14] performed diagnostic laparoscopy on sputum-positive pulmonary TB cases and found bands of adhesions, tubercles and hyperemia in 60% cases, intestinal adhesions in 24%, tubercles on fallopian tubes in 22% of women and adhesions in pouch of Douglas in 11% of women.

PATHOGENESIS

Tuberculosis is caused by the *Mycobacterium tuberculosis* complex (*M. tuberculosis, M. bovis, M. africanum* or atypical *Mycobacteria* spp.). Human disease in immunocompetent individuals is mostly caused by *M. tuberculosis*. Predisposing factors for TB are poverty, over-crowding with improper ventilation, inadequate access to healthcare, malnutrition, diabetes mellitus, smoking, alcohol abuse, drug abuse especially injectable drugs, end-stage renal disease, renal failure, hemodialysis patients and co-infection with HIV.[1–3,5,6] Genital TB almost always occurs secondary to pulmonary (commonest) or extrapulmonary TB, such as gastrointestinal tract, kidneys, skeletal system, meninges and miliary TB.[5–7] However, primary genital TB has been reported in women whose male partners had active genito-urinary TB by transmission through infected semen.[15] The site of involvement in primary genital TB can be cervix or vulva.[5,7] The spread of TB from lungs and other sites is usually by hematogenous or by the lymphatic route. Less commonly, direct contiguous spread from nearby abdominal organs like intestines or abdominal lymph nodes can cause genital TB. The various genital organs affected by TB in order of frequency are: fallopian tubes (90–100% of cases), endometrium (50–80% of cases) ovaries (20–30% of cases), cervix (5–15% of cases) and, rarely, vagina and vulva (1% of cases).[5–7]

Tuberculosis of fallopian tubes

Fallopian tubes are involved in almost all women with genital TB and the involvement is usually bilateral.[7] Depending upon whether it is hematogenous spread or direct spread from intestines, disease may start in the muscularis mucosa of the tube or on the peritoneal surface, but involvement of mucosa is always present. In order of frequency, ampulla is the commonest site to be involved followed by isthmus and the interstitial part of the tube (rare). The severity and the stage of the disease affect the gross appearance of the tubes. Initially, there is congestion of fallopian tubes, ovaries and peritoneum of the pouch of Douglas with flimsy adhesions and miliary tubercles on their surface. In later stages, thick and vascular plastic adhesions are formed between tubes and adjacent pelvic organs.[16] In more severe cases, there may be multiple adhesions in the peritoneal cavity with obliterated pouch of Douglas.[16] Varying grades of Fitz-Hugh-Curtis syndrome (violin string adhesions between liver and diaphragm or anterior abdominal wall) is often seen in up to 48% cases of female genital TB in the experience of the author.[17,18] Usually, the characteristic feature is the presence of yellowish-grey tubercles on the peritoneal surface of the tubes and mesosalpinx with fimbrial end of tube remaining open in half the cases.[19,20] In advanced stage, tubes become dilated, retort-shaped and loculated. The leakage of infected material from tube causes development of peritubal abscesses, TB peritonitis and ascites. In chronic cases, a fibrotic stage develops resulting into thickened, hard and beaded tubes with calcification and tubal blockade.[19,20] In TB of fallopian tubes, tubal damage is due to endosalpingitis, exosalpingitis or interstitial salpingitis. Tubo-ovarian masses are due to peri-oophoritis, hydrosalpinx, pyosalpinx or massive adhesion formation. On microscopic examination, appearances vary depending upon the severity and activity of the disease.[20] TB granulomas with Langhans giant cells and chronic inflammatory cells (lymphocytes) with or without caseation may be observed. However, tubal mucosa may be totally destroyed or there may be fusion of papillae in the endosalpinx making women more prone to ectopic pregnancy and infertility.[5,20]

Endometrial tuberculosis

Endometrium is involved in 50–80% of cases of FGTB.[7,21,22] Gross endometrial appearance may be unremarkable due to repeated menstruation minimizing the disease. Initially, there is no macroscopic disease but caseation and ulceration occurs later with progression of TB; in advanced stages, there is distortion of cavity, varying from slight distortion to complete obliteration due to adhesions.[20] Total destruction of endometrium may result in Asherman's syndrome resulting in amenorrhoea secondary to end-organ failure. We found genital TB to be an important cause of Asherman's syndrome in India leading on to secondary amenorrhoea and infertility with poor prognosis for treatment.[23] Microscopically, TB granulomas with or without caseation, epitheloid cells and Langhans cells may be seen, especially in the premenstrual phase and close to the surface of endometrium. However, typical granulomas may not always be seen due to repeated sheddings at the time of menstruation.[9] Some authors have suggested that even in absence of typical granulomas, endometrial TB may be diagnosed in the presence of a focal collection of lymphocytes with or without the presence of dilated glands and destruction of epithelium.[9,24]

Ovarian tuberculosis

Isolated TB oophoritis is rare. It is more often seen as part of TB peritonitis or with TB of other genital organs (tubes or endometrium). Depending upon the severity and stage of disease, there may be tubercles on the ovary, adhesions, caseation, tubo-ovarian cyst or mass formation.[5,21] Sometimes, the ovary may be completely destroyed by the disease.[20]

Peritoneal tuberculosis

TB may involve pelvic or abdominal peritoneum which can be disseminated TB with tubercles all over the peritoneum, intestines and omentum; it may cause ascites and abdominal mass and may masquerade as ovarian cancer as even CA 125 levels are raised in peritoneal TB. CT scan and MRI also give a similar picture and diagnosis may be made only on laparotomy done for suspected ovarian cancer. In such cases, ascitic fluid tapping for biochemical analysis and peritoneal biopsy may confirm the diagnosis of TB, thus avoiding a needless laparotomy.[25] We have collected about 25 laparotomy samples from various Delhi hospitals done for suspected ovarian cancer but which turned out to be abdomino pelvic TB (Sharma JB, Kumar S, Zutshi V, Roy KK, Rajaram S, Mittal S, Agarwal S, unpublished data). On laparotomy there may be vague masses without a line of cleavage with adherent loops of bowel or omental masses mimicking secondaries from ovarian cancer (Fig. 1). Rarely, genital TB may be associated with other gynecological pathologies like ovarian cancer, genital prolapse, fibroid uterus, *etc.*[26]

Cervical tuberculosis

Cervical tuberculosis may be seen in 5–15% cases of genital TB usually as a downward extension of endometrial TB; rarely, it may be a primary disease transmitted by the partner through infected semen.[5,15] It may masquerade as cervical cancer necessitating biopsy for confirmation of diagnosis.[27] Microscopic examination will differentiate between the two conditions showing granulomatous inflammation in TB. It may be diagnosed on Papanicolaou stain by the presence of multinucleated giant cells, histiocytes and epithelioid cells.[28]

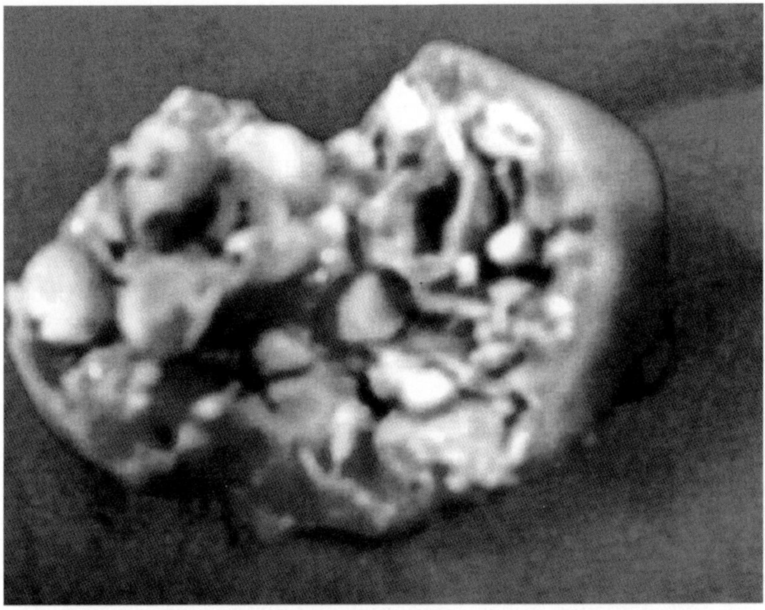

Fig. 1 Omental tuberculous mass simulating ovarian cancer on laparotomy.

Table 2 Symptoms in genital TB

Symptom	
Asymptomatic (up to 11%)	
General systemic symptoms	
	Fever with night sweats
	Anorexia
	Weight loss
	Poor general condition
Menstrual dysfunction	
	Puberty menorrhagia
	Menorrhagia
	Post menopausal bleeding
	Oligomenorrhea
	Hypomenorrhea
	Amenorrhea (primary and secondary)
Infertility (primary and secondary)	
Lump in abdomen	
Abdominal pain (may flare up after HSG or D&C)	
Chronic pelvic pain (may flare up after HSG or D&C)	
Acute abdomen (in rupture of tubo-ovarian abscess or flaring up of TB after HSG, D&C, coitus, exercise, menstruation)	
Abnormal vaginal discharge	
Unusual symptoms	
	Ulcers in vagina or vulva
	Labial swelling
	Retention of urine
	Urinary incontinence
	Fecal incontinence

Tuberculosis of vagina and vulva

Their involvement is rare (1–2%) and is usually secondary to extension from endometrium or cervix, but may rarely be primary due to transmission from an infected partner. There may be a hypertrophic lesion or a non-healing ulcer on the vulva or vagina mimicking malignancy. Biopsy and histopathological examination is usually needed to confirm the diagnosis and to rule out malignancy. Rarely, TB of the vagina can cause involvement of Bartholin's glands, vesicovaginal and rectovaginal fistula formation.[5,29,30]

Tuberculosis and infertility

Infertility is the commonest presentation of genital TB with the reported incidence of infertility being between 40–80% (Tables 2 and 3). Both primary and secondary infertility may occur. The average incidence of genital TB in infertility clinics world-wide is 5–10% and varies from 0.69% in Australia to 17.4% in India.[7] The reason for infertility is involvement of fallopian tubes (blocked and damaged tubes), endometrium (non-reception and damaged endometrium with Asherman's syndrome) and ovarian damage in TB.[7,11,23]

Table 3 Comparative symptomatology of female genital TB by different authors (percentages)

Reference	Women (*n*)	Infertility	Overall menstrual	Menorrhagia	Hypomen./ oligomen.	Amenor.	Vaginal discharge	Chronic pelvic pain	General symptoms	Past history of PTB/EPTB
Falk *et al.* (1980)[10]	187	12.8	41.2	NA	NA	NA	NA	24.6	NA, 11.2% asymptomatic	38
Bazaz-Malik *et al.* (1983)[9]	1000	47	NA	NA	NA	26	NA	2.4	NA	NA
Bobhate *et al.* (1986)[31]	337	58.6	NA	NA	NA	26.4	NA	NA	NA	NA
Bhide *et al.* (1987)[32]	71	35.2	NA	16.9	NA	19.7	NA	22.5	NA	66.2
Chhabra (1990)[11]	58	29.3	NA	15.5	34.5	18.9	NA	43.1	NA	NA
Saracoglu *et al.* (1992)[33]	72	47	NA	NA	NA	11	NA	32	NA	NA
Nagpal & Pal (2001)[34]	100	79	34	16	9	6	NA	54	36	NA
Jindal (2006)[12]	197	76.1	15.2	NA	NA	10.1	6.6	19.5	4.1	73.6
Sharma *et al.* (2007)**	86	63.4	70	22.5	37.5	7.7	9	30.5	12	37.5

**unpublished data

NA = data not available.
Hypomen. = Hypomenorrhea
Amenor. = Amenorrhea

Table 4 Signs in genital TB

No physical sign (common)	
Systemic examination	Fever
	Lymphadenopathy (TB in lymph nodes)
	Crackles and rales on chest examination (PTB)
	Other systemic signs depending on site of EPTB
Abdominal examination	Mass abdomen (vague or definite)
	Ascites
	Doughy feel of abdomen
Vaginal examination	Uterine enlargement (pyometra)
	Adnexal tenderness
	Adnexal induration
	Adnexal masses
	Tubo-ovarian mass
	Fullness and tenderness in pouch of Douglas
Unusual signs	Hypertrophic lesions in cervix, vagina or vulva
	Ulcerative lesions in cervix, vagina or vulva
	Labial mass (Bartholin swelling)
	Vesicovaginal fistula
	Rectovaginal fistula
	Tubovesical fistula
	Tuboperitoneal fistula
	Tubointestinal fistula
	Uterocutaneous fistula

CLINICAL PRESENTATION

The clinical presentation of genital TB depends upon site of involvement of genital organs as shown in Table 2. The comparative symptomatology of FGTB by different authors is shown in Table 3.[9–12,31–36] Up to 11% women with genital TB may be asymptomatic.[10,20] The age of presentation is the reproductive age group with 80% of women being 20–40 years old, especially in developing countries.

Clinical signs

The various signs of FGTB depend on the site of involvement of genital organs and are shown in Table 4.[5,10,30,36,37]

Differential diagnosis

As genital TB may manifest in different ways with no characteristic symptoms and signs, the differential diagnosis varies depending upon the clinical presentation and is shown in Table 5.[5,6,20]

Table 5 Differential diagnosis of genital TB which varies according to clinical presentation

For women presenting with pain and adnexal mass following possibilities should be considered

- Acute and chronic bacterial pelvic infections
- Ectopic pregnancy
- Ovarian malignancy
- Endometriosis
- Appendicitis

The differential diagnosis of granulomatous lesions in the pelvis after laparotomy should include the following possibilities

- Crohn's disease
- Actinomycosis
- Leprosy
- Granuloma inguinale venereum
- Syphilis
- Histoplasmosis
- Brucellosis
- Silicosis
- Schistosomiasis
- Filariasis

Ulcerative or hypertrophic lesions

- Vulval cancer
- Vaginal cancer
- Cervical cancer
- Bartholin abscess
- Condyloma acuminatum
- Condyloma lata
- Vulvar and vaginal warts
- Vaginal cyst

DIAGNOSIS

Being a paucibacillary disease, demonstration of *M. tuberculosis* is not possible in all cases: a high index of suspicion is required. The diagnostic dilemma arises due to varied clinical presentation, diverse results on imaging and endoscopy and availability of a battery of bacteriological, serological and histopathological tests which are often required to obtain collective evidence for the diagnosis of genital TB.[12,38] The diagnostic approach used is family history of TB or history of antituberculous therapy (ATT) in a close family member or a past history of TB or ATT in the patient which may show recrudescence of TB in the genital region. Detailed general physical examination for any lymphadenopathy, any evidence of TB at any other site in body (bones, joints, skin, *etc.*), chest examination (PTB), abdominal examination (abdominal TB), examination of external genitalia (vulvar or vaginal TB), speculum examination (cervical TB), bimanual examination (endometrial or fallopian tube TB) aids in the diagnosis of genital TB.

Not all tests are required for all cases of genital TB. The tests will depend upon the site of TB and its clinical presentation. The various tests performed are described below.

Complete blood count

Complete blood count with erythrocyte sedimentation rate (ESR) may show anemia, leukocytosis with lymphocytosis and raised ESR in TB. However, these are non-specific markers of TB and may be raised in many other conditions.

Chest X-ray

Chest X-ray (posterior–anterior film) to exclude or confirm co-existing respiratory TB.

Mantoux (Mx) or tuberculin test

Its role in genital TB is controversial as the positive reaction (more than 10 mm of induration) indicates that the person is, or has been, infected with *M. tuberculosis*, but does not prove that she is suffering from the disease. Moreover, with severe TB and or advanced immunosuppression, the tuberculin test may be negative in infected persons. In women with laparoscopically diagnosed genital TB, the Mx test was found to have only limited utility as it had a sensitivity of 55% and specificity of 80%.[39] Women with a positive tuberculin test may be subjected to more reliable interferon-γ immunological testing; however, this is expensive and not universally available.[1]

Serological tests

These depend upon the 38 kDa antigen of *M. tuberculosis* or monoclonal antibody based sandwich ELISA and can detect only about a half to two-thirds of the HIV-negative TB-positive patients with multibacillary extensive disease, but few in HIV-positive TB-positive cases and paucibacillary patients with genital TB.[40,41] Serological tests are not sensitive and specific enough to be of great value in the diagnosis of genital TB.

Endometrial biopsy, curettage or aspirate

Endometrial aspirate, biopsy or dilatation of cervix and curettage of endometrium in the premenstrual phase is the easiest and most commonly performed test for the diagnosis of genital TB. One part of the aspirate or biopsy specimen is sent in formalin solution for histopathological testing for granuloma formation. The other part of the specimen is sent in normal saline for acid-fast bacilli (AFB) smear, culture and guinea pig inoculation. Even polymerase chain reaction (PCR) can be done on the same specimen. Tuberculous endometritis has been observed in 13.6% of infertile women undergoing routine endometrial biopsy.[42] In the absence of typical epitheloid granuloma and caseation of TB, other features like dilatation of glands, destruction of epithelium and presence of inflammatory exudates in the lumen suggest tuberculous pathology.[9] Past history of TB or family history of TB with chronic inflammatory cells with proliferative endometrium also favor the diagnosis of genital TB. A negative biopsy does not rule out genital TB as TB endometritis is seen in only 50–60% of cases and there may be a sampling error.[5] Some authors recommend a second sampling if there is inadequate specimen obtained at the first attempt. Other reasons for false-negative results include non-representative tissue samples, technical failure on processing biopsy, period of specimen collection in relation to disease stage and effect of HIV co-infection.[43]

Mycobacterial smear and culture

Endometrial biopsy, aspirate, menstrual blood (within 12 h of onset of menses in unmarried girls), secretions from vagina or cervix, peritoneal fluid or peritoneal or tubal biopsy from tubercles are subjected to smear examination for AFB, culture on Lowenstein-Jensen (LJ) medium, and guinea pig inoculation which take 6–8 weeks to provide results. The positive yield of LJ culture was found to be 57% while guinea pig inoculation showed positive results in only 11% cases in endometrial TB cases.[44]

In a comparison of histopathological evidence of granuloma on endometrial biopsy and culture, the former gave higher results in most studies.[10,12,43] Falk *et al.*[10] in their study on 187 cases of genital TB found positive culture in only 29.4% of cases in contrast to a 69.5% positive granuloma rate. Jindal[12] observed positive culture on endometrial biopsy in only 15.6% cases in contrast to a 38.8% positive rate by histopathology. In a study on female genital TB in Ethiopia with high (45%) seropositivity for HIV, AFB staining, culture and histopathology for TB were found positive in 4%, 12% and 28% of cases, respectively.[43] Sheth *et al.*[45] have highlighted the lack of diagnostic value of guinea pig test for diagnosis of TB. While LJ culture has a low sensitivity (30–35%), the radiometric culture BACTEC 460 developed by Becton Dickinson based on the generation of radioactive carbon dioxide from palmitic acid has a higher sensitivity (80–90%) with quicker results (5–10 days). It is particularly useful for drug susceptibility testing and is suited to genital TB and multidrug resistant TB analysis.[46] Other rapid diagnostic methods are Mycobacteria growth inhibitor tube (MGIT, radioactive detection system using fluorochromes), MB/Bac T (colorimetric detection of bacterial growth), septi-chek system. The growth can be established by rapid methods based on lipid analysis and specific gene probes, PCR RFLP methods and ribosomal RNA sequencing.[46] However, all these tests are expensive, are not routinely available, and are only performed in the research setting or for culture sensitivity in MDR TB.

Polymerase chain reaction (PCR)

This is a rapid, sensitive and specific molecular biological method for detecting mycobacterial DNA in both PTB and EPTB samples from suspected TB patients. PCR assays targeting various gene segments including a 65-kDa protein encoding gene, the IS 6110 element and the *mpt64* gene.[46] In a study from our hospital (AIIMS, New Delhi), Bhanu *et al.*[47] studied samples from endometrial aspirates, endometrial biopsies and fluid from the pouch of Douglas from 25 women with infertility suspected to be suffering from genital

TB on laparoscopic findings for the presence of the *mpt64* gene of *M. tuberculosis*. Overall, PCR demonstrated *M. tuberculosis* DNA in 56% of cases compared to 1.6% smear-positive and 3.2% culture-positive cases. PCR was positive in all women with laparoscopic findings suggestive of TB, in 60% of those with probable diagnosis, in 33% of those with incidental findings and even in one case with normal laparoscopic findings.[47] Other authors have also observed PCR to be more sensitive than histopathology and culture.[12,43] Rozati *et al.*[48] observed PCR to be positive in 43.1% of suspected cases of FGTB in contrast to 5.2%, 7.8% and 11.5% detection rates with AFB staining, culture and histopathology, respectively. They recommended a combination of PCR with the other available techniques for achieving sufficient sensitivity and specificity for the diagnosis of FGTB. Microscopic examination of AFB requires the presence of at least 10,000 organisms/ml in the sample. Culture is more sensitive requiring as little as 100 organisms/ml while PCR may be positive with only 1–10 organisms/ml.[47] However, PCR has its own disadvantages. It can give false-negative results due to contamination with heparin or to a high salt concentration of the specimen which may interfere with PCR results. As it can not distinguish between live and dead bacilli, there is a small risk of false-positive results.[47] Some authors have advised that PCR should not be used for rapid diagnosis of TB. Because of insufficient reliability, results obtained by PCR should not be used to initiate or to stop ATT.[49] In the author's experience, false-positive rates by PCR are high as it can detect even single *M. tuberculosis* cells and may not be able to differentiate between infection and disease as most of Indian people may show positive PCR without suffering from the disease. It is our policy not to start ATT just on the basis of positive PCR unless there is some other evidence of FGTB on clinical examination, or the presence of tubercles or other stigmata of TB on laparoscopy.

Imaging methods

Ultrasonography (USG)

Being non-invasive and with no radiation hazard, USG can be used in the diagnosis of FGTB and may show bilateral solid adnexal masses with scattered small calcifications with free fluid in pouch of Douglas (Fig. 2).[5,6,20] However, in the absence of pelvic masses, USG has a very limited role in the diagnosis of genital TB.

Computerised axial tomography (CT scan)

This is a useful modality for pelvic and abdominal masses especially when the lesion may resemble malignant ovarian tumors. In TB, there is low-density ascites, multiple pelvic, abdominal, hepatic or splenic lesions with or without lymphadenopathy especially in young infertile women.[5,6,20] In fallopian tube TB or ovarian TB, CT scan may help in delineation of tubo-ovarian masses.

Positron Emission tomograhy (PETscan)

It's a useful modality as it demonstrates glucose intake by the diseased area, but the data available on its role in genital tuberculosis is sparse.

Magnetic resonance imaging (MRI)

MRI is used increasingly in modern gynecology in the presence of abdominal

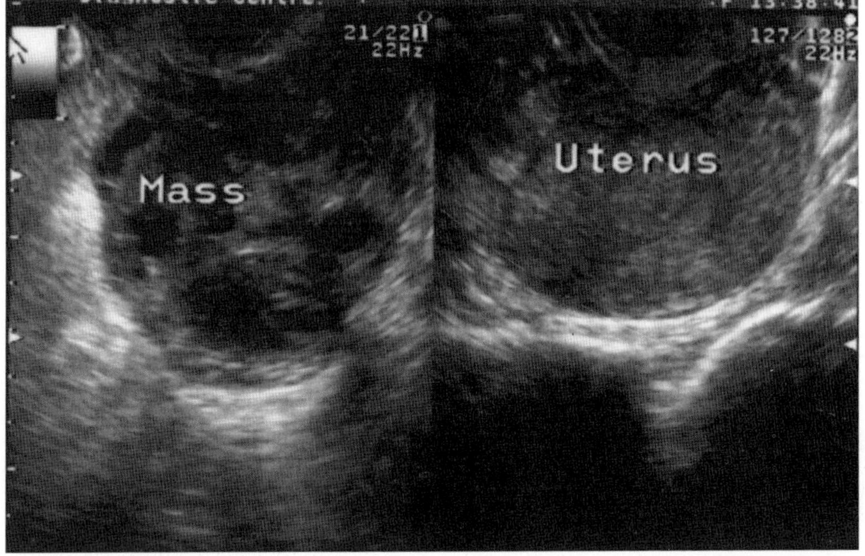

Fig. 2 Ultrasonography showing a tuberculous mixed echogenic mass on right side of uterus.

and pelvic masses. MRI has better resolution than a CT scan and may avoid the necessity of laparotomy as the differential diagnosis is usually from ovarian tumor. The presence of hypodense masses with rim enhancement abutting the pelvic walls are suggestive of TB (Fig. 3).

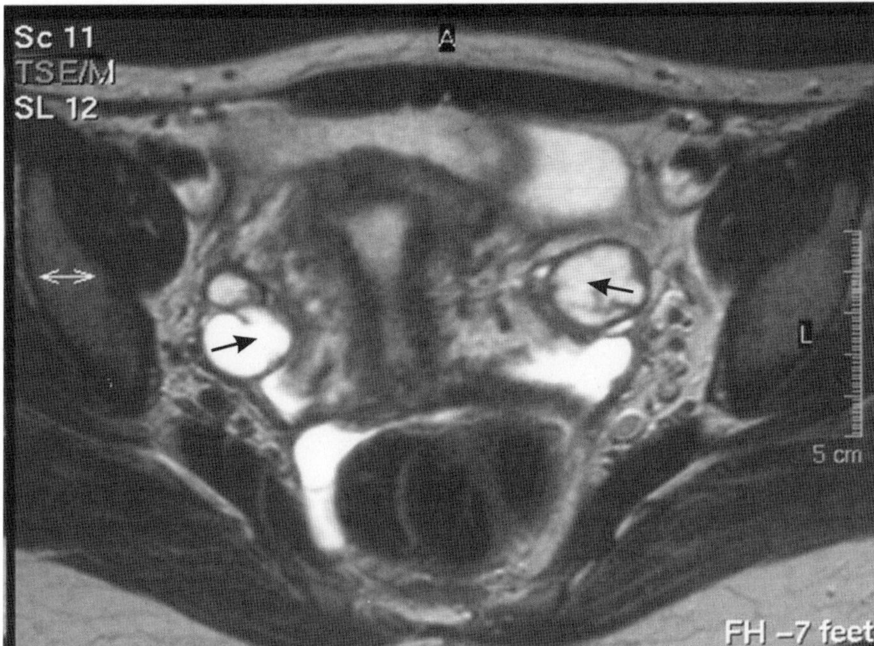

Fig. 3 MRI film showing bilateral tubo-ovarian masses in a patient of biopsy-proven genital tuberculosis.

Blood markers in genital TB

CA 125 is a useful tumor marker for epithelial ovarian cancer in which levels are markedly raised (normal levels < 35 U/ml). However, it is a non-specific marker and is also raised in endometriosis and in genital TB. Usually, the levels in genital TB are only moderately raised (usually < 200 U/ml). However, there have been case reports with very high levels of CA 125 in disseminated abdominal TB with as high as 18000 U/ml recorded in a proven pelvic TB with disseminated disease (Kumar S, personal communication). Hence, CA 125 is not a very reliable marker for diagnosis of FGTB.

Hysterosalpingography (HSG)

In a known case of genital TB, HSG is contra-indicated as it may flare up subclinical infection. Usually, diagnosis of genital TB is made retrospectively when HSG is performed for infertility patients without a suspicion of genital TB, a common scenario in India. It is an invaluable procedure for evaluating the internal architecture of the female genital tract and is the most helpful procedure in suggesting the diagnosis of genital TB in women being investigated for infertility. The various abnormalities depend upon the involvement of fallopian tubes and endometrium and the severity of the disease.[50,51] Endometrial TB causes non-specific appearances on HSG, commonly characterised by synechiae formation, a distorted uterine contour and venous and lymphatic intravasation (Figs 4 and 5).[50] The synechiae and

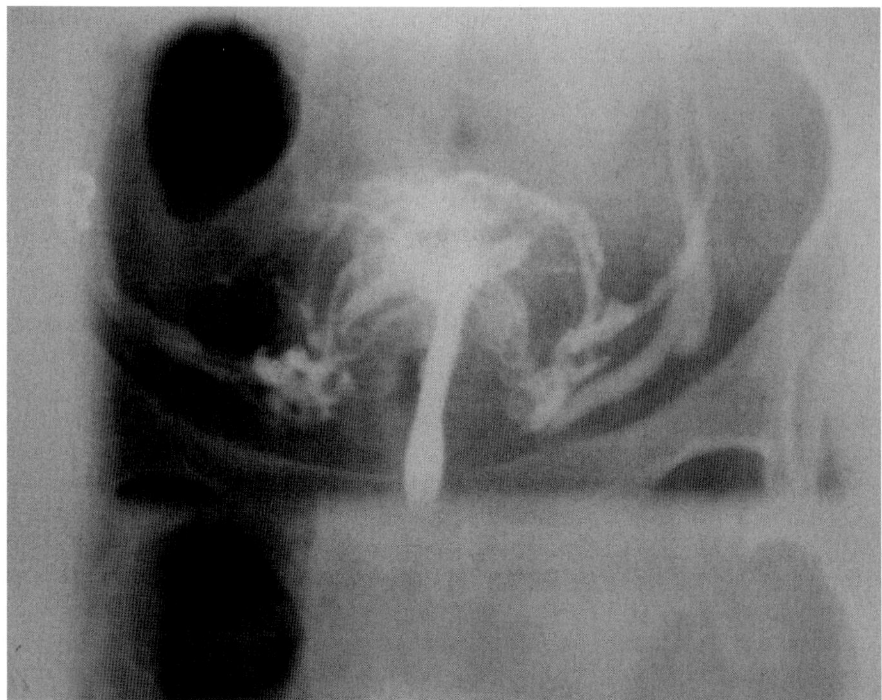

Fig. 4 Hysterosalpingography showing intravasation of dye in pelvic vessels with bilateral cornual tubal block in genital TB.

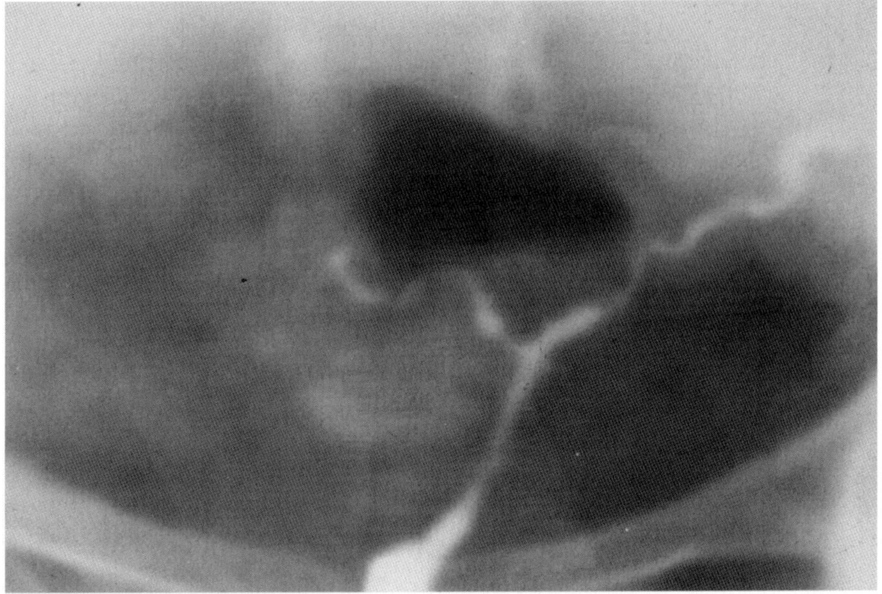

Fig. 5 Hysterosalpingography showing marked narrowing of uterine cavity with Maltese cross appearance of fallopian tubes with no spill.

intra-uterine adhesions in TB are characteristically irregular, angulated and stellate-shaped with well-demarcated borders. Unilateral scarring may cause obliteration of the uterine cavity on one side giving rise to a pseudo-unicornuate uterus. Scarring in TB may result in conversion of the triangular uterine cavity into a T-shaped cavity. An asymmetric, small-sized, uterine cavity is usually due to TB.[5,50] Venous and lymphatic intravasation is a good indicator of endometrial TB but is not very specific as it can happen in other conditions also (intra-uterine adhesions or tubal obstruction due to other etiologies).

The various diagnostic criteria established for diagnosis of TB of fallopian tubes from HSG by various authors are:[5,20,50,51]

1. Calcified lymph nodes or smaller, irregular calcifications in the fallopian tubes (adnexal area).
2. Obstruction of the fallopian tube in the zone of transition between the isthmus and the ampulla.
3. Multiple constrictions along the course of the fallopian tubes or beaded appearance (salpingitis isthmica nodosa).
4. Ragged and jagged tubal contour with small lumen defects and fistulous tracts.
5. Straight, rigid contour of the lumen with stem-pipe like configuration of the tube.
6. Golf-club appearance: only isthmus and proximal ampulla are visualised and the isthmic segment has a rigid, stove-pipe appearance.
7. Maltese-cross appearance: completely filled tube with rigid and irregular outline (Fig. 5).

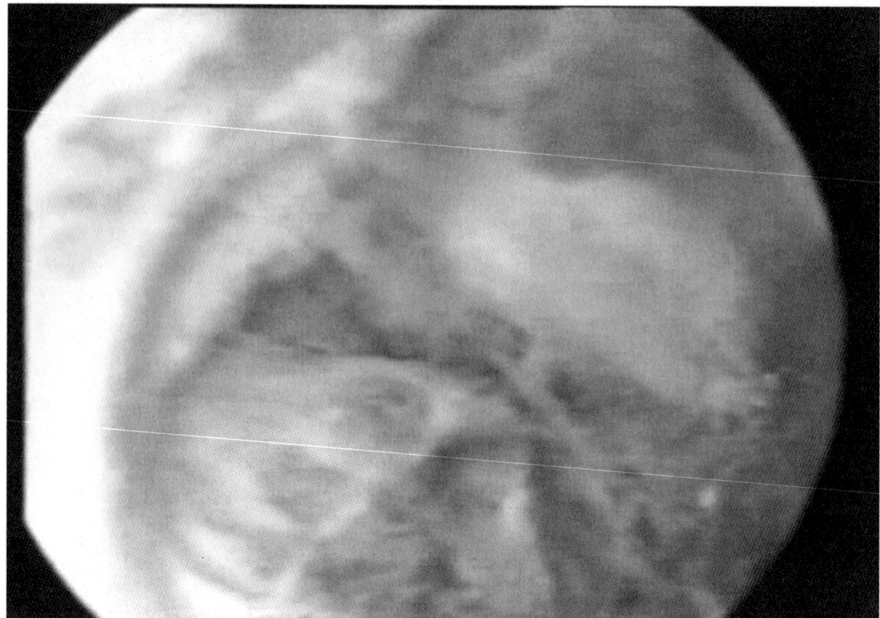

Fig. 6 Hysteroscopy showing shrunken uterine cavity with adhesions (Asherman's syndrome) in a case of confirmed endometrial TB.

8. Rosette type: the distal end of the tube is filled with dye giving a rosette-type image.
9. Leopard skin like speckled appearance of the ampulla due to the tube being partially filled with contrast.

Although the tubes are often blocked in genital TB, they may be patent in 37% cases of endometrial TB.[5] We found tubal calcification, irregularity of tubal wall, unilateral or bilateral cornual block, unilateral or bilateral hydrosolpinx, venous and lymphatic intravasation of dye in cases of genital TB in our studies.[16,51]

Endoscopy

Hysteroscopy

Endoscopic visualisation of the uterine cavity in genital TB may show a normal cavity (if no endometrial TB or early stage TB) with bilateral open ostia. More often, however, the endometrium is pale looking, the cavity is partially or completely obliterated by adhesions of varying grade (Fig. 6). There may be a small, shrunken cavity. One has to be careful when performing hysteroscopy in genital TB as the cervix is often constricted and dilatation is difficult with chances of perforation and false passage. It has been the author's experience over many such cases, that hysteroscopy is associated with difficulty, inability to do the procedure and increased chances of complications in women with genital TB. Hence, hysteroscopy in a patient with genital TB should be done by an experienced person. In case of inability to dilate the cervix, it may be advisable to perform the procedure under laparoscopic guidance to avoid false

Table 6 Laparoscopic findings in genital tuberculosis by different authors (percentages)

Reference	Women (*n*)	Normal findings	Tubercles on tubes/ peritoneum	Caseation/ granulomas	Beaded tubes	Blocked tubes	Adhesions	Hydro-salpinx	Tubo-ovarian mass	Encysted effusions
Bhide *et al.* (1987)[32]	71	NA	33.8	NA	NA	NA	46.5	NA	32.4	8.45
Rattan *et al.* (1993)[41]	15	NA	100	100	NA	NA	86.6	100	NA	60
Parikh *et al.* (1997)[52]	38	NA	NA	NA	NA	49.5	47.5	NA	15.3	NA
Kumari & Sinha (2000)[53]	11	0	100	NA	NA	NA	100	NA	NA	NA
Tripathy & Tripathy (2002)[54]	73	NA	56.1	NA	47.9	45.2	47.9	47.9	NA	NA
Jindal (2006)[12]	70	10	55.5	20.6	NA	NA	90	NA	54	NA
Gupta & Sharma (2007)[16]	40	0	32.5	32.5	32.5	NA	100	32.5	32.5	2.5

NA, data not available.

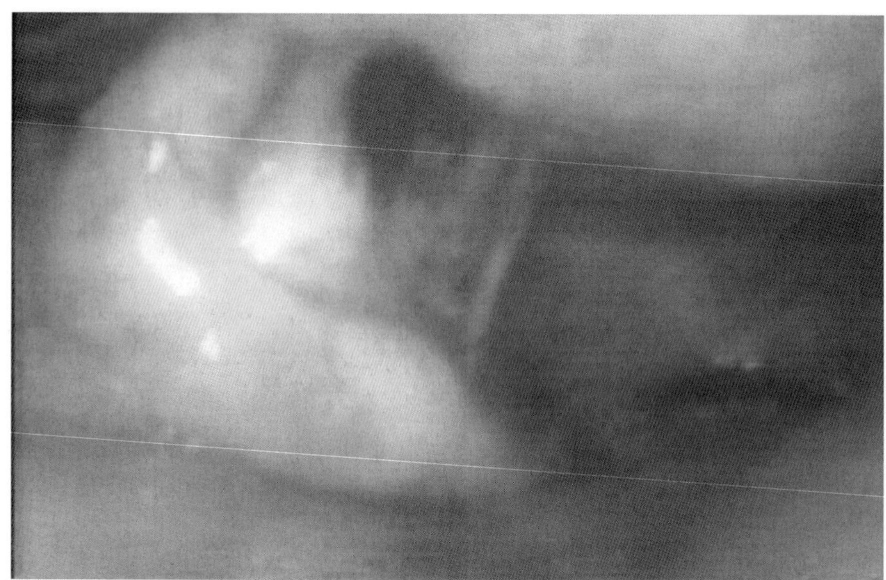

Fig. 7 Laparoscopy showing short, congested and swollen fallopian tube with adhesions in pouch of Douglas in a case of genital TB.

passage formation and injury to the pelvic organs. The abnormal findings on hysteroscopy in genital TB may be the presence of intra-uterine synechiae, granulomas and poor distensibility.[12] In an observational study on 20 women with genital TB where hysteroscopy was performed, we had to abandon the procedure in 2 (10%) cases due to perforation and inability to distend the cavity. Normal findings were seen in 6 cases (30%), difficult distension in 6 (30%), flimsy adhesions in 4 (20%), thick adhesions in 3 (15%) obliterated cavity and inability to see ostia or blocked ostia in 5 (25%) cases with more than one finding in many cases (Sharma JB, Roy KK, Kumar S, Malhotra N, Chawla P, unpublished data).

Laparoscopy

A laparoscopy and dye hydrotubation (lap and dye test) is the most reliable tool to diagnose genital TB especially for tubal, ovarian and peritoneal disease.[16,32] The test can be combined with hysteroscopy for maximum information. Morphological abnormalities of the fallopian tubes can be seen directly. Genital TB can be seen in 5–33.8% of cases of infertility on routine laparoscopy. The various abnormalities of genital TB on laparoscopy by different authors are shown in Table 6 and are summarized as follows.[12,16,32,41,52–54] In the sub-acute stage, there may be congestion, edema and adhesions in pelvic organs with multiple, fluid-filled pockets. There are miliary tubercles, white, yellow and opaque plaques over the fallopian tubes and uterus. In the chronic stage, there may be following abnormalities: (i) yellow, small nodules on tubes (nodular salpingitis); (ii) short and swollen tubes with agglutinated fimbriae (patchy salpingitis; Fig. 7); (iii) unilateral or bilateral hydrosalpinx with retort-shaped tubes due to agglutination of

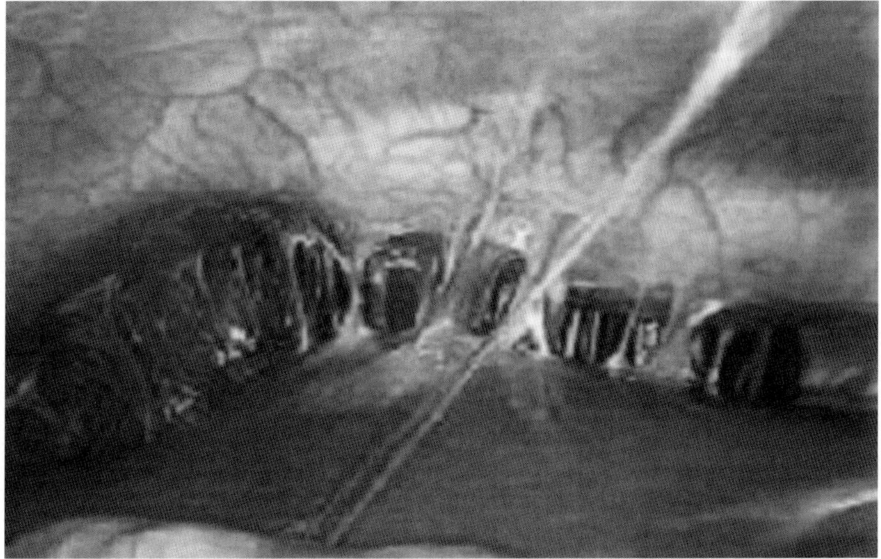

Fig. 8 Violin-string adhesions between liver and diaphragm (Fitz-Hugh-Curtis syndrome) in a case of genital TB.

fimbriae; (iv) pyosalpinx or caseosalpinx where the tube (usually bilaterally) is distended with caseous material with ovoid, white-yellow distension of ampulla with poor vascularization; and (v) various types of adhesions may be present in genital TB covering genital organs with or without omentum and intestines. The adhesions are usually vascular and it has been the author's experience that adhesiolysis in such women may be associated with significant bleeding and there is risk of injury to the bowel in the presence of dense adhesions. Even peritoneal biopsy from the lesions can cause excessive bleeding and needs careful hemostasis with cautery.

Various other abnormalities on laparoscopy in genital TB include adhesions, granuloma, plaques, exudates, tubo-ovarian masses and pelvic congestion in up to 88.6% of cases.[12] We observed dilated, tortuous and blocked fallopian tubes (32.5%), peritubal and peri-ovarian adhesions (45%), omental adhesions (45%) and bowel adhesions (37.5%) with more than one type of lesions in many women in 40 proven genital TB cases in our study.[16] We also observed very high prevalence (48%) of Fitz-Hugh-Curtis syndrome (Fig. 8) on laparoscopy in FGTB cases.[17,18]

In association with other diagnostic modalities like endometrial biopsy, PCR, HSG with or without other tests, laparoscopy has helped in making a correct diagnosis of genital TB in the majority of cases.[12] The final diagnosis is made from good history taking, careful systemic and gynecological examination and judicious use of diagnostic modalities like endometrial biopsy in conjunction with imaging methods and endoscopic visualization, especially with laparoscopy. Some authors have developed an algorithm for accurate diagnosis of FGTB by combining history taking, examination and investigations.[12]

Table 7 Category treatment regimens for tuberculosis including FGTB[4,58,59]

TB diagnostic category	TB patients	TB treatment regimens: Initial phase (daily or 3 times weekly)		Continuation phase (daily or 3 times weekly)	
1	New smear-positive pulmonary TB (PTB) patients. New smear-negative PTB with extensive parenchymal involvement. Severe concomitant HIV disease Severe forms of EPTB (FGTB included)	2 HRZE – dose: INH (600 mg), rifampicin (450 mg or 600 mg if > 50 kg), pyrazinamide (1500 mg) ethambutol (1200 mg) for 2 months		4 HR – dose: INH (600 mg), rifampicin (450 mg or 600 mg if > 50 kg) for 4 months	
II	Previously treated sputum smear-positive PTB. Relapse (FGTB included). Treatment after default (FGTB included). Treatment failure (FGTB included).	2 HRZES/IHRZE – dose: RHZE as in category I above. Injection streptomycin 0.75 g daily or thrice weekly (DOTS) for 2 months followed by 1 month of RHZE		5HRE – dose: INH (600 mg), rifampicin (450 mg or 600 mg if > 50 kg), ethambutol (1200 mg) for 5 months	
III	New smear-negative pulmonary TB (other than in Category I). Less severe form of EPTB	2HRZ		4HR	
IV	Chronic and MDR-TB cases (still sputum-positive after supervised re-treatment/or culture positive or histopathologically proven FGTB)	Standardized regimen (daily)			
		Drug	Dose (mg) if weight < 45 kg	Dose (mg) if weight > 45 kg	
		Kanamycin (IM)	500	750	6–9 months' intensive phase
		Ofloxacin (O)	600	800	
		Ethionamide (O)	500	750	
		Pyrazinamide (O)	1250	1500	
		Ethambutol (O)	800	1000	
		Cycloserine (O)	500	750	
		Ofloxacin (O)	600	800	18 months' continuation phase
		Ethionamide (O)	500	750	
		Ethambutol (O)	800	1000	
		Cycloserine (O)	500	750	

IM, intramuscular; O, oral; extrapulmonary TB, EPTB; pulmonary TB, PTB; female genital TB, FGTB.

TREATMENT

Medical treatment

Treatment and care should take into account each patient's individual needs and preferences and she, alone, should make an informed decision about her care and treatment. Good communication between the healthcare professional and patient is essential, supported by evidence-based information tailored to the needs of the individual patient. Treatment, care and information should be culturally appropriate and the carers and relatives should be involved in the process with the consent of the patient. Multiple drug therapy in adequate doses and for sufficient duration is the main-stay in the treatment of TB including FGTB. In the days before rifampicin, antituberculous therapy (ATT) was given for 18–24 months with significant side effects and poor compliance. The development of short-term, cost-effective chemotherapy for TB was a major achievement for clinical medicine. Short-course chemotherapy for 6–9 months has been found to be effective for medical treatment of FGTB.[12,55]

Directly observed treatment short course (DOTS) strategy treatment

The American Thoracic Society,[56] the British Thoracic Society and the UK National Institute for Health and Clinical Excellence (NICE) Guidelines (2006)[57] recommend that the first choice of treatment should be the 'standard recommended regimen' using a daily dosing schedule using combination tablets. They do not consider DOTS necessary in management of most cases of TB in developed countries who can adhere to treatment and recommend DOTS only for street- and shelter-dwelling, homeless people with active TB or patients likely to have poor adherence. DOTS was vociferously argued for by the WHO after declaring TB a global emergency in 1993. Poor compliance with standard, long-term treatment regimens compounded by over-crowding, poor living conditions in low socio-economic conditions has fuelled the epidemic of multidrug resistant (MDR) TB in parts of the world. To prevent MDR and for better results, the DOTS strategy has been proven to be cost effective throughout the world. The five components of DOTS are given in Table 1. The author strongly feels that all women with FGTB should be treated under the DOTS strategy throughout the world for best results. The patient is first allocated to one of the treatment categories and is then given treatment as per guidelines for national programs by the WHO (Table 7).[58] Genital TB is classified under category I as being seriously ill, extrapulmonary disease. As *M. tuberculosis* divides very slowly (18 h), thrice weekly treatment is as effective as daily treatment. However, it must be reiterated that intermittent treatment can only be given under direct observation as even one dose should not be missed to avoid development of MDR disease. After diagnosis of FGTB and decision to start ATT by the treating physician is made, the patient should be sent to a DOTS center near her area of residence (in India, the whole country is now under DOTS strategy). To ensure quality-assured drugs in adequate doses, a full 6-month course pack is booked for an individual patient in the DOTS center. As shown in Table 7, the woman is given a fixed drug combipack (FDC) of isoniazid (INH), rifampicin, pyrazinamide and ethambutol, 3 times a week for the first 2 months (intensive phase) under direct observation in front of a health worker at a DOTS center. Compliance is ensured by the DOTS center providers by contacting the homes of any defaulters. In the continuation phase, the patient is given a combination blister pack of isoniazid and rifampicin 3 times a week for the next 4 months with at least one of the weekly doses administered under direct observation; compliance is ensured by noting empty blister packs brought by the patient on each weekly visit.

Rarely, FGTB cases can have relapse or failure categorizing them into category II (Table 7). The diagnosis of all such cases should be made by the attending physician and should be supported by culture or histological evidence of current active TB in these cases. Such women are categorised as others in category II and are given treatment accordingly (Table 7) which includes 2 months intramuscular injections of streptomycin thrice weekly along with another four drugs (RHZE) of category I under direct supervision of a DOTS center health worker for the first 2 months followed by four drugs (RHZE) thrice a week for another month (intensive phase). The continuation phase is with three drugs – isoniazid (H), rifampicin (R) and ethambutol (E) – thrice a week for another 5 months with at least one of the three times a week dose being administered under direct observation.

Some clinicians treat minimal genital TB (asymptomatic except for infertility and diagnosed on endometrial biopsy culture) as category III by omitting ethambutol from the first 2 months' regimen, especially in areas where resistance to isoniazid is unlikely. As the exact prevalence of resistance to isoniazid in India is not known (but is probably high), it is the author's policy to treat all women with genital TB as category I under the DOTS strategy. The Revised National Tuberculosis Control Programme (RNTCP) of India has achieved a treatment success rate of up to 95% with DOTS for all types of TB including FGTB.[4]

Alternative treatment (non-DOTS)

The author does not recommend treatment out of DOTS especially in developing countries as this policy only provides best results in all types of TB including FGTB by ensuring consumption of quality-assured drugs in the right dosage and duration to the patients under direct supervision. This is very important for countries like India where drugs bought from the market may sometimes be spurious. Some women may feel the drugs bought from the market are superior to the drugs available free of cost at government DOTS centers, but they must be counselled and encouraged to get treatment under DOTS only.

However, some women obtain treatment from private sector doctors and may buy their medicines. In such cases, daily treatment should only be given, as intermittent therapy must be given as supervised therapy (DOTS strategy). Convenient commercial combipacks are available containing one capsule of rifampicin (450 mg), two tablets of pyrazinamide (750 mg each), one tablet of ethambutol (800 mg) plus isoniazid 300 mg (AKT-4; Lupin Laboratories, Mumbai, India: CX-5; Cadila Healthcare, Ahmedabad, India) at a very economic price (Rs. 15 per combipack equivalent to 30 US cents or 17 English pence per day). These have to be taken every day for 2 months followed by a combination of rifampicin (450 mg if body weight < 50 kg, 600 mg if > 50 kg) and isoniazid (300 mg; R-Cinex 600 or 450; Lupin: Rimactazid; Novartis, Mumbai, India) as a combipack to be taken daily at a very economic price (Rs. 7 per day).

It is strongly recommended to use the DOTS strategy even in developed countries for its proven efficacy. In the US and UK, unsupervised treatment can be given using a combipack of rifampicin, pyrazinamide, isoniazid (Rifater) with or without separate ethambutol (as isoniazid resistance is uncommon) for the first 2 months (initial phase) followed by a combination of rifampicin and isoniazid (Rifanah, Rimactazid) for a further 4 months (continuation phase).[56,57]

Monitoring

Most women tolerate ATT safely. They should be counselled about the importance of taking ATT regularly, maintain a good and nutritious diet during ATT, and should report any side effects of the drugs. Liver function tests are no longer done regularly unless there are symptoms of hepatic toxicity. Similarly, pyridoxine is not routinely prescribed with ATT unless there are symptoms of peripheral neuropathy with isoniazid. Rarely, hepatitis can be caused by isoniazid, rifampicin and pyrazinamide, optic neuritis by ethambutol, and auditory and vestibular toxicity by streptomycin. In such cases, the opinion of an expert should be sought for restarting the ATT in a modified form.

Treatment of chronic cases, drug-resistant and multidrug-resistant (MDR) FGTB

The risk factors for MDR are a history of prior TB treatment or prior TB treatment failure, contact with a known case of drug-resistant TB, residents of high-incidence areas and HIV-positive women. Resistance to either isoniazid or to rifampicin is termed 'drug resistance' (DR) while resistance to both isoniazid and rifampicin, the two main ATT drugs, is called 'multidrug-resistance' (MDR). Extreme drug resistance (XDR) is resistance to isoniazid, rifampicin, injectable aminoglycosides and floroquinolones. For isoniazid resistance, the ATT regimen used is 12 RZE for immunocompetent patients and 18–24 RZE for immunocompromised (HIV positive) cases. For rifampicin resistance, the regimen used is 18–24 HZE.

Although rare, MDR (resistance to both isoniazid and rifampicin) can involve any site including FGTB. Its treatment is like MDR PTB. It is treated as category IV (Table 7) with a DOTS Plus strategy using standardized or individualized regimen. The drugs are toxic and expensive highlighting the need of DOTS strategy for all drug-sensitive TB cases to prevent MDR. Treatment of MDR TB should be started in consultation with an expert. RNTCP uses a standardized treatment regimen (daily) comprising of 6 drugs for 6–9 months in the intensive phase followed by 4 drugs for the next 18 months in the continuation phase (Table 7).[59] As the drugs are very expensive, the WHO Green Light Committee can help in procuring second-line ATT drugs at a discounted price through collaboration with the pharmaceutical industry.[60]

Treatment of FGTB in HIV-positive women

HIV has had a disastrous impact on attempts to control TB in many countries and will continue to be a formidable challenge. TB is a leading cause of HIV-related morbidity and mortality, while HIV is the most important factor in fuelling the TB epidemic in high HIV prevalence populations; HIV is rampant in sub-Saharan Africa and present even in developed countries. There is a clear need for a new evidence-based international strategy to reduce the burden of TB and HIV. WHO has formulated an interim policy in collaborative TB and HIV activities for better management of co-infection.[61] In India, RNTCP and National AIDS Control Organization (NACO) work jointly to manage this dual epidemic better. There is need to expand the scope of the DOTS strategy for TB control in HIV-endemic areas and use measures to decrease HIV transmission (*e.g.* condom use and treatment of sexually transmitted infections), administer highly active antiretroviral therapy (HAART) and implement effective TB prevention and treatment. Treatment of TB including FGTB in HIV-positive women is the same as in HIV-negative women with best results being obtained through the DOTS strategy. Only thiacetazone (still used in certain poorer countries instead of the expensive ethambutol) is contra-indicated in HIV-positive women as it can cause severe skin rashes. Such women should be treated in consultation with a specialist in the management of HIV and TB, as rifampicin stimulates the activity of the cytochrome P450 liver enzyme system that metabolises protease inhibitors (PIs) and non-nucleoside reverse transcriptase inhibitors (NNRTIs) reducing their blood levels. Possible options for antiretroviral therapy in TB patients include:

- defer antiretroviral therapy until TB treatment is completed
- defer antiretroviral therapy until the end of the initial phase of treatment and use ethambutol and isoniazid in the continuation phase
- treat TB with a rifampicin-containing regimen and use efavirenz + 2 NRTIs (nucleoside reverse transcriptase inhibitors)
- treat TB with a rifampicin-containing regimen and use 2 NRTIs; then change to a maximally suppressive HAART regimen on completion of TB treatment.

Surgical treatment

Schaefer[7,19] had recommended surgical treatment in the form of total abdominal hysterectomy with bilateral salpingo-oophorectomy for persistent or recurrent disease or pelvic masses following medical treatment, persistent symptoms after treatment, recurrent pyometra, TB pyosalpinx, ovarian masses, non-healing fistulas and MDR disease. However, these recommendations were given in the pre-rifampicin era when lengthy and less effective treatment regimens with poor compliance were used. With modern, short-course chemotherapy, the need for surgery is very rare. Even fistulas heal spontaneously on ATT as has been the experience of the author.[30] Similarly, MDR disease needs treatment with the DOTS Plus regimen rather than surgery for best results. There are also much higher chances of complications during surgery in women with genital TB, including increased perforation rates in hysteroscopy, more bleeding during adhesiolysis on laparoscopy and excessive hemorrhage and non-availability of surgical planes at time of laparotomy with higher risks of injury to the bowel and other pelvic and abdominal organs. In a case of abdomino pelvic TB, bowel loops may be matted together with no plane between them and the uterus and adnexa may be buried underneath the plastic adhesions and bowel loops making them non-approachable. Even trying to perform a diagnostic laparoscopy or laparotomy in such cases can cause injury to bowel necessitating a very difficult laparotomy and resection of injured bowel as has been experienced by us and others (Mitra S, personal communication). It is the policy of the author to only take biopsies from representative areas and close the abdomen without pelvic clearance in cases of laparotomy done for suspected pelvic tumors but found to be tubercular at laparotomy and treating the women with short course chemotherapy under DOTS strategy. However, limited surgery such as drainage of pelvic or tubo-ovarian abscesses, pyosalpinx can be performed followed by ATT for better results. The American Thoracic Society[56] only recommends surgery (drainage) for residual large tubo-ovarian abscesses. It has been the author's experience that women undergoing surgery (laparotomy, hysterectomy, laparoscopic surgery, *etc.*) with pelvic and peritoneal TB bleed much more than other women. We recently performed a vaginal hysterectomy and pelvic floor repair in an elderly woman with third degree utero-vaginal prolapse. There was excessive hemorrhage at the time of surgery, but hemostasis was achieved. However, she needed an unexpected laparotomy after 48 h for hemoperitoneum from ooze from the tubo-ovarian pedicle. The histopathology of hysterectomy specimen turned out to be endometrial TB explaining the reason for excessive hemorrhage (Sharma JB, Kumar S, Roy KK, Pushparaj M, unpublished case).

Laparoscopic and hysteroscopic surgery

Some times, even after a full 6 months' course of ATT, women with genital TB with infertility do not conceive. In such cases, laparoscopy and hysteroscopy may be repeated to visualise any remaining disease. After treating many such women referred from all over the country, it has been our experience that fertility outcome for FGTB is only good when ATT is started early in the disease. However, cases of advanced TB, with extensive adhesions in pelvis and uterus, are usually untreatable with very poor prognosis for fertility.

Tuboplasty

After ATT for genital TB in infertility cases, tuboplasty by laparoscopy or laparotomy may be tried especially in women who cannot afford expensive assisted reproductive techniques (ART), such as *in vitro* fertilization and embryo transfer, and who insist on tubal surgery which is available free of cost in government hospitals in India. Unfortunately, there is usually permanent damage of tubes due to TB in these women. In spite of ATT, tuboplasty (laparoscopic or laparotomy) does not help much. There are chances of flare up of the disease and risk of ectopic pregnancy, should the women conceive.

***In vitro* fertilisation (IVF)**

Most women with genital TB present with infertility and have poor prognosis for fertility in spite of ATT. The conception rate is low (19.2%) with the live-birth rate also low (7%) in the Tripathy and Tripathy series.[54] Parikh *et al.*[52] found IVF with embryo transfer to be the only hope for some of these women whose endometrium was not damaged and a pregnancy rate of 16.6% per transfer was achieved. Jindal[12] observed IVF embryo transfer to be the most successful of all ART modalities in genital TB patients with a 17.3% conception rate in contrast to only 4.3% with fertility enhancing surgery. Dam *et al.*[62] found latent genital TB responsible for repeated IVF failure in young Indian patients in Kolkata presenting with unexplained infertility with apparently normal pelvis and non-endometrial tubal factors. We follow a policy at our hospital (AIIMS, New Delhi), where we cater to large number of such women referred from all over the country especially from high-risk areas like Bihar, that if, after ATT, their tubes are still damaged but their endometrium is receptive (no adhesions or mild adhesions which can be hysteroscopically resected) to refer them for IVF embryo transfer. However, if they have endometrial TB causing damage to the endometrium with shrunken small uterine cavity with Asherman's syndrome, we counsel them about the poor prognosis for fertility and advise them to consider adoption as the endometrium in such women is usually not receptive to embryo transfer.

TUBERCULOSIS AND PREGNANCY

The occurrence of pregnancy in women with TB is increasing in developed countries mainly in ethnic minorities, especially in recent migrants, giving an incidence of 252 per 100,000 deliveries in the UK.[63] In developing countries, TB is very common in the reproductive age group where pregnancy is also common; this double condition, tuberculosis and pregnancy, is further compounded by co-infection with HIV. Data on the exact incidence of TB in India is lacking. The US Centers for Disease Control (CDC) in Atlanta observed the incidence of TB during pregnancy as 5.7, 26.7 and 49.6 per 100,000 population in American whites, African-Americans and Asians, respectively.[64] PTB is the commonest lesion during pregnancy but EPTB like TB of lymph nodes, bones, kidneys, abdominal tuberculosis and rarely TB of meninges or miliary TB can occur in pregnancy.[65–67] In fact, the prenatal setting represents a missed opportunity for diagnosing and treating latent TB, especially in immigrants; this has been used in the US for non-US-born pregnant women by testing with the tuberculin skin test and treating the positive women with latent TB with isoniazid to prevent active TB.[68] There is no evidence that TB is more common during pregnancy.[69] The course of TB is usually unaffected by pregnancy. The lesions do not progress and there is no increased mortality in women compared to non-pregnant women. Pregnancy is not contra-indicated in women with TB unless advanced.

Clinical presentation of TB in pregnancy

The presentation of TB in pregnant women is similar to that in non-pregnant women but diagnosis may be delayed by the non-specific early symptoms of TB and the common occurrence of malaise and fatigue in pregnancy.[69] Women with PTB usually present with cough, expectoration, fever, malaise, fatigue and hemoptysis, but may be asymptomatic in up to 20% women.[67,69] Chest radiography should be performed using abdominal shield in suspected cases to avoid missing the diagnosis and treatment. Tuberculin skin testing can be done safely in pregnancy to diagnose latent TB. The bacillus Calmetté Guerin (BCG) vaccine being a live vaccine is contra-indicated in pregnancy and is given only following delivery after a second negative test. Women with EPTB presenting with signs and symptoms suggestive of TB of different organs, like lymphadenopathy (lymph node TB), abdominal pain and distension (abdominal TB) with fever and other constitutional symptoms, need specific investigations like fine needle aspiration cytology (FNAC) for confirmation of the diagnosis.

Treatment of TB in pregnancy

Women with latent TB can be treated with 6 months of isoniazid or 3 months of isoniazid and rifampicin. A woman with PTB or EPTB must be treated with a full course of short-term chemotherapy irrespective of gestation (even in first trimester) as per DOTS strategy (Table 7) using category wise treatment. All four drugs – isoniazid, rifampicin, pyrazinamide and ethambutol – are non-teratogenic and safe in pregnancy and should be given. Some clinicians avoid pyrazinamide in pregnancy as there are less data available on its safety in pregnancy. Streptomycin is avoided in pregnancy as it can cause ototoxicity in the fetus.

Perinatal outcome

Although some studies have demonstrated higher perinatal mortality (up to 6-fold) and incidence of prematurity (2-fold), small for gestational age babies and low birth weight babies (< 2500 g) in PTB mothers diagnosed later in pregnancy, the outcome of those diagnosed in early pregnancy was the same as in non-TB women.[65,69] In EPTB, Jana *et al.*[66] observed no adverse effect of lymph node TB on perinatal outcome, but found adverse effects on fetuses with a low Agpar score at birth; the proportion of low birth weight infants increased to 33% as compared to 11% in controls in other types of EPTB. Current thinking, however, is that TB (both PTB and EPTB), if diagnosed and treated in time, has no adverse effect on perinatal outcome.[63,67,69]

Maternal outcome

Maternal outcome varies with the site and severity of the TB. In PTB with late diagnosis, obstetric morbidity was 4-fold and preterm labor 9-fold higher, with an increased frequency of abortion, toxemia and intrapartum complications.[65] However, most other studies found no adverse effect of PTB and EPTB on maternal outcome.[63,67,69]

Treatment of MDR TB in pregnancy

Of the second-line drugs, kanamycin and amikacin (being aminoglycosides) can cause ototoxicity in the fetus. Ethionamide and prothionamide are potentially teratogenic and should be avoided in women of child-bearing age. Therapeutic abortion can be considered in the presence of MDR TB in a woman after proper counselling about the potential teratogenic effects of drugs. Those keen to continue the pregnancy must be treated for MDR with complete dosage of second-line drugs (Table 7).

Treatment of HIV and TB in pregnancy

The management of pregnant TB women in HIV-positive cases is the same (DOTS strategy) but may need appropriate adjustments to avoid drug interactions in consultation with an expert in the area

Congenital TB

Congenital TB is the infection of the fetus *in utero* through the hematogenous route via the umbilical vein or aspiration or ingestion of contaminated amniotic fluid through the placenta. Symptoms of congenital TB appear in the second or third week of life. Examination and culture of placenta for AFB is useful. Tuberculin skin test is usually negative initially, but may become positive in 4–8 weeks. As it is often difficult to obtain sputum from infants, *M. tuberculosis* is more easily cultured from gastric aspiration. It is a rare, but serious, condition with high (up to 50%) mortality which is usually due to delay in diagnosis and treatment. Treatment is with isoniazid (10–15 mg/kg), rifampicin (10–20 mg/kg), pyrazinamide (15–30 mg/kg) and ethambutol (15–25 mg/kg) for 2 months followed by isoniazid and rifampicin for 4–10 months.[67,69]

Management of new born of a TB patient

In the case of latent TB in the mother (positive tuberculin test) without active TB or sputum-negative active PTB, the risk to the infant is negligible. However, if she is sputum positive, then the infant needs evaluation for active TB with chest X-ray, gastric aspirate for AFB to rule out congenital TB. If no active TB is found, the infant should receive isoniazid prophylaxis for 3 months or until after the mother's sputum becomes negative. BCG vaccine is either postponed or given with isoniazid-resistant BCG vaccine.

With a tuberculin-positive infant, isoniazid prophylaxis should be given for 6 months after ruling out active TB. In the presence of MDR TB in the mother, INH prophylaxis has no role and should not be given. In such cases, the infant should receive 2 sensitive drugs of index case and BCG vaccination as it has been found to be protective. However, BCG is contra-indicated in HIV-positive child.

Lactation

Breast feeding is recommended regardless of the mother's TB status. If she is sputum positive, she should use a mask over her face while breast feeding the infant.

ATT and contraception

As rifampicin stimulates cytochrome P450 enzymes, the metabolism of oral contraceptives is stimulated and their efficacy is reduced. Alternative contraceptive should be used in such cases or, following consultation with a clinician, an oral contraceptive pill containing a higher dose of estrogen (35–50 μg) may be given.

FUTURE RESEARCH

There has been renewed interest in research into TB world-wide.[70,71] A new and improved BCG vaccine (γ BCG 30) and a recombinant-modified vaccinia virus Ankara (MVA) vector with added Ag 85 have entered phase I clinical trials in the US and UK.[70] New drugs are needed to treat TB because the current drug combinations have significant disadvantages.[71] New drugs, effective against strains that are resistant to conventional drugs and requiring a shorter treatment regimen are being developed by many pharmaceutical companies in collaboration with TB Alliance (a non-profit global alliance for TB drug development, New York), WHO Stop TB partnership, Global fund for AIDS, TB and malaria devising strategies for distribution of new drugs and making regimens affordable for developing countries.[70,71] Such drugs are SQ109, an ethambutol analogue by Sequella Incorporated (Rockville, USA), Pyrrole LL-3858 by Lupin Limited (Mumbai, India), a diarylquinolone called R207910 (Johnson & Johnson), moxifloxacin, gatifloxacin (already available for other indications), Nitroimidazole PA-824 (Chiron, TB Alliance), Diamine SQ109 (Sequella Inc.) and FAS20013 (Fasgen Inc.).[71] By controlling TB, FGTB can also be kept at bay and treated early to prevent development of short-term and long-term sequelae.

KEY POINTS FOR CLINICAL PRACTICE

- Tuberculosis has again become a major public health problem throughout the world due to migration of people from endemic areas to non-endemic areas, the HIV epidemic and the emergence of multidrug and extreme drug resistant TB.
- Though pulmonary tuberculosis continues to be a bigger public health problem due to its infectiousness, extrapulmonary tuberculosis is becoming more common due to HIV co-infection.
- Female genital tuberculosis prevalence varies in different countries being much more common in developing countries especially Africa and Asia and is usually a secondary infection from lungs and other sites like the abdomen.
- Female genital tuberculosis is responsible for up to 16% of infertility cases in developing countries, while infertility is seen in up to 40–50% cases of genital tuberculosis. Other main symptoms are menstrual dysfunction especially oligomenorrhea and amenorrhea, chronic pelvic pain and vaginal discharge.
- A high index of suspicion is required as many cases can be asymptomatic in the early stages when it can be treated without causing significant damage to genital organs; untreated female genital tuberculosis can cause permanent sterility through tubal damage and endometrial destruction (Asherman's syndrome).
- Diagnosis is by good history taking, thorough clinical examination and judicious use of investigations especially endometrial sampling for acid-fast bacilli culture, polymerase chain reaction and histopathological testing. Laparoscopy and hysteroscopy may be helpful in early diagnosis and to estimate the severity of disease for fertility prognosis.

KEY POINTS FOR CLINICAL PRACTICE *(continued)*

- Medical treatment using the Directly Observed Treatment Shortcourse (DOTS) strategy under direct observation and using quality assured ATT drugs in appropriate dosage and for adequate time is the main stay of treatment.
- Prognosis for fertility is poor. However, for tubal disease in the absence of endometrial disease, assisted reproductive techniques, especially *in vitro* fertilization and embryo transfer, give encouraging results. In cases of endometrial disease with shrunken cavity, prognosis for fertility is very poor even with *in vitro* fertilisation embryo transfer.
- Surgical treatment is rarely required and should only be done in exceptional circumstances in the form of limited surgery (laparoscopy, hysteroscopy and drainage of abscess, *etc.*) Surgery in genital and peritoneal tuberculosis can be difficult and hazardous.
- Pregnant women with pulmonary tuberculosis or extrapulmonary tuberculosis should be treated fully even in the first trimester using DOTS strategy using all four primary drugs with optimum maternal and perinatal outcome.
- Treatment of tuberculosis in HIV-positive woman is the same as in HIV-negative woman in consultation with experts in the field.
- Renewed interest in tuberculosis research world-wide and active collaboration by WHO, Stop TB Organization, TB Alliance is showing promising results and the emergence of newer and effective vaccines and antituberculus drugs.

ACKNOWLEDGEMENTS

The author thanks WHO Geneva, WHO Regional Office Delhi, Indian Council of Medical Research, New Delhi, TB Research Centre, Chennai, Stop TB Organization, TB Alliance and RNTCP for supplying study material for preparing this manuscript. I am also grateful to Prof. S. Mittal and Prof. S. Kumar (for their guidance and allowing me to have access to the patients of FGTB at AIIMS), Dr K.K. Roy (for his help in obtaining laparoscopy and hysteroscopy photographs of patients with FGTB), residents of obstetrics and gynecology at AIIMS (in collecting data on FGTB) and Dr Sangeeta Sharma, pediatrician at LRS Institute of TB and Respiratory Diseases, New Delhi for her help in preparing this manuscript.

References

1 Dye C, Watt CJ, Bleed DM, Hosseini SM, Raviglione MC. Evolution of tuberculosis control and prospects for reducing tuberculosis incidence, prevalence and deaths globally. JAMA 2005; 293: 2790–2793

2 World Health Organization. WHO Report on the TB epidemic. TB a global emergency. WHO/TB/94.177. Geneva: WHO, 1994
3 World Health Organization. Global Tuberculosis Control: Surveillance, Planning, Financing. WHO/HTM/TB 2006. Geneva: WHO, 2006; 362
4 TB India 2006. Revised National Tuberculosis Control Programme (RNTCP) Status Report. Central TB Division, Directorate General of Health Services. Ministry of Health and Family Welfare. Nirman Bhavan, New Delhi, India. <http:\\www.tbcindia.org>
5 Kumar S. Female genital tuberculosis. In: Sharma SK, Mohan A.(eds) Tuberculosis, 1st edn. Delhi: Jaypee, 2001; 311–324
6 Sharma JB. Female genital tuberculosis revisited. Obstet Gynaecol Today 2007; XII: 61–63
7 Schaefer G. Female genital tuberculosis. Clin Obstet Gynaecol 1976; 19: 223–239
8 Deshmukh KK, Lopez JA, Naidu TAK, Gaurkhede MD, Kashbhawala MV. Place of laparoscopy in pelvic tuberculosis in infertile women. Arch Gynecol 1985; 237 (Suppl): 197–200
9 Bazaz–Malik G, Maheshwari B, Lal N. Tuberculosis endometritis: a clinicopathological study of 1000 cases. Br J Obstet Gynaecol 1983; 90: 84–86
10 Falk V, Ludviksson K, Agren G. Genital tuberculosis in women. Analysis of 187 newly diagnosed cases from 47 Swedish hospitals during the ten-year period. 1968 to 1977. Am J Obstet Gynecol 1980; 138: 974–977
11 Chhabra S. Genital tuberculosis – a baffling diseases. J Obstet Gynaecol India 1990; 40: 569–573
12 Jindal UN. An algorithmic approach to female genital tuberculosis causing infertility. Int J Tuberc Lung Dis 2006; 10: 1045–1050
13 Roy A, Mukherjee S, Bhattarcharya S, Adhya S, Chakraborty P. Tuberculous endometritis in hills of Darjeeling: a clinicopathological and bacteriological study. Indian J Pathol Microbiol 1993; 36: 361–369
14 Tripathy SN, Tripathy SN. Laparoscopic observations of pelvic organs in pulmonary tuberculosis. Int J Gynecol Obstet 1990; 32: 129–131
15 Sutherland AM, Glean ES, MacFarlane JR. Transmission of genitourinary tuberculosis. Health Bull 1982; 40: 87–91
16 Gupta N, Sharma JB, Mittal S, Singh N, Misra R, Kukreja M. Genital tuberculosis in Indian infertility patients. Int J Gynecol Obstet 2007; 97: 135–138
17 Sharma JB, Malhotra M, Arora R. Fitz-Hugh-Curtis syndrome as a result of genital tuberculosis: a report of three cases. Acta Obstet Gynecol Scand 2003; 82: 295–297
18 Sharma JB, Roy KK, Gupta N, Kumar S, Malhotra N, Mittal S. High prevalence of Fitz-Hugh-Curtis syndrome in female genital tuberculosis. Int J Gynecol Obstet 2007; 99: 62–63
19 Schaefer G. Tuberculosis of the genital organs. Am J Obstet Gynecol 1965; 91: 714–720
20 Arora R, Rathore A. Female genital tract tuberculosis. In: Arora VK, Arora R. (eds) Practical Approach to Tuberculosis Management, 1st edn. Delhi: Jaypee, 2006; 113–119
21 Nogales-Ortiz F. Tarancon I, Nogales Jr FF. The pathology of female genital tuberculosis. A 31-year study of 1436 cases. Obstet Gynecol 1979; 53: 422–428
22 Oosthuizen AP, Wessels PH, Hefer JN. Tuberculosis of the female genital tract in patients attending an infertility clinic. South Afr Med J 1990; 77: 562–564
23 Sharma JB, Roy KK, Pushparaj M *et al*. Genital tuberculosis: an important cause of Asherman's syndrome in India. Arch Obstet Gynecol2007: In Press
24 Agarwal J, Gupta JK. Female genital tuberculosis – a retrospective clinicopathological study of 501 cases. Indian J Pathol Microbiol 1993; 36: 389–397
25 Barutcu O, Erel HE, Saygili E, Yildirim T, Torun D. Abdominopelvic tuberculosis simulating disseminated ovarian carcinoma with elevated CA-125 level: report of two cases. Abdom Imaging 2002; 27: 465–470
26 Sharma JB, Sharma S, Gupta S, Gulati N, Banga G. Bilateral serous cystadenocarcinoma of ovary with associated endometrial tuberculosis. J Obstet Gynaecol India 1990; 40: 613–614
27 Sharma JB, Malhotra M, Pundir P, Arora R. Cervical tuberculosis masquerading as cervical carcinoma: a rare case. J Obstet Gynaecol India 2001; 51: 184
28 Angrish K, Verma K. Cytologic detection of tuberculosis of the uterine cervix. Acta Cytol 1981; 25: 160–162

29 Dhall K, Dass SS, Dey P. Tuberculosis of Bartholin's gland [Letter]. Int J Gynecol Obstet 1995; 48: 223–224

30 Sharma JB, Sharma K, Sarin U. Tuberculosis: a rare cause of rectovaginal fistula in a young girl. J Obstet Gynaecol India 2001; 51: 176

31 Bobhate SK, Kadar GP, Khan A, Grover S. Female genital tuberculosis. A pathological appraisal. J Obstet Gynaecol India 1986; 36: 676–680

32 Bhide AG, Parulekar SV, Bhattacharya MS. Genital tuberculosis in females. J Obstet Gynaecol India 1987; 37: 576–578.

33 Saracoglu OF, Mungan T, Tanzer F. Pelvic tuberculosis. Int J Gynecol Obstet 1992; 37: 115–120

34 Nagpal M, Pal D. Genital tuberculosis – a diagnostic dilemma in OPD patients. J Obstet Gynaecol India 2001; 51: 127–131

35 Sharma S. Menstrual dysfunction in non-genital tuberculosis. Int J Gynecol Obstet 2002; 79: 245–247

36 Malhotra D, Vasishta K, Srinivasan R, Singh G. Tuberculous uteroenterocutaneous fistula – a rare postcaesarean complication. Aust NZ J Obstet Gynaecol 1995; 35: 342–344

37 Sutherland AM. The changing pattern of tuberculosis of the female genital tract. A thirty year survey. Arch Gynecol 1983; 234: 95–101

38 Jassawala MJ. Genital tuberculosis – a diagnostic dilemma. J Obstet Gynaecol India 2006; 56: 203–204

39 Raut VS, Mahashur AA, Sheth SS. The Mantoux test in the diagnosis of genital tuberculosis in women. Int J Gynecol Obstet 2001; 72: 165–169

40 Perkins MD. New diagnostic tools for tuberculosis. Int J Tuberc Lung Dis 2000; 4: 182–188

41 Rattan A, Gupta SK, Singh S *et al*. Detection of antigens of *Mycobacterium tuberculosis* in patients of infertility by monoclonal antibody based sandwiched enzyme linked immunosorbent assay (ELISA). Tuberc Lung Dis 1993; 74: 200–203

42 Mani R, Nayak KS, Kagal A, Deshpande N, Dandge N, Bhardwaj R. Tuberculous endometritis in infertility: a bacteriological and histopathological study. Indian J Tuberc 2003; 50: 161

43 Abebe M, Lakew M, Kidane D, Lakew Z, Kiros K, Harboe M. Female genital tuberculosis in Ethiopia. Int J Gynecol Obstet 2004; 84: 241–246

44 Seward PG, Mitchel RW. Guinea pig inoculation and culture for mycobacteria in tuberculosis in infertile women. A study of cost effectiveness. South Afr Med J 1985; 67: 126–129

45 Sheth SS. Lack of diagnostic value of guinea pig test for tuberculosis. Lancet 1991; 337: 124

46 Katoch VM. Newer diagnostic techniques for tuberculosis. Indian J Med Res 2004; 120: 418–428

47 Bhanu NV, Singh UB, Chakraborty M *et al*. Improved diagnostic value of PCR in diagnosis of female genital tuberculosis leading to infertility. J Med Microbiol 2005; 54: 927–931

48 Rozati R, Sreenivasagari R, Rajeshwari CN. Evaluation of women with infertility and genital tuberculosis. J Obstet Gynaecol India 2006; 56: 423–426

49 Grosset J, Mouton Y. Is PCR a useful tool for the diagnosis of tuberculosis in 1995? Tuberc Lung Dis 1995; 76: 183–184

50 Chavhan GB, Hira P, Rathod K *et al.* Female genital tuberculosis: hysterosalpingographic appearances. Br J Radiol 2004; 77: 164–169

51 Sharma JB, Pushparaj M, Roy KK, *et al.* Hysterosalpingography findings in female genital tuberculosis. Eur J Obstet Gynecol Reprod Biol 2007: In Press

52 Parikh FR, Nadkarni SG, Kamat SA, Naik N, Soonawala SB, Parikh RM. Genital tuberculosis – a major pelvic factor causing infertility in Indian women. Fertil Steril 1997; 67: 497–500

53 Kumari C, Sinha S. Laparoscopic evaluation of tubal factors in cases of infertility. J Obstet Gynaecol India 2000; 50: 67–70

54 Tripathy SN, Tripathy SN. Infertility and pregnancy outcome in female genital tuberculosis. Int J Gynecol Obstet 2002; 76: 159–163

55 Arora R, Rajaram P, Oumachigui A, Arora VK. Prospective analysis of short course

chemotherapy in female genital tuberculosis. Int J Gynecol Obstet 1992; 38: 311–314
56 American Thoracic Society, Centers for Disease Control and Prevention, Prevention/Infectious Diseases Society of America. Controlling tuberculosis in United States. Am J Respir Crit Care Med 2005; 172: 1169–1227
57 National Institute for Health and Clinical Excellence. Tuberculosis. Clinical diagnosis and management of tuberculosis, and measures for its prevention and control. Clinical Guideline 33. London: NICE, 2006. <www.nice.org.uk/CGO33>
58 World Health Organization. Treatment of tuberculosis. Guidelines for national programmes, 3rd edn. Geneva: WHO, 2003; 313. <WHO/CDS/TB/2003>
59 Revised National Tuberculosis Control Programme. DOTS – Plus Guidelines. Central TB Division, Directorate General of Health Services. Ministry of Health and Family Welfare. Nirman Bhavan, New Delhi, India, 2006
60 World Health Organization. Instructions for applying to the Green Light Committee for access to second line antituberculus drugs. Geneva: WHO/CDS/TB/ 2001; 286
61 World Health Organization. Interim Policy on Collaborative TB/HIV Activities. WHO/HTM/TB/2004. Geneva: WHO, 2004; 330
62 Dam P, Shirazee HH, Goswami SK *et al.* Role of latent genital tuberculosis in repeated IVF failure in Indian clinical settings. Gynecol Obstet Invest 2006; 61: 223–227
63 Kothari A, Mahadevan N, Girling J. Tuberculosis and pregnancy – results of a study in a high prevalence area in London. Eur J Obstet Gynecol Reprod Biol 2006; 126: 48–55
64 Centers for Disease Control. Leads from the MMWR. Tuberculosis in minorities – United States. JAMA 1987; 257: 1291–1292
65 Jana N, Vasishta K, Jindal SK, Khunnu B, Ghosh K. Perinatal outcome in pregnancies complicated by pulmonary tuberculosis. Int J Gynecol Obstet 1994; 44: 119–124
66 Jana N, Vasishta K, Saha SC, Ghosh K. Obstetrical outcomes among women with extra-pulmonary tuberculosis. N Engl J Med 1999; 341: 645–649
67 Sharma JB. Pregnancy complicated by tuberculosis: maternal and perinatal issues. Obstet Gynaecol Today 2007; In press
68 Sackoff JE, Pfeiffer MR, Driver CR, Streett SL, Munsiff SS, DeHovitz JA. Tuberculosis prevention for non-US-born pregnant women. Am J Obstet Gynecol 2006; 94: 451–456
69 Ormerod P. Tuberculosis in pregnancy and the puerperium. Thorax 2001; 56: 494–499
70 Friedrich MJ. Basic science guides design of new TB vaccine candidates. JAMA 2005; 293: 2703–2705
71 Hampton T. TB drug research picks up the pace. JAMA 2005; 293: 2705–2707

John Studd

Indications for different regimens of HRT

Two major well-publicised studies, the Women's Health Initiative (WHI)[1] and the Million Women Study (MWS)[2], have shaken the faith in the safety of HRT for doctors and post menopausal women alike in spite of the criticism of the design and conclusions of the WHI study[3–5] and the many anxieties about the MWS data collection.[6–8] It is now difficult to respond to the WHI study in an optimistic way and for this to be considered and published. Following the NAMS/NIH statement of October 2002,[9] many proscriptive guidelines from advisory bodies in Europe and North America have appeared, which advise prescribing hormone therapy at the lowest dose principally for menopausal vasomotor symptoms, and for the shortest time.[10] It was also recommended that it was not to be used as a primary treatment for low bone-density and that it has no place in the prevention of coronary heart disease. In view of later consideration of the data, both items of advice are questionable. There is no protest about the uncontroversial recommendation that the lowest dose should be used and the appropriateness of continuing HRT should be reviewed each year with full discussion of benefits and risks. However, the 'lowest dose' varies from patient to patient and should be one that is effective for a particular indication.

What is missing from statements from regulatory authorities is the understanding that treatment should be individualised for a particular patient, her expectations and her pathology. Such variation of therapy is sound clinical practice but it is notable that the great fault of the WHI study is that there was no individualisation with the assumption that one dose of Prempro fitted all patients regardless of age and general health even though they were, by their inclusion criteria, asymptomatic and did not require therapy.

The epidemiologists and investigators who designed the WHI were not aware of, or chose to ignore, the basic tenant of good practice relating to HRT. This is the knowledge that different women, require a different dose, by a

John Studd DSc MD FRCOG
Professor of Gynaecology, Chelsea and Westminster Hospital, 369 Fulham Road, London SW10 9NH, UK
E-mail: harley@studd.co.uk

different route, of different combinations, of different hormones, for different symptoms. This would also vary depending upon the surgical status, the age of the patient and there will also be a difference depending on the clinical needs of the woman. This paper is an attempt to correct that omission by stating the variations necessary for effective treatment with estrogens with the possible addition of progestogens and androgens.

AGE

Perhaps the most fundamental variation is one of age. The average age of the women in the WHI study was 63 years (range, 50–79 years) and 22% being recruited for therapy over the age of 70 years. The study demonstrated an increase in breast cancer and VTE, a decrease in colon cancer and fractures of the hip and spine as well as an unexpected increase in heart attacks and stroke.[1] However, it should be recognised that 97% of patients in normal clinical practice commence treatment below the age of 60 years and it is this age cohort of patients which is of particular interest to the prescribing physician.[11] The data from this age group are re-assuring, as a later report the WHI study in 2003 showed that the excess of cardiovascular events[12] occurred only in women starting estrogen and progestogen therapy 20 years after the menopause, and that there was a non-significant (HR 0.89) decrease in these events in women starting the therapy within 10 years of the menopause.

Similarly, the estrogen-only arm,[13] which was reportedly stopped in 2004 because of an excess of stroke, showed that in the 50–59-year-old age group there was a 42% decrease in coronary heart disease, being much the same as the protection found in the former case-control studies. There was also a 28% decrease in breast cancer, a 41% decrease in colorectal cancer, a 27% decrease in deaths and a 20% decrease in global index pathology. The 8% increase in stroke was in fact 19 patients in the control group and 19 patients in the active group. None of the considerable beneficial changes were significant but it does raise a question why this age cohort of the estrogen-only study was stopped as results could have confirmed the cardiovascular and colorectal benefits in the many earlier observational studies. It was a lost opportunity to solve this continuing controversy.

WHEN TO START?

There are clear differences concerning the correct time to start therapy. Most women start HRT in the post menopausal state but this can be soon after a normal menopause in the early 50-year age group or later in a > 60-year age group. Hormone therapy may also be required in younger women after a premature menopause[14] or following hysterectomy and oophorectomy.[15] These groups should all be treated in different ways. HRT may also be prescribed to peri-menopausal women in the transition phase before the periods have ceased if they have appropriate symptoms. These will require different doses of different hormones depending on the age and clinical needs and will be discussed in detail.

Essentially, older women need a smaller dose, and non-hysterectomised women may also require testosterone for specific symptoms.

INDICATIONS FOR STARTING HRT

The indications for HRT in this review are wider than those initially recommended by NAMS CSM and EMAS where the advice is a result of the 'one dose fits all' WHI study and the incomprehensible data collection of the MWS. An alternative view is that hormone therapy prescribed intelligently is safe and associated with considerable quality of life benefits.

In Europe, estrogen has been principally given for the treatment of climacteric symptoms and for the improvement of low bone-density. The symptoms may be due to the vasomotor instability of hot flushes and sweats with insomnia and tiredness or pelvic atrophy with vaginal dryness, dyspareunia, sexual dysfunction and the urethral syndrome.[16] The estrogen may also be given for the prevention or the treatment of osteoporosis in women with decreased bone density as estrogens, in the appropriate dose, have an anabolic as well as an anti-catabolic effect on the skeleton.[17]

More controversial indications would be for peri-menopausal depression[18,19] or premenstrual syndrome, particularly in the years of the peri-menopausal state.[20,21] Loss of energy and loss of libido in association with climacteric symptoms are distressing for the couple and should be indications for estrogen, sometimes with the addition of testosterone.[22]

The value of estrogen therapy in the prevention of coronary artery disease, Alzheimer's disease and stroke is now controversial and would not, with current knowledge, be recommended. Similarly, the belief that estrogens are of value in the secondary prevention of further coronary artery disease seems no longer valid. Thus, estrogen therapy for prevention of these chronic cardiovascular and neurological disorders is no longer recommended although many workers cling to the hypothesis of a window of opportunity for prevention if estrogen therapy is started in the first 10 years after the menopause before irreversible arterial and neurological degeneration has occurred. The different indications are discussed in more detail.

Vasomotor symptoms

These classical and the most common symptoms of the climacteric are the vasomotor symptoms of hot flushes, palpitations, night sweats with insomnia and headaches which all respond well to estrogen therapy. Patients with these symptoms require low-dose estradiol preparations either by an oral route, by gel or patch for 3 months or longer for the duration of symptoms. The commencing dose should be low but can be increased to a dose which alleviates the symptoms. Because of the anxiety about breast cancer, many other treatments (particularly herbal remedies, SSRIs or clonidine) have been used but none are as effective as estrogen in women who have these troublesome symptoms. The increasingly popular natural herbal remedies are usually no better than placebo but, even if pharmacologically active, they are uncontrolled, poorly investigated, of unknown estrogenic potency and not without serious side effects.

Those patients receiving estrogens will, of course, need cyclical or continuous progestogens if they have an intact uterus in order to protect the endometrium from hyperplasia or malignancy.[23] There is now much debate about the progestogen component, because this hormone, more than estrogen, seems to be implicated in the possible excess of breast cancer in the combined HRT preparations. There is also a problem in that progestogen reproduces PMS-type symptoms,[24] particularly in women who have progestogen intolerance.[25] This is a major reason why women discontinue therapy. These women should try a different gestogen, at a lower dose, or should consider the long cycle of progestogen every 3 months. A Mirena IUS delivering local progestogen within the uterine cavity should be considered.[26]

Another possibility is to have a shorter duration of progestogen every month. One regimen is for a progestogen (such as norethisterone 5 mg or MPA 5 mg) to be taken for the first 7 days of each calendar month which will bring about a withdrawal bleed on about day 10 of each calendar month. This will bring about 12 periods a year instead of 13 with fewer progestogenic symptoms of irritability, depression, tiredness and bloating. This option is an important concept because, following the demonstration of possible disadvantages of continuous progestogen, there is currently a risk of accepting the other extreme of unopposed estrogens,[27] without considering the compromise of a shorter 7-day monthly course of progestogen which has already been shown to be effective in preventing endometrial pathology in early work on this subject.[28]

Pelvic atrophy

Vaginal dryness like vasomotor symptoms should be easy to treat with estrogens. After the menopause, women lose collagen from the skin, ligaments, bone matrix, the genital tract and bladder which can be corrected with hormone replacement.[29] These patients with symptoms of pelvic atrophy should have the same low-dose estradiol, with the appropriate progestogen if necessary, for as long as it takes to eradicate the symptoms. Local vaginal estradiol or estriol can be used. Progestogen is not normally added to this therapy although endometrial proliferation and hyperplasia may rarely occur. If bladder symptoms of urgency and recurrent 'cystitis' are present, a higher dose may be required for a longer duration regardless of whether the route of administration is local oral or transdermal.

Premature menopause

Apart from the sadness of infertility, women with a premature menopause have a higher incidence of osteoporosis, coronary heart disease, stroke and also depression.[30] Indeed, it was this association which led to the concept of estrogens preventing these chronic diseases in older women. Estrogen therapy has been shown to increase the bone density and also to improve the histomorphometric parameters of strength of bone even in young women with Turner's syndrome.[31] They need HRT in the appropriate dose for these symptoms until at least until the age of 50 years, the time of the normal menopause. If there is to be a 5–10-year recommended limit for the duration of HRT, these treatment years should be counted from the age of 50 years, the age of natural menopause. In reality, these young women with their excess risk of chronic disease are having their estrogen therapy discontinued or not started due to the anxiety created by the common misinterpretation of the WHI data.

Post hysterectomy and oophorectomy

Women who have had a hysterectomy should have continuous estrogens without progestogens; thus treatment should be straightforward without bleeding and without PMS-type symptoms produced by gestogens, which often limit the acceptability of HRT. However, these women may need a higher dose than is usual for the vasomotor symptoms and, as the surgery usually occurs in premenopausal women, they may well, like those with a premature menopause, need estrogens for a longer duration for relief of symptoms.

If the ovaries have been removed, these women would have lost their ovarian androgens and be at risk of developing the female androgen deficiency syndrome (FADS) characterised by loss of energy, loss of libido, depression, loss of self-confidence and headaches.[32] These are frequent complaints in women who have had a hysterectomy with loss of ovaries and have been receiving a low dose of estrogens over the years. These symptoms can usually be eradicated by the addition of testosterone, either in the form of implants (licensed for women in many countries) or Testogel, which although effective will have to be used off-licence in women using about one-quarter of the dose recommended for men. However, the fact that it is not licensed in a particular country is not a good reason to deny women this important item of treatment. It should not be forgotten that testosterone is not only a normal female hormone but it is present in higher concentrations in young women than estradiol.

Estradiol and testosterone implants are the most effective and convenient route of administration for these women, with the pellets inserted into the wound on closure and repeated approximately every 6 months as a simple office procedure.[15] The fact that it is an old drug lacking in patent or profit or the benefit of costly licensing studies does not reduce its value in hysterectomised women or those with problems of loss of energy and libido or depression.

Peri-menopausal depression

There are many patients in their forties with severe recurrent depression, sometimes cyclical, who will respond well to transdermal estrogens. These patients with reproductive depression often reveal the changes of mood with changes in hormone levels because of a past history of post natal depression, premenopausal depression as well as the severe depression in the peri-menopausal years of the transition. Often, they state that they were last well during the last pregnancy many years ago. They then developed post natal depression which became cyclical as premenstrual dysphonic disorder (PMDD) when the periods returned having only about 10 good days per month free of PMS periods and menstrual headaches. The depression then becomes less cyclical and more constant.[33]

These peri-menopausal women respond well to moderately high doses of transdermal estrogens (either moderately high doses 100–200 μg), which not only suppress any residual cycle but have a mood-elevating effect. As these women with hormone-responsive depression are often progestogen intolerant, the continuous estradiol treatment should be supplemented with progestogen tablets for 7 days of each calendar month rather than the orthodox 14 days. A Mirena IUS is also useful, preventing the recurrent depression that often occurs with progestogen.

Estrogens do not convincingly help the depression of post menopausal women apart from the domino effect of removing night sweats/insomnia or vaginal atrophy and sexual dysfunction. It seems to have little significant effect in the absence of these classical menopausal symptoms.

Low bone density

Although the new, non-hormonal therapies for low bone density are currently more in favor, there is still a place for estrogen therapy which is the only treatment shown to decrease the risk of both vertebral and hip fractures. Estrogens are anabolic as well anti-catabolic to the bone and are most effective in older women or in women with an osteoporotic skeleton. The increase of bone density with estrogens is dose-dependent with a positive correlation between plasma estradiol levels and bone density. There is also a correlation between estradiol levels and histomorphometric changes of wall thickness, trabecular volume and new formation of matrix collagen.[17] No such data exist for bisphosphanates.

Plasma estradiol levels of 300 pmol/l are necessary for an increase in bone density in most patients. However, as most North American patients are prescribed conjugated equine estrogens, estradiol measurements have not been a feature of American practice.

The advice from the regulatory authorities that estrogens should not be first-line therapy for the prevention or treatment of osteoporosis particularly in otherwise healthy women under the age of 60 years has been questioned.[35] Regrettably, there has always been a conflict, almost a 'turf war', between bone physicians for whom the side effects of bleeding, mastalgia and PMS symptoms with progestogen is uncharted territory and gynecologists who are more familiar with the problems of gonadal hormones. This has been re-inforced by Banks *et al.*[35] of the MWS who claim that on cessation of estrogen therapy bone density 'rapidly' reverted to pre-treatment levels. This has been disputed,[36,37] but it does further demonstrate the design problem of this study which relied upon a single questionnaire. In reality, 10 years of moderately low-dose estrogen therapy will increase the vertebral bone density by approximately 10%. It is both counter-intuitive and certainly against clinical observations that this benefit is rapidly lost. However, it is cited as further justification to use non-hormonal therapy as first choice or to discontinue this therapy after a short course of estrogens in these younger women, in spite of the added quality of life benefits of hormone therapy.

Older menopausal women

Older women in the past have been shamefully neglected due to the belief that the osteoporotic skeleton did not respond to drugs which otherwise would increase bone density in younger women. In reality, the skeletal response to estrogen is greatest in women who had the lowest bone density and who are most years past the menopause.[38] It appears that this denial is occurring again following justifiable anxiety about the cardiovascular effects found in older women in the WHI study. These women require the lower starting dose of estrogens or bisphosphanates may be used as a first option. If older women are treated with estrogens, it is advisable to start on low-dose, unopposed therapy for the first 3 months using estradiol patches or gels or oral estradiol 0.5 mg daily. At 3 months after assessing the symptomatic response, a decision should be taken whether to continue to use low-dose, unopposed estrogens or to add a monthly low-dose, low-duration, progestogen component.

Bleed-free preparations

The desire to have estrogen therapy without a withdrawal bleeding opens up a large variety of therapeutic possibilities. The use of continuous estrogen and progestogen is effective, commonly used but is currently suspect because of the data from the WHI study. However, it continues to be with justification the most frequently used preparation for this purpose. Recently, there have been reports of low-dose or ultra low-dose continuous estrogens producing relief of symptoms and bone protection without bleeding.[27] Tibolone is a complex gestogen with estrogenic and androgenic properties, which by depressing SHBG levels[39] increases free testosterone thus having a beneficial effect on energy libido and depression.[40] The use of SERMS with their certain protective effect on breast cancer is being evaluated, although this drug does produce vasomotor symptoms as well as the desirable endometrial atrophy and amenorrhea.

SUMMARY AND CONCLUSIONS

The principles of hormone therapy for the menopausal or perimenopausal woman can be summarized thus. These items are not entirely consistent with the current advice of regulatory bodies but they do reflect a studied analysis of the available data as well as a long clinical and academic interest in the subject. Medical practitioners of all levels require guidance for the hormonal treatment of middle-aged women. These views should be considered, discussed and criticised as a fresh clinical approach is urgently needed. Currently, many women suffering severe hormonal disorders are being needlessly denied appropriate safe hormone therapy

1. Estrogens are safe when started below the age of 60 years, particularly if progestogen is not required and are positively indicated in women with a premature menopause It should be used for treatment of specific climacteric symptoms and low bone density and the advice that estrogens should not be first option for the prevention or treatment of osteoporosis in this age group is questioned. The dose and route will depend upon the symptoms and the age of the patient.
2. Women with a uterus need endometrial protection with progestogen. The usual duration is 14 days but, if the extra risk to the breasts from progestogen is confirmed, it would be sensible to reduce the duration to 7 days each calendar month. This shortened course is also useful in women with progestogen intolerance and is adequate for endometrial protection.

Alternatively, a Mirena IUS can be inserted. The long-term value and safety of low-dose, unopposed estrogen is unproven.

3. Estrogen-only therapy commenced before the age of 60 years is associated with a considerable, but non-significant, decrease in coronary heart diseases, osteoporotic fractures, colon cancer and deaths. These results are consistent with the previous case-control studies. There may also be a decrease in breast cancer in women receiving estrogens without progestogen.
4. Estrogens appear to have no place for the secondary prevention of cardiovascular disease but there may be a window of opportunity in 45–60-year-old symptomatic women who may show long-term cardiovascular and neurological benefits from early estrogen therapy. Estrogens commenced in older 69–79-year-old women may do 'early harm' before any benefit can be achieved and should be avoided if possible or started on very low-dose estrogens.
5. A moderately high dose of transdermal estrogens is useful for perimenopausal depression as well as premenstrual depression. Progestogen is necessary for endometrial protection and cycle control even though these patients may be intolerant to small doses and short duration of any gestogen.
6. Patients may wish to avoid bleeding by using low-dose estrogen and progestogen, Tibolone or have a Mirena IUS inserted.
7. If loss of libido and loss of energy remain a problem, the addition of testosterone to estrogen should be considered. Androgen as well as estrogen is often necessary after hysterectomy and bilateral oophorectomy. Hysterectomized women do not need progestogen.
8. A 5-year duration has been recommended but in reality women remain on HRT if they are feeling well with relief of symptoms. It is difficult to persuade these women to stop even after 10 or more years.[41] The need for estrogens should be reviewed each year for long-term users with clear discussion of current views on safety.
9. In spite of the re-assuring data from estrogen-only studies, the possible increase in breast cancer remains a problem. Until the controversy concerning breast cancer risk is clarified, it is probably advisable that regular mammograms should be performed each year and breast examination every 6 months although it is correct to recognise that many oncologists would doubt the value of these frequent examinations.

The optimistic recommendations in this paper are now supported by the latest publication from the WHI reporting the results of starting Prempro before age 60 years which results in 24% fewer cases of coronary heart disease and 30% decrease in total mortality.[42] Age is the most critical factor whether estrogen-only or estrogen plus progestogens was used. Both the North American Menopause Society[43] and the International Menopause Society[44] have now changed their guidelines recognising the efficacy for many indications for HRT outlined in this review and the long-term safety of such therapy. This belated conversion to the clinical realities of HRT have been warmly welcomed.[45]

References

1 Writing Group for the Women's Health Initiative Investigators. Risks and benefits of estrogen plus progestin in healthy postmenopausal women; principal results from the Women's Health Initiative randomised controlled trial. JAMA 2002; 288: 321–333
2 Million Women Study Collaborators, Beral V. Breast cancer and hormone-replacement. Lancet 2002; 362: 419–427
3 Studd JWW. Up to general practice to pick up the pieces – what pieces? A response to WHI and MWS. Maturitas 2003; 46: 95–96
4 Harman SM, Naftolin F, Brinton EA, Judelsopn DR. Is the estrogen controversy over? Deconstructing the Women's Health Initiative study: a critical evaluation of the evidence. Ann NY Acad Sci 2005; 1052: 43–56
5 Clark JH. A critique of Women's Health List of studies (2002–2006). Nucl Recept Signal 2006; 30: e023
6 Whitehead M, Farmer R. The Million Women Study: a critique. Endocrine 2004; 24: 187–193
7 Speroff L. The Million Women Study and breast cancer. Maturitas 2003; 46: 1–6
8 Genazzani AR, Gambacciani M. The sound of an international anti-HRT herald. Maturitas 2003; 46: 105–106
9 North American Menopause Society (NAMS) conference report. 2002
10 RCP (Edin) Consensus conference on HRT. 2003
11 Studd JWW. Second thoughts on the Women's Health Initiative study: the effect of age on the safety of HRT. Climacteric 2004; 7: 412–414
12 Manson JE, Hsia J, Johnson KC *et al*. Estrogen, progestin and the risk of coronary heart disease. N Engl J Med 2003; 349: 523–534
13 Anderson GL, Limacher M, Assaf AR *et al*. Effects of conjugated equine estrogen in postmenopausal women with hysterectomy. Women's Health Initiative randomized clinical trial. JAMA 2004; 291: 1701–1712
14 Nelson LM, Covington SN, Rebar RW. An update: spontaneous premature ovarian failure is not an early menopause. Fertil Steril 2005; 83: 1327–1332
15 Khastgir G, Studd JWW. Patients' outlook, experience and satisfaction with hysterectomy, bilateral oophorectomy and subsequent continuation of hormone replace therapy. Am J Obstet Gynecol 2000; 183: 1427–1433
16 Campbell S, Whitehead M. Oestrogen therapy and the menopausal syndrome. Clin Obstet Gynaecol 1977; 4: 31–47
17 Khastgir G, Studd JWW, Holland N, Alaghband-Zadeh J, Fox S, Chow J. Anabolic effect of estrogen replacement on bone in postmenopausal women with osteoporosis; histomorphometric evidence in a longitudinal study. J Clin Endocrinol Metab 2001; 86: 289–295
18 Montgomery JC, Appleby L, Brincat M *et al*. Effect of oestrogen and testosterone implants on psychological disorders in the climacteric. Lancet 1987; 1: 297–299
19 Watson NR, Savvas M, Studd JWW, Garnett T, Barnet RJ. Treatment of severe premenstrual syndrome with oestradiol patches and cyclical oral norethisterone. Lancet 1989; ii: 730–734
20 Soares CN, Joffe H, Steiner M. Menopause and mood. Clin Obstet Gynecol 2004; 47: 576–591
21 Schmidt PJ. Mood, depression and reproductive hormones in the menopausal transition. Am J Psychiatry 2006; 163: 133–137
22 Davis SR. The use of testosterone after menopause. J Br Menopause Soc 2004; 10: 65–69
23 Sturdee D, Wade-Evans T, Patterson MEL, Thom M, Studd JWW. Relations between bleeding pattern, endometrial histology and oestrogen treatment in menopausal woman. BMJ 1987; 1: 1575–1577
24 Magos AL, Brewster E, Singh R, O'Dowd T, Brincat M, Studd JWW. The Effects of norethisterone in postmenopausal women on oestrogen replacement therapy: a model for the premenstrual syndrome. Br J Obstet Gynaecol 1968; 93: 1290–1296
25 Panay N, Studd JWW. Progestogen intolerance and compliance with hormone replacement therapy in menopausal women. Hum Reprod Update 1997; 3: 159–171
26 Hampton NR, Rees MC, Lowe DG, Rauamol I, Barlow D, Guillebaud J. Levonorgestrel intrauterine system (LNG-IUS) with conjugated oral equine estrogen: a successful

regimen for HRT in perimenopausal women. Hum Reprod 2005; 20: 2653–2660
27 Ettinger B, Ensrud KE, Wallace R *et al*. Effects of ultralow-dose transdermal estradiol on bone mineral density: a randomized clinical trial. Obstet Gynecol 2004; 104: 443–451
28 Patterson ME, Wade-Evans T, Sturdee DW, Thom MH, Studd JWW. Endometrial disease after treatment with oestrogens and progestogens in the climacteric. BMJ 1980; 280: 822–824
29 Brincat M, Moniz CJ, Studd JWW *et al*. Long term effects of the menopause and sex hormones on skin thickness. Br J Obstet Gynaecol 1985; 92: 256–259
30 Oliver M, Boyd GS. Effect of bilateral ovariectomy on coronary-artery disease and serum-lipid levels. Lancet 1959; 2: 690–694
31 Khastigir G, Studd JWW, Fox SW, Jones J, Alaghband-Zadeh J, Chow J. A longitudinal study of the effect of subcutaneous estrogen replacement in bone in young women with Turner's syndrome. J Bone Miner Res 2003; 18: 925–932
32 Sands R, Studd JWW. Exogenous androgens in postmenopausal women. Am J Med 1995; 98: 76S–79S
33 Studd JWW, Panay N. Hormones and depression in women. Climacteric 2004; 7: 338–346
34 Stevenson J. Justification for the use of HRT in the long-term prevention of osteoporosis. Maturitas 2005; 51: 113–126
35 Banks E, Beral V, Reeves G *et al*. Fracture incidence in relation to the pattern of use of hormone therapy in postmenopausal women. JAMA 2004; 291: 2212–2220
36 Simon JA, Wehren LE, Ascott-Evans BH *et al*. Skeletal consequences of hormone therapy discontinuance: a systematic review. Obstet Gynaecol Surv 2006; 61: 115–124
37 Bagger YZ, Tanko LB, Alexandersen P *et al*. Two to three years of hormone replacement treatment in healthy women have long-term preventive effects on bone mass and osteoporotic fractures: the PERF study. Bone 2004; 34: 728–736
38 Lindsay R, Tohme JF. Estrogen treatment of patients with established postmenopausal osteoporosis. Obstet Gynecol 1990; 76: 290–295
39 Abdalla HI, Hart DM, Lindsay R, Beastall GH. Organon OD 14 (Tibolone) and menopausal dynamic hormone profiles. Maturitas 1986; 8: 81–85
40 Rymer J, Robinson J, Fogelman I. Ten years of treatment with Tibolone 2.5 mg daily: effects on bone loss in postmenopausal women. Climacteric 2002; 5: 390–398
41 Horner E, Fleming J, Studd JWW. A study of women on long-term hormone replacement therapy and their attitude to suggested cessation. Climacteric 2006; 9: 459–463
42 Rousseau JE, Prentice RL, Manson JE *et al*. Post menopausal hormone therapy and risk of cardiovascular disease by age and years since menopause. JAMA 2007; 297: 1465–1477
43 North American Menopause Society. Estrogen and progestogen use in peri- and postmenopausal women: March 2007 position statement of The North American Menopause Society. Menopause 2007; 14: 168–182
44 International Menopause Society. Climacteric 2007; In press
45 Genazzani AR, Gambacciani M, Simoncini T. The latest elaboration of the Women's Health Initiative data on hormone replacement therapy and cardiovascular disease in postmenopausal women. Gynecol Endocrinol 2007; 23: 183–185

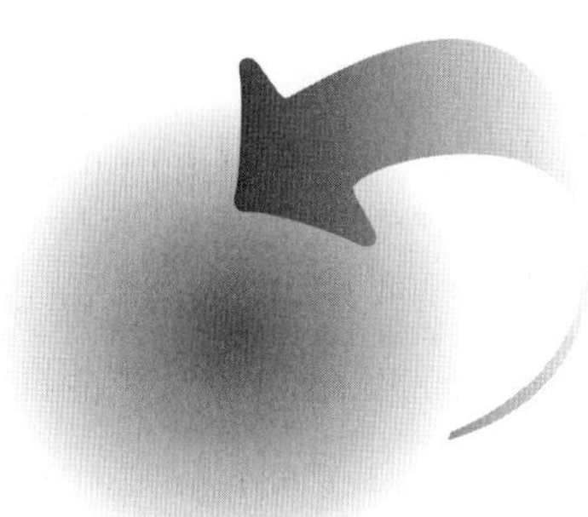

Index